1 MONTH OF
FREE
READING

at
www.ForgottenBooks.com

By purchasing this book you are eligible for one month membership to ForgottenBooks.com, giving you unlimited access to our entire collection of over 1,000,000 titles via our web site and mobile apps.

To claim your free month visit:
www.forgottenbooks.com/free102846

ISBN 978-0-483-12232-1
PIBN 10102846

end 1142

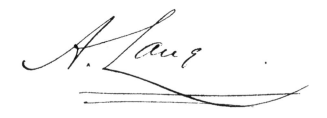

June 1876.

THE

INFLUENCE OF TROPICAL CLIMATES

IN

PRODUCING THE ACUTE ENDEMIC DISEASES OF EUROPEANS.

"Rerum cognoscere causas, medicis imprimis necessarium, sine quo, nec morbum curare, nec praecavere potest."

INFLUENCE OF TROPICAL CLIMATES

IN

PRODUCING THE ACUTE ENDEMIC DISEASES OF EUROPEANS:

INCLUDING

PRACTICAL OBSERVATIONS ON THE NATURE AND TREATMENT OF
THEIR CHRONIC SEQUELÆ, UNDER THE INFLUENCE OF
THE CLIMATE OF EUROPE.

BY

SIR JAMES RANALD MARTIN, C.B., F.R.S.,

PHYSICIAN TO THE COUNCIL OF INDIA; SURGEON BENGAL ARMY, RETIRED;
LATE PRESIDENCY-SURGEON, AND SURGEON TO THE NATIVE HOSPITAL, CALCUTTA;
MEMBER OF THE ROYAL ASIATIC SOCIETY OF GREAT BRITAIN AND IRELAND;
AND OF THE ASIATIC SOCIETY OF BENGAL, ETC. ETC.

Second Edition.

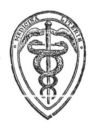

LONDON:
JOHN CHURCHILL, NEW BURLINGTON STREET.
MDCCCLXI.

LONDON:
SAVILL AND EDWARDS, PRINTERS, CHANDOS STREET,
COVENT GARDEN.

PREFACE

SECOND EDITION.

———————

ALTHOUGH but six years have elapsed since the first Edition of this work was published, the present is not produced as a mere reprint; on the contrary, it is hoped that additions and alterations have been made which may be regarded as improvements. The work differs also in the arrangement of the materials, the climatic, statistical, and hygienic departments of inquiry preceding those of the nature, causes, and treatment of tropical diseases, acute and chronic.

Limited to one volume, and to so many pages consequently, I am not permitted to amplify upon certain subjects, such as fever, the great disease of the world, and the most important branch of scientific medicine, to the extent that I could desire; but I trust that upon no question has any omission of importance occurred.

Since the publication of the former edition numberless additional examples of the sequelæ to acute tropical diseases have presented themselves to me, so as to test and illustrate the doctrines and practices set forth in my first work; and the result has been that I am more and more confirmed in the truths that if, in the Eastern Hemisphere, in treating Europeans in youth, and middle life, we would prevent the destruction of organs essential to life, we must overcome congestive and inflammatory diseases of extreme acuteness and danger with a high hand, whether in the use of depletory and emulgent means for the immediate arrest of dangerous disease, or in the use of antiperiodics for the control of malarious paroxysmal fevers; while, in the temperate Western Hemisphere, in treating returned Indians of more advanced age, we have to remove passive congestions and organic diseases of the

b

abdominal viscera, requiring gently eliminative and tonic means of a different and milder nature than such as were proper under the previous and opposite conditions of tropical climates.

Throughout this work I have held in constant view the fact, that a true pathological induction depends mainly on a careful observation of disordered function during the progress of disease, and not upon mere morbid anatomy : in other words, I have endeavoured always to rest pathological conclusions on a physiological basis. It is now felt, says an admirable writer on fever, Dr. Handfield Jones, generally by our best writers and practitioners that morbid anatomy, and even physical signs, are very unsafe guides to trust to exclusively in the treatment of disease. There are symptoms and external signs in fever, for instance, which are more declarative of the true quality of the disease, than sounds appreciated by the ear or *post-mortem* revelations. The adage adopted by Trousseau, that " *naturam morborum remedia ostendunt*" is to the clinical observer the most practically important.

As in the former edition, so in the present, I am under great obligation to Mr. Athol Johnson for his kindness in revising the work while being printed.

J. R. MARTIN.

24, MOUNT-STREET, GROSVENOR-SQUARE,
October, 1861.

PREFACE

FIRST EDITION.

WHEN, little more than twelve months ago, I was called upon to prepare anew the work composed by the late Dr. James Johnson and myself, in 1841, on the "Influence of Tropical Climates on European Constitutions," I felt that a mere reprint could not in justice be proposed as a Seventh Edition. Many years had elapsed since Dr. Johnson's original and admirable work on the subject first appeared. The additions in subsequent re-publications consisted chiefly of his able reviews of the labours and researches of other authors on tropical diseases, which appeared in the "Medico-Chirurgical Review." The work thus became in great part a collection of reviews, which, excellent as they were at the time, could not now be made to represent the advancing knowledge of the day.

I have therefore ventured to re-cast and re-write the entire work. Even the Introductory Chapter is entirely re-written—so much only of Dr. Johnson's observations being retained as appeared to me proper to the subject, and all beyond is exclusively my own composition.

I am well aware of the responsibility I have thus reluctantly assumed. Throughout the present Edition I have adhered to, and preserved the medico-topographic and statistical character of my original Official Reports, which were printed and circulated at the public cost in Bengal, by order of the Supreme Government of India, while I was serving under its orders. In doing so, I am actuated by the conviction that, next to the importance of physiological investigations, stand those which relate to the discovery of the EXTERNAL CAUSES OF DISEASE. By such a course of inquiry we shall, I think, most readily appreciate both the prevention and cure of those formidable diseases to which Europeans are subject in hot climates.

I have likewise continued, so far as the scope and intent of the work admits, an examination of the physiological influences of climate, both Asiatic and European, while every suggestion is offered which seemed to me likely to enhance the value and importance of PREVENTIVE MEDICINE.

For the discussion of the nature, causes, and treatment of tropical diseases, my opportunities, whether rightly or wrongly applied, have been both varied and extended. I served in various parts of India—in peace and war—amongst natives and Europeans —in hospital and in private practice—for two-and-twenty years, and during this time I did my best to collect materials in the ample field which came under my observation ; I wish much that I could command more leisure for the arrangement and completion of my subjects.

A treatise purporting to describe "The Influence of Tropical Climates on European Constitutions," which should not comprise some description of the sequelæ to tropical diseases, and of the counter-influences which, under an European climate, affect the health of persons who have resided long in warm regions, would be obviously incomplete. I therefore here reprint from "The Lancet" certain articles published by me during the last six years, on "The Nature, Causes, and Treatment of the Diseases of Europeans on their Return from Tropical Climates." The want of such a supplementary treatise was felt by my friend Dr. James Johnson, who urged me, on my return from India, to this under-taking ; and having now been several years in extensive observation of this class of invalids, I venture on the discharge of the duty which my friend proposed to me. In conclusion, I cannot refrain from offering a tribute of respect to the memory of the author of the "Influence of Tropical Climates on European Constitutions," originally published in 1813, from materials collected and arranged by him when he was not twenty-four years of age. Having served not quite three years in the Indian seas, as surgeon to a ship-of-war, he had at this time returned home with broken health, several abscesses having been discharged from the liver, rendering his life one of extreme suffering for years thereafter. By great native elasticity of mind and body, he overcame his distresses and difficulties, and ended his career as an esteemed and eminent physician of this metropolis.

Referring to the subject of the sixth edition of the work, composed jointly by Dr. Johnson and myself, in 1841, he observes, with a just pride, that " Although successive editions have received additions and improvements, yet very few of the Author's original doctrines have been subverted or practices exploded, during a period of more than a quarter of a century."

Few men in our profession could say so much ; and I speak but the general sentiment when I say, that fewer still have departed from us leaving a higher reputation for kindliness of feeling and high sense of honour than did Dr. James Johnson.

To his talented son, Mr. Athol Johnson, I am under much obligation for the aid he has given me in revising the work while being printed.

J. R. MARTIN.

GROSVENOR-STREET, GROSVENOR-SQUARE,
December, 1855.

CONTENTS.

PART I.

CLIMATE AND MEDICAL STATISTICS.

PART II.

PREVENTION OF DISEASE.

PART III.

ACUTE TROPICAL DISEASES AND THEIR CURE.

PART IV.

CHRONIC DISEASES OF EUROPEANS ON THEIR RETURN FROM INDIA, AND THEIR CURE.

PART I.

CLIMATE AND MEDICAL STATISTICS.

SKETCH OF THE PHYSICAL CLIMATE OF CALCUTTA,

WITH GENERAL REMARKS

ON THE CAUSES OF PHYSICAL CLIMATE IN BENGAL.

"L'ensemble de toutes les circonstances naturelles et physiques, au milieu desquelles nous vivons dans chaque lieu."—CABANIS.

"The best observations upon climate often lose half their value for want of an exact description of the surface of the country."—MALTE-BRUN.

WHOEVER considers climate with reference to its vast importance to human welfare, must feel some degree of disappointment at the meagreness in which the advanced state of knowledge in the nineteenth century has yet left this most interesting branch of inquiry.

On this all-important subject it is but too evident that, in the language of Sir John Herschel, we have not yet determined *"what ought to be observed,"* and thus it has happened, for want of "a right direction," that much of the labour of observation and minute investigation has been "but labour lost." In medical pursuits, we find continually that the apparent cause of sickness, or of death, is not the real cause; and so it is with the causes of physical climate. "When a thing is accounted for in two ways," says Fontenelle, "the truth is usually on the side most opposed to appearances."

One philosopher, for instance, will view climate as any space distant from the equator and poles; another, as nothing more than a well-arranged table of the winds, of the thermometric, barometric, and hygrometric degrees; a third, as having reference solely to elevation above the mean level of the earth's surface; a fourth, as consisting only of the internal heat of the globe; while a fifth, supposed to be better informed than all the rest, an authority who "seemed to have been in nature's cabinet council," pronounces climate to be influenced only by latitude and local elevation, and allows it to be but slightly affected by any other causes. We may, then, with some show of reason, exclaim with Dr. A. T. Thomson, "What is climate?"

That such partial views are unequal to the elucidation of the subject of climate, will at once be apparent by reference to the common geographical fact, of two places in the same elevation and degree of latitude possessing climates the most opposite. We must, then, look for the causes of climate elsewhere; and however much those may be influenced by elevation and latitude, we shall find other and powerful accessories which greatly influence health, and consequently human happiness. He must be a bold, if not a presumptuous man, however, who shall pretend to do full justice to a subject so elaborate, and which demands the application of such refined principles in physical science as climate; yet I cannot help thinking that much that is important may be done by a careful observation and comparison of facts, made at different times and places; for it is by such means that a complex science like that of climate can alone be perfected. A most interesting demonstration of the *local character* of climate is furnished by Mr. Glaisher of the Royal Observatory, Greenwich, in his remarks on the weather during the quarter ending September 30th, 1847. After showing from a most accurate series of observations, continuous and comparative, that the climate of Cornwall and Devonshire is not only different from every other part of England, but is far from being the same in different parts of these counties, this eminent meteorologist concludes:—"In fact, there seem to be several different climates in these counties, but all of them free from extremes and sudden changes of temperature." If this be true (and who that knows anything of the subject can doubt it?), how vast and various must be the climates over the great continent, the islands, and the extensive lines of coast of the East Indies, and how important must be the careful study of local influences throughout our empire there!

Whether we view the subject in a physical or medical sense, we shall do well to carry along with us the maxim of Professor Adam Fergusson, "that all observation is suggested by comparison." The value of all scientific facts depends in a great measure on their being comparable, and this in an especial manner applies to inquiries relating to medical topography and medical statistics. Speculation can here yield no profit; it is but throwing words in the air. Milton tells us that—

"To know
That which before us lies in daily life
Is the prime wisdom."

I am satisfied that, in a professional sense, it is impossible to take too extended a view of the subject of climate, and that he who succeeds best must follow the indication of Cabanis; "L'ensemble de toutes les circonstances naturelles et physiques, au milieu desquelles nous vivons dans chaque lieu;" for this much is certain, that the framers of elaborate tables of the winds and of the degrees of the thermometer, have as yet done little to inform our minds, or guide our inquiry. "Le climat n'est donc point resserré dans les circonstances particulières des latitudes, ou du froid et du chaud; il embrasse, d'une manière absolument générale, l'ensemble des circonstances physiques attachées à chaque local, il est cet ensemble lui-même; et tous les traits caractéristiques par lesquels la nature a distingué les differents pays entrent dans l'idée que nous devons former du *climat.*"

Medical men, to whom a right understanding of the subject is paramount, whether we consider the good or the evil to be derived from climate, are happily beginning to be aware of this fact; and it is with much satisfaction I find a late writer on medical topography in England declaring, in furtherance of the just and comprehensive views above quoted, that the character of a climate is much more faithfully indicated by such a natural test as its influence on vegetable products, "than by any instrumental or artificial means whatever."

Dr. Mason Good asserts, with truth, that it is no exclusive reproach to medicine that meteorology has hitherto been turned to so little practical advantage; "for, of all the subdivisions of general philosophy, there is none so little entitled to the name of science as meteorology itself. And, till the naturalist has explained the variations of the barometer, the physician need not blush at being incapable of turning to account the supposed influence of the planets, or unfolding the origin, or tracing the capricious courses of epidemics and pestilence." Difficult as is the subject, however, it ought to have its great attractions for the physician; for, assuredly, no other affords so free a scope for original observation and inquiry; and this applies in an especial manner to tropical climates. Dr. Watson observes justly, that "to ascertain the causes of any disease, and to display them before the public mind, are large steps towards the ultimate removal of such as human endeavours are competent to remove. To know the cause of a disease is sometimes to be able to *cure*, often to be able to *prevent* it." Medical officers who go to India may therefore rest assured that, in respect of the climates and their diseases, they will there acquire a real and practical amount of knowledge in exact proportion to the theoretical knowledge of them which they may take to that country. The mind of the young surgeon must be prepared by a careful previous study, so as rightly to distinguish between what may and what may not be analysed and reasoned upon with advantage. Such a course of preparation would be alike advantageous to those whom it will render better qualified to serve the State, and to the State which will be so much the better served.

Malte-Brun's division of Physical Climate shall here be adopted, because it marks the geographical points to which our inquiries may most profitably be directed, inasmuch as a consideration of the details, as given by that admirable writer, brings us at once to the discovery of such errors in the physical condition of any given place as may lead to its improvement, and the consequent prevention of disease—the great end of medical topography.

When, again, we look back to our native country, and boast of its pure and bracing air, let us not forget the important fact, "that it is man himself who has in a great measure created these salubrions climates. France, Germany, and England, not more than twenty ages ago, resembled Canada and Chinese Tartary, countries situated, as well as our Europe, at a mean distance between the equator and the pole."

" Whenever nature is more powerful than industry, whether for good or for bad, man receives from the climate an invariable and irresistible impulse ;" and so it is in Bengal, *"for bad,"* in consequence of the total absence of that " industry" which elsewhere moulds nature to the purposes of man, for his " good."

Physical climate, says Malte-Brun, comprehends the degree of heat and cold, the drought, the humidity, and the salubrity which occur in any given region of the earth.

The causes of physical climate he states to be nine in number :—

1st. The action of the sun upon the atmosphere.

2nd. The interior temperature of the globe.

3rd. Elevation of the earth above the level of the ocean.

4th. The general inclination of the surface and its local exposure.

5th. The position of its mountains relatively to the cardinal points.

6th. The neighbourhood of great seas and their relative situation.

7th. Geological nature of the soil.

8th. Degree of cultivation and of population at which a country has arrived.

9th. The prevalent winds.

To these perhaps may be added :—

10th. Position in respect to the equator.

11th. Position in respect to large rivers or lakes.

12th. Position in respect to forests.

By tracing these causes, and by uniting and arranging under general points of view, the results of particular local observations, we shall, according to Malte-Brun, arrive at an approach to climatology, in some measure corresponding to the present state of the other sciences.

ACTION OF THE SUN UPON THE ATMOSPHERE.

Of all the elements which constitute climate the subject of Heat is the most immediately important to the medical inquirer. Sennertus declares that "Physicians do not calculate the seasons by the sun's course, but by the temperature of the atmosphere."

"All observation," says Dr. Richardson, "leads to the inference that the sun, acting by means of caloric, is the source of all physical power. We have evidence of this in measuring the amount of life, animal and vegetable, throughout the world; for we find that the proportion of life and of motion, from the poles to the equator, corresponds with the heating power of the central luminary. Further, when we desire to supplement nature, we call caloric into action; as in the warming of our bodies at the fire; in the application of heat to the artificial forcing of flowers and fruits; in the employment of heat in the processes of the chemical laboratory or of the iron-foundry; and in the production of motion by the alternate expansion of water into steam and condensation of steam into water."

At all places between $20°$ and $23\frac{1}{2}°$ of latitude, the solar rays during two months fall at noon either perpendicularly, or at an angle which deviates from a right angle only by $3\frac{1}{2}°$ at most. The degree of temperature is also increased by the greater length of the longest days, which near the tropic are $13\frac{1}{4}$ hours. The application of these facts to the geographical position of our Eastern capital, during portions of May, June, July, and August, is sufficiently obvious, and would not seem to require the lengthened details offered by some writers.

The difference between sensible heat and that indicated by instruments, is nowhere more remarkable than within Calcutta during the hot months; where, from the length of time the houses, walls, and roads are getting heated by the sun, the first hours of the night are rendered even more oppressive than the day, from the copious radiation going on for some time after sunset. "The true indication of the force of the solar rays," says Herschel, "would seem to be, *not* the statical effect upon the thermometer, but their momentary intensity measured by the velocity with which they communicate heat to an absorbent body."

Professor Daniel's observations also go to show that the power of solar radiation in the atmosphere increases from the equator to the poles, and from below upwards.

Chowringhee and Garden Reach have a perceptible advantage over Calcutta, from their openness and the great extent of evaporation from trees, which tends so much to reduce temperature.

This delightful property in trees should always be turned to our advantage; and where the grounds are kept in proper order, a moderate number of trees will prove grateful and beneficial in every sense, but especially in the hot dry season. The influence of trees, like that of water expanse, is powerful in another way. By a process of nature, as yet unknown, umbrageous trees arrest the extension or neutralize the qualities of malaria.

In the rains, the evaporation from trees can add but little to the humidity already existing in the atmosphere. It has been computed, however, that a country covered with trees emits more vapour by one-third than one even covered with water, and it is this property that gives to the shade of vegetables a coolness so much more effectual and agreeable than that of rocks or walls.

In the sweeping condemnation by Dr. M'Culloch, of trees, &c. —down to the very flower-pots, he goes a length unwarranted by any known facts. It is surely unphilosophical to view everything in nature as made only for man's destruction.

The following table will exhibit the state of the atmospheric temperature in Calcutta, its weight and humidity, during the years specified. The thermometer in the open air is found to vary from 40° to 110° in this city.

YEAR.	INSTRU-MENT.	MAXIMUM.	MINIMUM.	REMARKS.	
1830	Therm. ...	90°·4	53°·3	Mean barometer.	During these years the observations were registered four times a day, at sunrise, 10 A.M., 4 P.M., and 10 P.M., hence the variations of the maximum and minimum are greater.
	Barom. ...	30 ·131	29 ·512	Wet bulb depression	
	Hygrom...	16 ·9	1 ·5		
1831	Therm. ...	95 ·8	57 ·8		
	Barom. ...	30 ·122	29 ·456		
	Hygrom...	14 ·5	1 ·5	Mean barometer.	
1832	Therm. ...	96 ·9	54 ·6	29°·764	
	Barom. ...	30 ·071	29 ·467		
	Hygrom...	15 ·2	1 ·6		
1833	Therm. ...	97 ·2	61 ·1	Mean temperature.	
	Barom. ...	30 ·095	29 ·485	78°	
	Hygrom...	17 ·3	2 ·3		
1834	Therm. ...	99 ·4	58 ·9		
	Barom. ...	30 ·022	29 ·470		
	Hygrom...	13 ·8	1 ·4		
		In the sun.	On the ground.		
1835	Therm. ...	110°·2	42°·0		Observations only registered at 10 A.M. and 4 P.M.
	Barom. ...	30 ·038	29 ·480		
	Hygrom...	13 ·9	3 ·2		
1836	Therm. ...	May 97°·9	Jan. 53°·5		
	Barom. ...	Jan. 30 ·087	Aug. at 9 h. 50 29°·569		
	Hygrom...	March 14 ·8	August 5 ·6		
1837	Therm. ...	June 98 ·2	not observed.	Each entry is the	
	Barom. ...	Jan. 31 ·101	July 29°·547	average of a month's	
	Hygrom...	April 20 ·4	July, Aug. 4°·2	observations.	

The mean temperature of each month in Calcutta may be seen by the following table.

January.	February.	March.	April.	May.	June.	July.	August.	September.	October.	November.	December.
66°·2	69°·8	80°·0	85°·4	85°·7	83°·7	81°·8	82°·0	82°·0	79°·2	74°·2	66°·6

The greatest range of temperature takes place in December and January, when it amounts to about 18°, the least range is in July, when it is about 6°. The mean hour of minimum temperature for the year is about sunrise; that of maximum temperature, 2 40 P.M.

" At a military station in Upper India the air some feet above ground was observed in the month of January to sink so low as the freezing point; while in July of the same year the temperature rose, at the same station, to 122° in a northern aspect and sheltered position. Here was a difference of 92°—an extreme instance; but in Western India an annual range of 70° to 80° is far from uncommon."—*Julius Jeffreys.*

INTERNAL HEAT.

Some philosophers have sought the cause of climate in the internal heat of the globe. The subject has engaged the attention of scientific men in various countries, but it is only of late that anything approaching to precise information has been obtained. From experiments recently made, it would appear certain that, in proportion to the depression below the earth's surface, so does the temperature steadily increase; and even where the depths were very small the elevation was quite perceptible. At the depth of 100 feet from the surface, the temperature of the earth is the average temperature of the climate, and differs with the latitude; thus at Walso, in Lapland, it is 36°; at St. Petersburg, 40°; in England, 52°; at Paris, 54°; at Rome, 61°; and at Cairo, 70°.— *T. Griffiths.*

It is stated, on the other hand, by Fourier, that at 100 feet below the surface the influence of the solar rays is extinct. The position where this takes place he calls the invariable stratum; all variations above this place are imputed to the influence of radiation, all below to the nature or primeval heat of the globe.

"It is obvious," says Professor Alfred Taylor, "that this increase of our temperature cannot be due to solar influence. 1st. Because the existence of a zone of invariable temperature shows that the power of the sun must be limited to that portion of the earth's crust which is above it. 2nd. Because, if the interior heat of the mass of the earth were due to external or solar influence alone, the thermometer should fall just in proportion as we descend below the invariable stratum. But the reverse of this is the fact, as we may presently be able to establish from the results of accurate observations. Hence we are irresistibly led to this conclusion —that in going below the invariable stratum, we are approaching some great source of heat, which must be situated within the interior of our globe. . . The experiments hitherto made lead to the following interesting results. Diurnal variations of temperature are not perceived beyond two or three feet. Variations depending on the months or seasons extend somewhat lower ; and annual variations are entirely lost at a depth of from 60 to 100 feet, varying slightly in different localities. The maximum depth at which the changes in the thermometer are perceptible, amounts to only 1-400,000th part of the earth's diameter! Upon the alternate heating and cooling of this film, which does not exceed the nine-millionth of an inch in a globe of three feet in diameter, depend all the vicissitudes of temperature in climates, seasons, and cycles of years. . . The extent to which the strata become warmed by the sun must depend,—1st, upon the directness with which the rays fall, hence it is greater in the tropics than in temperate regions, and greater in summer than in winter; 2ndly, upon the conducting power of the strata, which is subject to great variation. It is, however, obvious that the *depth* to which this solar influence extends may be determined by the thermometer. If below the surface of the earth we can find a stratum in which, after a long series of careful observations, made at all seasons of the year, and at all periods of the day and night, this instrument remains stationary, it is certain that we have reached a depth beyond which the power of the sun cannot extend. Such a stratum has been found, and it is called the stratum of INVARIABLE TEMPERATURE. . . One test which has been proposed for the invariable stratum is, that its temperature should correspond to, or differ but little from, the mean temperature of the climate in which the observations are made. On this principle, Boussingault fixed its position in the tropics at one-third of a metre, or rather more than a foot below the surface of the soil; but the recent experiments of Captain Newbold have shown that this is an error ; the *diurnal* variation at this depth amounting to as much as 2°·75 Fah. Captain Newbold found the thermometer to remain stationary, in a shady locality, at about four feet, *i.e.*, at that depth the temperature corresponded to the mean of the atmosphere. . . Whatever affects the mean temperature of a place must affect its position. The influence of the strata in altering the position of this zone was observed by Captain Newbold in the tropics. He found a constant temperature to exist at four feet depth from the surface in clayey soils, but in order to obtain it in light *sandy* soils, it was necessary to go much deeper."

The following is taken from the "Thermometrical Table" of Professor Taylor:—

				Fah.
Artesian well, Vienna, at	200	feet below the surface	. .	55°
Artesian well, Hanwell	290	,,	,, . .	55
Mines of Brittany	500	,,	,, . .	58
Deep mines, Europe	—	,,	,, . .	62
Cumberland coal mines	600	,,	,, . .	66
Durham coal mines	900	,,	,, . .	69
Cairo well	210	,,	,, . .	70
Monkwearmouth mine	1500	,,	,, . .	72
Artesian well, Grenelle	1300	,,	,, . .	73
Mexican mines	1650	,,	,, . .	75
Valenciana mine, Mexico	——	,,	,, . .	91
Grenelle well	1794	,,	,, . .	91

The temperature in mines rises on an average 1° for every 49·6 feet, while that of water in the wells rises 1° for every 54 and 55 feet; the average ratio of increase, in various parts of England and the continent, being about 1° for 46 feet in depth. In the Artesian well of Grenelle the temperature rises 9° in the last 500 feet.

The temperature of the deep sea, on the other hand, varies but little from the equator to the poles, while that on the surface varies considerably, being about 27° in the polar regions, and 88° under the equator.

The conclusions arrived at by the authority here referred to, on the important subject under discussion, are:—

1st. That the *temperature* of the surface of our globe, including that of the air, earth, and sea, depends exclusively upon the quantity of heat transmitted to it from the sun, the heat thus received being again lost, partly by radiation into space, and partly by conduction downwards through the superficial strata.

2nd. That the chief loss takes place undoubtedly by radiation, and that it is by the amount of this last we learn the temperature of the medium (space) in which our globe is floating.

3rd. That at a certain depth below the surface of the earth, there is a source of heat which progressively affects the thermometer as we descend.

4th. That this interior heat cannot be derived from the sun or from local chemical changes.

5th. That it does not directly affect climates or seasons, or perceptibly influence the temperature of the surface of the earth, the depths of the ocean, or the atmosphere floating above them.

6th. That the vicissitudes of climates, seasons, and cycles of years are due entirely to solar influence.

7th. That this influence, even at a maximum, does not penetrate to a greater depth than the 1-400,000th part of the earth's diameter.

8th. That although we have positive evidence of the existence of subterranean heat, we can neither measure its degree, nor, at present, determine its exact ratio of increase downwards into the interior.

9th. That there is not the slightest evidence to show that the earth is gradually cooling from a high temperature, or that, within the last two thousand years, its temperature has undergone any increase or diminution.

ELEVATION OF THE GROUND.

When we consider the accuracy and extensive knowledge we have arrived at in the position of points of interest on the surface of the globe, with regard to the co-ordinates of latitude and longitude, and how little has been done for the third co-ordinate of elevation, we shall have a field before us open to cultivation in many parts of our empire, and of the greatest interest within the Tropics—in the East and West Indies especially.

The importance, in a sanitary point of view, of attention to the subject of elevation, is exemplified in the fact that, plague in Egypt, yellow fever in the West, and marsh remittent in the East and West, have never been known to ascend to any considerable height. The limit of yellow fever, in the Island of Jamaica, was long ago observed by Robert Jackson, while it is notorious that the plague of Egypt confines itself to the low, damp, and marshy districts—never ascending so far even as Assouan, where the soil and, consequently, the atmosphere are dry. But so virulent is the malarious power in the East and West Indies, that an elevation of from two to three thousand feet is necessary to exemption from fever; while in Italy the same immunity is attained by a rise of about fifteen hundred feet above the marshy plains.

With the elevation of the land cold increases in a very rapid progression, being caused by the enlarged capacity which air acquires by rarefaction.

While in descending into the earth we obtain an increase of heat of one degree for about every fifty feet, we find that the rate of increase of cold is one degree for every three hundred and fifty feet of mountain altitude; and this latter beneficent appointment of nature considerably increases the number of habitable countries in the Torrid Zone :—" In ascending from Bengal to Thibet, we imagine ourselves in a few days transported from the equator to the pole."

The site of Calcutta is said to be, on the average, but little, if at all, above the level of the tides at Sägor : in the diplomatic language of Asia, "What more need I say?" as to the choice of our position !

GENERAL AND LOCAL ASPECTS.

The general aspect should be distinguished from the local aspect. The general declivity of a country, large in itself, does not exclude the most opposite local declivities. It may, however, be admitted as a general principle, that the positive sum of all the local aspects is in the same direction as the general aspect.

This principle can only be applied to spaces of great extent; for example, the entire tract of country through which a river flows. Every one knows of what effect as to temperature is the exposure of a soil relatively to the sun. A hill inclined 45° to the south, when the sun is elevated 45°, receives solar rays perpendicularly, whilst upon a plain the same rays strike the soil under an angle of 45°, that is, with one quarter less of force; and a hill inclined 45° to the north will be struck by the solar rays in a horizontal direction, which makes them glide along its surface.

Malte-Brun, speaking of the northern hemisphere, says that the south-south-west and south-west situations are the warmest of all; whilst, on the contrary, those of the north-east are the coldest. The general aspect of the valley of the Ganges is about east and west, with an inclination of the delta to the south.

POSITION OF MOUNTAINS.

Mountains act on climates in two ways. They attract the vapours suspended in the air; these vapours, by their condensation, produce clouds and fogs; often, also, these assemblages of watery substances, which the winds waft in every direction, are stopped in their devious course by chains of mountains, in the elevated valleys of which they continue to accumulate. These effects are still more sensibly felt, when a chain of mountains is crowned with extensive forests. In hot climates mountains of certain elevations secure two cardinal advantages, namely, purity of air and coolness.

The elevated lands in Bengal-Proper hardly merit the name of mountains, and are mostly situated in the districts of Bheerboom, Sylhet, Chittagong, and along the eastern boundaries of Tipperah. They are limited in extent, and exert apparently but little influence on the climate of Calcutta.

EFFECTS OF THE NEIGHBOURHOOD OF THE SEA.

The neighbourhood of the sea moderates the excess of temperature, besides contributing, according to Pouillet, through evaporation, one of the most important sources of atmospheric electricity.

In hot climates the maritime regions are not so warm as the
centre of the plains;—of this we have an annual example in the
marine current of the south-west monsoon.

" In the trade-wind regions at sea," says Lieutenant Maury,*
" evaporation is generally in excess of precipitation, while in the
extra-tropical regions the reverse is the case; that is, clouds let
down more water than the winds take up again; and these are the
regions in which the Gulf Stream enters the Atlantic.

" Along the shores of India, where experiments have been carefully made, the evaporation amounts to three-fourths of an inch
daily. Suppose it in the trade-wind region of the Atlantic to
amount only to half an inch, that would give an annual evaporation of say fifteen feet. In the process of evaporation from the
sea, fresh water only is taken up, the salts are left behind. Now,
a layer of sea-water fifteen feet deep, and as broad as the trade-
wind belts of the Atlantic, and reaching across the ocean, contains
an immense amount of salts."

In some parts of the earth the precipitation is greater than
the evaporation; thus the amount of water borne down by every
river that runs into the sea may be considered as the excess of
the precipitation over the evaporation that takes place in the
valley drained by that river. This excess comes from the sea;
the winds convey it to the interior, and the forces of gravity dashing it along in mountain torrents or gentle streams, hurry it back
to the sea again.

In other parts of the world the evaporation and precipitation are
exactly equal, as in those inland basins such as that in which the city
of Mexico, Lake Titicaca, the Caspian Sea, &c., are situated; which
basins have no ocean drainage. If it were not so, the Caspian
would in the one case overflow the surrounding countries, and in
the other it would dry up, leaving plants and animals to perish.
In the Desert of Sahara, again, there is neither evaporation nor
precipitation, and in it we find neither plants nor animals.

In his annual report of the Bombay Geographical Society, from
May, 1849, to August, 1850, Dr. Buist states, on the authority
of Mr. Laidly, the evaporation of Calcutta to be " about fifteen
feet annually; but between the Cape and Calcutta it averages, in
October and November, nearly three-fourths of an inch daily;
between 10° and 20° in the Bay of Bengal, it was found to exceed

* " Physical Geography of the Sea." By M. F. Maury, LL.D., Lt. U. S. Navy.

an inch daily. Supposing this to be double the average throughout the year, we should have eighteen feet of evaporation
annually.

"On the other hand, we have a rainless region about the Red
Sea, because the Red Sea for the most part lies within the
north-east trade-wind region, and these winds when they reach
that region are dry winds, for they have as yet in their course
crossed no wide sheets of water from which they could take up a
supply of vapour.

"Most of New Holland lies within the south-east trade-wind
region, so does most of inter-tropical South America. But intertropical South America is the land of showers. The largest rivers
and most copiously-watered country in the world are to be found
there; whereas, almost the exact reverse is the case in Australia.
Whence this difference? Examine the direction of the winds
with regard to the shore line of these two regions, and the
explanation will at once be suggested. In Australia, east coast,
the shore line is stretched out in the direction of the trades; in
South America, east coast, it is perpendicular to their direction.
In Australia, they fringe this shore only with their vapour, and
so stint that thirsty land with showers, that the trees cannot
afford to spread their leaves out to the sun, for it evaporates all
the moisture from them; their instincts, therefore, teach them to
turn their edges to its rays. In America, they blow perpendicularly on the shore, penetrating the very heart of the country with
their moisture. Here the leaves, as the plantain, &c., turn
their broad sides up to the sun, and court its rays."

Calcutta is situated about 100 miles from the sea, but so level
is the country that the tides ascend in the dry season as far as
Sooksägur, being 140 miles from Sägor Point.

In the beginning of March, when the south-west monsoon sets
in, the currents set up the Bay of Bengal, and gradually raise the
sea at its head several feet, raising the river Hooghly with it, and
that long before the freshes are felt. This continues till October,
when the pouring of the rivers into the bay, during the rains in
July, August, and September, and the changes of the monsoon to
north-east in the end of October, give the current a set in the
contrary direction, and gradually restore the sea and river to their
condition in the previous March. The effect of the two monsoons
upon the currents, and the height of the sea in the Bay of Bengal,
may therefore be considered as that of two long unequal tides
during the year—eight months of flood and four of ebb. From
the point of lowest low water in the dry season, to that of the
highest high water in the freshes is 20 feet 10 inches.

The greatest mean rise of the tide from low- to high-water mark
in the freshes is ten feet. The smallest mean rise of the tide in
the dry season, neap tides, is four feet. The "Bores" in the
Hooghly occur only in the highest, or alternate spring tides; their

appearance may with certainty be predicted by the season of the year and the parallax of the moon. They are greatest under the influence of the south-west monsoon, and are only felt in those portions of the river where the peculiar form of the sands, and the direction and set of the tides in any particular reach, actuate their rise.*

Persons who speak confidently, and enter into minute details on the tides and levels, assert that we are only protected from irruptions of the sea by the counter-currents of the rivers, and the friction of the tides against their banks. They state the tides in the Salt Lake to be but two feet above the mean level at Sägor, and consequently several feet, at flood-tide, below that at Sägor. Of the truth of some of these assertions we had a calamitous illustration on the 20th and 21st of May, 1833, when the sea, backed by a storm from the east-south-east and south-east overran the low countries along the coast from Balasore, along Hidgelee, and up to Tumlook and Diamond Harbour, making a breach over the Soonderbuns as far north as Calcutta, and extending its devastations as far east as Dacca. There have been many irruptions of the sea within fifty years, but none to equal this last in violence and extent. In some days the barometer stood at 28 inches and 8 decimals, being lower than it had been known for years; the thermometer averaged 84°.

The tide, which ran for seven hours, rose to a height of twelve feet above its ordinary level, destroying embankments and buildings of every kind, while the storm levelled the trees; nothing stood within the influence of tide and wind, and the loss of human life and destruction of cattle must have been enormous.

Sägor Island was covered seven feet deep; and out of a population of 7000 persons few escaped. The rains were nearly a month later than usual in setting in, and the ordinary cultivation was arrested from the saturation of the soil with salt. The starving survivors from these united calamities crowded about the outer suburbs of Calcutta, and were at last reduced to the necessity of supporting the parents' lives by the wretched and unnatural traffic in their children, the most emaciated of whom sold at last *for one rupee.*

Government did much to relieve the more pressing necessities of these poor people; but there was much that no power could relieve. Towards the end of August there broke out a severe epidemic fever, which, by the end of September, and during the drying process, ripened into terrible violence—carrying off, according to the reports of respectable natives, nearly three-fourths of the remaining population to the south and east of us. Neither did Calcutta escape; thousands of the natives died, particularly in the suburbs, nearest the land inundated in May; even the

---

* *Vide* the interesting paper by Mr. James Kyd, Trans. A. Society.

Europeans suffered severely, though there were not many casualties in proportion to the numbers attacked with the fever.

It is an object of interest to ascertain the surface temperature of the sea in different situations. The following is stated by Dr. Mitchell, on the authority of Aimé, to be the temperature of the Mediterranean at a distance of 100 to 2000 metres outside the port of Algiers, compared with the temperature of the air, from observations made between 1840 and 1845. Averages calculated for the seasons.

	Sea.	Air.	Difference.
Winter	57·92	54·32	+3·60
Spring	59·90	61·34	−1·44
Summer	71·96	73·40	−1·44
Autumn	69·03	68·00	+1·08
Annual averages	64·71	64·26	

" In winter and autumn, therefore, the surface temperature of the Mediterranean off Algiers is higher than the temperature of the atmosphere, but lower in spring and summer. In the waters of the Mediterranean outside the port of Algiers, the diurnal variations cease at a depth of about 60 feet, and the annual variations at a depth of 380 to 440 yards. Observations made in France and Belgium show that the diurnal variations of temperature of the crust of the earth cease at a depth of rather more than 4 feet, and the annual variations at about 80 feet."

It has been shown by the observations of Drs. Lloyd and Hennessy, that the mean temperature of the sea on the west coast of Ireland is four degrees higher than the mean temperature of the land. The winter temperature is as high as that of the southern shores of the Euxine, while, on the other hand, the great precipitation of vapour gives a summer heat as low as parts of Finland. These results are due to the warm current of water which flows from the Gulf of Mexico towards the British Islands and the north of Europe. This current, heated in the warm regions of its origin, exercises its influence very sensibly on the atmosphere, raising its temperature, and charging it with vapours which are known to give out a certain amount of heat.

On the general question, Dr. Lloyd states that, " According to the computation of Bessel, 25,000 cubic miles of water flow in every six hours from one quarter of the earth to another. The store of mechanical force is thus diminished, and the temperature of our globe augmented, by every tide. We do not possess the data which would enable us to calculate the magnitude of these effects. All that we know with certainty is, that the resultant effect of all the thermal agencies to which the earth is exposed has undergone no perceptible change within the historic period. We owe this fine deduction to Arago. In order that the date-palm should ripen its fruit, the mean temperature of the place must exceed 70° Fah.; and, on the other hand, the vine cannot be cultivated successfully when the temperature is 72° or upwards. Hence, the mean temperature of any place at which these two plants flourished and bore fruit must lie between these narrow limits, *i.e.*, could not differ from 71° Fah. by more than a single degree. Now, from the Bible we learn that both plants were simultaneously cultivated in the central valleys of Palestine in the time of Moses; and its then temperature is thus definitively determined. It is the same at the present time; so that the mean temperature of this portion of the globe has not sensibly altered in the course of thirty-three centuries."

GEOLOGICAL NATURE OF THE SOIL.

Whenever the natives of India speak of climate, they designate it by the terms "air and water." They have, indeed, no other definition of it. The circumstance is here mentioned to show that the popular impression on this important head, throughout Hindustan, is at least as well-founded in fact as some others that, in Europe, are entertained by philosophers.

The nature of the soil, which must of necessity influence the qualities of both air and water in an essential manner, remains unnoticed in most definitions, European and Asiatic; yet the geological nature of the soil would seem one of the most important of the causes of physical climate. Of this I became satisfied very early in my service in India. "Man," says Boudin, " is in more respects than one the mere expression of the soil in which he lives."

Clay lands, while they retain water and moisture of every kind, do not readily admit either heat or air, owing to their compact and adhesive nature. They are proverbially cold, as are also the chalky soils. Soils containing much carbonaceous or ferruginous matter, on the other hand, acquire a very high temperature under the solar rays, while they likewise cool more rapidly than other soils, especially when dry.

Dark soils, too, absorb heat more powerfully, and radiate heat more energetically than light-coloured soils, which reflect a great portion of heat. In short, a very slight attention to the effects of various qualities of soils will be sufficient to show that these last affect very powerfully both the temperature and the humidity of the atmosphere; and hence the vast importance of this branch of study.

The internal nature or composition of the soil must have an influence on climate in a variety of ways. All grounds are not heated equally soon. One soil quickly parts with its acquired heat, while another retains it for a long time. Exhalations, which vary according to the nature of the soil, rise into the atmosphere, and become identified with it. Clayey grounds, and those which are impregnated with salt, cool the atmosphere; extensive accumulations, when they are dry, augment the heat. The general soil of Bengal is clay, with a considerable proportion of silicious sand, fertilized by various salts, and by decayed substances, animal and vegetable. Both the upper and sub-soil are generally pervious to water, but at an average depth of twenty feet is found a tenacious clay; at this depth, too, brackish water is obtained. In sinking wells in the vicinity of Calcutta no springs of fresh water were reached at a depth of 480 feet.

In the old magazines and newspapers printed in Calcutta, I find very frequent mention of earthquakes; but in none of these does there seem to have been any material injury sustained, which looks as if the causes were remote from us.

In April and May, while marching to join the Ramghur battalion, over the abrupt mountain ranges which are crossed between Midnapore, in the province of Orissa, and Sumbhulpore, on the Mahanuddy river, province of Gondwana, I observed that throughout the entire extent of that country, so noted for the fatal character of its fevers, the soil was invariably ferruginous. During the whole march through this deadly country free electricity was noticeable in the air to an amount which I never observed anywhere else. Crackling noises and distinct flashes of light accompanied the passage of the comb through the hair.

The late Major Markham Kittoe, of the Bengal army—a fellow-sufferer from the destructive fevers of those countries—presented me with the following sketch from memory, when at home on sick leave, in 1842. The quality of the soil is given as the result of repeated personal examination :—

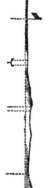

Calcutta and Fort William, on the Hooghly.

Tumlook. The Roopnarrain and Doomooda.

Midnapore on the Kossai.

High land of Midnapore between the Roopnarrain and Kossai rivers. Iron clay resting on decomposed primitive rock and lithomarge—soil and water strongly impregnated with iron oxide—cerebral fevers common here.

Seersa on the Subanreeka.

Shingle and sandy tracts—quartz and hornblende—oxide of iron—forests of stunted saul and Assina—fevers prevalent.

Granite, sienite, quartzose rocks, steatite, and serpentine hornblende—this is the first range running north and south, varying from 500 to 3500 feet, covered with dense forests of saul and other

LEVEL OF SEA

trees, and the climate deadly—water very scarce, impregnated with vegetable and mineral matter—iron ore in great abundance, the soil red with its oxide.

Keunjhur on the Byturnee.

This country is very deadly; the soil chiefly red from iron oxides.

300 MILES

Keunjhur and Mahagirri Hills, sienite, gneiss, talcite, hornblende, kidney-iron ore and iron in every shape—it affects the needle—deadly climate except on the heights, which vary from 1700 to 4000—gneiss—gold found in the rivers.

Bonaie on the Brahmini.

Beaumurra Hills—gneiss, quartzose, iron ore in abundance—some very fine falls of water strongly impregnated with calcareous matter, leaving stalactite—considered wholesome—height 1200 feet.

Height of this range about 300 feet above Sumbhulpoor, or 800 feet above the sea.

Gneiss formation, talcite—much iron, though less than in the other ranges—diamonds and gold worked for—matrix red clay and sand—height supposed to be about 500 feet—climate very unhealthy in the hot season—to strangers deadly.

Sumbhulpoor on the Mahanuddi.

In the " Madras Quarterly Medical Journal," for 1841, is published a very interesting report " On the Hill Fevers of the Southern Peninsula of India," by Dr. Heyne, of the Madras army. This officer, after describing the hill ranges, " which have rendered themselves known to Europeans for the malignity of the fever," and likewise those that are " as *constantly free of the hill fever*," goes on to state that here, the received opinions, as to the vegetable or marshy origin of fever, will not hold, for that the hills in question " are not more woody than in other healthy places ;—some, indeed, where the epidemic of 1808 and 1810, as well as the endemic, were most destructive, are quite naked of trees, as Dindigal, Madura, and the rocks west of Seringapatam.   .   .   .

Now, if it should be found that the fever exists *constantly* and *invariably* among *certain* description *of hills*, when others of *a different composition* are as *constantly free from the same*, would it not become reasonable to suppose that the *nature* or composition of the rock itself must furnish the cause of the calamity? The hills where it is found to prevail appear, at first view, to be quite harmless, as they are *granite*, which is the most common rock-kind on this globe. They contain, however, besides *quartz, felspar, and mica*, a great proportion of *ferruginous hornblende*, which, by its disintegration or separation from the rock, becomes highly magnetic, and *in which*, I suppose, the *cause resides* which produces this fever, besides a great train of other diseases. The iron hornblende occurs in such quantity that all the rivulets, public roads, indeed, all hollows along the hills, are filled with its *sand;* from which, also, all the iron in this part of the country is manufactured."

Dr. McClelland of Bengal, in his excellent "Medical Topo-graphy," draws a distinction which, if fully verified by future observation, may prove of importance in a sanitary point of view, namely, that between hilly districts composed of laterite—hard, rough, and much inclined, having but scanty vegetation—and the flat, low, wet lands, or laterite covered with sandy soil, always clothed with coarse rank grass, there is a difference as to season in manifesting their evil influences—especially in the production of fever.

" The character in common which the remittents of these late-rite districts present, and by which they are distinguished from the corresponding type of fever of the Tarai and Soonderbuns is, that while the fevers of the laterite districts prevail during the hot weather as early as March, those of the low districts, composed of light sandy soil, do not set in until after the rainy season has commenced, being above two months later.

" Again, the jungles of laterite districts do not become safe until the month of January—that is, three months after the rains have subsided; while those of the light soils of the flat plains become safe in November, within a month or six weeks of the breaking up of the rains."

In the districts referred to in my personal experience, it did not happen that, of two detachments of troops employed there in two different years, either found any difference in health between the hot and the cold season, both having proved equally obnoxious to fever.

In pursuance of my early observations, and referring also to those of Dr. Heyne, I obtained through the kindness of my friend Sir Charles Trevelyan, Secretary to the Treasury, a report on the quality of the soils of all the most unhealthy stations on the west coast of Africa, as well as samples of the several earths. These last, including the mud of the rivers, were, without exception, ferrugi-nous. Reports from Hong-Kong speak of "ferruginous-looking clay," and of "pestiferous mineral gas." The soil of this station proves on analysis to be ferruginous.

Captain Pemberton says that the ranges of hills stretching south of Chittagong, and forming a great portion of the prover-bially unhealthy country of Aracan, are composed "almost entirely of sandstone, with which a stiff ferruginous clay is frequently commingled." Here the army of General Morrison was destroyed by malignant fever chiefly, in 1825, Europeans and natives of Hindustan suffering alike.

In the "Excursions" of Mr. Featherstonhaugh into the Slave States of the American Union, we find "malaria" mentioned in continual connexion with the "ferruginous" soil of those countries, with the "red sandstone rock," and "the red mud of the Arkansas."

In the "Medical Topography of the West Coast of Africa," by Mr. Ritchie, surgeon R.N., it is stated that the rugged surface of the country around Freetown, Sierra Leone, is composed of a "scanty and red earth." Speaking of Bathurst, at the mouth of the Gambia, Mr. Ritchie says of the rainy season and its tornadoes, which are most prevalent at the commencement and termination of the rains :—"They always come from the eastward, and produce violent electrical phenomena. This period of the year is the most pregnant with disease."

My friend, Dr. M'William, in his admirable " Medical History of the Expedition to the Niger," speaks of "fever of a most malignant character" as having broken out in the Albert, within a short distance of the red cliff of Iddah. This cliff is composed of "ferruginous sandstone."

Sir William Napier, in his history of Sir Charles Napier's administration of Sindh, states that Dr. Kirke, of the Bengal army, who bestowed great attention upon the subject, attributed the fatal fever of that country, in 1844, "to exhalations from limestone rocks on which the barracks were built." Others again attributed the fever, so fatal to the 78th Highland Regiment, to neglect of the tanks ; but the sickness was more generally ascribed to "an unusually high and anomalous inundation, and an equally anomalous fall of the Indus, which brought an extraordinarily fertile but premature vegetation. The early and entire subsidence of the waters left this vegetation to be withered up by the sun, which produced, as it always does in Sindh, malaria."

Sir William Napier, referring to these several opinions, justly observes, that probably all the causes were here condensed. He adds, that "this and other epidemics which prevail at irregular periods in Sindh, arise from exhalations produced by volcanic action ; for the country, though alluvial, is so subject to sudden and extensive changes from earthquakes, that in 1819 nearly the whole surface of Cutch was changed."

But soils of various colours may be quite as ferruginous as the red soils—the difference being that, when dark, they retain organic matters, while, in the purely red earths, all organic substances have been more or less decomposed or dissipated. May not this decomposition by the iron, together with the magnetic phenomena elicited by heat and other agents, be productive of disease, and of fever especially, in certain climates and localities ?

I am aware of the numerous objections that may be urged to this, or to any other hypothesis ; but, in the absence of conclusive aids from chemistry and meteorology, we can do no better than have recourse to rational conjectures. " There is nothing so clear and obvious," says Biot, " as the discovery of yesterday : nothing so obscure as that of to-morrow."

"Whatever may be the cause," says Hennen, "it is certain that, in many countries, the malaria does not arise until all the surface-water has totally disappeared, and leaves the whole surface of the country, including the many courses of the winter streams, an arid desert."

The difference in the composition of the soil on the sea-coast and in the interior of the United States, is declared by Dr. Forcy to cause the vast difference observable in the prevalence of inter-mittent fever. On the coast, with a sandy soil, the rate of inter-mittent fever is but 36 per 1000 annually, while in the interior, where the soil is alluvial, composed of a rich vegetable mould from three to six feet deep, the fever is nearly six times as prevalent.

In the suburbs of London it is said that in places drained within the last few years the temperature has been raised, fogs have disappeared, and influenza, marsh fevers, rheumatism and neuralgic, pains have much diminished. The deaths also in the clay districts of the metropolis, compared with the " gravelly districts within a few miles of London, were as three to one."

M. Boudin, surgeon-general to the Military Hospital at Ver-sailles, speaking of the great importance of the nature of the soil in relation to public health, and how necessary it is that this should be an object of special attention on the part of military surgeons especially, observes :—" It may not be out of place at present to call to mind the connexion which the attentive ob-server remarks between the configuration and the geological cha-raeter of the soil. If we consider that other connexion which exists within certain limits between the geological nature of the soil and certain pathological conditions of man, we comprehend at once the important part reserved in future, in a medical point of view, for the study of physical geography. Thus the occur-rence of goitre and cretinism in the Alps and Pyrenees caused the existence of the same forms of disease in the Himalayas and Cordilleras to be foreseen a long time, and experience has verified the induction." The same able writer says justly, that the known effects of the marshes of the Italian rivers enable us to determine with certainty the character of predominant disease in the great deltas of the Blue and Yellow rivers in China ; the Zaire, the Orange, and Zambeza, in Africa ; the Amazon, the Orinoko, and the Rio del Norte, in America. " Finally," he says, " as under a dissimilar geological constitution, we see the forms of disease differ entirely at the mouth of the Po from those of the Arno, so we can predict a similar difference between the eastern and western coasts of America, and affirm safely the rarity of marsh fevers at the granitic embouchures of the Simpson, the Columbia, the Oregon, and the St. Francis."

The same authority remarks, that a reference to the geological map of England exhibits the sites of the largest of our towns on the hard red sandstone; while the smaller towns, and those of the agricultural districts, are situated on the chalks or oolites.

When we reflect on the vital importance of the cerebral and organic functions, and on the readiness and power with which these functions are influenced by the electric and malarious states of the atmosphere, we shall at once comprehend the vast interests connected with the subjects treated in this article. They form, indeed, the real and only excuse for its length.

It has long been known that animals waste and perish when they have been deprived of their positive electricity by being attached to the opposite pole of a galvanic battery. When the human body, on the other hand, has been for some time exposed to an atmosphere of a negative electricity, it is believed by many to become thus incapable of resisting the various causes of disease, as the exhalations from the earth, the force of epidemics, &c. The varying states of the earth's magnetism cannot fail of exercising powerful influences on human health, however little may be the present amount of our knowledge respecting the nature and operations of these influences.

In 1845 I obtained, through Sir Charles Trevelyan, samples of three kinds of earth from Sierra Leone;—viz. that of the Coast, of the Isles de Loss, and of Grand Cape Mount, as also of the rivers Sierra Leone and Pongos. The following replies to questions submitted by me were likewise received from the colony of Sierra Leone :—

" 1. What is the geological character of the soil in and around the settlement ?

" Above high water mark, red earth—specimen sent. Below high water mark, black mud—specimen·sent from Congo Creek. Flats and valleys, black earth—specimen sent from King Tom's Point.

" 2. Does ferruginous or red sandstone prevail, or red earth ?

" Red earth. Red sandstone in the strata (used for building) underneath—specimen sent from Freetown. Occasionally large blocks and some strata of blue granite (now used in building)— specimen sent from Fort Thornton.

" 3. Is the soil of the most unhealthy stations of a ferruginous nature ?

" I have never heard any one station in this colony called less healthy than another.

" 4. Does the soil of the valleys or flats partake of the ferruginous character?

" Yes.

" 5. Do the low lands emit any offensive gases or smells, and, if so, at what period of the twenty-four hours?

" The mud by the river banks smells when exposed to the sun at ebb tide.

" 6. Does magnetic iron exist, and, if so, is the variation of the compass affected by it?

" Yes—specimen sent from Tower Hill barrack-yard.

" 7. Has the nature of the soil in general, or of the most unhealthy localities in particular, been chemically analysed?

" Answer by Dr. Fergusson—So far as I know there has not been any minute analysis of the soil of this colony beyond the general one, that the soil is ferruginous; gravelly in some parts, loamy in others, in others sandy; but in all ferruginous."

For the following report on the qualities of the specimens of earth from Sierra Leone, I am indebted to Professor Bowman, of King's College, London. The numbers, as given below, do not correspond with those mentioned in the answers to queries; and one of the specimens reported on by Professor Bowman was from the colony of Hong-Kong:—

" I have now completed the estimation of the oxide of iron in the specimens of soil from Sierra Leone, and beg to hand you the following results. They are nearly all remarkable for the large quantity of ferruginous matter which they contain:—

"No. 1 contains   8·84 per cent. oxide of iron.
     2   ,,   26·00   ,,   ,,
     3   ,,   11·48   ,,
     4   ,,   23·20   ,,
     5   ,,   29·00   ,,
     6   ,,   46·12   ,,
     8   ,,   6·92   ,,
     9   ,,   11·56   ,,
Another, numbered 9, 12·48   ,,   ,,

This is described as "taken up at the rising of the hill below Mr. Melville's farm, not far from the Regent Farm road, and a fair specimen of the earth of the colony. That in the bottle, with no label, but which is probably No. 7, contains 11·00 per cent. oxide of iron."

Mr. Clarke, the colonial surgeon of Sierra Leone, states that " among the causes of unhealthiness of the climate the electric condition of the atmosphere, and the sudden alternations of temperature may be mentioned; but the latent cause of the atmospheric impurity has hitherto eluded the investigations of the chemist. Sulphuretted hydrogen, no doubt, plays a distinguished part in this infection of the atmosphere."

at the mouth of the Po from
a similar difference between
America, and affirm safe th
tic embouchures of the in
the St. Francis."

The same authority re
map of England exhibits
the hard red sandstone;
agricultural districts, ar

When we reflect on

and
these functions are in
of the atmosphere, we
connected with the
indeed, the real and

It has long bee
they have been
attached to the
human body, the virule
to an atmo ection
to become by comb
the
vary hot climates
po sea the dried

Humboldt, in the 5t
mentioning the fevers
around the two great
natives believe the pest
of the Raudales to
and wherever the Orin
Santa Barbara, pe
smooth black
matter does
granite contain
pearance is
by the n
that of
the
the
be

would be salubrious or agree-
an exercises so powerful an in-
d purity of the air.   By cultiva-
ıoxious elements from the earth,
rifies the atmosphere he breathes ;
ıı renders the soil and air impure

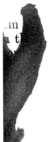

, thatanimalized vegetable matters in a
are coılensed and not decomposed by
t which ıe sand may be classed.   " In the
er putriddecomposition commences.   The
oduces ar condensed in the sandy soil of
¹, and in ·hich the dead repose.   When the
ature mıkes the ferments evaporate, man
ıerficia absorbent vessels, or by those of
piratin."
esertıountry, the rivers, abandoned to
ـd anıoverflow, and their waters serve
marshı.   A labyrinth of thickets and of
ıe mostertile hills.   In the meadows the
om and he useless moss choke the nutri-
ecome impnetrable to the rays of the sun ;
e putrid exalations of the trees which have
essure.of aə ; the soil, excluded from genial
ıth of air, exales nothing but poison ; and an
ıth gathers oⅴr all the country.   But what do
ıd perseveranceaccomplish ?   The marshes are
ers flow in theirlisencumbered channels ; the axe
ar away the foəsts ; the earth furrowed by the
d to the rays cˈthe sun and the influence of the
ıe soil, and the wɩers acquire by degrees a character
d vanquished naıre yields its empire to man, who
ountry for himsdˈ.
ed fertility of thsoil," says Dr. Southwood Smith,
e healthy by diıinishing its moisture and raising
One cubic footf water in the process of evapora-
·ee millions of ıbic feet of air of one degree of
n undrained fieⅼ growing rushes has a permanent
. four to six deⱳees lower than an adjoining field
ⱳing wheat. Ɓy draining and manuring, by
ıces, by remoⱳg trees, by clearing underwood,
the free aëratbn of the soil, the temperature of
l in the northɔf England has been permanently

The opinion here expressed refers, doubtless, to the report of Mr. Daniel, who was sent by the Admiralty to the west coast of Africa to analyse the sea-water along the coast between latitudes 15° and 16°. In it he found a large quantity of sulphuretted hydrogen, emanating from a soil of volcanic origin, or from the decomposition of sulphates in the sea-water by the carbonaceous matters arising from the decay of the immense masses of vegetable productions which grow down to the water's edge. For a long time past it has been observed that the copper sheathing of a ship will be more damaged during a nine months' cruise off this coast, than from a service of three or four years in other climates.

By some authorities it is deemed probable that, of all the matters evolved in volcanic eruptions, sulphur is the agent which, by its affinities, adds most to the intensity and virulence of malarious exhalations along the west coast of Africa—a region at all times so fatal to European settlers. "If sulphuretted hydrogen," says Dr. Aitken, "should hereafter be determined to be an element increasing the virulence of the disease [fever], it will be an interesting question whether it acts merely as a depressant, or whether, by combining with the poison, it augments its intensity."

In many hot climates the most deadly sites for encampments have been the dried-up beds of rivers, or their immediate vicinities.

Humboldt, in the 5th volume of his "Personal Narrative," in mentioning the fevers in the villages of Atures and Maypures, around the two great cataracts of the Orinoko, says that the natives believe the pestilent exhalations that arise from the bare rocks of the Raudales to be the cause :—"Among the cataracts, and whenever the Orinoko, between the missions of Corichana and Santa Barbara, periodically washes the granite rocks, they become smooth black, and as if coated with blacklead. The colouring matter does not penetrate the stone, which is coarse-grained granite containing a few solitary crystals of hornblende. The same appearance is seen in the primitive rocks of Syene, and was observed by the naturalists of Captain Tuckey's expedition in the 'Yallalas' that obstructed the Congo." Humboldt asks, "Can it be possible that, under the influence of excessive heat and constant humidity, the black crusts of the granite rocks are capable of acting on the ambient air, and producing miasmata with a triple basis of carbon, azote, and hydrogen ?"

INFLUENCE OF THE LABOUR OF MAN—GENERAL POPULATION.

Without cultivation few climates would be salubrious or agreeable, and it is by its means that man exercises so powerful an influence upon the temperature and purity of the air. By cultivation the husbandman eradicates noxious elements from the earth, and thereby warms, dries, and purifies the atmosphere he breathes; while by his neglect of tillage he renders the soil and air impure and unwholesome.

Parisot remarks justly, that animalized vegetable matters in a state of decomposition are condensed and not decomposed by porous bodies, amongst which fine sand may be classed. " In the mild and moist winter putrid decomposition commences. The subtle ferments it produces are condensed in the sandy soil of which Egypt is formed, and in which the dead repose. When the elevation of the temperature makes the ferments evaporate, man receives them by the superficial absorbent vessels, or by those of the lungs in the act of respiration."

Let us contemplate a desert country, the rivers, abandoned to themselves, become choked and overflow, and their waters serve only to form pestilential marshes. A labyrinth of thickets and of brambles overspreads the most fertile hills. In the meadows the unsightly wild mushroom and the useless moss choke the nutritious herbs; forests become impenetrable to the rays of the sun; no wind disperses the putrid exhalations of the trees which have fallen under the pressure of age; the soil, excluded from genial and purifying warmth of air, exhales nothing but poison; and an atmosphere of death gathers over all the country. But what do not industry and perseverance accomplish? The marshes are drained; the rivers flow in their disencumbered channels; the axe and the fire clear away the forests; the earth furrowed by the plough is opened to the rays of the sun and the influence of the wind; the air, the soil, and the waters acquire by degrees a character of salubrity; and vanquished nature yields its empire to man, who thus creates a country for himself.

" The increased fertility of the soil," says Dr. Southwood Smith, " renders it more healthy by diminishing its moisture and raising its temperature. One cubic foot of water in the process of evaporation deprives three millions of cubic feet of air of one degree of temperature. An undrained field growing rushes has a permanent temperature from four to six degrees lower than an adjoining field drained and growing wheat. By draining and manuring, by throwing down fences, by removing trees, by clearing underwood, and by promoting the free aëration of the soil, the temperature of large tracts of land in the north of England has been permanently raised three degrees. Thus that very culture of the earth by which it is made to yield the largest amount of food, increases its salubrity as an abode for man, and lessens at their source the main causes of epidemics."

Agriculture must be much improved in Bengal before the European, in the language of Malte-Brun, can be said to have created a country for himself. A Hindu field is described by Mill to be in the highest state of cultivation where only so far changed by the plough as to afford a scanty supply of mould for covering the seed, while the useless and hurtful vegetation is so far from being eradicated, that where burning precedes not, the grasses and steriles which have bid defiance to the plough cover a large portion of the surface. The same author concludes, that "everything which savours of ingenuity, even the most natural results of common observation and good sense, is foreign to the agriculture of the Hindus. Their ideas of improvement are very limited; they scarcely extend beyond the introduction of irrigation into land which was formerly cultivated dry. Each small proprietor is content to follow the customs of his forefathers; the same rude implements of husbandry, the same inferior race of cattle, and the same practices are still in operation, which have existed unchanged for centuries. As to any new experiments of general manuring, draining, differences in the rotation of crops, introducing new grain or vegetables, or new sorts of those already known, any attention to their breed of cattle, any adoption of a better and more combined system by which a smaller number of people could raise the same or a larger proportion of produce—all these are out of the question."

I cannot find that the example of Eurppean superiority has had much influence on the state of agriculture around the metropolis of India. It is certain that in the cold season the markets are supplied with excellent vegetables of every kind; but beyond this I believe matters are much the same as in the days of Job Charnock, the founder of Calcutta. The general crops are of rice. In the Appendix to the Parliamentary Reports of 1831, I find the population of the 24 Pergunnahs, suburbs, and city, rated at 1,225,000, which I have reason to think is over-estimated.

THE PREDOMINANT WINDS.

The united influence of all the elements which constitute physical climate is variously modified by the prevailing winds; and all their variations depend on the equilibrium of the atmosphere, the heat of one climate and the cold of another, exercising a continual influence on each other. Atmospheric currents prevent the accumulation in it of the noxious elements which are constantly emanating from the earth's surface. Winds are justly stated to control the temperature and humidity, to promote evaporation, and to possess individual unexplained peculiarities which affect both animal and vegetable life.

Mr. Atkinson, referring to the well-known influence of different winds on plants and insects—on the animal and vegetable fibre—observes, that " there is something in the atmosphere which, by change of wind, causes a simultaneous action in all living substances and structures. The pimpernel, ' the poor man's weatherglass,' and the chickweed," he says, " are both excellent natural barometers, opening their delicate structures on sunny days, and closing them against rain. So also the spiders prognosticate the north and east winds, which ' cause them to leave their webs and shelter themselves in holes.' " Mr. Hingeston suggests that the causes of the violence of the winds, if not their directions, are electro-magnetic, and that the partial rarefaction of the air by heat, and its condensation by cold, hitherto employed for explaining the force and current of the winds, are most likely only striking parts of terrestrial electro-magnetism.—Dr. Pickford's *Hygiene.*

The northern parts of a great continent will sometimes send forth their cold air towards the southern parts; and sometimes they will receive warm air in return. The monsoon always changes some time after the equinoxes, and constantly blows towards that hemisphere in which the sun is found. The action of this luminary on the atmosphere is therefore plainly one of their causes, the cold air from the mountains of Thibet following its course for half the year, and that from the southern seas during the other.

The south-west rainy monsoon, the most remarkable of our periodical winds, begins on the Malabar coast in May, and reaches Delhi by the end of June, extending to the north-eastern parts of Affghanistan, but greatly modified. It prevails more in the mountains than the flats of the Punjaub; the hills and valleys of Cashmere have their share of it, and it gradually loses itself westward in the valley of Peshawur, where it appears only in clouds and showers. On the Coromandel Coast it is retarded, the clouds brought by the south-west winds being detained by the Ghauts. It reaches Bengal by the 15th of June.

Owing to the arrest of the south-west monsoon by the mountains, and consequent accumulation of vapour, an extraordinary deposition of rain takes place on the Malabar Coast, being not less than 123—5 inches in the year in the latitude of $11\frac{1}{2}°$ north.

When not influenced by elevated lands, this monsoon generally prevails north of the Equator from April to October, accompanied by tempests, storms, and rain, while a north-east wind blows during the other six months. The periodical winds that prevail in the Bay of Bengal extend their influence over the flat country, until they are diverted by chains of mountains into another direction, nearly correspondent, however, with the course of the

Ganges. When the sun has passed into the southern hemisphere, the monsoon alters its direction; the mass of air which had been accumulated during the hot season and rains on the central platform of Asia, now bestirs itself, and moves towards the regions south of the Equator, where the atmosphere has been dilated and dissipated by the solar heat. Over most parts of the Indian Ocean this monsoon proceeds from the north-east, because the central platform lies to the north-east. On the other hand, as the seas of China, of Borneo, of New Guinea, of Java, have the centre of Asia to the north and north-west, the monsoon comes to them from these points.

In the south of Bengal the prevalent winds are north and south; in Behar east and west, and the same takes place in Assam, following the course of the Brahmaputra.

That the monsoons exercise a beneficial influence on health cannot be doubted, but especially the south-west, from its prevalence during the greatest heats, and from its greater power of thoroughly ventilating the country—" Qualis aer, talis spiritus." Stagnation would prove immediately destructive to health in a climate where so many and such abundant sources of noxious effluvia exist, ready to ripen into activity should such a cessation of wind occur as would admit of their accumulation, and that of heat, in any one place, or in such streets, for instance, as those of the native portion of Calcutta. Of the north-east monsoon I must limit my praises solely to its ventilating properties; for in every other respect it exercises an unfavourable influence on health to a degree not generally known; indeed, so far from it, that it is common to hear the accession of the cold season hailed by invalids who are ignorant of the many dangers it carries along. It is the true "Sirocco of the North."

The following table gives the direction of the winds at noon during the years specified :—

Years.	N. Days	NW. Days	W. Days	SW. Days	S. Days	SE. Days	E. Days	NE. Days	Calm Days	Unregistered days.
In 1832 the wind was	44	60	26	44	67	49	4	71	9	No regist. 1 day.
1833 ,, ,,	56	39	14	30	115	24	25	32	29	,, ,, 2 ,,
1834 ,, ,,	53	52	12	25	99	22	26	40	36	
1835 ,, ,,	41	65	31	84	41	45	12	31	7	,, ,, 8 ,,
1836 ,, ,,	67	58	88	38	46	7	23	20	12	,, ,, 6 ,,
1837 ,, .,,	83	26	77	43	76	6	21	13	7	,, ,, 3 ,,
1838 ,, ,,										
Total.........	344	300	248	264	444	153	111	207	100	No regist. 20 days.

The following table,* given by Mr. Smeaton ("Philos. Trans.,") and confirmed by Mr. Hutton ("Mathematical Dictionary,") ex-

* A. B. Maddock, M.D., on the "Influence of Air and Weather."

hibits in pounds avoirdupois the pressure which different winds will exert upon a square foot of surface exposed directly against them. The first column is a rough representation of the second :—

Velocity of winds.		Force on one square foot in pounds avoirdupois.	Character of the wind.
Miles per hour.	Feet per second.		
1			
2	1·47	·005	Hardly perceptible.
3	2·93	·020	Just perceptible.
4	4·40	·044	
5	5·87	·079	Gentle pleasant wind.
10	7·33	·123	
15	14·67	·492	Pleasant brisk gale.
20	22·00	1·107	
25	29·34	1·968	Very brisk.
30	36·67	3·075	
35	44·01	4·429	High winds.
40	51·34	6·027	
45	58·68	7·873	Very high.
50	66·01	9·963	
55	73·35	12·300	Storm or tempest.
60	88·02	17·1715	Great storm.
80	117·36	31·490	Hurricane.
100	146·70	49·200	Destructive hurricane.

THE RAINS—SOURCES OF AQUEOUS EXHALATIONS— HUMIDITY.

The eudiometric processes having failed of discovering in the atmosphere of places the most opposite, such as the narrow lanes of London and the summits of lofty mountains, any difference in the constituent properties of their permanent gases, it becomes a question of the highest interest and importance to ascertain the varying quantity of aqueous vapour in our atmosphere; for it is the only ascertainable fluctuating ingredient in its composition. To the medical topographer, a minute inquiry of the kind here suggested may lead to a knowledge interesting and important respecting the causes and cure of certain diseases, in so far as these may be connected with climate, and this is no small benefit from the proper application of instruments.

" The rain in falling," says Mülder, " carries with it everything that floats in the atmosphere and which is not essential to its constitution; which brings back to the earth what came from the earth; and which, while it thus purifies the atmosphere from these hurtful adulterations, restores to the soil these numberless volatile substances, where they have abundant opportunities of forming not only harmless but useful combinations." Mr. Hingeston states that during the fall of rain electricity is positive, and very often active; ánd that in damp weather the amóunt of animal electricity is the smallest, and the most easily parted with.

Without taking into view the expanse of the Bay, the *coup-d'œil* of a good map of Bengal will at once show how bountiful nature has been to that country, by means of her majestic rivers with their innumerable tributaries, in yielding the sources of aqueous exhalations; and it were gratifying to the medical topographer, could his description be limited to these.   There are not any lakes in Bengal resembling those of Scotland or Canada, but there is a profusion of extensive jheels, which may be either denominated shallow lakes or morasses.   A large proportion of these in the dry season contain little or no water, but during the rains present immense sheets, over which boats of the greatest magnitude may be navigated, and some are navigable to a certain extent through-out the year.   There is reason to believe that nearly all these stagnant sheets of water rest in what were, at a remote period, the channels of large rivers, which have since altered their courses and now flow in other directions.   The area of Bengal and Behar is 149,217 square miles, and with Benares not less than 162,000 square miles.   The following proportions of the surface are grounded upon many surveys, after making allowance for large rivers :—

	Parts.
Rivers and lakes (one-eighth)	3
Deemed irreclaimable and barren (one-sixth)	4
Sites of towns and villages, highways, tanks, &c., (one twenty-fourth)	1
Free land (three twenty-fourths) remaining liable to revenue	3
In tillage (three-eighths)	9
Waste (one sixth)...	4
Total	24*

According to another calculation, Bengal contains 97,244 square miles; if from this, that portion of Tipperah which is independent, the tract of the Soonderbuns and other wastes, equal to 13,244 miles, be deducted, the remaining inhabited country will be equal to 84,000 square miles; but the extent of waste and surface occu-pied by rivers, marshes, &c., seems here greatly underrated.

When all this is considered, along with the complete saturation, during five months in the year, of every inch of soil, even that which may not be actually inundated, the extent and sources of aqueous exhalation—the commerce of land and water—may be imagined.   It is ascertained that the capacity of the atmosphere for moisture varies with its temperature, so that at 113° it holds a twentieth part of its weight of moisture; at 80° a fortieth, and so on.

To a scientific officer well acquainted with the localities, I put the two following questions : " 1st.   Taking the area of the 24

* W. Hamilton.

pergunnahs to be 882 square miles, what proportion should you say the water surface bears to the land, on the 30th of May and the 10th of October, the first being just before the rains, and the latter just after? 2nd. What proportion does the cultivated land bear to the waste and jungle within the said area?"

Answer to 1st Question.—"I should say that on the 10th of June you might assume 1-20th part as the proportion of the water to the land; of course, I mean by water, ground from which exhalations could arise. *Answer to 2nd Question.*—The cultivated land may be about 14-20ths; water, 1-20th; roads and villages, 2-20ths; uncultivated, 3-20ths."

The subjoined table will show the annual fall of rain during the years specified. The average annual fall is about 60 inches.

RAIN.

						Inches.
1830	...	...	...	...	...	63·28
1831	...	...	...	...	...	57·50
1832	...	...	...	...	...	49·26
1833	...	...	...	...	...	60·56
1834	...	...	...	...	...	68·73
1835*	...	...	...	...	...	85·50
1836	...	...	...	...	...	45·39
1837	...	...	...	...	...	43·06
1838	...	...	...	...	...	,, ,,
Mean	...	...	...	...		59·228

The following are the average rates of evaporation for the dry months: January, three inches; February, five; March, seven; April and May, nine.

It is during the periods of the year when the drying process is in greatest activity that unhealthiness prevails with greatest severity, namely, the commencement and termination of the rainy season. In the former, or that called by the natives the lesser rain (Chota bursàt), common remittent fevers arise, and at the termination, or that from 15th September to the end of October, the severest forms of the same fever prevail, but chiefly amongst the indigent natives, and Europeans newly arrived.

The connexion of the rainy season with disease would, in such a climate as this, form a highly interesting subject of inquiry; but the absence of everything like statistical object in our older hospital reports prevents even an approach to accuracy on this, or indeed on any subject connected with climatorial influence.

The following statement is taken from the "Bengal Hurkaru" of September 6th, 1845.

"The Englishman is informed that seventy-four inches of rain fell in Arakan during the last month; and that fifty inches had fallen during the first twelve days of the present month. The whole fall during the monsoon, to the 15th August, was two hundred inches."

* Sixteen inches fell on the 10th of May in less than twelve hours.

The quantity of rain that occasionally falls in a brief space of time within the tropics, and especially near the equator, is enormous:—On the 10th of May, 1835, sixteen inches fell in Calcutta in twelve hours. But owing perhaps to the direction and elevation of the mountain ranges, and to the nearer approach to the equator, it is in the Burmese territories that we find the most surprising examples of great falls of rain. Those who served at Rangoon, and in Upper Ava, as the first European observers, will never forget the rainy seasons of those countries. The "Calcutta Review," in an article describing the Khasia Hills, says of the station of Chirra-Poonjee :—"Professor Oldham informs us that the fall during the year 1851 amounted to 592 inches, or to *eight fathoms and a quarter* of water; for it seems absurd to use a smaller unit in treating of such a quantity." This is the greatest fall of which as yet we have any record.

"The climate of Khasia," says Dr. Hooker, "is remarkable for its excessive fall of rain. Attention was first drawn to this fact by Mr. Yule, who stated that in the month of August, 1841, 264 inches fell, or twenty-two feet, and that during five successive days, thirty inches fell in every twenty-four hours. Dr. Thomson and I recorded thirty inches in one day and night; and during the seven months of our stay upwards of 500 inches fell; so that the total annual fall perhaps greatly exceeded 600 inches, or fifty feet, which has been registered in succeeding years. This unparalleled amount is attributed to the abruptness of the mountains which face the Bay of Bengal, from which they are separated by 200 miles of jheels and soonderbuns."

THE HOOGHLY RIVER—THE WESTERN BRANCH OF THE GANGES —THE BHAGIRATHI, OR TRUE GANGES OF THE HINDUS.

By some persons who have spoken of our climate, a large portion of the evils under which we suffer has been ascribed to the river—its supposed overflowings—its sluggish tides and foul waters—its muddy and slimy banks, and the action of a vertical sun upon them, &c., but I shall view the river in a different and more friendly light, *as the purifier of our city*.

Certain am I that, without this great scavenger, to whose tides we owe more than Captain Hamilton ever dreamt of, we should now be in a worse condition even than when he left us a hundred years ago. The truth is that, under moderate supervision on the part of the police, the river banks are inoffensive; and along their whole extent, although crowded with buildings for a space of nine miles, disease will be found less prevalent by far than in the interior quarters towards the east; in short, the causes of fever are to be traced to other and more palpable sources than the river-bank, which is the most elevated of all our grounds, being from three to four feet above the surrounding levels. The causes of unhealthiness in Garden Reach, after the salt-water inundation of 1833, could be readily traced to the state of the back-grounds— no one ever thought of looking for them in the river-bank. The annual rise of the Ganges and its branches, is in

				Feet.	Inches.
May	...	...	... ...	6	0
June	...	...	... ...	9	6
July	...	...	.. ...	12	6
Half of August	...	...	...	4	0
Total	...	...	...	32	0

From above 350 observations of temperature made by Mr. G. A. Prinsep, of which the details are given in the "Journal of the Asiatic Society," it would appear that "the mean temperature of the surface water exceeds 81° Fah., everywhere between Calcutta and the sea." In the dry season the mean rate of motion is less than three miles per hour; in the rainy season, and while the inundations are draining off, the current runs from six to seven, and even eight miles in particular situations.

The river is at its lowest in the beginning of March, and the freshes are at their height in September, when the tides are scarcely visible off Calcutta; and the river water is "perfectly sweet far beyond Saugor in the open sea."

The following table exhibits the depths of the river channel at the different seasons :—

	Dry season.
Minimum depth	8½ feet.
Maximum average depth of eleven of the shallowest places in the Hooghly, spring ebb	15¼ ,,
Maximum average depth over the same places, spring flood	31 ,,

	Rainy season.
Minimum depth	16 feet.
Minimum average depth of eleven of the shallowest places in the Hooghly, spring ebb	22¼ ,,
Maximum average depth over the same places, spring flood	32¼ ,,
Highest rise, ditto, ditto	36 ,,

Difference between highest and lowest, 20¾. Dry and rain.

THE SALT LAKE.

The situation and extent of the salt-water lake have already been described; and it only now remains to state the probable advantages of causing its area to be drained, filled up, and brought under cultivation. Owing to the shallowness of the lake generally, it is easy to drain it for the purposes of native agriculture; but to deprive the ground so drained of the sources of noxious exhalation is not so easy.

It is not sufficient to convert the ground into a state of soft low meadow land; for the most dangerous exhalations are those which are retained, and occasionally emitted from under a crust of earth during the drying process, whereby they would appear to acquire unusual concentration, and prove the origin of the worst fevers. It is necessary that the grounds *be thoroughly* drained, leaving none of the characters of the marsh, otherwise it had better be left as it is ; its present condition being one of far greater safety than such half-drained soil as that obtained from the marsh of Chartreuse, for instance, near Bordeaux, which caused in the year 1805 alone, 12,000 persons to be affected with fever within the city, of whom 3000 died within five months !

Two modes of effecting the drainage suggest themselves ; the one by letting in the river during the rains, and thereby gaining a succession of deposits of the river silt, so as gradually to fill the lake, and thereby bring it in time to a level with the surrounding land ; this would seem the easiest ; it imitates the simple operations of nature, and would be the cheapest ; but perhaps not the most conducive to health. Another mode is by a deep and well-constructed canal, so as to effect the drainage ; but, as even this must, to a certain degree, prove a receptacle for noxious matter, and offer a considerable surface for evaporation, a close line of umbrageous trees should, under the proposed plan, be planted along each side of the canal, as being powerfully attractive of marsh exhalation. This property in trees was practically known to the ancients,* and is now beneficially exemplified in Demerara, and other parts of Guiana, " where the humid heat constantly cherishes the seeds of disease."

The ground cleared from water should be well ploughed and cultivated, the ploughing to be done during the heaviest rain, so as to prevent exhalation ; for it is during a certain stage of the drying process that marsh exhalation is most concentrated, and it has been observed in many countries that the drying up of brackish water is more injurious than that of either salt or fresh alone. A succession of crops purifies and evaporates the soil, and thereby obviates exhalation ; but they should not be of rice, or such crops as require profuse irrigation. The want of attention to some of the precautionary measures above hinted at, has neutralized the advantages that would otherwise have resulted from extensive draining executed in some parts of France and Italy ; and I have only thus long dwelt on that of the Salt-water Lake, because I believe its proper performance to be a matter of great importance to this city, so far as regards the prevention of disease ; and I need not here insist on the superior efficacy of *preventive* measures, such as have advanced in our own country apace with our civilization, and altogether banished from us some of the severest calamities that have ever afflicted the human race.

* Regaud de L'Isle says of the malaria of Italy, that various obstacles form barriers which they cannot pass, and against which they deposit themselves.

THE WOODS AND MARSHES OF THE SOONDERBUNS.

The enormous extent of the Soonderbuns—covering a superficies of more than 20,000 square miles, and extending 180 miles to the South and East of Calcutta—is composed of marshy land, covered with forest and underwood, together with the numerous embonchures of the Ganges—a region from whence the solar light, the heat, and the air are excluded by the forest-trees, to the extinction of all minor vegetation. When we consider all these circumstances, and their common influences on all the conditions of the atmosphere necessary to health, we shall be at no loss to perceive how great must be the deteriorating influences of so vast a region on the climate of Calcutta. That "forest on the borders of the sea"—that "land of flood and forest"—must necessarily exercise a very powerful influence on the temperature, humidity, electricity, and freedom of circulation of the atmosphere in and around it, not to speak of the noxious exhalations generated within and disseminated without. It is evident that the electric condition of the air must be greatly affected by the combination of oxygen with the materials of living plants over so vast a surface, as also by the enormous extent of evaporation from it; and these are subjects deserving our most careful consideration.

How far the geological nature of the soil—the amount of evaporation—the presence of forests—the vicinity of seas, lakes, and rivers; how far, in fact, all the local circumstances noted in our topographic charts may affect the electrical states of the medium in which "we live, move, and have our being;" these are questions of the last importance to be observed and noted.

Humboldt, in describing the forests of tropical regions, says :— "Under the bushes, deep, green verdure of trees of stupendous height and size, there reigns constantly a kind of half daylight, a sort of obscurity, of which our forests of pines, oaks, and beech-trees afford no example; forming a carpet of verdure, the dark tint of which augments the splendour of the aërial light. The mould contains the spails of innumerable quantities of reptiles, worms, and insects. Wherever the soil is turned up we are struck with a mass of organic substances, which by turns are developed, transformed, and decomposed. Nature in these climates appears more active, more fruitful, we might say more prodigal of life.

"On fixing our eyes on the tops of the trees, we discovered streams of vapour wherever a solar ray penetrated and traversed the dense atmosphere, exhaling, together with the aromatic odour yielded by the flowers, the fruit, and even the wood, that peculiar odour which we perceive in autumn in foggy seasons. It might be said that, notwithstanding the elevated temperature, the air cannot dissolve the quantity of water exhaled from the surface of the soil and of the vegetation."

In the Bight of Benin, West Coast of Africa, a tract of forest land, covering a superficies of a hundred thousand square miles, presents an unbroken surface of densely-wooded alluvial soil, intersected by innumerable creeks and rivers. "At the distance of several miles from the coast," says Dr. Daniell, "the peculiar odour arising from swampy exhalations and the decomposition of vegetable matter, is very perceptible, and sometimes even offensive. The water also is frequently of a dusky hue, with leaves, branches, and other vegetable *débris* floating on the surface, brought down from the interior by innumerable narrow channels that empty their turbid streams into the open ocean."

Here, as might be anticipated, the atmosphere is truly pestilential. "It is under these climatic conditions," says Dr. South-wood Smith, "that the worst forms of epidemics are engendered; the most sudden in their attack, the most rapid in their development, the most general in their prevalence, and the most mortal." For the most part, adds the same author, these epidemics are strictly endemic, and are confined to the particular regions in which they are engendered.

That the clearing of the extensive surface of the Soonderbuns, or of any considerable portion of it, leaving belts and clumps of forest-trees, would tend greatly to improve the local climate in and around Calcutta there can be no doubt. The history of this city, and that of the effects of clearing marshes and forests in the neigh-bourhood of other cities in other countries, offer a demonstration of this fact.

Such a measure would open out the city to the more free influence of the sea-breezes, diminish the moisture of its atmosphere, and purify it. These are no speculative results.

The Soonderbuns, described by De Barros three hundred and fifty years ago as a well-peopled country, has since become what we have seen it. This desolation is stated by the best authorities, as quoted in the "Calcutta Review," to have resulted from the gradual process of silting at the heads of many of the rivers. Through this circumstance the influence of the tides prevailed a greater distance *north;* and the water consequently lost its sweetness, and became brackish. "The cause of the desertion by the people was the salt water." The Bengalee, whose system of agriculture is limited by extreme poverty, will squat on the banks, plant his fruit-trees, raise his homestead, and dig his tank so long as the water is meetah, or sweet.

It is found, contrary to the vulgar opinion, that in cleared and cultivated tracts the air is rendered drier and warmer in summer, and colder in winter, than in such as, from want of cultivation, remain, like the Soonderbuns, covered with wood and marsh.

"Earth-clouds" are commonly observed in the early morning to the east of Calcutta, over the borders of the Salt-water Lake and the cleared portions of the Soonderbuns. They are caused by the immense radiation of heat in the calm nights, and by the cooling of the earth's surface far below that of the air above—thus forming vast clouds, or mists, close to the earth's surface. If, then, to counterbalance the only disadvantage attendant on clearing—some little increase of temperature—we obtain more purity and dryness of our atmosphere, we shall still be very greatly the gainers; for it is not so much from the high rate of temperature we Europeans suffer, as from the excessive humidity that is conjoined with it for so many months in the year, and both which, commingled with the terrestrial exhalations, tend gradually, through their united influence, by inducing what may be termed a *Cachexia Loci*, to undermine the best and most robust of constitutions.

The clearing and draining immediately around the city, partial and imperfect as these are, have removed only some of the concentrated evil; but that emanation which was death within a few yards, cannot be other than insalubrious even at the distance of a few miles, and in a diluted form.

The general influences produced by trees on the climate of a country, or, as St. Pierre defines it, " the elementary harmonies of plants with the water and the air by means of their leaves and their fruits," have been ably summed up by Dr. Balfour of the Madras army as follows :—

" 1st. That the extensive clearing of a country diminishes the quantity of running water which flows over the surface.

" 2nd. That it is impossible for us to determine at present whether this diminution is owing to a smaller annual fall of rain, or to an increased evaporation of the surface-water, or to those two causes combined.

" 3rd. That it is, however, shown by various authors that rain oftener falls, and that more dew is deposited in well-wooded countries than where the country is naked ; and, drawing our conclusions from the meteorological facts collected in equinoctial regions, we may presume that the extensive clearing of a country diminishes the actual quantity of rain which falls upon it.

" 4th. That mountains, particularly when covered with their native forests, by an electric action on the atmosphere cause clouds to form around them, collect and condense the vapours of the air, and equalize the fall of rain.

" 5th. That the forest-trees which grow on mountain summits have a structure peculiarly fitting them to receive the waters of the clouds.

" 6th. That lands destitute of the shelter of trees allow of more rapid evaporation.

" 7th. That, independent of the preservation of surface-water, forests husband and regulate its flow.

" 8th. The authors alluded to also show that in all forest-tracts the temperature of the air is more equable throughout the year; that in tropical regions the atmosphere around trees is cooler, and contains more moisture than the air on the open glade; that the atmosphere of a tropical country without trees has an arid dryness in it totally dissimilar to the cool softness of a well-wooded one; that lands covered with trees are cooler and moister than those which are exposed; that in hot climates the destruction of forest trees, by inducting aridity, destroys vegetation; and that forests and trees afford the shelter from violent winds which is absolutely essential to the health of the vegetable creation.

" 9th. That springs draw their supplies from sources in their immediate vicinity; that the presence of trees near these sources seems to prevent the dissipation of the supply of water.

" 10th. That in clearings which are purely local, springs may disappear without there being any ground to conclude that the annual quantity of rain has diminished.

" 11th. That the tenacious clayey under-soil found in forests is peculiarly adapted for preserving the surface and subsoil waters.

" 12th. That there is a difference in the condensing power of trees, but by means of the vegetable creation a valuable supply of moisture is collected from fogs, and from the atmosphere in the form of dew.

" If the facts detailed warrant these deductions, it may be confidently asserted that Southern India would be greatly enriched and its climate ameliorated by the introduction of arboriculture."

POSTSCRIPT.

Referring to the influences of all the physical and geographical circumstances detailed in the foregoing notes as affecting the electricity of the atmosphere, I would call attention to the conclusions arrived at by Dr. Pallas of the French army in Algeria, offering them here only as subject-matter for examination and test in other hot climates.   Dr. Pallas considers :—

" 1st. That, just as light and air are the essential agents of vision and respiration, so electricity is the functional agent of innervation.

" 2nd. That the greater number of diseases, and especially those which belong to the class of neuroses, are occasioned by the exaggerated influence of general electricity, of which clouds, storms, and marshy regions are the most fruitful sources.

" 3rd. Marshes, in their geographical constitution, and in the effects which they produce upon the economy, present the greatest analogy to the galvanic pile.   Thus their action is much the more baneful, as they contain certain proportions of water, and their activity is considerably increased when the water contains organic or saline matters in a state of solution.   This explains why salt marshes and such as are near maritime rivers are the most insalubrious. The drying up or submersion of marshes produces analogous conditions to those of a galvanic pile deprived of humidity, or which is under water, and the effects of which are then insignificant.

" 4th. The researches of philosophers and physiologists have shown that the electricity produced by our machines exerts a special action upon the nervous system. Experience and rigorous observation of facts prove that the diseases which are produced by a marshy atmosphere are primarily nervous, and become inflammatory only by the re-action of the nerves upon the vascular system, inducing consecutive, local, or general irritation.

" 5th. The neuroses are occasioned generally by the effects of electricity, and intermittent fevers have a similar origin ; that is to say, they are due to the electrical emanations of the marshy pile, which are very active in hot countries, and not to miasmata, which have never been met with."

Professor Schönbein considers, on the other hand, that the physiological importance of electricity has, upon the whole, been much exaggerated, that agent, in comparison to heat and light, acting but an inferior part in the economy of organized beings. " Electricity," he says, "would affect neither the sense of taste nor smell, if atmospheric air did not contain oxygen and nitrogen ; and the phenomena of sound and light, perceived during electrical discharges, are due to the vibrations into which the particles of air are thrown by the electrical discharges, electricity having directly nothing to do with them."

MEDICAL CLIMATE AND THE INFLUENCE OF SEASON.

"Si l'histoire naturelle a besoin d'une bonne géographie physique, la science de l'homme a besoin d'une bonne géographie médicale."—CABANIS.

PHYSICAL EFFECTS OF CLIMATE.

UNDER this head I shall offer some cursory observations on what is usually called by physicians "medical climate;" meaning thereby the physiological forces which act perceptibly upon our organs. I desire also to submit some brief notices of the geography of disease, as connected with our Bengal climate and seasons.

Temperature and humidity being the elements that give activity to terrestrial emanations and all the external causes affecting health, derived from locality, I shall now consider them apart from the subjects above classed; remarking generally that the heat of Hindustan, as compared to that of other regions, is more characterized by its duration than by its intensity. On the other hand, where the cold is excessive, the rise of temperature in spring and summer is sudden and intense, while again in those countries where the range is more limited, the seasons glide gradually and imperceptibly into each other. It has been well observed that the most poisonous gases, mephitic emanations, malarious, miasmatic, and paludal exhalations, the products of putrefactive changes of *organic* and *vegetable* origin, are extricated by heat, and dissolved and retained in the atmosphere by moisture. In Bengal, throughout the hot season, the rivers become shallow, the tanks dried up, the water impure and scarce, while the air is rendered thick and hazy by the quantity of impalpable matter floating in it.

Speaking of the average of men, the terms hot, warm, cool, cold, as applied to the surrounding air, are regulated by the sensations produced; and if the heat be carried off as fast as it is generated, and no faster, no particular sensation is felt—the bodily powers being neither stimulated nor exhausted. Supposing then that no extraordinary exertions are made, the equilibrium is maintained when the thermometer stands at 62°, or thereabouts; and this point in the scale is therefore called *temperate*. All degrees above that point, up to 70°, are reckoned *warm;* all above 70°, *hot*. Descending again in the scale, we speak of the temperature denoted by any degree between the 60th and the 50th as being *cool,* and any lower degree of temperature as *cold*. Changes of temperature seem to be as readily felt at one part of the thermometric scale as at the other, and in whichever direction they take place. Captain Parry found that a rise in the thermometer from 13° below zero to 23° caused discomfort to his men. " I may possibly incur the charge of affectation in stating that this temperature was much too high to be agreeable to us; but it was nevertheless a fact that everybody felt and complained of the change." On the other hand, the fall to from 40° or 50° at night in Bengal, during the cold season, might seem to an European as both agreeable and salutary; but a very brief experience teaches him the contrary. Much has been said and written on the superior capabilities of adaptation to climate in man over the lower animals; but if the power and just application of the arts of civilization be deducted, I am disposed to think, with Dr. James Johnson, that the difference would be but small; for, even with these aids, we find that in this climate "many die suddenly, others droop, and all degenerate," very much as with the lower animals of more temperate regions; and all we can hope to learn is, how best to conquer by obeying nature. It is thus that man, the weakest of animals, is, in reality, the strongest; and it is under circumstances apparently calculated to overwhelm and destroy his vigour that he finds the means of developing new faculties and resources, which excite even his own astonishment.

Gibbon, after stating that the Roman soldiers, from their " excellent discipline," maintained " health and vigour in all climates," adds, that " man is the only animal which can live and multiply in every country from the equator to the poles. The hog seems to approach the nearest to our species in that privilege." It is true, as stated by the historian, that men do " live" in other than their natural climates, but their existence is very unlike to the health and vigour of the Roman soldier, whose habit and discipline did not allow his manly character and physical energy to be dissolved in indolence.

" The truth is," says Dr. Johnson, " the tender frame of man is incapable of sustaining the degree of exposure to the whole range of causes and effects incident to, or arising from, vicissitudes of climate, which so speedily operate a change on the structure, or at least the exterior of unprotected animals. The object of these remarks, which at first sight might seem irrelevant, will now appear. Since it is evident that nature does not operate more powerfully in counteracting the ill effects of climate on man, than any other animal, it follows that we should not implicitly confide, as too many do, in the spontaneous efforts of the constitution, but on the contrary, call in to its aid those artificial means of prevention and amelioration which reason may dictate and experience confirm. In short, that we should study well the climate, and mould our obsequious frames to the nature of the skies under which we sojourn."

Although the physical effects of climate, in forming or influeueing the differences by which the varieties of tribes of the human species are characterized, are foreign to the present inquiry, still one cannot help remarking that, if the native of Bengal Proper is to be classed among the Caucasians—the standard of the human race—the effects of climate and locality must indeed be great and remarkable.

No climates exist that are uniformly hot and dry, hot and moist, cold and dry, or cold and moist; yet certain countries have such a preponderance of one or other of these qualities, as to give a very marked character to the physical and moral nature of man; and physicians would do well to observe these results of climate more closely than has yet been done:—" Si l'histoire naturelle a besoin d'une bonne géographie physique, la science de l'homme a besoin d'une bonne géographie médicale."

The moral as well as the physical influences of climate have been considered so powerful by some philosophers, as to make some persons doubt whether a people situated as our Asiatic subjects are capable of receiving the impress of European knowledge and institutions. There is in hot climates, it has been well observed, a *vis inertiæ* which indisposes men to change their customs, or to cope with abuses; and the indolence which the climate occasions conduces to the stability of their barbarous institutions.

" The astonishing rapidity of political revolutions in Asia," says Montesquieu, " arises out of one fact which is really dependent on its physical geography. In that part of the world, weak nations are opposed to strong; people warlike, brave, and active border upon those who are effeminate, idle, and timid; the one must necessarily be conquerors, the others conquered. Here we have the principal reason of the liberty of Europe and the slavery of Asia." Malte-Brun, commenting on the above observations, says: " It is necessary to combine this just remark with another truth proved by physical geography, namely, that Asia has no temperate zone, no intermediate region between very cold and very hot climates. The slaves inhabit the hot, and the conquerors the elevated and cold regions."

In European countries, a certain amount of injury is caused to public health by the agitations of ceaseless competition, commercial speculation, religious controversy, and party politics; and though these influences are not apparent in India generally, we cannot altogether overlook them, or the many causes arising from long ages of civil and sacerdotal domination, and other abuses of native government which, with difference of race and of religion, produce so remarkable a distinction between the moral and physical constitution of the Asiatic and European, rendering the latter so much more liable to be affected by tropical climates.

The hot and dry season in Bengal extends from the beginning of March to the middle of June, during which the winds are steady and strong from south and south-west. The temperature rises gradually from 80° to about 90°—95° in the shade, and reaches to 100°—120°—130° and upwards in the open air. Notwith-standing the high temperature, this season is rendered far less oppressive to the feelings than might be supposed, by means of the moisture carried along with the monsoon in its passage over the Bay of Bengal, and likewise by the frequency of refreshing storms, accompanied by rain, lightning, and thunder. Of Calcutta at mid-day, in April, May, and part of June, it may be said, however, with truth, that it is "a city of stone, in a land of iron, with a sky of brass;" the soil of the surrounding country being "rent and riven as if baked over a volcano," often emitting noxious vapours. The local newspapers of May, 1851, speak of the heat as more intense than it had been for years. "The thermometer in the coolest rooms stands at 92° to 94°, and the breeze which should bring refreshment at the close of the sultry day, has been as the breath of a furnace."

The intensity of light at different places differs greatly, and it is a matter of regret that there is no ready means of measuring it, as the results would certainly prove interesting. According to Herschel, that of the Cape of Good Hope, compared with that of a bright summer's day in England, is as 44° to 17°.

"There is," says Dr. Mitchell, "a health-giving influence in a bright atmosphere and a cloudless sky, which is not fully appre-ciated. Light has a higher power on the functions of the animal economy than we are apt to think; and proofs are not wanting. Deprive the tadpole of the influence of light, and nourish it as you like, it remains the tadpole still. This agent is essential to its development, and it is arrested when deprived of it. Again, disease among the soldiers who lived on the dark side of an exten-sive barrack at St. Petersburg, was uniformly in the proportion of three to one compared with that on the side exposed to a strong light.

"But it is in the vegetable that we have the clearest manifes-tations of its markings. In plants we find the secretions developed 'in greater perfection according to its intensity.' Deprived of it, we find them flowerless, fruitless, and with small and stunted leaves, while on branches of the same plant 'which grow towards the light we have full-sized leaves and perfect flowers and fruit.' Had we no other, we should be authorized in inferring that that which is so potent on vegetable is not inert on animal life. The physiology of the two kingdoms is ever more or less closely related; and that which stimulates the flower to expand its petals—giving a welcome, as it were, to the vivifying influence—is also, though perhaps more obscurely, a stimulus to man. But the operation of no stimulus must be continued or uninterrupted. And that of light is no exception: hence darkness and light alternate." Well may Boudin declare that light exercises an influence as powerful as it is varied on entire nature.

The most ordinary and simple effects of the Bengal season just described are—determination of the fluids generally to the surface of the body, the blood being venalized in proportion to the elevation of temperature; and respiration being less perfectly carried on, owing to the rarefaction of the air, and the consequent diminution of its oxygen in a given bulk, a vicarious decarbonization of the blood is established in the increase of the biliary secretion; while, at the same time, the urine is surcharged with saline impregnation, and much diminished in quantity. Recent experiments render it probable that, as temperature rises, the quantity of oxygen consumed in respiration is less, while the amount of carbonic acid exhaled is less also; and hence lassitude, diminished muscular power, and diminished change of matter. At this season, too, it is believed that both the relative and absolute quantity of carbonic acid exhaled is diminished. There seems at length some reason to hope that the vicarious nature of the relations existing between the depurative functions of the liver, kidneys, mucous surfaces, skin, and lungs may receive demonstration from chemistry; meanwhile we know that there is not a function of the body the integrity of which does not depend on that of respiration.

"Vierordt has made a very extensive series of observations, with the view of ascertaining the connexion between the temperature and the pulse, the respiratory movements and the volumes of air expired, and of carbonic acid, in one minute. His experiments were made at every degree of temperature between 37° and 76° Fah.

"From a table of observations, we see that elevation of temperature is accompanied by a diminution of the number and of the depth of the inspirations; its effect on the excretion of carbonic acid is, to a certain degree, of an indirect nature, since the diminished number and depth of the expirations must have a considerable influence; but inasmuch as the diminution does not merely show itself in the total quantity excreted, but also in the per centage of carbonic acid in the expired air, it seems obvious that the elevation of temperature has a more direct influence on the excretion of carbonic acid than could be accounted for by the modified respiratory action.

"The degree of atmospheric moisture, to a certain degree, influences the respiratory functions and the excretion of carbonic acid. Lehmann, some years ago, experimented on this subject with pigeons, greenfinches, and rabbits. The quantity of carbonic acid exhaled in a moist air was much greater than in a drier atmosphere. . . The researches of Vierordt on the influence of atmospheric pressure, show that this also is by no means an unimportant element. . . Vierordt and Baral agree in the opinion that more carbonic acid is excreted in winter than in the summer.

"The excretion of carbonic acid is very considerably diminished during sleep. This is most decisively proved by the experiments of Scharling, who found that a man, during one hour of the night, exhaled only 22·77 grammes, who, during an hour of the next day, immediately after a meal, exhaled 33·69 grammes; and who, in another case, found that the horary excretions of carbonic acid during the night and during the day were as 31·39 : 40·74.''— *Brit. and For. M. C. Rev.*, July, 1854. The alternations here mentioned cannot fail of being important in relation to European health within the tropics. It has been observed in all malarious countries, that to night exposure, and to the condition of sleep, is the greatest danger—a lowering of the nerve-power, and a consequent vascular debility occurring in the night time. These physiological alternations may be more or less immediately connected with the circumstance of the hours of 3 and 4 A.M. being the minima of atmospheric electricity, and of atmospheric pressure likewise.

THE HOT SEASON AND ITS EFFECTS.

Dry heat causes a very rapid evaporation, a high degree of electric tension, and a generally stimulating effect. These effects, however, vary according to age and individual temperament, whether sanguine or leucophlegmatic.

It appears to me that the physiological action of heat is exhibited, first, in its temporary stimulation of both the ganglionic and cerebral systems of nerves, and in the increased manifestation of all those functions governed by them; and secondly, in its sedative and more lasting influence on the same systems of nerves, in the progress of years, and in diminished manifestation, consequently, of all those functions governed by them. This last result is strikingly exemplified in the diminished muscular powers of both the heart and uterus. Heat may be regarded for a time, and for a short time only, as the universal chemical quickener of the various functions. Besides its direct effects, heat is in fact the great moving power of all other subordinate sources of disease, whether these last be neglects in public or personal hygiene.

Bearing in mind these important and interesting facts, as they appear to me, we shall at once perceive how it is that for a certain time the respiration, circulation, the hepatic function, and that of innervation itself, are unnaturally excited, and how the newly-arrived European is exhilarated in mind, and so prone also to acute inflammatory and congestive abdominal diseases. But, as this state of over-excited or exalted function cannot be maintained beyond a certain limited term of years without danger to the power and equable functional action of the source—the ganglionic nerves—we see how, along with a feeble respiration and circulation, diminished power of generating heat, and torpor of the hepatic function eventually succeed;—all tending to congestion and other dangerous forms of more passive disease. Again,

we perceive how the long-continued operation of alternate stimulation, and of subsequent depressive and sedative influences on the
functions of the organic and animal systems of nerves, produces
and confirms that eventual bodily and mental inertness and indisposition to healthy action, which not even the most powerful of
Europeans can hope always to resist, beyond certain defined limits
as to time.

The anæmic states of the system induced by a lengthened
exposure to the influences of heat, moisture, and malaria are frequently referred to, more or less in detail, in the course of this
work ; and all I would say is, that the existence of this morbid condition should be constantly held in recollection by the medical officer
when called upon to treat Europeans suffering from tropical disease,
and who may have resided long in hot climates. . Old Indians may
occasionally prove of plethoric habits ; but the asthenic condition
of the system is by far the more general among that class.

The hot season swells the exterior and produces that general
chubbiness of appearance which is so remarkable in the torrid zone,
even where the weight of the body is sensibly diminished : it increases the animal heat, and accelerates the pulse, accompanied by
a prodigious increase of the pulmonary and cutaneous transudations : it produces nervous excitability varying in degree in most
persons—an exaltation of the general sensibility : eruptive diseases,
latent during the cold season, become actively developed ; and the
cutaneous vessels, even in healthy persons, are excited to the extent
of producing the distressing eczema solare, known in the tropics by
the name of prickly-heat.   In ordinary seasons, we find that here,
as in the West Indies, the most healthy months are from February
to May inclusive ; while in the seasons of epidemics (cholera in
particular) these are the months in which the disease is most fatal
and long-continued ; indeed, it seldom vanishes till the setting in
of the rains.

Under exposure, excessive fatigue, mental depression, or neglect
of temperance in diet, results ardent fever, with some serious local
determination, and that very frequently to the cerebral organs—
occasionally to the liver ; but though this is admitted, under the
measures of precaution dictated by common sense and experience,
the very hottest are yet the healthiest of our seasons, and of our
stations also,* which goes far to prove that it is not heat alone that
does all the mischief, but something else in the climate and in the
constitution and habit of the stranger European, not common to
the native of the country.   From the results of personal observations in active field service both in India and in Ava, I am led to
conclude that mere heat, unless long continued, and combined with

* At Agra, the hottest of our stations, the per-centage of death has not been two,
or one in fifty per annum, out of a garrison of one thousand men ; a more favourable
result than shown in any table hitherto prepared in India.—*Asiatic Researches.*
Major Henderson.

intemperance, with chills, and other untoward circumstances, is very rarely the direct cause of disease.

Edwards states it as a fact that the quantity of cutaneous exhalation from the human body is sometimes ten times greater in dry than in moist air, and that it is doubled in the mere passing from 32° to 64° F.

I have seen men of the Bengal Pilot service, persons who lived and laboured in the sun during their youth and manhood, in whom the functions of the skin appeared at length to have been exhausted. They exhibited a permanent dryness, roughness, and scaliness of the whole surface of the body, from which they experienced distress in the cold season of Bengal, and more in the English winter and spring. One old pilot's skin was so furfuraceous that he would often say: " I could write my name with my nail on any part of my body and limbs." With these men the functions of the kidneys were always disturbed also.

The troops from Bengal and Madras were exposed, in the expedition to Egypt, to an excessive heat in crossing the Desert from Kosseir to the Nile ; yet they enjoyed excellent health, because they were not exposed to extreme fatigue or to excesses, and their minds as well as their bodies were kept in activity. The service, too, was not protracted.

The superior power of enduring heat, *under a sudden effort, or while the mind is keenly occupied,* possessed by Europeans in India, even beyond the natives, has often been exhibited in other climates. It would seem to arise from the same causes that enabled the natives of the southern countries of Europe, according to Larrey, to bear the cold of the Russian winter, during the French retreat from Moscow, " better than the natives of the Northern and - moister climates—such as the Hanoverians, the Dutch, the Prussians, and the other German people : the Russians themselves, from what I learned at Wilna, suffered more from the cold than the French." These last suffered also in Holland, in 1799, much more from cold than the British with whom they co-operated, as observed on the spot by Robert Jackson.

The inhabitants of the temperate regions of the globe, it is supposed, having their constitutions matured by genial climates, are able to bear the extremes of both heat and cold, during a short time especially, better than those whose frames have been weakened either by the severities of the arctic, or the relaxations of tropical climates. Robert Jackson, speaking of the first American campaigns, says :—" Bad effects from the greatest exertions in the hottest weather of summer were extremely rare in that country, after the campaign had been continued for a few days."

These remarks must be understood to apply only to sudden efforts or brief exposures ; for it is now well known that to the duration of heat more than to its intensity—to the long-continued exposure to an unnatural and uniformly high range of temperature, more than to the temperature itself—must be referred much of the injurious influence of tropical climate on European constitutions. Dr. Armstrong says of the unnaturally extreme climate of the polar regions, that "Men are less capable of resisting cold in the second year in the climate than they are in the first, and so on for every subsequent year of their sojourn."

The equable determination to the surface consequent on the progressive increase of temperature, seems to exercise an agreeable as well as a favourable influence on general health, especially in the old Indian; and even a new comer seems to bear without complaint or apparent injury the great augmentation of the sensible perspiration. It is only the opposite condition—the total suppression of it in our cold season—that is felt by all as unnatural as it is unhealthy:—indeed, we then become aware of the effect of long-continued exposure to a high range of temperature, through our extreme predisposition to be injuriously influenced by cold.

Miscarriages, frequent at all seasons in India, occur yet more frequently in the hot season, and the recovery is more protracted, owing to the increased force and frequency of the circulation, especially in those of plethoric habits.

There are two classes of persons to whom our climate seems genial, the weak-chested, as they are called in England, who are of a scrofulous habit, but in whom pulmonary disease has not actually declared itself. These are saved by going to India; and I have known many persons in the curable stage of consumption—that is, labouring under the preceding stage, or that of "tuberculous cachexy"—enjoy good health in Bengal, and survive their brothers and sisters at home. The greater expansion of the lungs produced by the warmth and rarefaction of the air would appear to aid the other influences already mentioned. The soft and moist air of marsh-districts, also, as long ago remarked by Dr. Harrison of Lincoln, may exercise a beneficial influence. The fate of those, on the other hand, who go to the East with suppurating tubercles, or even in the softening disorganization approaching it, is only precipitated. Persons of phlegmatic habit also, with dyspepsia, languid circulation and cold extremities, seem to have better health there than in Europe.

The climate of India tends, in fact, powerfully to the production of disease within the abdominal cavity; while that of Europe tends as powerfully to the production of disease within the thoracic cavity. That catarrh, bronchitis, and pneumonia will occasionally arise among British soldiers in India, when exposed to cold and damp while marching and campaigning, and when sleeping on the ground, is well known; but that such diseases are either generally prevalent, or often fatal, is equally well known as not being the case.

As the two hemispheres are divided, the eastern from the western, by the meridional line, so the diaphragm separates the two
great cavities of the body, in one of which, the thoracic, is manifested very generally the morbid results of the Western, while in
the other, the abdominal, are generally manifested the morbid
results of Eastern climates. Thus, as the globe is divided into
two hemispheres and great climates by the meridian, so, to a great
extent, the influences of those climates on health are marked and
bounded in the cavities on each side by the diaphragm; the line
of demarcation being as determinate in the one instance as in
the other: the climate in each instance determines with accordance and correspondence of effect the cavity of the human body
in which disease shall manifest itself. Again, speaking in reference
to particular tissues, we find that in the acute diseases of temperate
climates inflammations of the serous membranes occur frequently,
while in tropical climates it is the mucous surfaces that are involved
in disease.

Out of 1000 deaths in England and Wales, mortality occurs
from the following causes, and in the following proportions :—

From diseases of the cerebral cavity	144
,, ,, ,, thoracic	302
,, ,, ,, abdominal, including childbirth, &c.	87
,, other diseases	430
,, violent deaths	37
Males and females at all ages	1000

Out of 1000 deaths (males) in London, mortality occurs from the
following causes, and in the following proportions (age 15 to 35
included) :—

Diseases of cerebral cavity	80
,, thoracic	559
,, abdominal	74
Other diseases	202
Violent deaths	85
	1000

The returns from the East Indies include soldiers only, men of
the mean age of twenty-six years; and the British military returns
comprehend the same class. But the returns of the civil population of England and Wales by the Registrar-General include
persons of all ages and of both sexes; and here, under the head of
diseases of the abdomen, we have included all diseases of the
uterus and urinary organs.

Besides the protecting influences already mentioned, an antagonism of phthisis and intermittent fever is believed by some
observers to exist; and the fact that tubercular disease is much
less frequent in marshy districts than in any others, has been
insisted on by certain physicians of France and Italy, supported
by statistical details, the results of experience in many of the

E

marshy quarters of those countries. But, like the influence of heat, the malarial influence must, they say, be sufficiently intense and continued in its action to produce the marshy cachexia, or, in other words, the antagonism to phthisis.

In Algeria the French surgeons found phthisis a rare disease. Out of 1480 French soldiers in hospital, M. Haspel found but three cases of pulmonary disease, and only one death was caused by it out of 138 deaths. A general report gives but thirteen phthisical cases out of a total of 8485 patients, and but ten deaths from pulmonary disease out of a total of 871 deaths. But the infrequency of pulmonary consumption in Algeria is not, as supposed by M. Boudin, the consequence of malarious fevers and their efficient causes, so much as from peculiar climatic circumstances.

It may, then, be asserted, on the ground of statistical evidence of the most extended nature, that climates and employments that induce sweat, or that induce a gentle perspiration not subject to check, are unfavourable to the existence of scrofula or consumption. It may be inferred also that the curative virtue of marshy countries, as respecting phthisis, resides less in the miasmata themselves than in the uniformity of temperature, the heat of the atmosphere, a moderate degree of moisture, and the absence of dry sharp winds. Even in the favoured Nice—the resort of thousands of sufferers from thoracic disease—the Cimios, those unrivalled hills where old Rome sent her convalescents, are still the chosen spots.

There is, on the other hand, a malarious cachexy, or *cachexia loci*, generally observable in Europeans who have resided long in the more unhealthy districts or stations of tropical climates, even when they have escaped actual visceral disease there. But when the contrary holds—when organic disease within the abdomen *has* resulted—the condition of the blood here referred to forms a serious complication. It renders the cure difficult and tedious, the system being cachectic, the blood dissolved, there being a general anæmia, in short.

To give a more concentrated view of the physical circumstances above related, it may be said that in hot climates, the air being expanded, less oxygen is taken in at each inspiration; and thus the changes effected by respiration on the blood are diminished. The necessity for hydro-carbonaceous food is therefore lessened. Less of the "elements of respiration" ought to be taken in the food than would be taken in colder climates. In consequence of the internal increase of temperature, less internal heat is required—the supply of and demand for animal food depending, in fact, on the external temperature.

Exercise increases the heat of the body by increasing the rate of circulation and respiration. In a very hot climate all increase of heat is undesirable. Moreover, the excessive heat renders muscular action impossible, because the circulation is chiefly directed, in consequence of the activity of the skin, to the surface, in order that fluid may be furnished for evaporation, to keep down the heat of the body, to prevent the parching of the surface, which otherwise must ensue.

In consequence of the lessened muscular action, less of the albuminous constituents of the food are required to supply the waste of the muscles.

Hence, in hot climates, less of both kinds of food should be taken, and nature points this out, in the absence of appetite; to force an appetite stimulants are taken, and then the system is overloaded with nourishment. The excessive perspiration requires an excess of liquids; but, instead of water alone, sugar and spirit, the elements of respiration, are taken with the water as beer, and the spirit, by its stimulating properties, is doubly injurious.

The excessive flow of blood to the surface (the consequence of the high temperature) no doubt prevents for a time the evils resulting from an excess of the two kinds of food. The chemical changes and evaporation going on in the skin draw the circulation to the surface of the body, just as the flame of the lamp draws the oil up the wick. Whilst the high temperature lasts, this increased action of a flow to the surface is kept up. It is probable that the action of the heart is thereby made feeble by the excessive suction of the skin, as we see it frequently is, temporarily, by the perspiration bath. As soon as the temperature falls, the blood ceases to flow in excess through the skin. According to the degree of cold, it is almost driven from the surface. It accumulates within, and congestions and inflammations are produced. Free action on the inner or outer surface of the body for a time relieves the congestions, and enables the circulation to proceed.

After such alternations for years, the resident in the hot climate returns to a far colder home. There no heat leads the blood to the surface; it accumulates in the enlarged capillaries of the internal viscera. The outward appearance is that of anæmia; whilst in reality an internal plethora frequently exists.

The more frequent and severe the temporary congestions of the viscera have been, whilst in the hot climate, the more permanent does the internal congestion become, when the surface is constantly exposed to cold. Though the surface and extremities may look void of blood, the capillaries of the liver and spleen will often be full; and the enlargement of the internal capillaries which was the effect of temporary congestion for years, becomes permanent when the coldness of the atmosphere leaves the blood to be circulated by the enfeebled heart alone.

The consideration of the effects produced by migration, during a state of disease, from a cold to a warm and moist climate, says Dr. Copland, is of the utmost importance. Keeping in mind its influence on the healthy frame, chiefly in exciting the functions of the skin and liver, and diminishing those of the lungs, we are led to prescribe it in various diseases.

In hæmoptysis this change is obviously beneficial, especially as a warm and moist atmosphere, by this mode of operation, lessens the activity of the pulmonic circulation and the disposition to sanguineous exudation from the surfaces of the bronchi ; bronchitis and tubercular phthisis are also often benefited, and the progress of the latter much delayed by this change of atmosphere, especially when adopted early.

Chronic rheumatism is sometimes cured by this measure, seemingly owing to its influence in promoting the biliary and cutaneous functions.

Dropsies, particularly anasarca and hydrothorax, have been, in a few instances, removed by a change to a warm climate ; but whilst a moist state of the air is most serviceable in pulmonary and hæmorrhagic diseases, dry warmth seems more beneficial in dropsies, dyspeptic affections, and hypochondriasis, evidently from its effects in augmenting the insensible perspiration and the pulmonary exhalation, and imparting tone to the capillary circulation.

Besides these, he adds, gout in its early stages, *dysmenorrhœa*, and *scrofula* in nearly all its forms, are benefited by a change to a warm or even a mild atmosphere.

THE RAINY SEASON.

Although medical authorities have not been able accurately to estimate the effects of moisture, either acting simply or in combination with heat, yet it is certain that this last union is more injurious than either applied separately.   In warm and moist climates, obesity and laxity of frame are induced—a fact which was very early observed ; thence the proverbial acuteness of the Athenians, and the sluggishness and stupidity of the Bœotians.   On the other hand, countries where it seldom rains are generally the healthiest —fevers of the malarious type being almost unknown in them.

The effect of situation upon the habit may in some degree depend also on the gravity or weight of the atmosphere connected with locality.   When the barometer is high, we feel vigorous and cheerful ; when it sinks, languor and low spirits oppress us. Bichat states that, " accumulations of fat are said to take place in some animals in a few hours, in certain states of the atmosphere. During a fog of twenty-four hours' continuance, thrushes, wheatcars, ortolans, and red-breasts are reported to become so fat that they are unable to fly from the sportsman."

In Bengal, as on the West Coast of Africa and other unhealthy climates, the heat and moisture combined cause a vast increase of minute vegetable and animal life, while the decomposition of dead animal and vegetable matter is equally rapid, showing the aptitude of all sustances to pass from the inorganic to the organic, and *vice versa*. The oxidation of metals proceeds with immense rapidity also during the rainy season.

During the first month of this season, the temperature falls considerably, accompanied by a freshness of the air delightful to the senses, after the previous excessive and dry heat. The monsoon is steady and veers to the south and south-east; vegetation springs up with all the exuberance of a tropical climate, promoted, as is supposed, by an electric current of increased activity between the atmosphere and the earth; and the dust, so offensive at all other seasons, subsides and is washed away. In the rainy season, but especially on its subsidence, the rapid growth and rank health of the vegetation may, in neglected, ill-drained and impure localities, be taken as a kind of measure of the sickness and mortality prevalent in them. We find that even in the temperate climate of England, and in a beautiful village in Hertfordshire, scores of its inhabitants have within a few years perished from fever, owing to the want of clearing, draining, and other most obvious measures of sanitary regulation. Let those who may be in charge of stations and cantonments throughout India reflect on these simple facts, and on the evidences of the disastrous consequences of igno-rance and neglect of sanitary precautions, as exhibited in every page of this work.

From the 15th July to 15th October, and as the rains advance, we live in an atmosphere having all the properties of a tainted vapour-bath; and when the wind comes sifting through the Soon-derbuns at south-east, we experience many of the inconveniences ascribed by Hennen to the sirocco of the Mediterranean, which, "*without affecting the thermometer or barometer in any remarkable degree*," yet inflicts on the delicately sensitive human frame a feel-ing of indescribable languor and oppression, with an exhausting perspiration, much like what we suffer from in Bengal during the latter portion of the rainy season, and which a West Indian lady, speaking of the sirocco, described as giving "*the feel as if she had been bathing in a boiler of syrup*; while a Bishop of Calcutta said that in the rainy season he felt "*like a boiled cabbage.*"

This is the moist sirocco of Bengal. The mind, too, seems to partake in the general relaxation, being unfitted for vigorous or sustained effort; in short, we here perceive the *capiplenium, lan-guor, et expletio* remarked by Petronius amongst the luxurious and dissolute Romans of his time. The muscular system, including the heart, is relaxed and weakened; so that, and after a time, it becomes irritable and very defective in tone. These circum-stances, together with the influences of malaria on the nervous system, appear to me to occasion the intermitting pulse so com-mon to the old Indians.

At this season, through the saturation of the atmosphere, the perspiration by evaporation is suppressed, but that by transudation is enormously increased, thus rendering the system susceptible of the least impression from cold or malarious exhalation, with a strong tendency to congestion in the abdominal vessels, while at the same time absorption is increased, and all the excretions diminished. The excessive watery discharge from the skin, during this season, must also, and of necessity, have the effect of rendering the venous blood unnaturally dense, and thus cause the European to be more liable to congestive forms of disease. Dr. J. B. Williams refers the disposition to liver complaints, dysentery, and cholera, to the stimulating properties of the blood, deprived, as we have seen, of more than usual of its water, and less of its hydro-carbon.

Such is the rainy season, and such are some of the reasons for its proverbial unhealthiness in all tropical climates. If it be true that an individual in health ought to be in that state of perspiration in which it is insensible, what are we to think of the exhausting drain flowing from the pores of an European during this and the preceding season, though differing in their modes of action? When, during the rainy season, the temperature ranges as high as, or higher than, that of the human body, and when, at the same time, the atmosphere is saturated with moisture, we find the accumulated animal heat carried off by becoming latent in the then extraordinary transudation which covers the whole surface of the body. Evaporation being now at its lowest point, we have here a beautiful illustration of the wonderful power of nature in establishing an immediate and effectual compensation, without which life would speedily be endangered.

As in the sirocco, we here experience an extreme oppression of the nervous energy, and consequent muscular lassitude, with disinclination to active exertion of mind or body, the body *seeming* more bulky and *feeling* heavier to the individual; the hair looks dank and greasy, while the scalp is covered with furfuraceous eruption, and exudes an unpleasant acid odour. "The walls of houses, stone-floors, and pavements," says Hennen, "invariably become moist when the sirocco blows. I have seen the stone-floors at Corfu absolutely wet without any rain having fallen, and gentlemen who made hygrometrical experiments state to me, that the instrument has frequently fallen from ten to twenty degrees during the prevalence of this wind—wine bottled in a sirocco is greatly injured, and often destroyed. Meat taints astonishingly soon during its prevalence. No prudent housekeeper ever salts meat at this time, for it either taints at once, not taking the salt, or else it keeps very badly. Drains emit more putrid smells in a sirocco than at any other period. No carpenter uses glue in the sirocco, for it does not adhere. No painter willingly works during its prevalence, for his paint will not dry. Bakers diminish the quantity of their leaven during the sirocco, as dough is found to ferment sufficiently without. It is a remarkable fact that wounds and ulcers, and the discharge from mucous surfaces generally, deteriorate during the prevalence of the sirocco, and it is equally certain that if vaccination or smallpox inoculation be performed at this period, they are both extremely liable to fail ; and if they succeed, the progress of the pustule is often suspended, and it is frequently ten or-twenty days in reaching the state usually attained in six or eight." When we come to the influence on vegetable life the parallel ceases. Hennen says that, though "the sirocco is so charged with moisture, vegetables, especially that part of them exposed to it for any length of time, appear quite shrivelled and burnt up, and very frequently they are destroyed altogether."

The whole of these observations, in so far as they relate to the human frame, were annually verified in the surgical wards of the Native Hospital under my charge; and we had the same discomforts in perhaps a severer degree whenever a calm of any duration existed during the rains : in former times, ulcers used to assume a gangrenous condition, but vigorous measures of prevention entirely obviated these occurrences in latter times.

I know nothing I should dread so much as a long calm at this season in Calcutta. It might not be followed by plague as in London, Nimeguen, and Vienna, in former times ; but in the result, as affecting human life, I think we should not fare better than did those cities.

Amongst Europeans the diseases of the rainy season assume a character of diminished vital action ; the ardent fever, with burning skin and racking head, of the hot season, degenerating into the congestive form, with a moist cool skin, indicative of an extreme atony in the sudatory vessels, and an oppressed pulse ; the complications are generally abdominal. Dysenteries, as well as fevers, become more frequent, severe, and complicated, as the rainy season advances, the former implicating the whole of the abdominal organs ; but the most severe cases, especially amongst newly-arrived Europeans, are at the commencement and termination of the rains. During the former, or that called by the natives Chota-Bursat, which leaves some days of sunshine between the falls, fevers of a severe and complicated form arise, and during the drying process which terminates the season, they are even more so : occasionally these last are attended with a yellow suffusion of the skin; but I have only once seen anything like black vomit.

The greater liability of the human frame to fever, during natural sleep, may be referred to the diminished power of generating heat in the system during the time of repose—a time when the circulation is comparatively languid, tending farther to diminish the power of generating heat, and consequently to increase the morbific power of both cold and malaria on the system. But may not this greater susceptibility to disease be also promoted by the known increase of putrefaction in dead animal and vegetable substances during the night, resulting from the rapid abstraction of heat from the earth's surface by radiation, and the consequent production of moisture in the form of vapour, dew, or water—all productive within the tropics of vast increase of decomposition? That persons who have undergone fatigue, been exposed to great solar heats, and been subjected to its peculiarly debilitating influences, are greatly more liable to be affected by malaria, and by the cold or poisoned night air, is a fact often observed in various countries.

The abortions of the rainy season appear to arise from simple congestion and relaxation, aided and promoted by diminished nervous power—the natural results of an excessive and exhausting humidity joined to a high temperature.

Humid air, says Dr. Edwards, at an equal or even superior temperature, produces a peculiar sensation of cold which differs, not in its intensity, but in its nature. It is more profoundly felt, and seems to penetrate the whole system, and particularly disposes to paleness and shivering. By these characters I could not mistake a species of refrigeration, which consists in the diminution of the power of producing heat.

In dry air, on the contrary, a sensation is experienced which is called a *sharp cold*, and which designates rather the nature than the degree of sensation; moreover, it is superficial, and when the reduction of temperature is not too great, an increase of activity is experienced; the skin reddens, and in extreme cases the limbs have a tendency to stiffen, instead of yielding to the irregular and involuntary motions, which constitute shivering. It may be seen by this comparison, and by what we have stated above, that damp cold must tend to produce in individuals whose power of developing heat is rather feeble, the series of actions which constitute the accession of an intermittent fever, especially if they are exposed to that action during sleep. The confirmation of this will be found in the study of medical topography. In the greater number of cases these fevers are ascribed to marsh miasmata in fine weather, but others occur in places and at seasons at which the atmospheric constitution which we have mentioned predominates. "As a general rule, the merits of a dry atmosphere are superior to those of a moist one. It is obvious that man was not intended to live in an atmosphere *saturated* with vapour, since, if so constituted, it would be unable to carry off the aqueous exhalations for which it is palpably the intended medium. A perfectly dry atmosphere—whether cold and dry or hot and dry—would only be less objectionable. We have seen that it is prejudicial to vegetable life. It would be to the skin what a purgative is to the mucous membrane of the intestines, and in its stimulating action would subject it to an increasing and exhausting drain. Nor would this 'simply involve the drinking of a pint or more of extra fluid,' according to Dr. Forbes Watson, since the function of the skin being complex or manifold, it would not be stimulated to

hyperaction in one direction and remain unaffected in the others."
—Dr. Mitchell's *Algeria*.

A familiar but emphatic illustration of the effects of our climate may be seen in its influence on the habitations of Calcutta. Constructed of the finest known materials, whether of wood or mortar, and of such solidity that in England they would endure for centuries, and in Upper Egypt for a thousand years, they are here, through the destructive influence and severe alternations of climate alone, rendered in a score of years, or less, fit habitations only for crows; in much less time, indeed, they may be seen reduced to a heap of rubbish covered with vegetation. " A deserted village is overflowed by the forest like the waves of the sea, in course of two wet seasons, and the traces of man are buried by the exuberant productions of nature"—all mark of human labour, industry, and art being obliterated in the East, by the influence of climate, in an incredibly short time.

Of all the causes which thus render household and other property so surprisingly perishable, heat, humidity, and the exuberant vegetation caused by them would seem the most influential.

The peepul tree (*Ficus Indicus*) is the great enemy of buildings in Bengal. " No wonder," says Colonel Sleeman, " that superstition should have consecrated this tree, delicate and beautiful as it is, to the gods. The palace, the castle, the temple, and the tomb—all those works which man is most proud to raise, to spread, and to perpetuate his name—crumble to dust beneath her withering grasp. She rises triumphant over them all in her lofty beauty, bearing high in air, amidst her light-green foliage, fragments of the wreck she has made, to show the nothingness of man's efforts."

THE COLD SEASON.

I believe it was Charles the First who described the best climate as that in which a man could bear exposure during the greatest number of hours at all seasons. On this view our climate of Calcutta is assuredly one of the worst, for even during the cold weather, from the end of October to the beginning of February, an European cannot be exposed for any length of time with impunity; the hot sun and cold parching wind, with its evening and morning rawness, causing the most uncomfortable feelings of external dryness and internal fulness, unless it be in persons of youth and robust health, and under exercise sufficient to determine moisture to the surface. But, with all its disadvantages, this is the season during which the European soldier should be initiated into the climate of Bengal, and of India generally. This truth is now beginning to be understood by the authorities; and let us hope that we may never again witness the arrival of recruits from England, as of old, in the month of May, the hottest of the year. It was a cruel and destructive custom.

The unfavourable influence which the north-east monsoon exercises on the general health of persons of a feeble constitution, or
who are ailing, may in part be ascribed to its relatively low electric
state, or its being in a negative state, thus attracting the positive
electricity of the animal frame, as well as that of the soil. If the
powerful physical agent of electricity is that which, through the
system of organic nerves, influences the various secretions, how
much must our climate, and consequently our health, be influenced
by those causes, whether general or local, which affect the proportions of electricity in our atmosphere, always greater and more uniform than in European climates. Coming down upon us directly
from the frozen platform of Central Asia, the temperature of the
monsoon is also relatively reduced so as to absorb much of our terrestrial heat, while, at the same time, its hygrometric capacity is
much increased, parching up the soil along with the animal and
vegetable fibre.

"The temperature of the blood is about 98°, at which it is sustained, with some slight variations, even when the body is immersed
in an atmosphere of 29°, or of a still lower temperature. But the
heat that is lost by the lungs and the skin is so great, that it is not
supplied with sufficient rapidity in the very young and the old ; who,
to use a common expression, do not ' stand the cold' so well as men
in the prime of early manhood. The above numbers show that the
power of cold on life varies according to definite laws ; thus the
mortality by cold (35) is twice as great under the age of 20 as the
mortality (18) at 20—40 ; but after that turning point the power
of resisting cold decreases every year, and men of 90 and men of
30 have suffered from the cold that we have experienced in the
proportion of 100 to 1 (or of 1749 to 17·5)."—Dr. *Farr*, February
27th, 1855.

People, on coming into Lower Bengal from the Upper Provinces during the cold season, perceive an extraordinary change
in the condition of the atmosphere on first approaching the Delta
of the Ganges ; the bracing elastic cold of Upper India is exchanged for that of a damp cellar, and thus they invariably describe it.

At the commencement of the cold season, in October, the temperature and the winds are variable, the drying process is in full
activity, and the unhealthiness is great. In General Sir Alexander
Tulloch's " Statistical Report on the West Indies," it is stated
that, though the months previous to the cold ones have the most
sickness, yet "the principal mortality is during the cold dry weather
which generally prevails at Christmas." In Aracan also, during the
first Burmese war, it was found that, "in September and October,
when the rain began to abate, the fever was equally prevalent, and
still more fatal than in the preceding months ; and in November,
when little or no rain fell, the disease appears to have been at its
height."

From the 1st of November to the end of February the weather is settled, and agreeable to persons in health; but to the delicate and sickly the altered balance of circulation and nervous function occasions much discomfort. The monsoon keeps steadily to north-east, the atmosphere during the day is dry, and a slight rise takes place in the barometer—the thermometer ranging from 45° to 75°; the nights are damp as well as cold during this season, the dewing process being excessively productive; and the fogs which prevail occasionally are of a nature more dense than I have anywhere seen, except in Pegu.

On the other hand, during the day, the cold north-east wind absorbs moisture with extraordinary rapidity from every object, animate and inanimate, over which it passes. Furniture, although made of the most seasoned wood, foreign or native, warps and cracks audibly; plaster newly laid falls from the wall through rapidity of evaporation; the old Indian becomes goose-skinned and shrivelled, with a sense of dryness in the palms of the hands, so uncomfortable as to give to some persons of irritable habit, and in whom the power of generating heat may be diminished by a long residence in India, a constant sense of nervous uneasiness of the whole sentient surface not to be described. "I can bear the chilling blasts of Caledonia," says a Scotchman, quoted by Ward, "but this—this cold, I know not what to do with it;" indeed, it requires a degree of equilibrium of health not commonly enjoyed by persons of long residence in Bengal, to take kindly to the alternation from copious and incessant discharge from the surface, to its total suppression, and consequent abdominal and cerebral engorgements.

By the older British residents it has long been matter of observation that the fall of heat a few degrees below the mean warmth is more productive of disease than the highest rise above the mean heat even of the hot season. Under direct exposure to such reduction of temperature the morbid results become at once manifest. "The first night the regiment spent in Sindh," says Dr. Arnott, of the Bombay European Fusiliers, "was upon the open bunder; most of the men and officers marched about the whole night to keep themselves warm, being without tents, bedding, or shelter of any kind. They felt the cold severely; and six of the deaths that occurred during the following twelve months were traced to the exposure of that night. For some years afterwards it was spoken of in the regiment as having given rise to its subsequent bad health."

It is only to the sound of constitution, in fact, who are temperate in all ways, and thereby able to bear the cold-bath, or to such as are recently arrived from Europe, that our cold season is either agreeable or healthy. But here I would observe, that the degrees of health and disease are not always to be measured by the thermometer, taken singly—such observations in connexion with health affording little information to the medical inquirer; and it has been well observed in our own country, that the influence of the weather on the human frame is not to be thus estimated. An east wind, with the thermometer at 56°, will impress the body with a more chilling effect than a south-west wind, when that instrument indicates a temperature 10° lower; and a foggy atmosphere, in like manner, much more injuriously than a clear one of equal cold. In the " Statistical Report on the West Indies," already quoted, it is stated that in Jamaica the lowest mortality throughout a long range of observation was in the three months prior to June, 1827, when twelve deaths only were reported through the whole quarterly returns. The next quarter, remittent fever broke out, and among a diminished force the deaths amounted to 252 in the same period, without the thermometer indicating any further increase of temperature than about 3°, and without any remarkable change in the weather.

The diseases more peculiar to the cold season in Bengal are— congestive fever of the continued form; intermittents, with the sequelæ of tumid or indurated liver or spleen; hepatic insidious sub-acute inflammation, terminating rapidly in abscess, if not promptly and vigorously treated; dysentery, frequently complicated with hepatic congestion—all more or less acute, according to individual habit or length of residence in India. Catarrhs and bronchial affections are not so severe or so prevalent as the contrasted nature of the season would lead us to suspect. Hæmorrhoids with many persons follow immediately on the drying up of the surface, and consequent fulness of the internal vessels. It results also from the cold season that the blood is more venalized, a larger quantity of oxygen being consumed in the maintenance of the temperature of the body; and this condition of the blood, aided by congestion, would seem to dispose to apoplexy, the most fatal forms of which that have come under my observation in Bengal having occurred at this season; and paralytic affections are not unfrequent amongst the aged and infirm. Chronic eruptions, in an active state of development during the previous hot season and rains, now become suddenly repelled, accompanied by headache and vertigo.

In old residents, the appetite fails, accompanied by an oppressive sense of abdominal fulness; and when this state is not met by a suitable change of diet, clothing, and some medicine to act upon the skin and bowels, visceral congestion, œdema of the lower extremities, or some more active disease may ensue. New-born infants suffer materially from, and are sometimes destroyed by, the impression of our cold season on the unguarded and delicate surface. The abortions of the cold months have always appeared to me connected with acute venous congestion; and the intermitting states of the pulse and epigastric pulsations common to old Indians at this season are increased by this state of the great venous trunks.   The kidneys act during the continuance of the cold weather with diabetic violence, the urine being limpid, and they only cease to do so on the return of a warmer season, and consequent equability of circulation, causing moisture of the surface.   The biliary excretion, in excess during hot and rainy seasons, is here diminished, as indicated by the whitish or clay-coloured state of the alvine discharges, following the reverse order of what takes place in the instance of the kidneys.   The function of the liver, indeed, is now depressed and depraved.

The reader will not fail to observe that *congestion* has repeatedly been mentioned as participating in the most dangerous of our diseases.   The blood is thrown inwards so as to be retained and accumulated in the abdominal organs, whose vascular structures have been variously affected, and whose functions have been most disturbed during the previous hot and rainy seasons.   Congestions of those organs, by intropulsion, is now the consequence of the cold season.   That the peculiar climate of Bengal has a principal share in producing this unfavourable state there can be no doubt; but, admitting this, we must consider also that the absence of all exhilarating exercise of mind and body, with their animating, varied, and healthful influences on all the functions, predisposes much, when aided by a too full and stimulating diet, to this end. Unhappily, too, the European resident in tropical climates has no sufficient remedy against the evils of this double inaction, excepting the moderation in diet, which he will not adopt; for, during the hot and rainy seasons, the amount of exercise necessary to health in temperate regions would here be impossible, and would be hurtful even if possible.   Those who would preserve their healths, therefore, must be temperate,* use such bodily exercise as each season will admit of, and relieve their minds from the monotony of routine official duty by the inexhaustible resources of European science and elegant accomplishment.   It is only thus that health, happiness, and reputation can be ensured under the disadvantages of our position in India, where too commonly the whole time is given up to business.

From the sketch now given of the locality and climate of Calcutta, it will be seen that, without taking the specific or malarious influences into account, we are there exposed to atmospheric changes to an extraordinary degree;—to an extreme of heat and dryness—extremes of heat and moisture—cold and moisture—cold and dryness.   The European exile may well join in the "complaint of the Black Knight" of Chaucer:

> "Nowe hote as fire, nowe colde as ashes ded;
> Nowe hote for colde, now colde for hete again;
> Nowe cold as yse, and now as coles red,
> For hete I brenne."

---

* It has been shown by experiment, that when alcohol has been introduced in large quantities into the circulation, "the arterial blood retains the venous colour."   It is

That these various influences of extremely contrasted seasons alternately excite and depress the vital processes must be evident; and it is to their long-continued application (even where disturbance of function does not amount to actual disease), that we must refer the attenuated condition and general feebleness of the old Indian.

"Bengal has received a bad character for insalubrity," says Malte-Brun, "and certainly it is in an eminent degree exposed to a succession of violent extremes and vicissitudes; at one time to excessive rain, at another to hurricanes; then to scorching heat, and frequently to thick fogs; yet the English have, by dint of prudent regimen, accommodated themselves to the climate."   In the time referred to by Malte-Brun—the time when English youths went to India "to make a fortune or die of fever"—I fear there was not much of that "prudent regimen" to which he ascribes such happy results; but let us hope that it is now about to be attained—that it may no longer be a reproach to us that, not satisfied with choosing the worst localities, we also adopt habits of life the worst calculated for the accommodation of our constitution to them and their climates;—that it may no longer be said of the Englishman, as in the days of Clive—that he returned from the East with a tawny complexion, a bad liver, and a worse heart.

If Bichat could propound with justice the axiom that, in our native climate of Europe, life is but the assemblage of functions which resist death, what are we to think of the health-history of Europeans in the East Indies during the last hundred years!   I confess that to me the exhibitions of their bodily and mental energies, at all times, but as displayed in 1857-1858 especially, under highly unnatural influences of climate, exposure, mental anxieties, and exertions, have shown a wonderful power in the white man to resist death in the climate of the dark races: yet it is a power that ought not to be overtaxed, if we are to hold India with a firm hand becoming the superior race.

The Government of British India has never bestowed any attention on the subject of the injurious influences of climate in that country, or on the means of preventing them.   It is true, nevertheless, that the Anglo-Celtic race has there made some advance, by its own unaided action, towards moulding itself to the climate, without succumbing to the enslaving civilization of the East.

As illustrative of the conservative influence of good habits of life, it is worthy of remark that, of the European officers on the Bengal establishment, there died, on an average of eight years, of the unmarried class, 3·77 per cent. annually; while of the married class the mortality for the same term was but 2·74.   Of the

doubtless through the contamination of the blood chiefly, and through the resulting congestions, that the abuse of ardent spirits proves so baneful in hot climates especially.

European soldiery, again, there died annually, during the period here referred to, 7·38 per cent.   This wide difference in sickness and mortality is referable almost solely to the difference of habits of life ; for, in the important circumstances of age and constitu. tion, the private soldier, on an average, has the advantage.   On entering the service he may be taken generally to be of a stronger frame than the commissioned officer ; and he very rarely serves to so advanced a period of life as the latter.   With the exceptions of coarser diet, a habitation inferior to the officer, and harder work on actual service, circumstances which do not generally tell much on the amount of sickness and mortality, the soldier has thus some real advantages over the officer—excepting in the all-important one of *habits of life*.

Referring, lastly, to the influence of habits of life and of climate, in preventing thoracic diseases, I would quote Dr. Atkinson of Wakefield, and others, who infer, that by the use of alcoholic liquids, "a state of the blood is produced opposite to that which obtains in tuberculosis, and may thus prevent the development of it."   This view is supported by Dr. Atkinson in a numerical statement, showing a mortality from phthisis, amongst the adults of Wakefield, "of rather less than one in three, and in publicans of one in twelve and a half."   Publicans are here placed in con. trast with the general community as affording examples of hard. drinking persons ; but a moderate supply of alcoholic liquids, with a generous diet, is what Dr. Atkinson recommends as a prophy. lactic.   This gentleman regards phthisis as "characterized by an excess of oxygen circulating in the system, and that when the blood becomes too highly carbonized from various diseases, tubercles are not deposited."

If further observation should confirm this view of tuberculosis and its causes, we may receive from it some assistance towards elucidating and determining the actual physiological operation of tropical climates in preventing the development of pulmonary con. sumption.   It has been seen that, during the hot weather and rains especially, the blood is venalized, and malaria may perhaps be regarded as having a somewhat similar influence ; so that the antagonism alleged by the French military surgeons to exist in Algeria may, after all, have more of foundation than did at first appear.

THE SOL-LUNAR INFLUENCES.

1. Many of the great medical authorities of antiquity were clearly of opinion that the celestial bodies exercised a marked influence upon the bodily and mental functions ; and Galen, adopting the Hippocratic notion, declared that the exacerbations of particular diseases were connected with the lunar periods.   The critical days, or *crises*, as they were termed, were said to correspond with the

interval between the moon's principal phases.   There seems no reason to doubt, also, that sol-lunar influence is much more powerful within the tropics than in other parts of the world.   Dr. Forbes. Winslow records an alleged case of moon-stroke, in the instance of an officer in India who had slept for several hours in the rays of a full moon.   The results were headache and gastric irritation, followed by permanent impairment of memory.

2. The subject is one of medical as well as meteorological and philosophical interest, and cannot justly be passed over in an inquiry respecting the causes of climate.   The difficulty of explaining lunar influence appears to be the great obstacle which, in modern times, has stood in the way of the belief in its existence and general prevalence; yet twenty-three medical philosophers, British and foreign, are named by Dr. Forbes Winslow as authorities on the subject.*

3. But, notwithstanding the investigations of the authorities indicated, the subject has still to be investigated systematically by persons possessing that preliminary amount of mathematical, astronomical, and meteorological science indispensably necessary in order to arrive at satisfactory results, with leisure also beyond what is enjoyed by medical men in general.   Although we would concede much to those eminent men who have patiently investigated this interesting branch of philosophic inquiry; still, it must be confessed that, in common with medical meteorology, it has not yet assumed that character of exactness and of demonstration for which we may eventually hope.

4. The doctrine of periodicity, as exhibited in the phenomena of life, is not of modern origin.   The ancients, masters in the science of pure observation, have not overlooked the fact.   The phenomena of menstruation were the subjects of particular observations in all ages, and the singular and well-marked periodical character of this function was attributed to the operation of causes acting independently of those organic laws supposed to regulate the special functions of life.

5. The same character of periodicity was observed in a large class of febrile affections, particularly in the bilious remittents, in intermittents of warm latitudes, in the diseases termed neuroses, in all spasmodic and convulsive diseases, particularly in epilepsy and its allied affections, in many forms of insanity, and in the diseases classed under the term exanthemata.

6. The author referred to in the foot-note considers that Dr. Laycock has made observations of great value on the philosophy, physiology, and pathology of this subject; not confining himself to the phenomena of periodicity as exhibited in disease, but with the hand of a master tracing the operation of the same law in the

* *Vide* "Contributions to Medical Jurisprudence of Insanity," *Lancet*, 1855— admirable Essays, which are here largely quoted.

animal and vegetable, as well as in man in his normal and abnormal state.

7. Dr. Radcliffe is also justly praised as having, in a philosophic spirit, suggested to the physiologist and pathologist the important question—whether the phenomena of periodicity, natural and morbid, result from the operation of causes exterior to the body, or should be considered as the effect of certain laws of organic life yet undefined and unexplained by modern physiologists.

8. Dr. Radcliffe agrees with the ancients, and with Mead and many of the moderns, in seeking for the causes of periodicity in sol-lunar influence; and he sees days, months, and years reflected in the lives of plants and animals; but he also considers this evidence in a new point of view, and elicits a new conclusion. In his opinion, this evidence shows that sol-lunar influence is *necessary* to the life of animals as well as of plants, and most necessary in proportion as the vital principle loses that independency which is characteristic of the higher animal, and approximates to the dependency of the plant; and because it shows this, he concludes that all the changes which are found to take place in the sol-lunar influence *must* be accompanied by corresponding changes in vital manifestations. In other words, there must be signs of periodicity, and these signs must be most marked where the vital principle is least independent—in the plant more than in the animal, in woman more than man.

9. For the same reason, he supposes there must be more marked signs of periodicity in cases where the vital energy is impaired by disease; and it is in this impairment, and in this only, that he thinks the true explanation of these signs is to be sought for. Such is the lesson which Dr. Radcliffe deduces from the evidence. The question of lunar influence is not indeed specially gone into; but the whole tenor of the argument is to show that the moon *must* exercise a great influence on the body.

10. There can be no doubt as to the obscurity of the evidences of periodicity, even where that obscurity is the least, as in epilepsy and the affections allied to it; but there can be no doubt also as to the existence of these evidences. Thus, on looking at a number of cases, it is found that convulsion and spasm occur more frequently at night than in the day, more frequently about the time of new moon than full moon, and more frequently in the winter months than in the summer months. Of these evidences of diurnal, monthly, and annual periodicity the diurnal are the most frequent and the best established; but all are sufficiently frequent and obvious to any one who will take the trouble to seek after them for himself. There is, in fact, much in the recorded observations of Drs. Laycock and Radcliffe, as well as in the valuable treatises of Mead and of Balfour of Bengal, to strengthen the presumption that the periodicity referred to arises directly or indirectly from sol-lunar influence.

11. Mead proceeds to demonstrate, as he conceives, on the foundations of the Newtonian philosophy, by how much more powerfully the moon influences the atmosphere than the sea, and that the tides of the air, from lunar attraction, are much greater than those of the ocean. After considering the effects of certain unnatural states of the atmosphere upon the barometer, and then the connexion between certain states of the barometer and special as well as epidemic diseases, he developes his views as to the mechanical influence of certain conditions of the atmosphere on the respiratory organs. " It will not," he says, " be difficult to show that these changes in our atmosphere at high water, new and full moon, the equinoxes, &c., must occasion some alterations in all animal bodies, and that from the following considerations :—

" *a*. All living creatures require air of a determined gravity, to perform respiration easily and with advantage, for it is by its weight chiefly that this fluid insinuates itself into the lungs. Now, the gravity, as we have proved, being lessened by these seasons, a smaller quantity than usual will insinuate itself; and this must be of smaller force to comminute the blood and forward its passage into the left ventricle of the heart; whence a slower circulation ensues, and the secretion of the nervous fluid is diminished.

" *b·* This effect will be the more sure in that the elasticity of the atmosphere is likewise diminished. Air proper for respiration must be, not only heavy, but also elastic to a certain degree; for as this is by its weight forced into the cavity of the thorax in inspiration, so the muscles of the thorax and abdomen press it into the most minute ramifications of the bronchia in expiration; where the bending force being somewhat taken off, and springy bodies, when unbended, exerting their power every way in proportion to their pressures, the parts of the air push against the sides of the vesiculæ and promote the passage of the blood. Therefore the same things which cause any alterations in the property of the air will more or less disturb the animal motions. We have a convincing instance of all this in those who go to the top of high mountains; for the air is there so pure (as they call it)—that is, thin—and wants so much of its gravity and elasticity, that they cannot take in a sufficient quantity of it to inflate the lungs, and therefore breathe with great difficulty.

" Lastly—All the fluids in animals have in them a mixture of elastic aura which, when set at liberty, shows its energy, and causes those intestine motions we observe in the blood and spirits, the excess of which is checked by the external ambient air, while these juices are retained in their proper vessels. Now, when the pressure of the atmosphere upon the surface of our bodies is diminished, the inward air in the vessels must necessarily be enabled to exert its force in proportion to the lessening of the gravity and elasticity of the outward : hereupon the juices begin to ferment, change the union and cohesion of their parts, and stretch the vessels to such a degree as sometimes to burst the smallest of them. This is very plain in living creatures put into the receiver exhausted by the air-pump, which always first pant for breath, and then swell, as the air is more and more drawn out; their lungs at the same time contracting themselves, and falling so together as to be hardly discernible, especially in the lesser animals."

12. Making allowance, says Dr. Forbes Winslow, for the absolute terms used by Mead, as well as for the state of physiological and pathological science of his epoch, the reader will be able to detect, in the language which he adopts to enunciate the theory of lunar influence, the germs of some great truths which have subsequently been confirmed, in all quarters of the globe, by appeals to the great book of nature. Mead has undoubtedly laid himself open to the charge of attempting to prove too much; but are not all ardent and zealous cultivators of science exposed to the same imputation?

13. The well-known " Collection of Treatises on the Effects of Sol-Lunar Influence in Fevers," by the late Dr. Balfour of Bengal, is then reviewed by Dr. Winslow. Balfour devoted great attention to the consideration of this subtle and disputed point of science. The first part of his work is a regular logical synthesis, proceeding from facts observed and collected by himself to the discovery of certain prevailing tendencies of nature, and thence to axioms or general laws. The second part is an analysis, in which these axioms or laws are employed to explain some of the most remarkable phenomena of fevers. The third part is an application of the principles of this theory to form general rules for practice. With a view to the satisfactory elucidation of his principles, Balfour placed himself in communication with all his brother officers of note of the three Presidencies of India, and obtained from them the results of their observations on the subject.

14. Balfour maintains that every type of fever prevalent throughout India is, in a remarkable manner, affected by the revolutions of the moon. Whatever may be the form of fever, he says that he has invariably observed that its first attack is on one of those days which immediately precede or fall on the full of the moon, or which precede or fall on the change of the moon, so that the connexion which prevailed between the attack of the disease and the moon at or during the time referred to was most remarkable: relapses, in cases of fever, are also said frequently to occur at such times.

15. Balfour had observed in Bengal, during fourteen years, this tendency to relapse at the full and change; and in particular cases he was able to prognosticate the return of the fever at these periods with almost as much confidence as he could foretel the revolution itself. The putrid, nervous, and rheumatic fevers of India, as he termed them, were equally under the influence of the moon.

16. In attempting to explain these phenomena, he says that, along

with the full and change of the moon, there is constantly recurring some uncommon or adventitious state or quality of the air which increases fever and disposes to an unfavourable termination or crisis; and that along with the intervals there is constantly recurring a state or quality of the air opposite to the former, which does not excite but diminishes fever, and disposes to a favourable crisis.

17. In the early part of Balfour's service in the East (1783-4), he had charge of a regiment of sepoys in Cooch Behar. The prevalent diseases were fevers, or "fluxes attended with fevers." In the first month some four hundred men fell ill, the greater part of whom became convalescent in course of the eight days that intervened between the full and change of the moon; but during the remaining months of his stay in the district, the diseases just mentioned increased to almost double their extent at every full and change of the moon, falling down again to their former standard during the eight days which intervened between these two periods.

18. With regard to smallpox prevalent in India, Balfour satisfied himself that the full and change of the moon interfered with the eruption, and increased the accompanying fever to a dangerous degree.

19. Balfour collected a vast body of valuable evidence in support of his lunar theory, establishing, says Dr. Forbes Winslow, beyond all dispute that in tropical climates the regular diurnal and septenary changes observed in the character of the fevers of India, are coincident and correspondent with periodical sol-lunar conditions. Mason Good thinks there can be no question that, *"under certain circumstances,* and especially in tropical climates, many diseases are influenced by lunation, as we are sure they are, in all climates, by insolation." Dr. Balfour, he adds, is of opinion "that the influence of the sun and moon, when in a state of conjunction, which is named sol-lunar influence, produces paroxysms or exacerbations in continued fever, in all cases in which a paroxysmal diathesis (for such is his expression) exists; and as this influence declines, in consequence of the gradual separation of these luminaries from each other, and their getting into a state of opposition, a way is left open to the system for a critical and beneficial change, which is sure to take place, provided the critical disposition is at the same time matured. In other words, paroxysms and exacerbations in fever may be expected to take place, and do in fact take place, at spring-tides, and crises at neap-tides."

20. Balfour, in his Treatise I., offers the following propositions:—

" (1.) That in Bengal fevers of every denomination are in a remarkable manner connected with, and affected by, the revolutions of the moon.

" (2.) That in Bengal a constant and particular attention to the revolutions of the moon is of the greatest importance in the cure and prevention of fevers.

" (3.) That the influence of the moon in fevers prevails in a similar manner in every inhabited part of the globe, and consequently, that a similar attention to it is a matter of general importance in the practice of medicine.

" (4.) That the whole doctrine of the crisis of fevers may be readily explained from the premises established respecting the influence of the moon in these disorders at the full and change."

21. In his Treatise II. he presents the following axioms :—

" (1.) That the force of sol-lunar influence is much greater during the meridional periods than their respective intermeridional intervals, and seems to be somewhat greater during the nocturnal than their respective diurno-meridional periods ; and somewhat greater during the evening than the morning intermeridional intervals.

" (2.) The force of sol-lunar influence is much greater during the lunar periods, than their respective interlunar intervals; and during the novilunar and plenilunar periods it is very nearly the same ; and also during their respective interlunar intervals, at the beginning and end of which it seems greater than in the middle.

" (3.) The force of sol-lunar influence is considerably greater during the equinoctial periods than their respective inter-equinoctial intervals ; and somewhat greater during the autumno-equinoctial than the verno-equinoctial periods."

22. The fevers of most unhealthy or malarious countries, as of Gondwana, Aracan, Sindh, Guzerat, and of certain districts in Persia, would appear to present the most marked relations to the lunar changes :—in other words, where the terrestrial causes of fever are most concentrated, there the influences of the moon's changes would appear to be most clearly manifested.

At the meeting of the British Association for the Advancement of Science, held in Dublin, 1857, Mr. J. P. Harrison announced a law of temperature depending upon lunar influence :—" The author commenced by saying that, although the question of lunar influence on the atmosphere of our planet was very generally considered as set at rest by the investigations of M. Arago, yet he felt very confident that he was in a position to prove the law he was now about to announce without fear of contradiction. He had reduced and thrown into the form of tables and of curves 280 lunations, with the corresponding mean temperatures ; and the laws at which he had arrived were, first, between the first and second octant the temperature immediately after the first quarter, both on the average and also, with rare exceptions, in each individual lunation, is higher than the temperature shortly before the first quarter; secondly, and more particularly the mean temperature of the annual means of the second day after the first quarter (or the tenth day of the moon's age) is always higher than that of the third day before the first quarter (or the fifth day of the lunation). The tables and curves accompanied the essay, which illustrated these laws at great length."

"An undoubted heat effect" was observed in the elevated points of Teneriffe by Professor Piazza Smyth, although the moon was at the time of observation "in a low declination, so as to have a meridional altitude of only 42."

Balfour regards the influence of the moon, in malarious fevers, as more clearly manifested between the 13th and 26th degrees of north latitude.

He also regards the vernal and autumnal periods, or those between 20th March and 21st June, and between 23rd September and 22nd December, as those in which periodical fevers are most severe; while those diseases were, in his experience, less frequent and less severe in what he termed the equinoctial intervals. The question of the intensity of malarious fevers has been carefully investigated by Mr. Francis Day, of the Madras army, in the records of 423 cases, among the native troops of that Presidency serving in Mysore and in the Deccan. The result proved "that the most severe cases did occur at the two equinoctial periods."

This talented officer sums up the results of Dr. Balfour's observations as follows :—

"(1.) That the influence of the moon is less apparent in Madras than in Bengal, but may be traced over every portion of our Eastern possessions.

"(2.) That the lunar influence is thus exerted :—the first attack of fever almost invariably commences on one of those days preceding the full or new moon, or on one of those three which immediately follow them ; but that the three last are the most violent in their effects.

"(3.) That the new moon is more injurious than the full.

"(4.) That during these times the most severe as well as the greatest number of cases take place, but that when they occur at other periods they are less severe and of shorter duration.

"(5.) That these laws are as applicable to relapses as they are to primary attacks ; so much so, that the author was often able 'to prognosticate the return of the fever at these periods, with almost as much certainty as he could foretel the revolution itself.'"

Mr. Day sums up the results of carefully prepared statistical observations as follows :—

"(1.) That no decided preponderance in the admissions for malarious fever is observed at the time of the new moon.

"(2.) That a decided preponderance is observed at the time of the full moon.

"(3.) That more admissions occur in the three days preceding the full moon than in the three days subsequent to those changes.

"(4.) That a slight increase in the admissions may be present about the first and third lunar quarters.

"(5.) That the cases admitted at the time of the new moon are generally slightly more severe than the average admissions.

" (6.) That the cases admitted at the time of full moon are much more severe than the average admissions.

" (7.) That at times increased severity is also apparent at the first and third lunar quarters.

" (8.) That the cases admitted during the three days preceding these changes are more severe than those admitted in the three subsequent ones."

From the entire series of cases, Mr. Day arrives at the probability that " *there is a sol-lunar influence,* which is greater in the equinoctial period than in the respective equinoctial intervals; and considerably more so in the autumn than in the vernal equinoctial period; that this force is greater at the full and new moon than at the intervals, and much more so at the full than at the new; that it is greater during the meridional period than at the intermeridional intervals, and much more so at the diurno-meridional than at the nocturno-meridional periods."

THE ELECTRICAL CONDITION OF THE ATMOSPHERE.

If we attentively regard the agencies operating in health, and the disturbances of them which produce disease, we shall, with Dr. Habershon, recognise the fact that in the exercise of its functions the human body presents the manifest action of the same physical forces within itself which are in operation without the body; that the chemical forces obey the same laws in the living body as in the laboratory; that gravitation and attraction, the forces of heat, and electrical or galvanic force also, are in constant exercise, and with them is probably associated another correlated in some manner, which has been called nervous. All these are in constant operation in life, and the disturbance of them may be the cause of disease.

Some of the ablest of our physiologists, past and present, have come to the conclusion that " some, if not all, the organic actions which take place in the living body are accompanied with the manifestation of electric action."*

" Starting," says Dr. Carpenter, " with the abstract notion of force, as emanating at once from the Divine Will, we might say that this force, operating through inorganic matter, manifests itself in electricity, magnetism, light, heat, chemical affinity, and mechanical motion; but that, when directed through organized structures, it affects the operations of growth, development, chemico-vital transformations, and the like; and is further metamorphosed, through the instrumentality of the structures thus generated, into nervous agency and muscular power."

Dr. Laycock says that " without light and heat plants do not grow; without heat chemical affinity ceases, and animals perish.

* F. Baxter, on " Organic Polarity."

This correlation of physical and vital forces is, in fact, a necessary deduction from the correlations of the physical forces with each other.   Hence the forces set free during the changes in the blood and tissues upon which the fundamental phenomena of life depend, are convertible not only into motion, but also into heat, electricity, magnetism, and chemical affinity."

I here quote from the interesting communications of Dr. Maddock on " The Influence of Air and Weather upon the Mind and Body :"—

" Electricity," he says, " like caloric and light, pervades every element around us, varying in quantity according to the condition of the atmosphere; and although its existence is not perceptible any more than theirs, till the equilibrium of its distribution is destroyed, it has, probably, even in its latent state, a very considerable influence on the actions of organized beings.   Positive and negative electricity may be said to stand in the same relations to each other as heat and cold—as light and darkness; that is to say, it is the former alone which has any existence, and in no degree of negative electricity are plants and animals quite withdrawn from the influence of this principle.   It is, however, only in its sensible state that this agent can be recognised; and in this condition there are few or none, except caloric, which can compare with it in its universality of action, since every irritable organ appears to be subject to its agency.

" Very formidable difficulties attend all explanations of electrical phenomena, for to the question—What is electricity?—no categorical answer can yet be returned. The question, however, may be set aside, as not demanding to be answered before the effects of certain electrical states of the atmosphere are considered.   Of the real nature of light and heat, as well as of magnetism, we are, in truth, quite ignorant; but we do not hesitate to discuss the varied changes which matter undergoes when illuminated, heated, or magnetized, without waiting till our theories relating thereto are perfected; and in like manner can we do the same in regard to electricity, provided we adopt some provisional theory as to its nature, which shall supply us with appropriate terms for describing the phenomena, although it may be quite inadequate to account for them. Experience is in most cases our sole, if not sufficient, instructress, and the constant conjunction of phenomena, as exhibited in her lessons, is the sole ground for affirming the necessary connexion between them.   If we go beyond this, and come to inquire the manner *how*, and attempt to discover the mechanism by which these things are effected, we shall find everything around us equally mysterious, equally incomprehensible,—from the stone which falls to the ground to the comet traversing the heavens— from the formation of a mite in cheese, or a maggot in putrid flesh, to the production of a Newton or a Franklin.   'If,' as a modern writer remarks, 'we perceive an useful end, and means adopted to that end, we perceive enough for our conclusion. If these things be clear, no matter what is obscure, the argument is finished.' This is the language of a man of sound sense and sober understanding; but, unfortunately, there are many persons who found their pretensions to wisdom on their readiness to scout everything that cannot be proved by mathematical demonstration, not considering that the nature of the subject may preclude the possibility of attaining to any stronger evidence than reason and analogy can supply.

" The relative intensity of terrestrial electricity of various parts of the earth is a point worthy of the highest consideration, for it doubtless exercises a most marked effect on physical, chemical, and vital phenomena. Although our knowledge of this subject is too confined to admit of any practical application of it in the choice of a climate, it has been incontestably proved that in dry and cold states of the atmosphere an accumulation of positive electricity takes place, which brings about an increased activity in all the functions, and that thereby the nervous and circulating systems acquire an increased energy and tone, the respiration is more complete, and animal heat is more quickly generated to replace that which has been carried off by the surface of the body; on the contrary, we find intense and humid atmospheres are extremely oppressive, the lungs do not play freely, and the whole system is prostrated by lassitude and languor. It is to relieve this state of the air that the lightning plays, the thunder rolls, when nature at length recovers from her swoon, and again appears relieved, cheerful, and gay. A proper play, therefore, of the electric affinities is evidently and intimately connected with a salubrious atmosphere, and, in truth, when it glides freely along the nervous cord its discourse is health; but when the atmospherical electricity is impeded, or imperfect, the equipoise of humidity is prevented, and the elements of disease are disseminated.

" Mr. Mather, an intelligent meteorologist, has endeavoured to show, from his own observations as well as from the experiments of other scientific men, that the presence of cholera is invariably attended by marked electrical derangements in the atmosphere, and that when electricity is negative, vitality is depressed, and when positive, excited. In corroboration of these views, Mr. Mather states that when the cholera was so prevalent at Paris, in 1849, the deaths rapidly increased till the 8th of June, on which day they numbered 623. On that evening a great thunderstorm shook the city nearly to its foundation. Next day the cholera began to decrease; in ten days there were little more than 100 deaths in a day, and in twenty days no more than 30. ' In the same year,' says Mr. Mather, 'when cholera of a very fatal character was in this district [South Shields], I made daily observations, sometimes twice a day, with a magnet which, in its normal condition, carried about 2 lbs. 10 oz., varying with the virulence of the disease.   My hygrometer indicated at the same time an atmosphere nearly saturated with moisture.'   Mr. Mather adds, that 'in the north, in the year 1853, when the cholera was so very prevalent, the old choleraic atmosphere became as marked as it was in 1832 and 1849.'   That a thunderstorm must necessarily exercise a considerable influence on the animal economy may be readily imagined, when it is remembered that not only does it tend to promote a more equable diffusion of heat and moisture, and introduce nitrous acid gas to check the evolution of noxious miasmata by effecting their decomposition; but, from some experiments made by Signor Libri, of Florence, on odoriferous bodies by currents of electricity, it may be inferred that the direct and immediate agency of the storm may be the destruction of subtle emanations.   The electricity of the atmosphere may be also materially affected, since ammoniacal gas may be expanded into double its former volume by a current of electric sparks passed through it.   But I cannot say that Mr. Mather's experiments (although deserving serious attention) accord with the results of my own inquiry, which incline me to the belief that the density and temperature of the air operate on choleraic poison only as they affect its power as a carrier, or a sort of interventional medium, and there is no actual connexion between cholera and negative electricity.   It may be remarked, *en passant*, that it is a curious fact that in London, diarrhœa and summer cholera sprung, in 1846, into much greater than their former activity, and have continued to produce a much greater mortality; whence it seems not unreasonable to infer, as Dr. Farr remarks, that there has existed, during the whole of the last nine years, an increased tendency to the disease, which rose into paroxysms in 1849 and 1854.   An inquiry into this point might be usefully extended to other places.

"The singular circumstance of high mountains in the Northern hemisphere producing reverse effects upon the travellers ascending them, to those in the Southern, have been attributed to the fact of electricity occupying the upper parts of bodies in the former, and the lower part thereof in the latter.   Dr. Cunningham, R.N., who was, I believe, the first to direct attention to this interesting subject, states, that at high elevations in the Northern hemisphere (such as the top of Mont Blanc) there is a strong determination of blood to the head, indicated by swelling and lividity of the face and lips, sleepiness, and bleedings from the mouth, nose, eyes, and ears; while at similar elevations in the Southern hemisphere there is an equally strong determination of blood in the contrary dircetion, indicated by paleness and shrinking of the features, sleeplessness, giddiness, faintness, and vomiting; apoplectic symptoms thus characterizing the first, and all the usual accompaniments of fainting the second.   The treatment affording relief in each is also diametrically opposite (with the exception of the horizontal posture, which is useful in both), the stimulant drinks and the stimulant applications to the external parts, such as the mouth, nose, and ears, so beneficial in the southern affection, being hurtful in the northern. The apoplectic symptoms experienced upon Mont Blanc, and other high northern mountains, have been hitherto ascribed to the great rarefication of the air, whereby the soft parts of the human body are permitted to be expanded by the reduction of the atmospheric pressure upon them; but as no such effects, but, on the contrary, effects of an opposite nature, are produced by similar elevations in the Andes of South America, we must consequently look to some other cause than atmospheric rarefication to account for them. Dr. Cunningham refers these peculiarities of the respective hemispheres to the circumstance of the electric polarities of bodies being the *reverse* in the southern to what they are in the northern; a very curious fact, for the observation of which we are indebted to Lieutenant Lecount, R.N., when employed at the Island of Ascension, during the period of Bonaparte's detention at St. Helena. Thus electricity being found to occupy the *upper* portions of bodies in the northern hemisphere, and the *lower* portions in the southern, will consequently tend to propel the blood towards the head in the first, and towards the feet in the second; thereby giving rise to an apoplectic tendency in the one, and a tendency to fainting in the other; the symptoms in both being necessarily mitigated by the horizontal posture, whereby the electricity is more equally distributed throughout the body, in consequence of its occupying the latter longitudinally instead of transversely. A remarkable circumstance relating to this subject was noticed by Dr. Cunningham—viz., that travellers in the Andes seldom experience any unpleasant feeling as long as they remain on horseback, when they are in a great measure insulated from the electric influence of the earth, by the non-conducting sheepskin paddings placed under the saddles in Peru."

Sir Henry Holland states that, " though unable to affirm any one disease to be actually produced by electricity, yet, considering the subject in its whole extent, it is impossible not to see the likelihood of its influence on the body in many ways hitherto undistinguished, or not understood. If a stroke of lightning can in an instant destroy muscular irritability throughout the system, and prevent the natural coagulation of the blood, either directly or indirectly, by hastening putrefaction, it is clearly to be inferred that lesser degrees of the same action must have definite effects, bearing proportion to the intensity of the electric changes or transference taking place. The conclusions best warranted by the facts we possess would direct us towards the blood and nervous system generally as the parts of the animal economy most liable to be thus affected. The influence of atmospheric electricity on the latter is shown in the various effects already mentioned on sensations and muscular power; and the proof is greatly strengthened, though indirectly, by the numerous experiments which prove the influence upon these two functions of electric action from different sources applied directly to the nerves themselves.

"The quantity or tension of the agent, as affecting the body through the air, may be less, and its application not so direct on the nervous system. The low average intensity of animal electricity, as ascertained experimentally, must also be taken into account. But, with all these allowances, it is impossible that the effect should be wholly absent or different in kind; and circumstances may often greatly augment its degree, disordering in the same ratio that balance which is most conducive to the general well-being of life. The same reasoning applies equally to its influence on the blood; and though this part of the subject is even more obscure, yet is there presumption that here the effects occur which are of greatest importance in the history of disease. All that chemistry has recently done to determine the nature and relation of parts in the blood (concurrently with that great fact which has now been established of the identity of electrical and chemical action) justifies the belief that every material change of the balance between the electricity without and that within the body must have effect on the state of the circulating fluid; transient and wholly inappreciable it may be in the great majority of cases; in others, possibly, of longer duration and more extensive in degree."

It is, moreover, the opinion of Sir Henry Holland, quoted by Dr. Pallas, that "electricity may be concerned in favouring the generation of malaria, whatever its nature, or it may induce a state of the body more liable to be affected by this, or by other causes of disease in activity at the time. We have no proofs on which even to approach towards assurance, but presumption from several sources that this great agent cannot be wholly inert as respects either of the conditions in question."

"It has been stated," says Dr. Pickford, "on the authority of Mr. Glaisher and of Mr. Hingeston, that epidemic or pestilential diseases are associated with an absence or deficiency, and their presence with an increase in the amount of positive electricity. The latter gentleman believes it ' all but incontestable that what is called negative electricity goes with diseases called asthenic, while the positive belongs to such as are sthenic or inflammatory;' and that ' the former is coincident with mild and moist weather—the latter with the cold and frosty, or the hot and dry.' The kind of electricity, again, is certainly connected with the amount of daylight. There is less light on those days on which the negative electricity prevails than on the bright, when the electricity is, with few exceptions, positive. The public health is seldom favourable when the sky is grey, the air moist, the temperature low, the daylight diminished, and the electricity negative. On the contrary, it is good when the season is open, the clouds distributed in masses, the moisture condensed in showers, the electricity positive, and the solar rays abundant."

In an elaborate work, the result of years of careful observation, " On the Influence of Variations of Electric Tension, as the remote Cause of Epidemic and other Diseases," by Mr. Craig of Ayr, the author has endeavoured to establish the following propositions :—

" 1. That nervous power can be substituted by electricity, to produce not merely muscular action, but also the more vital internal operations.

" 2. That the nervous system necessarily depends on the ingesta for the material of which it is composed.

" 3. That it is shown whence are produced the supply and the source of the power by which nervous action is produced.

" 4. That diseased action is produced by an abstraction of nervous power, and consequent derangement of the corporeal operations.

" 5. That cholera prevails in all countries, but is most frequent and virulent in countries within the torrid zone. That it arises from a low state of electric tension, produced either by speedy evaporation, or those occult influences which are the results, sometimes of volcanic actions, sometimes of deviations of terrestrial currents. That this low state of electric tension causes abstraction of nervous power, and produces enervation of the capillary system, and inverted action of the bowels.

" 6. That yellow fever is peculiar to those countries which have a high temperature—where there are successively great drought, heavy rains, and speedy evaporation, producing a low electric tension. That the negative state of the soil thus produced abstracts from the human being nervous power both speedily and copiously, and deprives the secreting, excreting, and other vital organs of that which is indispensable to their healthy and efficient action. That this is followed by vitiation of the blood, clogging up and bursting of the capillaries, and breaking up of some of the internal organs.

" 7. That plague has its origin from the same instrumentality, operating, however, less powerfully. That the heat is less intense, and the evaporation less copious, in the localities which are visited by this pestilence. That in those countries in which this disease is endemic the variations of electric tension are neither so sudden nor so great as in those countries where yellow fever prevails. That in plague, the slower but more continuous evaporation causes a more slow and gradual abstraction of nervous power from the animal body. That, as in yellow fever, so in plague, the blood becomes vitiated, but less hurriedly, and its altered consistence renders its progress through the capillaries difficult, causing their rupture where weakest, giving rise to internal lesions and external ulcerations.

" 8. That intermittent fever is produced by a still smaller amount of nervous abstraction. That it has the same origin as the previously mentioned disease. That the localities in which this disease is endemic are marshes, or in circumstances analogous, and maintain a slower and more persisting evaporation, and a proportionally slow abstraction of nervous power.

" 9. That the views here taken of the pathology of pestilential diseases satisfactorily account for the difficulty of treating them, especially when they are once established.

" 10. That the treatment, to be successful, ought to be commenced at the time of the earliest manifestation.

" 11. That those living in pestilential regions should have their habitations dry and well elevated, and their beds insulated by good non-conductors, and should be as little out of doors as possible during the absence of sunshine, unless the soil be thoroughly dry.

" 12. That fever on board ship is caused by continuous evaporation, and consequent low state of electric tension.   That on this account ships ought to be kept as dry as possible, and with no water in the hold, especially in hot climates.   That care ought to be exercised not to take a moist cargo on board.   That in an unhealthy locality the seamen ought never to be on shore at night.

" 13. That a high situation is favourable, and a low one unfavourable to health, arises from the more elevated one being drier, and having less provision for evaporation.

" 14. That authors have long considered that electricity had some connexion with the production of disease, but never have given definite ideas of its *modus operandi.*

" 15. That in proportion to the amount of ozone found in the air, so is the locality in an electro-positive condition."

THE INFLUENCE OF ATMOSPHERIC PRESSURE.

The average pressure of the atmosphere is represented by Dr. Maddock* and others to be the same, or very nearly so, at any one place from year to year, notwithstanding the various temporary alterations arising from meteorological causes; but it is not yet accurately determined in a sufficient number of places to settle the question whether it is the same either at heights or at the level of the sea, throughout the globe or not.   It is obvious indeed that it must always be difficult to determine whether there is an observed difference in the mean height of the barometer at two places from difference of level, or from the atmosphere itself.

If the temperature of the higher and lower stations were uniform in all localities and in all times, and if the force of gravity were

---

* *Vide* a series of interesting articles on the Influence of Air and Weather, "Medical Circular," from which this and the previous section are principally prepared.

precisely the same at all heights, one formula would serve for all times and for different places, if the heights of the barometer re-mained invariably the same at the same height above the sea. In such a case, one observation made in London a hundred years ago, combined with one made at Quito in the present time, would serve to settle the point; and, even as it is, the mean height of the barometer at the two places, when known, would be sufficient for the purpose. But, when only one or two observations can be made at each place, the difference of temperature and other influ-ences must be noted and allowed for ; and this necessity renders the numerical operations connected with the solution of the pro-blem more intricate than they otherwise would be.

" The fluctuations of atmospheric pressure, as shown by the rise and fall of the barometric column, are extremely complicated, though very minute. In winter it is found that the column attains a maximum height at nine in the morning; it falls from this hour until three in the afternoon; it then begins to rise, and attains another maximum at nine in the evening. In summer, the hour of the first maximum is eight in the morning, and that of the minimum four in the afternoon; that of the second maximum being eleven at night. In spring and autumn this maximum and minimum take place at intermediate hours. The hours are not exactly the same for all countries, and the extent of variation is also different in different places; but the rise and fall in the twenty-four hours is a universal occurrence. Between the tropics these variations are very slight, not extending to much above a quarter of an inch ; but beyond the tropics they are very great, and the barometer has a range of three inches. It is presumed that the abundant aqueous precipitations which take place on each side of the tropics are the cause of these extensive fluctuations.

" A great connexion has been remarked between the pressure of the air, or the height of the barometer, and the direction of the wind. The barometer generally falls during east, south-east, and south winds ; passes from falling to rising during south-west ; rises with west, north-west, and north winds ; and has its greatest rise with north-east winds. It is also a general law, between the amount of vapour and the height of the barometer, that they change in opposite directions. In summer, when the quantity of vapour is greatest, the pressure of the air is least; and in the winter time, the vapour being least, the weight of the air is greatest. Even in the daily fluctuations of these two quantities this opposition is perceivable. The mean pressure of the atmo-sphere at London, as deduced from twenty years' observation by Luke Howard, is 29·8655, or very nearly $29\frac{9}{10}$ inches."

Huxham, referring to the effects of the barometric variations on the phenomena of epidemics, and more especially of inter-mittent fevers, expresses his belief that these last are influenced by the varying pressure of the atmosphere upon the veins. The inquiry is replete with interest, and Dr. Maddock entertains nò doubt that facts favour the supposition of Huxham, whose views are recognised, among others, by Sir David Barry, in the following terms:—"It being now evident that the blood in the veins is placed under the influence of atmospheric pressure, it would be curious to trace the connexion which appears to exist between disease generally—intermittent fever for example—and the daily atmospheric variations."

All persons are sensible of the effects of atmospheric pressure, and more especially invalids, who are generally susceptible to very slight changes in this respect—as, for instance, the hurried respiration, quickened circulation, and tendency to bloody expectoration which attend the ascent of high mountains; the oppression felt in the diving bell; the diarrhœa incident to those who remove from low to very high situations—these are all familiar examples of the more extreme effects of increased and diminished atmosphere.* So great indeed is the influence of atmospheric pressure, that if we could dig a shaft down into the earth to a depth of forty-two miles, the air at the bottom of it would be as dense as quicksilver. On the other hand, if we could ascend to the height of 4000 miles, and there let loose a cubic inch of air, it would become so excessively rare, and so widely diffused, as to fill a space equal to Saturn's orbit: this will give us an idea of the lightness and diffusibility of the air.

We cannot be surprised at the great effects produced by atmospheric pressure upon the health, when it is remembered that our bodies bear a weight equal to the cylinder of the air, the base of which corresponds with the superficies of our bodies: every square inch of the superficies sustains a quantity of air equal to 15 lbs.; so that, if the superficies of a man's body were to contain 2000 square inches, which is very near the truth, he would support, at the level of the sea, a weight of 15×2000 or 30,000 lbs., or nearly fourteen tons! Hence, so far from it being a matter of astonishment that we sometimes suffer in our health by a change in the weather, it is the greatest miracle we do not always do so. When we consider, too, that the variations in density are so considerable that the mercury in the barometer may indicate a pressure of nearly a ton and a half more weight at one time than another, and that these differences are often very sudden, it may seem wonderful that the vessels of our bodies, being so much acted on by an increased pressure, do not stagnate the blood up to the very heart, and altogether stop the circulation.† Such indeed would be the inevitable consequence, did not the pressure of the atmosphere act *equally* in all directions—not downwards only, or on the upper

* The fall of one-tenth is equal to a diminution of 62 lbs. pressure on the surface of a man's body.

† At Nice, as in tropical climates, the atmospheric pressure varies only slightly during the year, the variation being but one inch and a half.

surface of the body, as might at first be imagined, but on every part of the body in contact with the air, as explained by Lardner.

The fluids which fill the entire vascular system are exposed, as well as the surface of the body, to the pressure of the atmosphere, which enters the lungs and all the cavities and open parts of other organs. These fluids transmit that pressure to all the minor parts of the body, so that the skin and integuments are pressed by them *outwards* by a force exactly equal to that with which the air presses the external surface of the skin *inwards*. These outward and inward pressures are necessarily always equal, because, in fact, they are one and the same pressure—*i. e.* that of the air—the pressure on the external surface acting inwards being the immediate action of the air, and the pressure of the internal fluids acting outwards being the same pressure of the air transmitted by those fluids to the inside of the skin and integuments.

Dr. Maddock (*opus citat.*) considers that a knowledge of the existing barometric condition of the atmosphere cannot fail to prove of service to the practitioner when treating the different disorders of his patients, inasmuch as it produces peculiarities of constitution which, under disease, demand remedies, if not opposed to each other, still very importantly varied. It will generally be observed, he says, that diminished atmospheric pressure has the effect of relaxing the fibre and reducing the vigour of the muscular system, and thereby of occasioning great fatigue. This debilitating influence will be more or less felt according to the state of the general health; those persons who are of a weakly habit will therefore be most susceptible.

Lieutenant Wood, in his "Journey to the River Oxus," re-marks that, when at an altitude of 15,000 feet above the level of the sea, he˗ and his comrades suffered so much from muscular weakness, that even conversation could not be maintained without great exhaustion. The influence of diminished pressure on the circulation is still more extensive and important than on the muscnlar system. Lieut. Wood observing : " I felt the pulses of my party whenever I registered the boiling point of water; for I found the circulation of the blood to be, in fact, a sort of living barometer, by which a man acquainted with his own habit of body can, in great altitudes, roughly calculate his height above the level of the sea." The fact of the bloodvessels being thus influenced may probably be attributed to the air contained in the blood expanding under diminished pressure, and thereby rendering the vessels turgid; the heart and blood-vessels becoming relaxed, they are then more dilatable, and the blood is accordingly circulated with greater rapidity but with less vigour.

If this theory be correct, it is but natural to suppose that such an altered condition of the circulation may induce sanguineous effusions, more especially in those persons in whom the vascular system is already disordered. Apoplexy may thus be produced;

but the air-tubes and lungs being the most permeable to the air, are more particularly susceptible of deficient atmospheric pressure, which, by promoting congestion of their blood-vessels, either originates or conduces to the return of bronchial and pulmonary complaints.

On the other hand, an increased pressure of the atmosphere is also frequently found troublesome to patients suffering from asthmatic and other affections of the respiratory organs, by over-powering the already diminished resistance of the air-tubes, and thereby augmenting the dyspnœa. The influence of this condition of the atmosphere upon the nervous system is also frequently evident in depressing the energies, in debilitating the mental powers, and in lowering the spirits; and hence Dr. Maddock has observed that it is almost invariably accompanied by an increase in the number of suicides. These facts, according to Shute, tend to show that affections of the mind are more influenced by the condition of the blood, which is connected with respiration, than is generally imagined.

If the nervous and arterial influences be the same things; if they are both to be regarded as certain modifications of the air; if the mind be influenced by the state of the nervous system (a fact which is proved in syncope, inhaling nitrous oxide, &c., &c.), may we not hope to influence the action of the brain through the medium of the respiratory organs, and thus to acquire some power over mental ailments? May we not, concludes Dr. Maddock, hope to account rationally for the influence of the air upon a variety of diseases?—*Medical Circular*, October 17, 1855.

"Of the number of cases of apoplexy which occurred in the years 1850-51," says Dr. Moffat, "50 per cent. took place on days of decreasing readings of the barometer, and 50 per cent. happened on days after such readings: 100 per cent. occurred with *fall of temperature*, and they all took place with a direction of the wind from S. E. and S. W. points of the compass; and of seven *sudden* deaths, five occurred with wind from N. W., with *hail showers*."

The high state of the barometer during certain epidemics has been observed as a remarkable characteristic by several persons. The late Dr. Prout, speaking of the high barometric range in London, in February, 1832, says:—"There seems to be only one mode of rationally explaining this increased weight of the air of London, which is, by admitting the diffusion of some gaseous body through the lower regions of the atmosphere of this city considerably heavier than the air it displaced. About the 9th of February, the wind, which had previously been *west*, veered round to the *east*, and remained chiefly in that quarter to the end of the month. Now, precisely on the change of the wind, the first cases of epidemic cholera were reported in London, and from that time the disease continued to spread. That the epidemic cholera was the effect of the peculiar condition of the atmosphere is more, perhaps, than can be safely maintained; but reasons which have been advanced elsewhere lead the writer to believe that the virulent disease termed cholera was owing to some matter which produced the additional weight of the air. The foreign body diffused through the atmosphere of London in February, 1832, was probably a variety of malaria."

Mr. Glaisher, speaking of the three visitations of cholera in London, says :—" The three epidemics were attended with a peculiar state of atmosphere, characterized by a prevalent *mist*, thin in high places, dense in low.   During the height of the epidemic, in all cases, the reading of the *barometer was remarkably high*, and the atmosphere thick. In 1849 and 1854 the *temperature was above* its average, and a *total absence of rain*, and a stillness of air, amounting almost to *calm*, accompanied the progress of disease on each occasion.   In places near the river the night temperatures were high, with small diurnal range, a dense, torpid mist, and air charged with many impurities arising from the *exhalations of the river* and adjoining marshes, *a deficiency of electricity*, and, as shown in 1854, *a total absence of ozone*, most probably destroyed by the decomposition of the organic matter with which the air in these situations is strongly charged."

The stagnation of the atmosphere, which, in a great city, must mean of itself much impurity, had doubtless given here, as in many noted epidemics, great force and activity to the disease ; but Mr. Glaisher, nevertheless, guards the reader against the conclusion that cholera was to be referred exclusively to atmospheric influences, however powerful and extensive they may have been. Sir Henry Holland, speaking of the feeling caused by what are termed, in misplaced or even inverted sense, lightness and heaviness of atmosphere, says that it is difficult to declare through what organ or function this feeling is chiefly conveyed; but probably it is a compound effect of the changes in circulation, in which the sensorium, the lungs, and the muscular system all participate.

" On a general view," he says, " of the circumstances stated, there is reason to conclude that the influence of different degrees of atmospheric pressure in disturbing the bodily functions and general health is derived from the frequency of fluctuations, rather than from any state long continued, either above or below the average standard ; that of the two conditions suddenly incurred in any extreme degree, the human frame is better capable of withstanding a rarefied than a condensed atmosphere ; and that, in every case, the previous health and proneness to disorder in particular organs, are greatly concerned in determining the results on the body." In proof of the correctness of these opinions, the author quotes the results of Mr. Green's frequent ascents by balloons, in company with four hundred persons at different times. In September, 1838, he and Mr. Rusk ascended to the height of 27,136 feet, or 5⅐ miles above the level of the sea, yet neither suffered inconvenience, excepting from cold, and from the toil of discharging ballast and gas. During the ascent the barometer fell from 30°·50 to 11°, and the thermometer from 61° to 5°. The first 11,000 feet were passed through in about seven minutes.

STATISTICS OF THE INFLUENCE OF CLIMATE AND SEASON IN PRODUCING SICKNESS AND MORTALITY IN CALCUTTA.

SICKNESS.

It now remains to trace, in a more special and statistical manner, the influence of season in producing sickness and mortality; for this purpose I have prepared several tables; and the first, exhibiting this influence on the mortality of natives, was got up, at my request, by Dr. Duncan Stewart; the period it comprehends is seven years—viz., from 1831 to 1837 inclusive:—

Months.	Of 1000 deaths there occurred in different months.	Of 1000 living Hindoos there died in different months.	Of 1000 living Mussulmans there died in different months.	Total natives. Of 1000 living, there died in different months.
In 7 Januarys	92½	27½	9½	22½
7 Februarys	67⅓	12½	8⅘	16½
7 Marches	65½	18½	8½	15⅘
7 Aprils	69½	19½	8½	16⅓
7 Mays...............	63⅔	17½	9	15⅓
7 Junes	54½	14½	8⅘	13
7 Julys...............	70¾	18	11½	16⅓
7 Augusts	90½	26	10½	21½
7 Septembers	98	28	12⅖	23⅘
7 Octobers	104½	30	12½	25⅓
7 Novembers	116½	34⅓	11⅗	28
7 Decembers.........	106½	31⅓	11⅓	25⅖

This table exhibits in a remarkable manner the fatal influence of the months from September to January inclusive, and which would be even more striking if we possessed the means of deducting the deaths by cholera in the months of March, April, May, and June, so as to show only the ordinary endemic influence; as it is, however, the table is instructive and interesting.

The following table I have had collated from the records of the vestry; it exhibits burials in the Protestant burial-ground for twenty years, from 1819 to 1838 inclusive, and arranged in months :—

Months.	Under five years of age.	Above five years of age.	Total.
In 20 Januarys	53	257	310
20 Februarys	41	165	206
20 Marches	70	260	330
20 Aprils	105	307	412
20 Mays	104	421	525
20 Junes	99	298	397
20 Julys	104	285	389
20 Augusts	87	389	476
20 Septembers	74	379	453
20 Octobers	84	368	452
20 Novembers	60	379	439
20 Decembers	53	349	402
Total	934	3857	4791

Thus it appears that, though the greatest number of deaths occurred in the Mays—the worst of the cholera months—the period of greatest general mortality has been from August to January inclusive; and if the deaths by cholera during the hot months could be excluded, this result would appear very striking.

With a view to exhibit the simple endemic influence in the fairest manner, I again had recourse to the vestry records, from which the following table of Protestant burials has been framed for the twenty years just previous to the appearance of cholera as an epidemic, namely, from 1796 to 1815 inclusive:—

Months.	Under five years.	Above five years.	Total.
In 20 Januarys	28	216	244
20 Februarys	26	153	179
20 Marches	31	164	195
20 Aprils	33	178	211
20 Mays	25	235	260
20 Junes	22	209	231
20 Julys	34	219	253
20 Augusts	44	288	332
20 Septembers	42	296	338
20 Octobers	32	293	325
20 Novembers	32	331	363
20 Decembers	23	311	334
Total	372	2893	3265

Thus it appears, that in twenty years Novembers were the most fatal months, and that the five months from August to December inclusive were more fatal than the whole seven months besides.

But further to ascertain the influence of season on the health and mortality of the European soldiers and seamen, I have prepared the following table from a document furnished by the Medical Board :—it exhibits the totals of admissions and deaths in the Presidency General Hospital in each month during twelve years ; the item "*other diseases*" has some awkwardness in it, but that I cannot help :—

RANGE OF OBSERVATIONS IN MONTHS.	TOTAL ADMISSIONS.					TOTAL DEATHS.				
	By acute diseases.	By chronic diseases.	By surgical diseases.	By "other diseases."	By all diseases.	By acute diseases.	By chronic diseases.	By surgical diseases.	By "other diseases."	By all diseases.
In 12 Januarys	899	64	261	245	1,469	89	10	5	8	12
12 Februarys	557	46	185	150	938	67	6	2	13	88
12 Marches	456	38	163	132	789	55	5	5	7	72
12 Aprils	619	42	138	175	974	50	6	6	12	74
12 Mays	722	70	161	178	1,131	67	11	7	12	97
12 Junes	791	63	184	186	1,224	64	4	4	11	83
12 Julys	843	38	176	127	1,184	104	6	11	24	145
12 Augusts ....:	732	42	180	146	1,100	88	9	9	8	114
12 Septembers	683	69	148	174	1,074	112	8	11	3	144
12 Octobers	764	48	229	182	1,223	114	4	10	18	136
12 Novembers	1142	120	282	325	1,869	97	4	5	10	116
12 Decembers	948	87	247	233	1,515	109	8	7	27	151
Total	9156	727	2354	2253	14,490	1016	81	82	153	1332

It appears from the "Medical Board's Table," from which the above is framed, that, out of 1704 Europeans who died in the twelve years, 372 died of cholera ; 304 of dysentery ; 58 of diarrhœa ; 465 of remittent fever ; 66 of intermittent ; 50 of hepatitis ; 88 of phthisis, so-called, but more than half were probably bronchitis ; 19 of rheumatism ; 6 only of splenic disease ; 8 of apoplexy ; 9 of delirium tremens ; 6 of smallpox ; leaving 270 deaths from "other diseases."

The total admissions in twelve years are 15,293, and the deaths 1704.

The proportions of deaths to cases treated are as follows :—

Of remittent fever, 5116 admissions and 465 deaths, or one in . 11
Of dysentery, 1877 admissions and 304 deaths, or one in . . $6\frac{1}{9}$
Of cholera, 853 admissions and 372 deaths, or one in . . . . $2\frac{1}{3}$
Of diarrhœa, 608 admissions and 58 deaths, or one in . . . . $10\frac{1}{2}$
Of intermittent fever, 501 admissions and 66 deaths, or one in . $7\frac{7}{13}$
Of hepatitis, 446 admissions and 50 deaths, or one in . . . . $8\frac{9}{10}$
Of spleen diseases, 58 admissions and 6 deaths, or one in . . . $9\frac{3}{3}$
Of delirium tremens, 124 admissions and 9 deaths, or one in . $13\frac{7}{9}$
Of apoplexy, 27 admissions and 8 deaths, or one in . . . . $3\frac{3}{8}$
Of "other diseases," 2253 admissions and 153 deaths, or one in $14\frac{3}{4}$

Average of deaths from all diseases, is therefore nearly one in nine.

Of a hundred British soldiers who die in Bengal, Dr. Burke states that 26·8 do so from fever ; 7·3 from hepatitis ; 30·5 from dysentery and other bowel complaints ; 19·5 from cholera ; 4·6 from pulmonic diseases, 1·9 of which is from phthisis pulmonalis ; leaving only 11 whose deaths are caused by other diseases.

From the " Medical Board's Table of Seasons" it appears that the most healthy months comparatively are February, March, April, and May ; that from June to January, the admissions range high, these also being by far the most fatal months. These results correspond nearly with observations on the climate of Jamaica, and others of the West Indian colonies, wherein the most unhealthy as well as fatal months of the year extend from August to December inclusive ; the months comparatively healthy being from January to June. Such observations would seem to apply to most parts of the Northern hemisphere, which generally possess the same character of climate : they also accord with the ancient maxim in the south of Europe which held the summer and autumnal to be the most sickly seasons.

Celsus, writing of the influence of season in the malarious city of Rome, says, " Igitur saluberrimum ver est ; proxime deinde ab hoc, hyems; periculosior æstas; autumnus longe periculosissimus."

From the researches of statistical writers, it appears that all over Europe the maximum of deaths occurs towards the close of winter, and the minimum towards the close of summer.

In order that the table should express only the result of ordinary season and endemic influence, I have not included cholera, which epidemic is found to prevail chiefly in the months of April, May, and June.

October, November, December, and January are the months in which there occurred the largest proportions of remittent fever cases, and the same applies to dysentery, diarrhœa, and acute hepatitis ; while September alone gives more intermittents than the whole of the other months besides.

In order to account for the unusual mortality under all heads of disease, it is proper to mention that the descriptions of persons treated in the General Hospital are as follows :—European soldiers belonging to detachments from Her Majesty's and the Honourable Company's regiments ; recruits for ditto ; the sick of all regiments returning from service, as for instance, during the Burmese war, &c.; European and American seamen from the shipping; townsmen, paupers, generally seamen ; invalid soldiers on their way to England, &c. &c. ;—in short, a class of persons, many of whom, besides being diseased and worn out, are away from that salutary control which leads to prompt measures both for the prevention and cure of disease. It thus happens that the earlier stages of acute illness are neglected ; an irrecoverable loss, and which must necessarily imply a larger proportionate mortality.

The following table exhibits the admissions and deaths, in each month, during the period included between 1827 and 1838, in the hospital of Her Majesty's regiment in the garrison of Fort William.

MONTHS.	TOTAL ADMISSIONS.					TOTAL DEATHS.				
	By fevers.	By hepatitis.	By bowel complaints.	By " other diseases."	Total by all diseases.	By fevers.	By hepatitis.	By bowel complaints.	By " other diseases."	Total by all diseases.
In 12 Januarys......	231	24	249	539	1,043	7	3	20	10	40
12 Februarys....	266	51	263	627	1,207	1	2	16	5	24
12 Marches	323	64	286	606	1,279	9	1	16	10	36
12 Aprils.........	303	66	318	708	1,395	6	2	19	9	36
12 Mays......—	418	53	330	726	1,527	8	2	22	12	44
12 Junes	488	57	253	698	1,496	5	2	18	13	38
12 Julys	403	68	314	586	1,371	16	5	28	10	59
12 Augusts	427	38	321	609	1,395	18	4	25	8	55
12 Septembers...	446	42	256	557	1,301	18	4	30	10	62
12 Octobers......	404	33	250	541	1,228	23	0	21	6	50
12 Novembers ...	423	39	203	574	1,239	19	4	25	9	57
12 Decembers ...	311	20	202	550	1,083	16	1	16	10	43
Total......	4443	555	3245	7321	15,564	146	30	256	112	544

It thus appears that in the 12 years there were 15,564 admissions by all diseases, and 544 deaths, or one death in every 28$\frac{2}{3}$ patients treated, being less by two-thirds than the general average afforded by the General Hospital returns for the same period—an emphatic example of the value of that internal discipline and economy in corps to which so much preventive and curative result is ascribed by all military and medical authorities. Out of 544 deaths, 256 are by bowel complaints—146 by fever, and 30 by liver disease, leaving 112 deaths by other diseases. If from the column of deaths we abstract for the hot months those by cholera, the comparative fatality of the months from September to January inelusive, will be rendered very remarkable.

The proportions of deaths to cases treated are as follows :—

By fever, 4443 admissions and 146 deaths, or one in 30 and two-thirds, nearly: by bowel complaints, 3245 admissions and 256 deaths, or one in 12$\frac{1}{2}$, nearly: by hepatitis, the very large proportion of 555 admissions and 30 deaths, or one in 18$\frac{1}{2}$: by other diseases, 7,321 admissions and 112 deaths, or one in 65 and $\frac{1}{3}$rd, nearly.

The winter, all over Europe, is the season of the greatest mortality ; and not only is this a proved fact in statistics, but a mild winter is found to be attended by a diminished mortality, comparatively. In the first quarter of 1846, the winter was unusually mild throughout England, and " the rate of mortality was lower than in the corresponding quarters of eight previous years."

In the first quarter of 1847, on the other hand, the temperature was below the average, the severity of the weather being throughout unusually great. The mortality corresponded, being " 6035 above the corrected average," for the 117 districts only comprised in the quarterly returns of the Registrar-General.

"Winter," says Dr. Farr, " appears to be the season in which it is most natural to man to die." The same authority justly observes, that "as man progresses in life, the more necessary does warmth become to him; while the summer lengthens, the winter shortens his days."

Dr. Mouat, of the 13th Light Dragoons, states that, while serving in the Madras Presidency, out of 3394 cases of disease treated in the Regimental Hospital, 1372 soldiers imputed their illness to cold, while only 62 ascribed theirs to exposure in the sun.

The influence of atmospheric pressure on sickness and mortality has not been observed in India; but the subject is one of much interest and importance. Professor Casper of Berlin founds the following position on numerous statistical tables, ranging over seven years' observation in the Prussian capital : " *In nearly all the seasons of the year a high atmospheric pressure increases, and a low pressure diminishes the rate of mortality.*"

MORTALITY OF THE VARIOUS RACES—EUROPEAN AND NATIVE.

"Man is not born, does not live, does not suffer, does not die in the same manner on all points of the earth. Birth, life, disease, and death all change with the climate and soil, all are modified by race and nationality. These varied manifestations of life and death, of health and disease, constitute the special object of medical geography."—*Boudin.*

In any inquiry as to the duration of life, and into the causes of mortality amongst the natives of Bengal, we must consider, not only that general climate exercises a powerful influence on the longevity of different races, by accelerating or retarding the development of the human system, but that, along with one of the worst of climates, all the institutions and habits of life of the Bengalis tend materially to abbreviate the term of existence— their premature decay being in perfect accordance with their early and forced development. The law of correspondence of the period of puberty with the whole term of life is subject to few exceptions, and has been well expressed by Bacon, by " Nature's finishing her periods in larger circles."—*Hist. Vitæ et Mortis.*

It is well known that the proportional number of individuals who attain a given age differs in different climates, and that the warmer the climate, other circumstances being equal, so much the shorter is the average duration of human life. Even within the limits of Europe the difference is very great, being one death in twenty-eight in the Roman States, and one death in forty-six in England annually. According to Moreau de Jonnes, the rate of mortality in some instances, and inversely the duration of life, differ by nearly one-half from the proportions discovered in other examples.

In approaching the Equator we find the mortality increase, and the average duration of life consequently diminished.

The same authority observes, that the comparatively low degree of mortality among the men of colour in the West Indies, and the Javanese and Parsees, in countries where those races are either the original inhabitants, or have become naturalized by an abode of some centuries, is remarkable. " It would seem that such persons are exempted, in a great measure, from the influence of morbific causes which destroy prematurely Europeans and other foreigners. That the rate of mortality should be lower among them than in the southern parts of Europe, is a fact which, in the present state of our knowledge, is difficult to explain."

The following tables and remarks were found by me amongst the records of the Committee for the Improvement of Calcutta, and were handed to the late Mr. James Prinsep, who published them in the eighty-second number of the " Journal of the Asiatic Society."

Mortality among all Classes in Calcutta for Twenty Years; but for the Native Population only Five Years.

Years.	Protestant burials.		Catholic burials, D. Rozario.	Catholic burials, Boitockannah.	Greeks.	Armenians.	Indo-Armenians.	Native Christians.	Natives.
1817	216		313	169	4	10	3	...	
1818	272		211	159	2	20	3	...	
1819	275		284	158	...	23	3	...	
1820	281		282	136	...	17	1	...	Native deaths for five years.
1821	246		277	172	...	16	3	...	
1822	324	Scotch	294	140	...	16	2	...	Hindus 8,299
1823	270	burying	277	156	...	10	2	...	Mussulmans 1,009
1824	278	ground	282	188	...	21	1	...	——— 9,308 in 1832
1825	297	began	285	154	1	12	10	....	Hindus 15,138
1826	275	1826.	309	145	2	19	17	...	Mussulmans 2,385
1827	254	11	308	174	...	15	16	4	———17,523 in 1833
1828	256	19	250	170	2	15	12	3	Hindus 11,167
1829	184	21	209	146	3	12	16	2	Mussulmans 1,900
1830	224	26	236	138	1	14	15	...	———13,067 in 1834
1831	186	29	236	122	3	17	19	8	Hindus 6,873
1832	217	25	269	121	1	17	16	1	Mussulmans 1,229
1833	302	30	288	204	2	23	14	5	——— 8,102 in 1835
1834	281	35	257	199	2	16	17	4	Hindus 6,366
1835	233	18	233	115	1	7	16	4	Mussulmans 1,515
1836	197	26	188	104	0	15	13	3	——— 7,881 in 1836
	5065	240	5288	3070	24	315	199	34	55,881
	20	10	20	20	12	20	20	9	5
Average	253	24	264	153	2	15¾	10	3⅓	11,178

Statement of the Average Rate of Mortality per Cent. among the different Classes of Inhabitants in Calcutta per Census and Table of Mortality.

Denominations.	Number of Inhabitants.	Total.	Average mortality per annum.	Average mortality per cent.	Proportion.
English......................	3138				
Eurasians..................	4746				
		7884	277	3½ per ct.	1 in 23
Portuguese	3181				
French	160				
		3341	417	12¼ ,,	1 in 8
Western Mahomedans ...	13,677				
Bengal Mahomedans ...	45,067				
Moguls	527				
Arabs	351				
		59,622	1607	2¾ ,,	1 in 36
Western Hindus	17,333				
Bengal Hindus............	120,318				
Mugs........................	683				
Low Castes	19,084				
		157,418	9553	6$\frac{1}{12}$,,	1 in 16
Armenians ......:........	...	636	25¾	4$\frac{1}{12}$,,	1 in 25
Native Christians.........	...	49	3½	7$\frac{1}{7}$,,	1 in 14
Chinese.....................	...	362			
Jews.........	...	307			
Parsees.....................	...	40			
Madrassees	...	55			

" The great difference in mortality between the Hindus[*] and Mussulmans is striking, while the difference to be observed between the Portuguese, as compared with the English and the Eurasians, is equally so.

" Here is much room for speculation, and it cannot be said that as yet we have as good means of getting correct information upon this subject as they possess in Europe; nevertheless, we may approach as near as we can to the point we wish to ascertain, and we may hope to improve in such statistical records.

" The Portuguese, among whom so great a mortality is shown, are a suffering race, very subject to the catalogue of complaints enumerated in these papers; while the English and Eurasians are far more prosperous in life, and enjoy comforts and happiness in a very high degree, as compared with the former section of society. The mortality of English and Eurasians, 3½ per cent. per annum, while that of the Portuguese being 12½ per cent., is very great. In 1830 I ascertained, and published in the ' Gleanings of Science,' the burials in Calcutta of Protestant Christians from the year 1820, to show at that time that, although the Euro-

[*] The difference of mortality amongst the Mahomedans and Hindus may be accounted for by the circumstance that the Hindus of Calcutta, consisting of families, include a much larger proportion of infant life. The same circumstance will explain the great difference between the average mortality amongst the Portuguese and the Europeans of Calcutta.—Ed. *Journal Asiatic Society.*

pean population must have greatly increased, yet, that the deaths and burials had not increased; and now that the same population is acknowledged to have increased very materially indeed, yet we see, upon referring to the first column of one of the tables, giving the Protestant burials for the last twenty years, no increase of deaths. The years 1833-4, the two years following the sea inundations, show the greatest mortality of late years; while among the native population those two years show an extraordinary mortality. The two last years show in both European and native population that healthiness is restored. The mortality among the other columns of society, the Catholic, Greek, Armenian, Hindu, and native Christian, are for the last twenty years, and I believe them to be nearly correct. The Chinese and Jews keep no account of their burials; I of course could not include them, and they form a minute portion of the population of this city."

" The native soldiers of Bengal," says Colonel Henderson, " are very healthy under ordinary circumstances. It has been found, on inquiry, that only one man died per annum out of 131 of the actual strength of the army. So injurious, however, is Bengal Proper to this class of natives, as compared with the Upper Provinces, that though only one-fourth of the troops exhibited are stationed in Bengal, the deaths of that fourth are more than a moiety of the whole mortality reported."

That the climate of the country of the great waters, the Delta of the Ganges, was not less fatal to our Mahomedan predecessors, is evident from Gladwin's translation from a Persian document:—
" In former reigns, Bengal, on account of the inclemency of the air and water, was deemed inimical to the constitution of Moguls and other foreigners, and only those officers who laboured under the royal displeasure were stationed there; and this fertile soil, which enjoys a perpetual spring, was considered a strong prison, as the land of spectres, the seat of disease, and the mansion of death."

" The Mussulman invaders," says a native writer, " of the west of Hindustan, who afterwards established themselves on the throne of Delhi, considered this country, Bengal, to be Dojakh, or an infernal region; and whenever any of the Ameers or courtiers were found guilty of capital crimes, and the rank of the individuals did not permit their being beheaded, while policy, at the same time, rendered their removal necessary, they were banished to Bengal. The air and water of Bengal were considered so bad as to lead to the certain death of the criminal."

In the " Journal of the Asiatic Society of Bengal," vol. vii. Sept. 1838, there is an interesting paper, drawn up with much care by Mr. H. T. Prinsep, on the Mortality of the Indo-British children in the Lower Orphan School of Calcutta. From a comparison of the mortality at each year of life from 10 to 20 with what occurs in London at the same ages, he draws the following deductions :—" The decrement in India is, as might be expected from the climate, greater from birth than in London, but the favourable years are the same—viz., from 9 to 14 ; and it will be observed, with due allowance for insalubrity, and for not perhaps the most favourable rearing in a large school like our Orphan Asylum, that there is a general correspondence in the results up to the age of six."

By a statement forwarded by the Medical Board to the Committee for the Improvement of Calcutta, it would appear that, during the thirty years from 1st January, 1808, to 31st December, 1837, there were, of admissions and deaths, amongst the European patients of the Presidency General Hospital, as follows :—

$$\text{Total admissions} \quad . \quad . \quad . \quad . \quad . \quad . \quad . \quad 35,119$$
$$\text{Total deaths} \quad . \quad . \quad . \quad . \quad . \quad . \quad . \quad . \quad 3,607$$

This, for thirty years, gives a mean ratio of $10\frac{27}{100}$ deaths per cent. of the admissions.

The quinquennial ratios are as follow :—

Years.	Admissions.	Deaths.	Ratio of deaths per cent.
From 1808 to 1812..............	2713	299	11
1813 1817..............	4360	450	$10\frac{32}{100}$
1818 1822..............	6425	657	$10\frac{22}{100}$
1823 1827..............	9560	1039	$10\frac{76}{100}$
1828 1832..............	6315	585	$9\frac{26}{100}$
1833 1837..............	5746	577	$10\frac{5}{100}$
Mean	$5853\frac{1}{3}$	$684\frac{2}{3}$	$10\frac{27}{100}$

That is all that the Medical Board could furnish ; for it was not till 1808 that any records were used, even of admissions and deaths.

The following table exhibits both the sickness and mortality of the British troops in garrison at the Presidency, together with the proportion of deaths to cases treated, of the three principal endemic diseases of Bengal; viz., fever, dysentery, and hepatitis :—

Table of Admission into Hospital and Deaths, during 17 *Years, of the European Troops in Garrison of Fort William.*

Years.	Strength.	Admissions.	Deaths.	Ratio per 1000 of strength.	
				Admitted.	Died.
1822	866	1,303	75	1,594·62	86·60
1823	828	1,687	51	2,037·24	61·59
1824	736	2,268	103	3,082·32	139·94
1825	902	2,542	110	2,818·18	121·95
1826	863	1,826	96	2,115·87	111·23
1827	893	1,336	56	1,496·08	62·71
1828	913	1,776	42	1,945·23	45·00
1829	885	1,995	58	2,253·67	62·14
1830	808	1,722	59	2,131·78	73·02
1831	831	1,061	57	1,276·77	68·59
1832	771	1,024	59	1,728·14	76·52
1833	687	1,387	64	2,018·92	93·15
1834	608	1,166	57	1,917·76	93·15
1835	743	1,211	33	1,629·87	44·41
1836	734	1,245	25	1,696·18	34·06
1837	709	899	26	1,267·98	36·07
1838	633	694	22	1,096·36	34·75
Total	13,410	25,142	497	... ...	... ...
Average ...	$788\frac{14}{17}$	$1,478\frac{16}{17}$	$29\frac{4}{17}$	1,833·33	73·26

The ratio of deaths to cases treated was, during ten years, as follows :—

In fever . . . . one in $28\frac{46}{198}$
dysentery . . . . " $12\frac{144}{166}$
hepatitis, acute and chronic . . . . . " $8\frac{1}{4}$

The mortality by all diseases in every hundred deaths of Euro-peans serving in the Presidency of Bombay, between 1830 and 1846, was as follows :—

Dysentery . . . . 28·527
Fevers . . . . 23·054
Cholera . . . . 10·320
Hepatic diseases . . . . 9·597
Diarrhœa . . . . 3·914
Pulmonary diseases . . . . 5·807
Other diseases . . . . 18·697
Lost in calculation . . . . ·084
Total . . . . 100·000

Table of Admission into Hospital and Deaths, during 12 *Years, of the European Troops at Chinsurah (Depot),* 18 *Miles distant from Calcutta.*

Years.	Strength.	Admissions.	Deaths.	Ratio per 1000 of strength.	
				Admitted.	Died.
1826	1083	818	86	755·31	79·40
1827	814	1,329	80	1,632·67	98·28
1828	200	542	20	2,710·00	100·00
1829	132	571	24	4,325·75	181·81
1830	366	822	24	2,245·95	65·57
1831	927	1,412	51	1,523·19	56·01
1832	737	1,182	41	1,603·79	55·63
1833	577	1,155	54	2,001·73	93·58
1834	784	1,308	32	1,668·36	40·81
1835	832	872	17	1,048·07	20·43
1836	743	1,428	39	1,921·93	52·35
1837	765	1,322	32	1,728·10	41·83
Total.......	7960	12,761	500	.. ...	... ...
Average ...	663⅓	1,063$\frac{5}{12}$	41⅔	1,930·40	73·72

The ratio of deaths to cases treated was, during three years, as follows :—

In fever . . . . one in 25¼
dysentery. . . . . „ 7$\frac{25}{88}$
hepatitis, acute and chronic . . . . „ 8$\frac{8}{10}$

The above must be taken as the mortality on the spot only, and does not include the invalids, who died on their passage to England, or shortly after their arrival there, amounting to 3¼ annually. If, as is well known also, the medical returns be taken at the highest strength in the course of the year or quarter, or a tenth part higher than it ought to be, instead of the mean monthly strength, the ratio of mortality will be greatly increased. It is believed that a correction of all errors would bring the annual mortality to more than eighty per thousand.

That in India, as elsewhere, age materially influences the ratio of mortality will be seen from the following tables for the officers of the Bengal army, and those of the Civil Service. Out of 1184 deaths among officers, the proportion occurring annually in each rank, and at each age, has been as follows :—

Percentage of deaths.	Colonels, average age 61.	Lieutenant-Colonels, average age 51.	Majors, average age 40.	Captains, average age 36.	Lieutenants, average age 18 to 33.	Cornets and Ensigns, average age 18 to 33.	General average at all ages.
Died annually per thousand of each class	59·4	48·4	41·0	34·5	27·5	23·4	31·2

The mortality among the civil servants, for a period of forty-six years, from 1790 to 1836, exhibits almost precisely the same results ; viz.—

Percentage of deaths.	Above 50 years of age and 30 of service.	Age 40 to 50, service 25 to 30.	Age 40 to 45, service 20 to 25.	Age 35 to 40, service 15 to 20.	Age 30 to 35, service 10 to 15.	Age 25 to 30, service 5 to 10.	Age 20 to 25, service 1 to 5.
Died annually per thousand of each class...............	48·6	36·4	35·4	23·4	16·6	20·8	19·9

Between ten and fifteen years' service is the period when leave of absence is allowed to those who choose to return to Europe for three years, which of course must have a material tendency in reducing the mortality of that class. With this exception, the results are uniform for both civil and military servants, and they are no less so when extended to the officers of the other Presidencies.

The official results in regard to the mortality at each age among the military officers and civil servants of the Bengal Presidency, afford a convincing proof that in the East Indies no advantage has hitherto been derived from length of residence. As those individuals are never employed out of India, and generally arrive there about the age of eighteen or twenty, their respective ages and ranks may be assumed as a criterion for estimating their length of residence in the country. On that principle, then, we find, taking equal numbers of each rank, that the mortality among the ensigns, for the most part youths but recently arrived, is only twenty-three ; while that of the lieutenants, who must have been at least three years longer resident to have attained that rank, is twenty-seven ; and that of the captains, who must have been about twelve or thirteen years longer, is thirty-four per thousand, and so on in a corresponding proportion with the higher grades. In case it should be objected that this does not exhibit the precise operation of mortality during the first year or two of residence in the country, when the influence of acclimation is supposed to be most strongly manifested, the following information in regard to the civil servants in the Bengal Presidency will supply that defect :—

Years of residence.	Numbers alive.	Deaths in first year.	Ratio of deaths per thousand of living.
1st year of residence	975	19	19·5
2nd ,, ,, ...	933	22	23·5
3rd ,, ,, ...	906	18	20·0
4th ,, ,, ...	874	19	22·0

Here, then, we have traced the same individuals through four successive years of residence, with the liability to mortality constantly augmenting; and unless we are to suppose that a different law regulates the mortality among Europeans in the tropical climates of the eastern and western hemisphere, we are inevitably led to the same conclusions which we have already demonstrated from the previous numerical results.—*Statistical Reports.*

The result of all inquiry goes to establish the truth of the declaration of Boudin, " that man possesses faculties of acclimation essentially limited, though varying notably according to race. The theory of acclimation, as aptly described by Lord Herbert, would persuade us that a man who suffers from illness in his first year of residence in an unnatural climate recovers his health by remaining there, and that he thus becomes a strong, hale man. The meaning of such a theory is that, if a thing is unwholesome to the constitution, we have but to go on with it." In point of fact, diseases originating in ill habits of life, or in exposure, may often be speedily cured on the spot; but the physical degradation resulting from long residence in a hot and pestilential country, such as the plains of India, cannot be cured, excepting by a protracted removal to the cool climate of the mountain regions there, or to Europe.

The following table exhibits the annual rate of mortality, and the influence of length of residence in tropical countries, on European troops, from January 1st, 1830, to 31st March, 1837 :—

Stations.	18 to 25.	25 to 33.	33 to 40.	40 to 50.
Jamaica........	70·0	107·0	131·0	128·0
Mauritius.........................	20·8	37·5	52·7	86·6
Ceylon.............................	24·0	55·0	86·4	126·6
Bombay............................	18·2	34·6	46·8	71·1
Bengal	23·8	50·3	50·6	83·3

The subject of statistics is one that has been altogether neglected by the medical authorities of the Bengal Presidency; and though the example of the hospitals of her Majesty's army, from which very complete · reports are made, has now been many years before them, this important branch—the very central point of medical science—can scarcely be said, until very recently, to have been approached. It is the deficiency here complained of that has caused the omission in this work of all mention of the hospitals of Calcutta, and of the General Hospital in particular ;—an institution that has existed for more than seventy years, and in which tens of thousands of European soldiers have been treated under three or four different medical systems, yet no one fact, out of the numerous and important observations made during that long time is known to any one of us. Its surgeons, and those of the other public institutions—many of them able and ex-

perienced officers—have, through the neglect of the controlling
medical authorities, been rendered, in respect to us and to science,
no more than a set of dumb actors in the circle of a routine duty.
Dr. John Macpherson forms a very honourable exception, his
statistical investigations prepared at the General Hospital of Calcutta being works of standard value.   All this official neglect and
want of discipline has been repeatedly complained of by me in what I
thought the right quarter, and in the most emphatic manner ; but
though my proposition met with no very flattering reception, I
have yet the satisfaction to know that I produced some action with
the civil authorities, tardy perhaps, yet such as will lead to some
ultimate improvement.   We are in India continually kept in mind
of that law of our nature by which old men are disinclined from
undertaking anything, however excellent, of which they cannot be
expected to see the end.   Through the operation of climate also,
we have too often to lament the premature display of the contracting influences of age on the moral and physical constitution
of man, to the prejudice no less of public welfare than of private
happiness.
    From the circumstance that no general mode of registering
and recording has existed till lately, on statistical principles,
which all should adopt, the great majority of experience in India
has hitherto perished with individuals, and the valuable materials of a long and active life have been thus for ever lost to
the public service.
    The labour of analyzing observations which have been irregu-
larly kept is immense—to some men impossible ; while by order
a habit of observation is fostered and kept alive through the increasing facility in the process, and the interest excited by the
subject.   Such are the opinions of some of the ablest writers in
England ; but they have as yet found no echo in our Bengal Medical
Board, where we have still to regret the leaden influences of an
exclusive seniority principle of promotion.
    To ensure precision and uniformity in reports, the nomenclature
of hospitals is systematic and strictly ordered in the royal army,
and this is one of the many advantages its plan of arrangement
possesses over ours.
    As to the constantly recurring questions, do we not live under
an improved climate; and is not the mortality of Europeans greatly
diminished of late years ? it is not very easy to speak satisfactorily,
owing to the absence of older statistical record.   That the climate
of the actual site of Calcutta is improved to a certain extent, there
can be no doubt ; and that European general mortality is likewise
diminished, amongst the better classes especially, I believe to be
true ; but the chief cause will be found in the improved habits of
the latter class ; for, with the troops in garrison, notwithstanding
the improved discipline and interior economy of modern times,

it would not appear that mortality is much diminished, and the same may be said of the nearest military station of former times—Berhampore.*

The decrease in the proportional mortality of British troops in our various colonies is stated by Robert Jackson to be only of recent date; and he adds, that it would not be safe to pronounce positively whether it is owing to improvement in medical management, with improvement in military economy, or to contingent and temporary change in the nature of morbid causes, producing a less aggravated form of disease than belonged to other times. The soldiers did not die in greater numbers in Germany and Holland in the war of 1793, 94, and 95, than they did in the war of 1803. Further, he says, that the mortality was not greater, *cæteris paribus*, in North America in the war of 1756, than in the revolutionary wars of 1775—or in the late war of 1813. It is in the navy, he might have added, that a great and progressive reduction in mortality has been effected by the measures of preventive medicine instituted in 1779.

Mortality has been nearly equal at all times in the West Indies, viz., in the war of 1756, in the war of 1778, the war of 1793, and the war of 1803.

Of the earlier health history of the European troops in Bengal we have little or no information.

I had a table prepared with a view to exhibit the mortality of European troops in garrison at Fort William from 1790 to 1810, both inclusive. It afforded an average of deaths of 76·40 per 1000 per annum. A similar table for Berhampore, Bengal, from 1788 to 1810, gave an average of deaths at that station of 90·69 per 1000 per annum.

Comparing these figures, which represent the deaths on the spot only, with the most recent returns, as prepared by Sir Alexander Tulloch, a great improvement must have taken place, if not in the climate of Bengal, at least in the sanitary condition of the troops now serving there.

The following table has been prepared from the admirable " Analysis of the later Medical Returns of the European Troops serving in the Bengal Presidency," by Hugh M. Macpherson Esq. :—

---

* Making the corrections stated at p. 87, the table for Fort William will give 88·40, and that for Berhampore 102·69, as the ratio of deaths per 1000. All the tables of the military have been framed from four official sources—viz., the Adjutant and Auditor-General's Office, that of the Inspector-General and the Medical Board ; and where they differed I took the estimates of the Audit Office. More deaths were recorded in the Adjutant-General's returns than in any of the others. Slight errors have been made by the writer in calculating some of the tables, but they in no manner affect the general accuracy of the whole.

Table showing the Ratio of Sickness and Mortality per 1000 of the Strength of Officers, Soldiers, Women, and Children of the European Troops in the Bengal Presidency.

	OFFICERS.		SOLDIERS.		WOMEN.		CHILDREN.	
Periods of observation	8 years { From 1st April, 1846, to 31st March, 1854.				4 years { From 1st April, 1850, to 31st March, 1854.			
Aggregate strength	5708		156,189		7941		9255	
DISEASES.	Treated.	Died.	Treated.	Died.	Treatd.	Died.	Treatd.	Died.
Fevers	450·1	5·6	814·1	11·2	638·0	11·0	322·8	17·8
Eruptive fevers..................	4·4	·3	2·4	·6	3·9	·6	62·5	5·4
Diseases of organs of re-spiration......	49·4	1·9	70·4	4·3	27·3	3·9	30·6	4·2
„ „ heart and blood-vessels........	3·0	·2	6·6	·4	3·1	·6	·3	·1
„ „ brain & nervous system	27·5	3·2	40·0	5·2	23·0	·2	27·1	15·9
„ „ alimentary canal	321·1	6·0	413·9	23·4	295·1	15·5	169·1	20·7
Cholera	7·4	1·2	17·4	7·1	15·9	5·0	12·0	4·8
Dropsies.........................	1·2	·2	2·2	·5	1·5	·5	·6	·2
Diseases of urinary organs ...	5·1		3·6		1·6		·3	
Venereal affections	128·2		220·6		1·4		·8	
Rheumatic „	55·9		93·0		23·0		·5	
Abscesses and ulcers	107·4		92·5		26·5		14·6	
Diseases of bones, joints, &c...	·7		2·7		·5		·1	
„ nutrition	2·1	·7	9·9	2·6	2·1	1·3	13·1	6·2
„ the eyes	14·0		87·0		57·5		75·5	
„ the skin	7·0		9·3		3·3		2·8	
„ the ear...............	10·3		7·1		3·1		1·5	
Punishment	...		3·8		...		...	
Ebrietas.........................	3·0		40·5		8·6		·1	
Anomalous diseases	7·9		24·9		17·3		6·7	
Wounds and injuries	116·8	1·9	81·7	·9	16·5		11·0	·5
Complaints peculiar to women	...	...	...	...	98·9	4·2	...	
„ „ children	...	...	...	...	...	...	36·1	8·2
Total	1322·5	21·2	2043·6	56·2	1268·1	44·6	788·1	84·1

For the following important and interesting General Abstract of Admissions and Deaths by the principal Diseases among the European troops in Calcutta, Chinsurah, and Berhampore, in Bengal Proper, I am indebted to my friend Sir Alexander Tulloch —

Diseases.	Calcutta for 10 years, viz. from 1827 to 1836 each inclusive. Aggregate strength, 7823.			Chinsurah for 8 years, viz. from June, 1826, to June, 1827, and from 1830 to 1836 inclusive. Aggregate strength, 6531.			Berhampore for 10 years, viz. for 1823, and from 1826 to 1834 each inclusive. Aggregate strength, 11,077.		
	Admissions into hospital.	Deaths.	Proportion of deaths to admissions.	Admissions into hospital.	Deaths.	Proportion of deaths to admissions.	Admissions into hospital.	Deaths.	Proportion of deaths to admissions.
Feb. intermittens.	747	6	1 in 124½	227	4	1 in 57	1,044	11	1 in 95
„ remittens ...	706	63	1 in 11	278	26	1 in 10⅔	1,467	120	1 in 12¼
„ cont. com....	2,390	53	1 in 45	1,413	24	1 in 59	5,324	90	1 in 59¼
Pneumonia.........	202	8	1 in 25	103	4	1 in 26	235	4	1 in 59
Hæmoptysis	11	3	1 in 3⅔	4	3	1 in 1⅓	10	1	1 in 10
Phthisis pulm. ...	14	9	1 in 1½	15	9	1 in 1⅔	31	25	1 in 1¼
Catarrhus	554	24	1 in 23	217	4	1 in 54	532	8	1 in 66½
Hepatitis, &c.......	490	21	1 in 23	228	19	1 in 12	636	34	1 in 18⅔
Enteritis............	43	11	1 in 4	8	...	0 in 8	22	7	1 in 3
Dysenteria	1,603	137	1 in 11⅔	1,381	119	1 in 11⅔	2,472	191	1 in 13
Diarrhœa	974	26	1 in 37½	475	24	1 in 19¾	1,593	18	1 in 88
Colica	358	3	1 in 119	200	1	1 in 200	356	1	1 in 356
Obstipatio	142	...	0 in 142	90	...	0 in 90	117	...	0 in 117
Cholera morbus...	240	75	1 in 3¼	235	64	1 in 3⅔	642	169	1 in 4
Apoplexia	18	12	1 in 1½	17	4	1 in 4¼	38	34	1 in 1⅛
Paralysis	12	...	0 in 12	14	2	1 in 7	7	1	1 in 7
Amentia............	3	...	0 in 3	2	...	0 in 2	...	...	
Mania...	8	1	1 in 8	...	...	...	2	...	0 in 2
Delirium tremens.	37	...	0 in 37	56	3	1 in 18⅔	100	15	1 in 6⅔
Epilepsia............	43	3	1 in 14⅛	26	2	1 in 13	49	4	1 in 12
Hydrops	23	8	1 in 3	20	4	1 in 5	40	12	1 in 3⅓
Rheumatisms......	632	4	1 in 158	420	4	1 in 105	665	...	1 in 665
All other diseases.	4,556	26	1 in 175	3,799	12	1 in 316½	6,774	18	1 in 376
Total............	13,806	493	1 in 28	9,228	332	1 in 27¾	22,156	763	1 in 29

From this record it appears that, out of an aggregate force of 25,431 British soldiers, stationed during ten, eight, and ten years respectively, between 1823 and 1836, at Calcutta, Chinsurah, and Berhampore, all in Bengal Proper, there occurred of sickness as follows:—

Fevers, remittent, intermittent, and continued	13,596
Dysentery and diarrhœa	8,499
Hepatitis	1,354
Cholera	1,117
Total cases of four acute tropical diseases . .	24,566

There was a total of admissions into hospitals, on account of all diseases, of 45,170 cases, and a total of deaths from all diseases of 1588 soldiers. It is true that these men were British soldiers, differing in habits from the higher classes of Europeans residing in the same localities—worse fed and lodged also, and that some out of the few survivors of the Burmese war may have been admitted into the hospitals. But, making due allowance for all these circumstances, and for the bad climate of Lower Bengal comparatively, the actual sickness and mortality, not to speak of the proportionate invaliding, were enormous.

Out of that portion of the inhabitants of George Town, British Guiana (a country somewhat resembling Lower Bengal in its medical topography and climate), who were likely to resort to public hospitals—the total population of the town amounting to 20,000—there were admitted into the Colonial Hospital, from June, 1846, to June, 1847, 2938 cases of remittent and intermittent fevers; and the annual consumption of quinine in Demerara and Essequibo averaged 3000 ounces. But mere figures convey only a very faint impression of the calamities attending upon and resulting from tropical fevers and other acute diseases of hot climates. To realize the full powers of such endemics we should be presented with the sequelæ of broken constitutions, and consequent invalidings, amongst British soldiers, and amongst all who are exposed to the widely-extended and unnatural influences here spoken of.

The following most valuable information is given in evidence before the Royal Commission ordered to inquire into the Organization of the Indian Army, by Sir Alexander Tulloch:—

Return showing the Ratio of Mortality per Thousand of the Strength at the under-mentioned Periods of Life among the Non-commissioned Officers and Privates of White Troops serving at the following Stations from 1st January, 1830, to 31st March, 1837.

STATIONS.	Under 18.*	18 to 25.	25 to 33.	33 to 40.	40 to 50.	Average of all ages.
Household cavalry ..) United {	8·4	14·7	11·4	16·3	22·8	14·5
Cavalry of the line ... { Kingdom {	4·4	13·9	14·0	17·3	26·7	15·3
Foot guards ....) {	6·1	22·3	22·5	17·7	27·5	21·6
Gibraltar ......)	10·0	18·7	23·6	29·5	34·4	22·3
Malta .... } Mediterranean. {	16·0	13·0	23·3	34·0	56·7	22·3
Ionian Islands) (	6·6	12·2	20·1	24·4	24·2	19·3
Mediterranean stations generally...	10·0	15·5	22·2	28·1	33·0	21·0
Bermudas.........) North)	...†	16·0	42·0	42·0	76·0	28·9
Nova Scotia, &c. } America. {	9·0	14·0	22·5	30·8	41·5	20·3
Canada............) (	...†	19·7	27·8	37·8	35·0	25·7
Windward and Leeward command...	4·0	50·0	74·0	97·0	123·0	67·0
Jamaica	57·0	70·0	107·0	131·0	128·0	91·0
Cape of Good Hope	14·0	9·0	20·6	29·7	32·0	17·6
Mauritius	11·0	20·8	37·5	52·7	86·6	34·6
Ceylon ....·............	23·3	24·0	55·0	86·4	126·6	49·0
Bombay	...†	18·2	34·6	46·8	71·1	33·1
Madras ....·......	...†	26·0	59·3	70·7	86·5	52·2
Bengal	...†	23·8	50·3	50·6	83·3	44·5

* No correct deductions can be drawn from the ratios under 18, as the numbers are so few, and the results consequently irregular.
† Not given.

" Return showing similar Results for the Ten Years from 1st April, 1837 to 31st March, 1847, at the under-mentioned Periods of Life, and at the following Stations.

STATIONS.		Under 20.	20 to 24.	25 to 30.	30 to 35.	35 to 40.	40 and upwards.	Average of all ages.
Household cavalry		7·5	11·7	10·3	13·3	8·4	13·4	11·1
Cavalry of the line	United Kingdom.	8·1	11·8	14·3	14·6	15·3	18·3	13·5
Foot guards ...		11·1	21·6	21·1	19·5	22·4	26·2	20·4
Infantry of the line		13·0	17·8	19·8	19·8	21·0	23·4	17·8
Mediterranean stations		...	16·3	15·1	16·4	25·4	34·4	16·4
Canada and Nova Scotia		14·8	13·1	17·7	19·2	20·3	35·6	17·0
Jamaica...............		37·0	60·0	50·0	73·0	83·0	97·0	59·0

The same result applies to officers as well as men, civil as well as military, as will be seen from the following calculations.

" Out of 1184 deaths among officers in the Bengal Presidency, the proportion occurring annually in each rank and at each age has been as under :—

RATIO.	Colonels, average age 61.	Lieut.-Cols., average age 51.	Majors, average age 40.	Captains, average age 36.	Lieutenants, average age 18 to 33.	Cornets and ensigns, average age 18 to 33.	General average at all ages.
Died annually per 1000 of each rank......	59·4	48·4	41·0	34·5	27·5	23·4	31·2

" This extends also to the civil servants, the mortality among whom, for a period of forty-six years, from 1790 to 1836, exhibits a modification of the same results, viz. :—

RATIO.	Above 50 years of age and 30 of service.	Age 45 to 50, service 25 to 30.	Age 40 to 45, service 20 to 25.	Age 35 to 40, service 15 to 20.	Age 30 to 35, service 10 to 15.	Age 25 to 30, service 5 to 10.	Age 20 to 25, service 1 to 5.
Died annually per 1000 of each rank...............	48·6	36·4	35·4	23·4	16·6	20·8	19·9

" Thus there can be no question that the longer any one stays in India the more likely is his health to be deteriorated.

" It follows as a natural consequence of these results, that if regiments of the line serving in India are relieved at proper intervals, say every ten years, their loss while serving there must generally be less than that of any European corps permanently resident, because they will, as a body, be younger men—hence a strong reason for the employment of the former force in preference to the latter.

" Those who contend for a local European army in preference to troops of the line, probably do so on the supposition that it would materially reduce the expense of reliefs, forgetting the important change which has been brought about by the Limited Enlistment Act now coming into operation in the Indian army.

" If the men thus enlisted wish to come home they must be discharged at the end of ten years, being the same period I propose for the relief of regiments of the line. If they do not wish to come home, they would be just as likely to continue in the service by the facility of volunteering into a newly arrived regiment of the line, to complete their second period of service, as if they had originally enlisted into a local European force. Besides, it appears very questionable whether, during the excitement of a war in Europe, young men would be disposed to enlist to the required extent in any local corps for remote service, and still more questionable whether it would be good policy on the part of the Government at such a time to encourage their doing so; but if the whole European force in India were composed of corps of the line, second battalions could be raised without reference to their ultimate destination; some of these might then be sent to India to replace the first battalions, which could be brought to the theatre of war, with all the experience acquired by their previous service, while the newly raised men would do just as well in India, where the ' white face' is all that is wanted.

" By this arrangement, in the event of war, India would add to our military strength, whereas any local European army would tend seriously to reduce it, by keeping back so large a proportion of our trained soldiers, whose services could not be made available elsewhere without a new engagement.

" It forms another weighty consideration, militating against the employment of any such force distinct from our troops of the line, that soldiers not returning home periodically, and serving under different conditions from the rest of the army, must always, to a certain extent, have local interests, and be subject to local influence. Some question of pay, allowances, or coveted advantages, granted to one branch of the service but denied to another, may with such a force some day create another mutiny. On such questions both officers and men of the Indian army have before now been nearly, if not altogether, in that state; but were any such feeling ever to arise among regiments of the line, the very first suspicion of its existence would lead to immediate removal to some other foreign station—a remedy which would be impracticable with any localized force. This danger becomes, of course, the greater the larger the army, as it must necessarily give confidence to the disaffected to know that they make their own terms from the utter impossibility of sending any adequate force against them.

Table showing the Mortality in each of the Presidencies for a Period of 39 Years, as extracted from the War Office Returns.

YEAR.	BENGAL.		MADRAS.		BOMBAY.	
	Strength.	Deaths.	Strength.	Deaths.	Strength.	Deaths.
1817	7,284	622	9,092	548	2,607	143
1818	6,203	384	9,306	903	3,645	352
1819	6,219	483	7,656	637	3,417	270
1820	6,156	439	7,043	411	3,076	404
1821	5,732	399	6,989	396	2,907	262
1822	5,899	365	6,949	491	3,164	318
1823	6,584	496	6,838	386	3,082	224
1824	6,894	937	7,388	1,068	2,562	147
1825	6,669	1,086	6,919	1,187	3,178	357
1826	7,877	1,312	6,405	1,081	2,936	344
1827	8,035	583	7,061	656	3,063	171
1828	8,284	633	7,602	434	3,222	209
1829	8,555	618	7,680	290	3,978	117
1830	8,325	406	7,408	219	3,914	160
1831	8,347	431	6,976	268	3,845	94
1832	8,031	346	6,773	418	3,723	79
1833	7,569	403	6,241	571	3,583	129
1834	7,340	394	6,086	444	3,426	134
1835	7,655	272	5,881	215	3,415	102
1836	7,541	369	6,646	254	3,465	139
1837	6,878	355	6,078	362	3,226	148
1838	5,401	327	5,493	269	3,319	141
1839	7,645	499	5,792	405	3,422	380
1840	8,581	1,268	6,255	265	4,402	296
1841	9,438	1,020	5,411	223	5,418	601
1842	12,593	1,698	6,101	292	6,106	668
1843	11,003	1,028	7,699	427	6,066	468
1844	11,280	984	7,850	276	6,323	824
1845	11,108	2,213	7,535	351	4,710	337
1846	11,007	1,103	5,772	264	7,197	681
1847	12,349	781	6,040	225	5,556	139
1848	11,502	1,190	5,321	125	6,208	179
1849	14,703	1,306	5,014	159	6,619	310
1850	17,307	911	4,838	110	5,872	165
1851	17,070	849	4,162	88	5,774	194
1852	16,659	1,186	4,548	304	5,688	194
1853	16,190	950	4,598	215	5,306	102
1854	17,087	782	4,357	143	4,104	90
1855	14,980	532	3,209	80	4,423	80
1856						
Totals.	377,980	29,970	249,012	15,462	165,947	10,152

Summary of the preceding Table.

						Per 1000.
Bengal . .	strength	377,986	. .	deaths	29,970	. . ratio 79·2
Madras . .	,,	249,012	. .	,,	15,426	. . ,, 62·9
Bombay . .	,,	165,947	. .	,,	10,152	. . ,, 61·1
Total		792,939			55,584	70·0

"These losses include some 200 or 300 men killed or dead of their wounds during the Mahratta, Pindaree, and other campaigns prior to 1824; also 3750 who perished in the first, and about 1000 in the second Burmese war, chiefly from sickness; also nearly a whole regiment lost at Cabul; likewise the casualties during the campaigns of Scinde, of the Sutlij and the Punjaub, about 2000 in all; and nearly 1200 who died in the first Chinese war, all from sickness with very few exceptions. The loss arising from the climate of stations now usually occupied on the continent of India may therefore be reduced by about 8000 or 9000 men, or to an average of 60 per thousand annually, though the total loss from all causes has been at least 70 per thousand.

" In addition to the latter rate, which must of course form our estimate of the number to be replaced, the proportion invalided annually may be taken at about 25 per thousand more, and of time-expired men not renewing their engagement nearly the same proportion (the last, of course, is altogether conjectural, as the effect of limited enlistment is only coming into operation). These totals would make in all a decrement of 120 per thousand, or 9600 annually; whereas the average number of recruits raised by all the recruiting districts throughout the United Kingdom, from 1845 to 1849 inclusive, which may be fairly assumed as an average for a period of peace, amounted to rather less than 12,000 annually; so that, unless means can be adopted to reduce the mortality and invaliding, the force in India alone would absorb nearly all the recruits raised under ordinary circumstances for the whole army, of which the requirements are not now likely to be less than 20,000 men a year—probably more.

"It has been ascertained by experience that in all tropical climates, whether in the East or West, localities may be found where the mortality to which European troops are exposed does not very much exceed that which takes place in their native country. Returns extending over a great number of years show that at Bangalore, or in the Neilgherry hills in the Madras Presidency, and at Poonah, or the Mahableshwar hills in the Bombay Presidency, European troops may be located without sustaining a greater loss than about 3 per cent. annually, a considerable portion of which arises from disease contracted at other stations more unfavourable to health. There can be little doubt that in the Upper Provinces of the Bengal Presidency, at elevations of from 3000 to 4000 feet, situations of equal salubrity might be found adapted for large bodies of troops; but, judging from the results given in the following abstracts and summary, which extend over a period of many years, the selection of stations there does not appear to have as yet been fortunate, probably because strategic may have hitherto overcome sanitary considerations."

Abstract showing the Sickness and Mortality of the Troops of the Line at the under-mentioned Stations of the Indian Presidencies, as nearly as can be ascertained from the Returns forwarded to the Medical Board from 1817 to 1836 inclusive.

STATIONS.	Period of observation.	Strength.	Admissions into hospital.	Deaths.	Ratio per 1000 of Admissions.	Deaths.
BENGAL.	Yrs.					
Fort William	17	12,855	23,967	885	1863	68·82
Chinsurah	7	4,155	6,930	224	1667	53·91
Dinapore	9	6,845	14,251	484	2081	70·70
Ghazeepore	14	10,936	16,888	449	1554	41·05
Cawnpore	19	25,701	46,471	1495	1808	58·16
Agra	4	2,701	3,671	49	1359	18·14
Berhampore	14	13,342	26,494	853	1985	63·93
Meerut	19	27,328	35,949	862	1315	31·54
Kurnaul	6	5,314	5,252	137	988	25·78
Hazareebaugh	2	1,368	2,308	78	1687	57·01
Boglipore	4	2,564	4,338	224	1691	87·36
MADRAS.						
Fort St. George	18	13,606	26,009	671	1911	41·96
Cannanore	18	12,809	18,402	420	1436	32·80
Trichinopoly	19	15,317	27,394	681	1788	44·46
Secunderabad	18	13,939	35,555	854	2555	61·26
Bangalore	21	21,870	34,538	672	1579	30·73
Quilon	6	4,846	6,576	146	1357	30·1
Wallajahbad	5	2,398	4,480	242	1868	100·9
Bellary	10	7,504	14,911	355	1987	47·3 ·
Arnee	5	3,136	4,518	140	1440	44·3
BOMBAY.						
Colabab and Bombay	16	11,907	22,195	763	1864	64·08
Poonah	16	19,974	36,140	495	1819	24·78
Belgaum	10	6,332	10,814	175	1707	27·63
Deesa	4	2,682	2,879	144	1073	53·69
Kirkee	10	6,207	9,447	162	1521	26·09
Kairah	8	4,059	10,108	500	2490	123·18

Abstract showing the Sickness and Mortality of the Troops of the Line at the under-mentioned Stations of the Indian Presidencies, as nearly as can be ascertained from the Annual Sanitary Reports forwarded to the War Office from 1838 to 1856 inclusive.

STATIONS.	Period of observation.	Strength.	Admissions into hospital.	Deaths.	Ratio per 1000 of	
					Admissions.	Deaths.
BENGAL.	Yrs.					
Fort William	7	4,683	7,735	272	1652	58·08
Chinsurah	2	859	2,235	60	2601	69·96
Dinapore	13	10,915	20,158	903	1847	82·73
Ghazeepore...............	5	3,002	5,638	276	1878	91·94
Cawnpore	10	8,985	20,473	799	2278	88·90
Agra	8	5,847	13,833	355	2365	60·71
Meerut	14	14,512	24,522	639	1690	44·03
Kurnaul...................	5	3,434	8,051	268	2344	78·04
Hazareebaugh	2	1,054	1,710	36	1622	34·15
Allahabad	2	938	2,325	108	2479	115·14
Loodianah	2	1,251	2,826	159	2259	127·10
Umballah	10	13,773	20,627	850	1497	61·71
Kussowlie	7	5,040	6,160	247	1222	49·01
Ferozepore...............	5	4,445	7,817	245	1759	55·12
Jullundur	5	4,273	7,380	160	1727	37·44
Lahore	7	5,232	14,901	473	2848	90·40
Rawul Pindee	4	3,359	6,276	146	1863	43·46
Peshawur	5	8,182	26,384	588	3225	71·86
Wuzeerabad	4	6,889	11,436	408	1660	59·22
Dugshai	3	2,618	3,726	69	1423	26·36
Subatho	3	935	1,524	29	1630	31·02
MADRAS.						
Fort St. George.........	16	11,858	20,804	343	1754	28·93
Cannanore	17	15,416	24,832	488	1611	31·65
Trichinopoly	11	7,628	14,599	237	1913	31·07
Secunderabad............	8	7,133	12,243	405	1716	56·78
Bangalore	17	17,133	24,016	418	1402	24·39
Kamptee	7	6,014	12,440	287	2068	47·72
Tennasserim Provinces	9	9,165	16,218	302	1770	33·00
Bellary	7	5,290	10,259	257	1939	48·60
BOMBAY.						
Colabah and Bombay...	7	3,606	7,806	219	2165	60·73
Poonah	13	13,663	28,541	451	2089	33·01
Belgaum	10	7,244	11,909	299	1644	41·27
Deesa......................	7	7,473	12,262	250	1641	33·45
Kirkee	14	9,131	17,218	234	1886	25·63
Kurrachee...............	12	12,410	23,662	585	1907	47·14
Ahmednugger	3	1,154	2,765	66	2396	57·19
Hyderabad...............	4	1,744	4,352	74	2495	42·43
Aden	8	3,983	4,934	138	1239	34·64

Summary of the two preceding Periods.

STATIONS.	Period of observation.	Strength.	Admissions.	Deaths.	Ratio of admissions per 1000.	Ratio of deaths per 1000.
BENGAL.						
Fort William :—	Yrs.					
First Period	17	12,855	23,967	885	1863	68·82
Second Period	7	4,683	7,735	272	1652	58·08
Total	24	17,538	31,702	1157	1807	65·92
Chinsurah :—						
First Period	7	4,155	6,930	224	1667	53·91
Second Period	2	859	2,235	60	2601	69·96
Total	9	5,014	9,165	284	1827	56·64
Dinapore :—						
First Period	9	6,845	14,251	484	2081	70·70
Second Period	13	10,915	20,158	903	1847	82·73
Total	22	17,760	34,409	1387	1937	78·09
Ghazeepore :—						
First Period	14	10,936	16,888	449	1554	41·05
Second Period	5	3,002	5,638	276	1878	91·94
Total	19	13,938	22,526	725	1616	52·01
Cawnpore :—						
First Period	19	25,701	46,471	1495	1808	58·16
Second Period	10	8,985	20,473	799	2278	88·90
Total	29	34,686	66,944	2294	1930	66·13
Agra :—						
First Period	4	2,701	3,671	49	1359	18·14
Second Period	8	5,847	13,833	355	2365	60·71
Total	12	8,548	17,504	404	2048	47·26
Meerut :—						
First Period	19	27,328	35,949	862	1315	31·54
Second Period	14	14,512	24,522	639	1690	44·03
Total	33	41,840	60,471	1501	1445	35·87
Kurnaul :—						
First Period	6	5,314	5,252	137	988	25·78
Second Period	5	3,434	8,051	268	2344	78·04
Total	11	8,748	13,303	405	1521	46·30

Summary—continued.

STATIONS.	Period of observation.	Strength.	Admissions.	Deaths.	Ratio of admissions per 1000.	Ratio of deaths per 1000.
BENGAL—continued.	Yrs.					
Hazareebaugh :—						
First Period	2	1,368	2,308	78	1687	57·01
Second Period	2	1,054	1,710	36	1622	34·15
Total	4	2,422	4,018	114	1659	47·07
MADRAS.						
Fort St. George : —						
First Period	18	13,606	26,009	671	1911	41·96
Second Period	16	11,858	20,804	343	1754	28·93
Total	34	25,464	46,813	1014	1838	39·82
Cannanore :—						
First Period	18	12,809	18,402	420	1436	32·80
Second Period	17	15,416	24,832	488	1611	31·65
Total	35	28,225	43,234	908	1531	32·17
Trichinopoly :—						
First Period	19	15,317	27,394	681	1788	44·46
Second Period	11	7,628	14,599	237	1913	31·07
Total	30	22,945	41,993	918	1829	40·00
Secunderabad :—						
First Period	18	13,939	35,555	854	2555	61·26
Second Period	8	7,133	12,243	405	1716	56 78
Total	26	21,072	47,798	1259	2268	59·74
Bangalore :—						
First Period	21	21,870	34,538	672	1579	30·73
Second Period	17	17,133	24,016	418	1402	24·39
Total	38	39,003	58,554	1090	1501	27·94
Bellary : —						
First Period	10	7,504	14,911	355	1987	47·30
Second Period	7	5,290	10,259	257	1939	48·60
Total	17	12,794	25,170	612	1959	47·80
BOMBAY.						
Colabah and Bombay:—						
First Period	16	11,907	22,195	763	1864	64·08
Second Period	7	3,606	7,806	219	2165	69·73
Total	23	15,513	30·001	982	1933	63·30

Summary—continued.

STATIONS.	Period of observation.	Strength.	Admissions.	Deaths.	Ratio of admissions per 1000.	Ratio of deaths per 1000.
BOMBAY—*continued.*						
Poonah :—	Yrs.					
First Period	16	19,074	36,140	495	1819	24·78
Second Period	13	13,663	28,541	451	2089	33·01
Total	29	33,637	64,681	946	1923	28·12
Belgaum :—						
First Period	10	6,332	10,814	175	1707	27·63
Second Period	10	7,244	11,909	299	1644	41·27
Total	20	13,576	22,723	474	1674	34·91
Deesa :—						
First Period	4	2,682	2,879	144	1073	53·69
Second Period	7	7,473	12,262	250	1641	33·45
Total	11	10,155	15,141	394	1491	38·80
Kirkee :—						
First Period	10	6,207	9,447	162	1521	26·09
Second Period	14	9,131	17,218	234	1886	25·63
Total	24	15,338	26,665	396	1738	25·82

" These results do not exhibit the loss at all the Indian stations during the 39 years included in the first Table, but at those only where regiments have been stationed for the whole or the greater part of a year ; they are also exclusive of the loss on long marches, which is often very heavy ; but it has been considered more advisable thus to found the results on incomplete data, than to incur the risk of adopting what might prove to be incorrect."

STATISTICS OF THE INFLUENCE OF CLIMATE

AND

SEASON IN THE PRESIDENCY OF MADRAS.

MADRAS PRESIDENCY.—In an admirable " Report on the Sickness and Mortality among the Troops serving in the Madras Presidency," prepared from a " General Topographical and Statistical Account of each of the Military Divisions of the Presidency," printed by order of the Madras Government, Dr. Graham Balfour, of the Grenadier Guards, classifies the stations occupied by the troops, European and native, as follows :*—

1. Those situated on, or immediately adjacent to, the sea-coast.
2. Those on the plains between the coast and the mountain ranges.
3. Stations on the table lands.
4. Stations peculiar from position, and from being depôts for recruits or for pensioners, but which are not included among the first three, with a view to avoid erroneous conclusions.

FIRST CLASS, OR STATIONS ADJACENT TO THE SEA COAST.—" On examining the relative proportion of admissions and deaths of Europeans by each class of diseases, it will be seen that fevers and diseases of the bowels furnish a third of the admissions, and that the latter and inflammation of the liver are the cause of half the deaths. *To the prevention of these three classes, therefore, the attention of medical officers in India should be particularly directed.* Fevers, although from their prevalence a source of considerable inefficiency, are by no means very fatal, the proportion of deaths not greatly exceeding that among troops in this country, and being even a fraction under that of sepoys at the same stations.

" In this respect there is a striking contrast between the East and the West Indies; fevers in the latter occupying the most prominent position, both as regards admissions and deaths. Inflammation of the liver, however, is comparatively a rare disease, and productive of little loss in the West Indies, while in the East it gives rise to a large proportion of sickness and mortality. The troops appear, on the other hand, to enjoy a remarkable exemption from diseases of the lungs, compared with any of the places of which the statistics have been investigated, a subject to which we shall hereafter more fully advert.

" To enable us to compare the amount of disease and its effects upon the native soldiers in India with other troops serving in their native country, we have annexed the ratios of sickness and mortality among the cavalry in the United Kingdom and the Cape native mounted rifle corps, being the only available information on the subject. The results show a most extraordinary uniformity in the mortality, which amounts to—

    15   per thousand for sepoys,
    14   per thousand for cavalry in England, and
    11·9 per thousand for the Cape corps; or, deducting epidemic
        cholera, to—
    12·8 per thousand in England,

* The records here referred to were prepared throughout Madras, in furtherance of the general plan proposed and carried out by me, in 1835, when in Bengal, for requiring from the medical departments "Topographical, Statistical, and Sanitary Reports on Districts, Stations, and Cantonments throughout the three Presidencies of India, and the Dependencies to the Eastward." The manner in which this call was answered in Madras reflects great credit on the medical department of that Presidency.

12·2 per thousand in Madras, and

10·9 per thousand at the Cape of Good Hope.

The class of diseases which has been most prevalent and most fatal amongst the sepoys has been fevers, for which, on the aggregate of the stations on the coast, 222 were admitted, and 3·1 died per 1000 of the strength. But this has been materially affected by the stations of Masulipatam and Chicacole. Omitting these two stations, the admissions by fevers would amount only to 129, and the deaths to 2 per 1000 of the strength; which, however, are higher ratios than in the United Kingdom, or among the native troops at the Cape.

"The next class of diseases in point of importance has been those of the bowels, which have caused 45 admissions and 2·6 deaths per 1000 among the native troops. The ratio appears remarkably low in a country where, among Europeans, this class of diseases occupies so prominent a place; but the constitution of the Indian and the nature of his diet no doubt tend to his exemption.

"Cholera has proved a source of considerable mortality, and has displayed, as usual, great irregularity in its prevalence at different stations, the deaths varying from 0·3 at Mangalore to 16·3 per 1000 at Ramnad. It has, however, fully maintained its fatal character, 217 out of 429 cases having died.

"The exemption from diseases of the lungs, which we remarked in the case of Europeans, has been enjoyed to a still greater extent by the native troops; among whom, also, diseases of the liver, which were a source of considerable sickness and mortality among the former, are of very rare occurrence.

"Beriberi, included in the class of dropsies, deserves especial notice, as having been almost entirely confined to Masulipatam, Vizagapatam, and Chicacole. The admissions at the first of these stations were 130, and the deaths 22; at the second 21, of whom 6 died; and at the last 243, and 16 deaths. Beriberi is chiefly confined to situations near the coast, being rarely seen on the high lands, and is supposed to be of malarious origin, which derives corroboration from its great prevalence at Masulipatam and Chicacole, where the troops were more exposed to that cause of disease than at any of the other stations. It is seldom met with in Europeans."

SECOND CLASS, OR THOSE ON THE PLAINS BETWEEN THE COAST AND THE MOUNTAINS.—From a table of sickness and mortality in the stations on the plains between the sea-coast and the mountain ranges, Dr. Balfour, speaking firstly of Europeans, says :—If we deduct the deaths by cholera, which, from the irregularity of its visitations, and in the amount of mortality to which it gives rise on different occasions, may fairly be omitted in estimating the influence of the climate, we find a remarkable similarity in the ratios, being respectively 32·4 and 33·3 per thousand.

The classes of diseases, however, by which the admissions and deaths have been produced are somewhat differently distributed, fevers having been more prevalent and fatal at Trichinopoly than at the coast stations, probably owing to the extent to which irrigation is carried on around it, and the consequent artificial production of marsh; while it has enjoyed a considerable exemption from diseases of the bowels; and also, though not to so great an extent, from inflammation of the liver. The comparative immunity from diseases of the lungs, which we formerly noticed, is enjoyed to quite as great an extent at this station, being only a very small fraction above that from pneumonia and catarrh alone among the cavalry in the United Kingdom, and less than a third of that from the whole of the diseases of this class.

THIRD CLASS, STATIONS ON THE TABLE LANDS.—By a well-arranged table the sickness among European troops is shown to have ranged between 1673 at Bangalore, and 2438 at Kamptee, and the mortality between 22·7 at Bangalore, and 82·1 at Secunderabad and Jaulnah, the average of all the stations on the table lands being 2082 admissions and 41 deaths per 1000 of mean strength. The mortality at Secunderabad, however, has been more than double that of any other station; omitting it from the calculation, the average amounts only to 29·2, being very little higher than that of the Mauritius or the Bermudas. The excess at Secunderabad has been caused chiefly by dysentery, which, during the period under review, gave rise to a higher rate of mortality than that from all causes at the other stations on the table lands. This disease has been a source of great sickness and mortality among the Europeans ever since Secunderabad was first occupied in 1804, and committees have at different times been appointed to investigate into the causes of it, but without any satisfactory result. The unhealthy character of the station has been attributed by some medical officers to "an endemial malarious condition of the atmosphere, occurring at a season when the vicissitudes of climate and the diurnal ranges of temperature are very great." It is worthy of remark, however, that the great excess of dysentery has occurred among Her Majesty's regiments, while the European artillery have been comparatively exempt from it. Thus, out of an aggregate strength of 7561 of the former, during ten years, 2100 cases of this disease were admitted and 306 died, being at the ratio of 278 and 40·5 respectively; while among the Hon. Company's artillery, out of a strength of 1382, only 262 admissions and 21 deaths took place, or 190 of the former and 15·2 of the latter per 1000 of mean strength.

Other observers attributed the sickness of the troops to the situation and faulty condition of the barracks. Considerable alterations were, in consequence, made in them, and the drainage was improved, apparently with some benefit at first; but in 1843,

Her Majesty's 4th Regiment suffered to as great an extent as any that preceded it. The position of the barracks, nearly surrounded by high land, which intercepts the free current of air, and on the border of a low, swampy plain interspersed with tanks, stagnant pools, and rice-fields, all fertile sources of malaria, seems the most probable cause of the unhealthiness of the troops. This opinion is much strengthened by the fact that the cavalry quartered at Bowen, fully two miles north of the cantonment, have generally been very healthy; but we have no specific returns on the subject.

The troops at Kamptee have suffered considerably from fever, which prevailed to a considerable extent in 1834. There is nothing in the position of the cantonment to which this can be attributed. The source to which it is generally referred is the dense and extensive tracts of jungle by which the station is surrounded, although at a distance of upwards of ten miles.

The results of the stations on the table lands generally are satisfactory, as showing that posts may be selected where European troops shall be exposed to a rate of mortality in a tropical climate not greatly exceeding that to which they are subject at home. Even Kamptee, although less favourable than others, illustrates the advantage of a judicious selection of a site. When the subsidiary force was first sent into this country, they were quartered close to the capital; but the situation proving very unhealthy, they were moved to Kamptee, and have suffered less from sickness than at their first station.

The native troops suffered to a greater extent at Secunderabad than at any of the other stations, and, as with Europeans, Kamptee has stood the next in point of mortality. They have enjoyed the same marked exemption from hepatic inflammation, which has already been shown to exist on the coast and plains, and which, with dysentery, forms the most striking point of contrast with the Europeans. The immunity from pulmonary disease, which is one of the most remarkable features in the sanitary condition of the troops in India, exists even in a more marked degree than at the stations already examined. The general results show the same favourable condition of the native army, the mortality from all causes amounting only to 14·2, or within a fraction the same as among troops in the United Kingdom, and, exclusive of cholera, only 11·4 per thousand of mean strength.

Omitting the consideration of four "stations peculiar from position, and from being depots for recruits and pensioners," we come to the aggregate summary of Dr. Balfour on the more prevalent diseases of Europeans at all the various stations above severally noticed.

FEVERS.—From an elaborate table, it appears that among both European and native troops fevers have been more prevalent and fatal at stations on the table lands than at those on the coast, or on the plains—a circumstance which shows that in India a certain moderate elevation above the level of the sea is not of itself sufficient to secure exemption from this class of diseases. On the coast stations, and among British soldiers, ephemeral and continued fevers predominated in the proportion of three-fourths, and at stations on the plains, of five-sixths of the admissions by this class of diseases ; while on the table lands two-fifths of the cases have been paroxysmal fevers.

Of the stations on the table lands Bangalore is comparatively exempt from fevers ; while the proportion is very high at Bellary, Secunderabad, and Kamptee. There is, however, this marked difference between the latter, that at Bellary one-third only of the cases are of a paroxysmal type, but at Secunderabad three-fourths, and at Kamptee five-sixths are of that character. This difference would appear to be explained by reference to the description of these stations ; the ground around Bellary being free from marshy ground, with the exception of the tank to the south-east of the fort ; while Secunderabad has been shown to abound in all the alleged causes of fever. The cause of paroxysmal fever at Kamptee is not so obvious, unless it arise from miasm generated in the numerous ravines and running waters by which the country is intersected.

A review of these stations will show why, at Secunderabad, no improvement in health has resulted from barrack and hospital amendments ; for such improvement can only be effected by removal to a healthy locality. At Bellary, on the other hand, mere structural arrangements may be expected to be followed by diminution of fever and mortality.

The excess of fevers among Europeans, compared with the natives, is not so great as to lead to the supposition that it is a disease peculiarly affecting immigrants—persons not indigenous to the country. There is, however, a very marked difference in the prevalent type in the two races. At the stations on the sea-coast two-thirds of the cases among the natives have been paroxysmal fevers, while among the Europeans they have scarcely amounted to one-fourth : on the plains the proportion has been three-fourths among natives, and about one-sixth among the Europeans ; and on the table lands the relative proportions have been three-fourths and three-fifths respectively. Thus the prevailing form appears to be paroxysmal among the natives, and, with the exception of the table lands, continued among the Europeans. It is interesting to observe that the relative amount of paroxysmal fevers among the natives is very nearly the same in all the three classes of stations, and that the intensity of these diseases also very closely approximates —the proportion of deaths to admissions by fevers of all types ranging from one in seventy-two and one in seventy-six.

Dr. Balfour concludes the subject of fever by stating that the above results tend to disprove the theory which would refer the fevers of the West Indies to excessive heat and moisture ; for that, were these alleged causes adequate, we should have the worst fevers in the East, the heat and moisture being greatest there, and many of the Madras stations being remote from the refreshing influence of sea-breezes.

During five years the admissions of Europeans on account of eruptive fevers was only 1 per 1000 of the strength.

DISEASES OF THE LUNGS.—The ratio both of admissions and deaths among European troops from this class of diseases is lower than when serving in their native country. The mortality has been lowest on the table lands, and highest on the coast stations, especially at Madras, where it has been double that of the other stations. This, however, has been caused by the numbers of invalid soldiers assembled there, awaiting embarkation for England. Omitting Madras, the mortality at the coast stations amounts to 2·3 per 1000, or almost the same as on the plain. There is no British colony which appears so suitable or so likely to prove bene-ficial to the class of consumptive men as the East Indies.

DISEASES OF THE LIVER.—In this class of diseases a remarkable diversity is shown, both in the prevalence and mortality of inflam- . mation of the liver among the Europeans as compared with the native troops. Among the latter this disease is of such trifling prevalence as scarcely to require notice, while it is more prevalent and fatal among the Europeans than in any other of our colonies. The same fact holds in respect to our troops in the West Indies, where the negroes enjoy a considerable exemption compared with Europeans. These results may be influenced to some extent by the mode of living and by the habits of the two classes of troops, especially as regards the use of intoxicating liquors ; but this is by no means adequate to explain the difference. The proportion of cases among the Europeans has been very nearly the same on the table lands as on the sea-coast, and the deaths have been even higher. Among the native troops the exemption has been enjoyed alike in all the divisions.

DISEASES OF THE BOWELS.—This class of disease, though less prevalent than fevers amongst Europeans, is more fatal, causing more than two-fifths of the mortality. The great majority of cases consist of dysentery and diarrhœa, and it will be observed that these have proved most fatal at the stations on the table-lands—a result attributable to the great prevalence and fatal cha-racter of dysentery at Secunderabad. During the five years 1834-38, the admissions at that station by dysentery alone amounted to 1591, and the deaths to 235, being in the ratio of 327 and 48·3 per 1000 of mean strength. If the deadly station of Secunderabad be omitted in the calculation, the admissions at the other stations on the table lands by dysentery and diarrhœa amount only to 186, and the deaths to 8·6 per 1000 of the strength.

Among the coast stations dysentery is nearly twice as fatal at

fatal at stations ɑ the table lands t
on the plains—a:ircumstance whicl
moderate elevatin above the levcl
sufficient to seeuz exemption from t
coast stations, an among British sol(
fevers predominted in the propor
stations on the pins, of five-sixths (
of diseases ; whii on the table lan(
been paroxysmal'evers.

Of the statioɪ on the table land
exempt from fevɩs ; while the propoɪ
Secunderabad, ad Kamptee. Thcr·
difference betwcɩ the latter, that at
cases are of a paɔxysmal type, but at
and at Kamptcc vc-sixths are of thaɩ
would appear tɩbc explained by rc.
these stations ; tc ground around Bcl.
ground, with thc xception of the tank tɩ
while Sccundcraad has been shown tɩ
causes of fcvcr. Ɫhe cause of paroxysm
so obvious, unlcɩ it arise from miasm g
ravines and runnɩg waters by which the

A review of tɔsc stations will show wɩ.
improvement in ɩealth has resulted froɩ.
amendments ; fɩ such improvement can
removal to a hɩlthy locality. At Bellɩ
mere structural rrangements may be ɩ
diminution of fɩvr and mortality.

The excess offevers among Eur
natives, is not ɩ great as to ɭɩ·
disease peculiarlɩnffecting iɪ·
the country. Tɭrc is ·
prevalent type inɭ
two-thirds of t'
fevers, while
to one-fourt
among natɩ
the table
and three-
be paroxy
table lanɩ
observe ·
natives ɩ
and tha
—the ɩ
rangin

Dr.
abovɩ

fevers of the West In[dies]... contained in my
were these alleged ca... here to adduce so
in the East, the heat a... he tables on pp.
of the Madras sta... [b]oth European and
of sea-breezes.

During five years the... [eruptive] fevers was only 1 per l...

DISEASES OF THE L[UNGS].—I... [B]RITISH SOLDIERS
deaths among Europe[an]... ON FOREIGN EX-
than when serving in... [VA]RIOUS ENEMIES.
been lowest on the ta...
especially at Madras, ... says that, leaving
stations. This, however... [an] army of 100,000
invalid soldiers assemb... [fiel]d on a campaign,
Omitting Madras, the m... of some months, if
2·3 per 1000, or almost... [n]umbers of patients
British colony which a... [u]pon a third being
ficial to the class of c... [fi]rst fifteen years of
DISEASES OF THE LIV[ER].—h... [se]venth part of the
diversity is shown, both in... two hundred and
mation of the liver a... i.e., twenty-three
native troops. Among... [ca]ses of the French
prevalence as scarcely... [a]ccidents of war,
and fatal among the... [p]roportions were
The same f...

-a result
dys ntery at ...
admission

Cannanore as at any of the others, and has of late years been on the increase.

The concluding observations of Dr. Balfour are eminently deserving of notice, as bearing out certain of the objects which I had in view in advancing the original plan of medical reports.

The facts contained in the preceding paper, he says, point out the necessity for a careful attention to the selection of the site for a cantonment. It has been shown that there are stations in India where the mortality among European soldiers is but little higher than in their native country, and that even where this is not the case, different localities within a short distance of each other possess very different degrees of salubrity. It is true that military and political reasons do on rare occasions exist, which render the occupation of an insalubrious spot necessary; but where this is not the case, competent medical officers should be directed to investigate and report upon the sanitary condition of any place which is intended to be occupied as a military station.

The utility of a system of periodical reports from all medical officers must be obvious, as affording information to the authorities on the state of the health of the army, and bringing under their notice any extraordinary amount of sickness and mortality that may occur in it. An opportunity is thus afforded, also, of directing inquiry into the origin and progress of the particular disease by which it is produced, and, if practicable, of removing or mitigating its causes.

The attention of medical officers would thus likewise be more constantly directed to the sanitary state of the troops, and the system of reporting would further be attended with a progressive improvement in their professional acquirements; but to render such reports of practical avail, they must be brought to the notice of responsible authority in a condensed form, and without any delay. Humanity and economy alike require such management of an important subject; for a little just calculation will prove that the expense of preserving the soldier in health and efficiency is much less than that of replacing him, and that in this, as in most other cases, prevention is better than cure.

The documents from which the present report has been prepared were printed by order of the Madras Government, but not published. Dr. Balfour's object has been to make the results of the investigation generally known, in the hope of directing a larger degree of attention to the important subject of the soldier's welfare—the first step towards which is, the ascertaining with accuracy what diseases he is most liable to, and to what extent, in the different districts, stations, and cantonments in which he may be called on to serve. It is highly desirable, also, that all such information should be gratuitously placed at the disposal of the officers of the army, for their information and benefit. The public should likewise have free access to it.

All these suggestions of Dr. Balfour's are contained in my original plan; and I am happy in being able here to adduce so able a witness to its desirableness.

In conclusion, I quote from Dr. Balfour the tables on pp. 120, 121, exhibiting the sanitary condition of both European and native troops.

CAUSES OF SICKNESS AND MORTALITY OF BRITISH SOLDIERS AND SEAMEN IN DIFFERENT CLIMATES, ON FOREIGN EXPEDITIONS, AND IN CONFLICTS WITH VARIOUS ENEMIES.

M. Meyne, surgeon in the Belgian army, says that, leaving out the influence of epidemics and battles, an army of 100,000 men may, by the sole act of having entered on a campaign, have 10,000 men in hospital. "At the end of some months, if some engagements have taken place, and the numbers of patients have increased, as is usual, we must count upon a third being placed out of service by disease. During the first fifteen years of the occupation of Algeria by the French, one-eleventh part of the forces was annually carried off by disease, and a two hundred and sixty-fifth part only by the casualties of war—*i.e.*, twenty-three times as many." The same author adds, that the losses of the French army in the Crimea were 16,000 deaths by the accidents of war, and 53,000 by disease—*i.e.,* 16 to 53 ; and the proportions were much the same for the Sardinian and the English. Of 25,000 French who marched from Bayonne to Lisbon, in 1808, an enormous but unascertained number perished on the road from fatigue and the scorching sun, no enemy having yet been encountered.

In land battles, the ordinary proportion is said to be one killed to every five casualties. Of the wounded, owing to the greater amount of attention and comforts which the officers, by their position, are enabled to secure, the proportion of deaths from wounds amongst them is found generally to be one-twelfth, while that amongst the rank and file is one-eighth.

The following summary deductions are made by M. Budin, in his admirable "Statistics of the Sanitary Condition and Mortality of Forces by Land and Sea, as influenced by Season, Localities, Age, Race, and National Characters."

These subjects are of such vast interest and importance, to naval and military surgeons especially, that I hope to stand excused for here republishing the conclusions of our worthy fellow-labourer of the French army :—

"1. The losses of armies from disease greatly exceed those in time of war from the sword and fire of the enemy. In the Walcheren expedition, in 1809, the mortality of the English army amounted to 16·7 deaths by wounds, and 332 by diseases per 1000 of the strength.

"2. The most trifling losses are experienced in general by troops

TABLE I.—*Showing the Admissions and Deaths among the European Troops serving at the following Stations in the Madras Presidency, from 1829 to 1838 inclusive.*

Years.	Cannanore, Calicut, and Mangalore.			Madras.			Trichinopoly.			Bangalore.			Bellary.			Secunderabad, &c.			Kamptee.		
	Str.	Admit.	Died.	Streng.	Admit.	Died.	Str.	Admit.	Died.	Streng.	Admit.	Died.	Str.	Admit.	Died.	Streng.	Admit.	Died.	Str.	Admit.	Died.
1829	998	1,534	43	2,002	2,632	53	895	1,789	31	1,638	2,448	57	923	1,890	13	1,223	2,676	42	785	1,764	30
1830	960	998	13	2,433	3,924	69	944	1,276	26	1,380	1,845	32	919	1,482	19	1,210	2,347	59	948	1,916	21
1831	899	845	33	2,006	3,775	121	875	1,246	29	1,533	2,199	45	876	1,621	21	1,181	2,181	43	918	2,348	43
1832	778	861	25	1,556	2,712	65	855	1,234	67	1,465	1,875	28	853	1,396	19	1,090	1,911	59	855	1,971	33
1833	749	856	20	1,470	3,028	71	850	1,431	41	1,503	3,560	92	867	1,784	58	991	2,471	62	999	2,717	62
1834	823	1,396	49	1,020	2,541	58	825	1,496	24	1,540	3,460	42	762	1,386	29	758	2,531	77	1052	3,414	42
1835	700	1,413	17	894	1,715	38	885	1,850	39	1,554	2,676	31	930	1,924	20	884	2,307	59	969	2,946	27
1836	720	1,492	26	950	2,084	25	921	1,535	22	1,736	2,869	44	995	1,770	37	1,102	2,338	62	1001	2,280	35
1837	675	1,510	41	886	1,905	75	964	1,614	44	1,628	2,232	32	1038	2,043	42	1,124	2,157	138	1024	2,015	50
1838	657	1,282	33	754	1,741	25	908	1,673	28	1,613	2,261	34	857	2,216	27	994	2,014	63	1023	1,721	34
Total.	7959	12,187	300	13,971	26,057	600	8922	15,144	351	15,590	25,425	437	9020	17,992	285	10,557	22,933	664	9574	23,092	377
Ratios.																					
1829			43·1			26·5			34·6			34·8			14·1			34·3			38·2
1830			13·5			28·4			27·5			23·2			20·7			48·7			22·1
1831			36·7			60·3			33·1			29·3			23·9			36·4			46·8
1832			32·1			41·8			78·4			19·1			22·3			54·1			38·6
1833			26·7			48·3			48·2			61·2			66·9			62·6			39·9
1834			59·5			56·8			29·1			27·3			38·0			101·6			39·9
1835			24·3			42·5			44·1			19·9			21·5			66·7			27·8
1836			36·1			26·3			23·9			25·3			37·2			56·3			34·9
1837			60·7			84·6			45·6			19·6			40·5			122·8			48·8
1838			50·2			33·2			30·8			21·1			31·5			63·4			33·2
Mean		1,531	37·7		1,865	42·9		1,697	39·3		1,631	28·0		1,995	31·6		2,172	62·9		2,412	39·4

TABLE II.—*Showing the Sickness and Mortality among the Native Troops serving at the following Stations in the Madras Presidency, from 1829 to 1838 inclusive.*

| | SEA COAST. | | | | | | | | | TABLE LANDS. | | | | | | | | |
| | Cannanore, Mangalore, and Calicut. | | | Madras. | | | Mysore Division. | | | Bellary and Cuddapah. | | | Secunderabad and Jaulnah. | | | Kamptee. | | |
YEARS.	Streng.	Admit.	Died.	Streng.	Admit.	Died.	Streng.	Admit.	Died.	Streng.	Admit.	Died.	Streng.	Admit.	Died.	Streng.	Admit.	Died.
1829	5,930	2,552	47	7,956	3,454	62	7,095	3,214	81	4,774	1,596	53	9,860	4,266	75	5,828	2,715	47
1830	5,601	3,019	75	9,546	3,619	63	6,586	2,546	54	4,998	1,431	37	9,036	3,649	96	5,364	2,677	43
1831	5,008	2,367	37	7,658	3,370	64	6,204	4,209	140	3,879	1,354	55	8,694	3,387	87	4,952	2,833	73
1832	4,569	2,006	54	7,025	3,033	58	7,459	4,785	133	3,222	1,595	45	8,656	3,573	129	5,066	2,869	73
1833	2,853	1,442	34	7,704	3,652	112	7,291	5,137	145	3,532	1,745	136	8,052	4,437	165	4,604	3,117	82
1834	3,098	2,076	51	4,863	2,305	65	5,980	6,037	113	3,009	2,221	28	5,425	6,361	149	4,636	4,533	60
1835	2,703	1,756	43	3,918	1,642	34	8,053	6,032	90	3,361	2,552	22	7,980	6,731	113	4,542	3,843	70
1836	2,502	1,465	29	3,755	1,837	42	7,617	5,238	71	2,739	1,707	21	7,885	4,646	88	4,631	2,752	58
1837	3,535	3,027	36	3,930	1,628	79	7,073	4,936	79	3,150	1,252	39	7,829	3,571	121	4,491	2,596	61
1838	3,944	2,958	101	3,787	1,404	82	6,658	4,842	85	3,335	2,251	145	7,625	5,857	184	5,199	2,830	52
Total..	39,743	22,668	507	60,142	25,944	661	70,016	46,976	991	35,999	17,804	581	81,042	46,478	1207	49,313	30,765	619
Ratios.																		
1829	...	430	7·9	...	434	7·8	...	453	11·4	...	334	11·1	...	433	7·5	...	466	8·1
1830	...	539	13·4	...	379	6·6	...	387	8·2	...	286	7·4	...	404	10·6	...	499	8·
1831	...	473	7·4	...	440	8·3	...	678	22·6	...	349	14·2	...	389	10·	...	572	14·7
1832	...	439	11·8	...	432	8·2	...	641	17·8	...	495	14·	...	413	14·9	...	566	14·4
1833	...	505	11·9	...	474	14·5	...	705	19·9	...	494	38·5	...	551	20·5	...	677	17·8
1834	...	670	16·5	...	474	13·4	...	1,010	18·9	...	738	9·3	...	1,172	27·5	...	978	12·9
1835	...	650	15·9	...	419	8·7	...	749	11·2	...	759	6·5	...	843	14·2	...	846	15·4
1836	...	586	11·6	...	489	11·2	...	688	9·3	...	623	7·7	...	589	11·2	...	594	12·5
1837	...	856	10·2	...	414	20·1	...	697	11·1	...	429	12·4	...	456	15·4	...	578	13·6
1838	...	750	25·6	...	371	21·6	...	727	12·8	...	675	43·5	...	768	24·1	...	544	10·
Mean..	...	570	12·7	...	431	11·0	...	671	14·1	...	495	16·1	...	573	14·9	...	624	12·5

serving in their native country; and they augment in European remies in a direct ratio as these approach the equator. The inverse takes place with negro troops, among whom mortality increases obviously in the direct ratio of their removal from the tropics.

" 3. Even during a residence in their native country, European armies are subject to a mortality exceeding, in a sensible manner, that of the civil population at a corresponding age. In certain tropical countries, Sierra Leone for example, the mortality of the soldier (483 deaths per 1000) surpasses the proportion of deaths which occurs in England among the male population at the age of 100 and upwards (454 per 1000).

" 4. In localities bordering closely upon each other, the mortality often differs in a very marked degree. This ought to be seriously·considered in the selection of military stations and places for garrisons, as well as in the choice of sites for barracks and hospitals.

" 5. In tropical regions the annual number of deaths ranges within very wide limits from one year to another, so that the mortality of a single year cannot serve as a basis for estimating the mean mortality of these countries.

" 6. In the most unhealthy tropical climates the judicious choice of good positions on elevated grounds will often secure to armies, composed of men of the Caucasian race, a perfectly healthy condition, worthy of the most favoured regions of temperate climes. The degree of elevation required varies in a marked manner with the geographical latitude and longitude of the place. Residence on the high grounds is fatal to negro troops.

" 7. The geological nature of the soil exerts a decided influence, not only on the sanitary condition and mortality of armies, but also on the presence or absence of certain defects which render a man unfit for military service.

" 8. The increase of the mortality of armies, especially in warm climates, is determined in a great measure by the marshy character of the localities occupied.

" 9. The mortality of the army in the different quarters of the world considerably exceeds that of the navy.

" 10. In the temperate region of Europe, the density of the population in garrison towns tends to affect the sanitary condition, and augment the mortality of the troops. The relative density of the population of the different quarters and streets of a large town should be seriously considered in selecting sites for barracks and hospitals.

" 11. Numerous facts militate against the hypothesis of a progressive amelioration in the sanitary condition of European troops in warm climates in general, and particularly in tropical regions, as an effect of length of residence.

" 12. In a military point of view, the knowledge of the pathogenic march of the seasons in different parts of the globe, and of the relation of the sanitary condition of armies with the different meteorological influences, is of immense interest, and has not yet received the attention it deserves.

" 13. The pathogenic influence of the seasons is in a strict dependence upon the quality of the soil, the latitude, longitude, and elevation of the places, their position in the northern and southern hemispheres, and the nationality and race of the soldier.

" 14. In all countries where the influence of age has been studied, the lowest mortality has been found to be that of soldiers from eighteen to twenty years of age.

" 15. Nationality and race favour or neutralize the pathogenic action of climate, so that, under precisely similar circumstances, troops of different races and nations may suffer and die in different proportions and of different diseases."

To the above we may add, of our own experience :—

16. That, in the first expedition to Rangoon, the mortality of British soldiers, in the first year of service, 1824-25, amounted to 35 deaths from wounds, and 450 by disease, per 1000 of strength ; while in the second year, 1825-26, the losses in action and by disease were about one-half of what occurred in the first, making a total mortality by wounds and by disease of $727\frac{1}{2}$ per 1000 of strength in the two years.

An expedition to Rangoon having been determined on in January, 1824, cattle were marched to Calcutta from distant stations, and slaughtered in the month of February, under a degree of heat so high that, before the process of salting could be established, some degree of decomposition must have commenced in the meat intended for the use of the soldiers. War was declared on the 5th of March, 1824. " From the middle of June," says Sir A. Tulloch, " the troops had nothing to subsist on but salt beef and biscuit of very inferior quality, and were without vegetables of any kind to counteract the effects of such a diet."

17. The other British expedition employed against Burmah, in 1825-26, and employed in the province of Aracan, under General Morrison, became speedily ineffective from the malignant fever of the country. Five thousand five hundred soldiers, European and native, were soon struck down with the disease, without reckoning the sick of the public establishments, and of the camp followers :—soon, indeed, " every one who was not dead was in hospital."

" The Bengal infantry sepoy suffered the most ; in fact, they disappeared altogether." Of the original European force three-fourths perished, and the miserable survivors were ruined in constitution—none living long thereafter.

18. It has been seen that in the first expedition to Rangoon, 1824-25, owing to the neglect of every sanitary precaution, " the deaths nearly equalled the number of British soldiers originally

employed on this service, and that but for the seasonable reinforcements which arrived, the whole must speedily have been annihilated."

To show, however, that governments, like individuals, are slow
to derive lessons from experience, we have cattle again marched
to Calcutta, and slaughtered in the same heats of February, as
stated by Colonel Hough, with the same consequences to the
European troops employed in China, in 1840-42. It was the
horrors of Rangoon over again.

" The attempt to improve the Calcutta salted meat by fresh
brine at Singhapore did not answer; and thus, in the island of
Chusan, between the 5th of July and the 22nd of October, 1840,"
" out of three thousand six hundred and fifty troops, only two
thousand and thirty-six were fit for duty"—the 26th Cameronians
and the 49th Regiment being the chief sufferers. These fine
regiments, says Colonel Hough, were reduced " to a perfect
skeleton;" and, in the short space of three months, the former
corps was reduced from upwards of nine hundred strong to two
hundred and ninety-one.

There was here, in addition to the neglects of the Government,
neglect and grievous ignorance in the officer placed in command
on the island of Chusan. " The sickness was comparatively mild
amongst the officers, who had means of living on more generous
diet." This, it must be confessed, reads very badly of the officer
in command, who seems to have lived well, while he neglected the
comfort and welfare of the soldiers.

As a contrast to our former arrangements in Burmah, in 1825-26,
and in China, in 1840-42, may be cited the following:—" The
Marquis Wellesley began early in the cold season of 1800 to prepare for the expedition to Egypt, which sailed in April from Calcutta." The circumstance here recorded ought to be remembered
to the honour of our great Indian statesman, as should also the
admirable arrangements of the Marquis Dalhousie for the conduct
of the last Burmese war.

Referring to the comparative circumstances of military service
in various countries and in different climates, it may not prove un-
interesting here to quote the results of some battles, sieges, and
campaigns in the East Indies, as compared to similar results in
Europe. In Marlborough's battles the losses were as follow:—

1704. Blenheim	1 in	5
1706. Ramillies, about	1 „	16
1708. Oudenarde	1 „	36
1709. Malplaquet*	1 „	5

Allied armies included.

At Waterloo,† the Duke of Wellington lost in the proportion of . 1 in 6

---

* In this desperate battle "the total loss of the Allies was not less than 20,000
men, or nearly a fifth of the number engaged."

"The proportion of the Allied loss in officers to their total loss was, at Ramillies, one
in ten, which is the same proportion as that of the British army at the battle of the
Alma."—Colonel Macdougall's *Theory of War*, 1856.

† In the battle of Waterloo, out of a British force of 36,273, there were killed 1417,

The Indian returns show the following ratios :—

1803. Assaye	. . . .	1 in	3
1804. Dieg	. . . .	1 ,,	4½
1817. Mehedpore	. . . .	1 ,,	6
1817. Sitabuldy	. . . .	1 ,,	4½
1818. Korygaum	. . . .	1 ,,	3¼
1845. Maharajpore	. . . .	1 ,,	6
1846. Battles of the Sutlej	. . . . . .	1 ,,	5
1848. Chilianwallah	. . . .	1 ,,	7

" Here," says the *Edinburgh Review*, No. 197, " is no proof of cowardice on the part of the defeated, whose loss in every affair, except perhaps the last, greatly exceeded our own."

During the siege of Seringapatam, in 1799, it was stormed and captured " by 4376 men, in two columns." The loss in the assault was as follows :—

	Killed.	Wounded.	Missing.
European officers	22 . . .	45 . . .	—
,, N.C.O. and soldiers . .	181 . . .	122 . . .	22
Native soldiers	119 . . .	420 . . .	100

Making a total, killed, wounded, and missing, of 1031 men.

Of the above officers, . twenty-five were killed and wounded in the assault.

Lord Lake, with an original force of 9000 men, augmented after the second storm by the force from Bombay, according to Colonel Hough, appeared before Bhurtpore in January, 1805. During four successive assaults, each increasing in desperation, Lord Lake was repulsed with the losses on each occasion, and, in the aggregate, as follows :—

First assault	456	men killed and wounded.	
Second ditto	573	,,	,,
Third ditto	894	,,	,,
Fourth ditto	987	,,	,,
Total	2910	,,	,,

There were of officers killed, 15, and 95 wounded, making a total of officers killed and wounded, 110. " Major Thorn gives the loss in all the operations at 3100 men and 102 officers, killed and wounded."

During the expedition to Walcheren, in 1809, 1·67 per cent. of the entire force was killed in action, and 32·2 per cent. perished by disease, making a grand total of 34·69 per cent. in that fatal and ill-directed attempt.

Of our losses in the earlier campaigns of the French revolutionary war, we receive but the following general statements :—

In 1794, says Dr. William Fergusson, the French army in Flanders, composed principally of mere boys, many of them of

making about 3·9 per cent. ; but, including 362 men killed of the King's German Legion, the ratio rises to 4·9 per cent. The total force, British and Allied, under the Duke of Wellington,. amounted to 69,686, out of which there was a total killed of 2947, or a grand total killed of 4·2 per cent., British and Allied.

five feet three or four inches in height, " kicked us before them like a foot-ball through Flanders and Holland into Germany, destroying in their course full three-fourths of our army." The same authority, speaking of the same campaign, says that " by disease, by famine, by the rigour of the season, and by the sword, out of a host of fully 30,000 men, when the retreat from Flanders first began, scarcely 8000 remained to witness its completion."

Figured statements more in detail would be desirable in respect of so important an operation as that described by Dr. Fergusson, but they are not now procurable ; and in respect of the Continental wars of 1745 and of 1756, as well as of the first American war, it were in vain to expect any accurate record.

The hospital arrangement of the British army, in 1794, was very defective, and the experienced regimental surgeons were set aside by order of " an old, broken-down court physician of London—an apothecary from Weymouth, chosen by George III. to direct and administer the complicated and difficult medical and sanitary affairs of immense armies, constantly engaged in active warfare, in various countries. He purposely superseded men like Robert Jackson, and placed over them " graduates of the English Universities." The consequences were such as might have been foreseen. . . . Disorderly hospitals," says Dr. Fergusson, " will destroy an army faster than it can be recruited." We may infer, also, that in those days the sanitary general arrangements were on a par with the hospital management ; and where both these are deficient together, there can be no hope for the safety of any army.

In the Peninsular army, again, under the Duke of Wellington, taking forty-one months during which the war was carried on with the utmost vigour, an annual mortality of about 4 per cent. occurred in battle and from wounds, and 12 per cent. was from disease, " being nearly 16 per cent. of those employed ;" whereas, in the first year of the first Burmese war, $3\frac{1}{2}$ per cent. of the British troops were killed in action, and 45 per cent. perished by disease, " making a total loss of $48\frac{1}{2}$ per cent., consequently each person employed throughout that year encountered more risk of life than in three Peninsular campaigns."

In the second year of the Burmese war, as already stated, the losses in action and by disease were about one-half of what occurred in the first, making a total for two years of $5\frac{1}{4}$ per cent. killed in action, and $67\frac{1}{2}$ by disease, or a grand total for the two years of $72\frac{3}{4}$ of the European force employed under Sir Archibald Campbell. The official records exhibit a loss of 61 officers of Her Majesty's army alone, killed, wounded, and died of disease—" a very heavy loss, indeed," says Sir A. Tulloch, " considering that the average number of officers present did not probably exceed 150."*

* War Office Statistical Report. Presented to both Houses of Parliament by command of Her Majesty.

The expedition to Rangoon, during the first Burmese war, was therefore the most fatal of which we have, as yet, any record.

This result of a war with a savage race is the most remarkable circumstance of all, and it is well worthy of notice. The Burmese are held in light estimation as soldiers by the Europeans, but without reason. Warring in their natural fashion, in well constructed stockades, they inflicted on British troops almost the same proportionate amount of loss as did the legions of Napoleon commanded by the marshals of France. Speaking of the destruction of the European force on this occasion, Sir A. Tulloch makes the following just observations :—" It seems essential to bring such facts as these prominently to notice, because there is no mode of estimating the severity of military service except by comparison, and it is of importance that the authorities with whom rests the ultimate reward of the soldier should have some means of knowing the risk of life and peril of constitution by which his pension has been earned."

A national mode of warfare always makes itself felt. It does not imitate what, from foreigners, is so easy to copy—the only thing that is always imitated—that which is bad. National modes of warfare are not, therefore, subject to the moral inferiority, the weaknesses, inabilities, and incapacities resulting from the systematic imitative routine of organized bodies, so cramping to the physical and moral energies of men. When the princes of India set aside their hordes of 80,000 to 100,000 horsemen, and imitated Europeans in forming brigades of disciplined infantry, and in stand-up fights, it was easy to foresee the speedy destruction of their armies, and the fall of their empires.

The Highlanders, in 1745, were sneered at by British officers, and especially by those of the cavalry, who, as usual, made the least respectable figure in that remarkable contest. The British army was then, as now, officered by gentlemen, and disciplined on the Prussian system. The formation of general lines and movements in lines, combining freedom of action with rapidity of movement, were then, as now, its characteristics ; yet, in conflict with peasants led by country gentlemen, it was first quickly routed, and then destroyed. Even at Culloden, where the mountain peasant was led in the usual manner, the result was the same.

" The Scottish Highlanders," says Robert Jackson, " were badly provided with arms ; they, notwithstanding, defeated the regular and experienced troops of the Crown, both at Prestonpans and at Falkirk ; and there are grounds to believe, from the decided experiment that was made upon Barrel's regiment at Culloden, that they would have defeated them a third time, had there been union in council and accord in action."

These various circumstances of service and statistical records are worthy the careful consideration of the military surgeon ; as, for the conduct of his difficult and toilsome duties, it is not enough that he should have some foreknowledge of the probable amount of his sick, but he should also prepare some estimate of the probable amount of his wounded men.   He should know with what results men have fought in the hot climates of the East, as in the temperate regions of the West.   " It is necessary that a medical chief calculate," says Robert Jackson ; " and he cannot calculate justly without experience of things."   This kind of general and special tact in calculation forms, indeed, one of the requirements of an effective administrative medical officer ; and records of the kind here presented prove not only of present value, but they constitute useful means of comparison for other times and other occasions.   An accurate knowledge of what *has* happened goes far to forewarn of what *may* happen again, under like circumstances.

Nor are the results of statistical investigations confined to military operations.   On the contrary, they may be rendered subservient to, and suggestive of vast improvements in civil communities, as remarked by Sir A. Tulloch in the following important observations :—

" To ascertain the races of men best fitted to inhabit and develope the resources of different colonies is a most important inquiry, and one which has hitherto attracted too little attention, both in this and other countries.   Had the Government of France, for instance, adverted to the absolute impossibility of any population increasing or keeping up its numbers under an annual mortality of seven per cent. (being that to which their settlers are exposed at Algiers), it would never have entered on the wild speculation of cultivating the soil of Africa by Europeans, nor have wasted a hundred millions sterling with no other result than the loss of 100,000 men, who have fallen victims to the climate of that country. In such questions, military returns, properly organized and properly digested, afford one of the most useful guides to direct the policy of the Colonial legislator ; they point out the limits intended by nature for particular races, and within which alone they can thrive and increase ; they serve to indicate to the restless wanderers of our race the boundaries which neither the pursuit of wealth nor the dreams of ambition should induce them to pass ; and proclaim, in forcible language, that man, like the elements, is controlled by a Power which hath said, ' Hither shalt thou come, but no further !' "

The worst enemy to the soldier has everywhere, and at all times, been disease.   Out of 1000 deaths in the hospitals at Scutari, for instance, 575 were caused by dysentery and diarrhœa, 173 by fever, and 55 by wounds ; but the last numbers do not represent those who died within a fortnight of being struck.

" Civilians, however, think that shot kills most soldiers ; but Colonel Queach, a Peninsular officer of some experience, and an authority upon the subject, having served throughout the Peninsular campaigns with the old 95th Rifles, says, that 40,000 men

were killed in action or died of wounds—120,000 died of disease,
a great deal of which was rendered fatal by the want of proper
medical attendance ; whilst 120,000 more were, by disease, rendered unfit for service."

It is a principle in modern war, well understood by the great
Marlborough, that the more rapid its course the more humane the
result ; and Frederick of Prussia held that "all wars should be
short and rapid ; because a long war insensibly relaxes discipline,
depopulates the state, and exhausts its resources." During the
protracted operations of previous wars, the destruction of men " by
famine and the ague" was horrible beyond description.

The losses in the great battles of Marlborough do not appear so
heavy when we consider the unusual nature of the obstacles to be
overcome, the numbers opposed to him, and the obstinate nature
of the defence.   This first of British commanders was careful, in
an especial manner, of the health and comfort of his men.   It was
the restless energy, the genius, the daring, and the impetuous
spirit of Napoleon, which allowed no repose to his own troops or
to those of his enemies, that completed the establishment of a
system which set all tardy rules and practice at defiance.   He
brought his men to make forced marches and to bivouac under
every extremity of season—his principle being that " legs win more
battles than arms."

Judging by the mortality records of our several wars, down to
that of the Crimea, no perceptible increase of mortality would
appear to have resulted from the improvements in the construction
of fire-arms, and the relative efficiency of different weapons—
subjects to which hardly sufficient attention has been directed.
From a return furnished by the surgeon of the Scots Fusilier
Guards, it appears that of that regiment 120 men were hurt at
Inkermann, of which 7 were bayonet and 79 were gun-shot wounds.
This conflict, in which the regiments of guards had a loss of 594
out of 2382 casualties suffered by 26 battalions, or parts of
battalions, has been held as specially won by the bayonet, and the
Russians have termed it an embittered bayonet contest; yet only
7 in 120, or about 58 in 1000, were hurt by the bayonet.

Again, in the cavalry encounter at Balaclava, where the British
heavy brigade was opposed to cavalry, of 106 casualties by sword
and lance only nine were fatal; whereas, of 281 among the light
brigade, who suffered from cannon and musketry, as well as from
hand-to-hand contest, 160 were fatal, or more than half, the
ordinary proportion being one death to five casualties.

The proportion killed of private soldiers was much the same in
the wars of 1793-1815, and in the Crimean war of 1854-55, being
in the ratio of 193 to 1000 wounded in the former, to 190 to 1000
wounded in the latter.   The ratios of deaths among the wounded
officers appear to have been nearly the same in 1793-1815 and in
the Crimean campaign; but the proportions returned as killed

K

Date	Battles	Nature of.	British — Total strength in officers and men engaged.	British — Casualties — Killed.	British — Casualties — Wounded.	British — Casualties — Total.	British — Casualties — Per 1000 engaged.	British — Estimated deaths. — Total.	British — Estimated deaths. — Per 1000 engaged.	British and Allies — Total strength in officers and men engaged.	British and Allies — Casualties — Total killed and wounded.	British and Allies — Casualties — Per 1000 engaged.
1801. March 21	Alexandria	Defensive	14,000	243	193	1,436	103	393	28·1	§	§	§
1806. July 4	Maida	Offensive	5,675	45	282	327	58	87	15·3	§	§	§
1808. Aug. 21	Vimiero	Defensive	19,200	135	534	669	35	215	11·2			
1809. Jan. 16	Coruña	Defensive	16,700	158	634	792	47	257	15·4			
,, July 28	Talavera	,,	22,000	801	3,913	4,714	213	1,455	65·8	56,000	6,268	112
1810. Sept. 27	Busaco	Offensive	27,800	106	500	606	22	183	6·6	57,000	1,300	23
1811. March 5	Barosa	Defensive	5,230	202	1,040	1,242	237	360	68·8	4,500	1,610	111
,, May 5	Fuentes d'Onore	Defensive	22,900	170	1,043	1,213	53	379	16·6	35,200	439	42
,, ,, 16	Albuera	,,	9,900	882	2,672	3,554	395	1,358	151·0	37,000	6,500	176
1812. July 22	Salamanca	,,	30,500	388	2,714	3,102	102	770	25·2	54,200	4,964	92
1813. June 21	Vittoria	Offensive	42,000	501	2,807	3,308	79	890	21·2	95,800	4,829	50
,, July 25 to Aug. 2	Pyrenees	Defensive	30,000	559	3,693	4,252	142	1,197	39·9	65,000	6,540	101
,, Nov. 10	Nivelle	Offensive	47,600	277	1,777	2,054	43	675	14·2	90,600	2,621	29
1814. Feb. 27	Orthes	,,	27,000	210	1,411	1,621	60	404	15·0	4,800	2,200	50
,, April 10	Toulouse	,,	26,800	312	1,795	2,107	79	582	21·7	54,400	1,641	85
1815. Jan. 8	*New Orleans	,,	6,000	386	1,516	1,902	317	625	104·2			
,, June 16	{ Ligny, Quatre Bras, Wo.	{ Defensive, Offensive, ,,	49,900	2,126	8,140	0,286	206	3,245	65·0	230,600	36,590	159
,, 18												
1854. Sept. 20	Alma	Offensive	26,800	353	1,619	1,972	74	559	20·9	55,000	3,545	64
,, Nov. 5	Inkermann	Defensive	9,000	632	1,878	2,510	279	883	98·1	§	§	§
			...	8,486	39,161	47,647					83,077	
Estimated deaths among the wounded				4,894	...	2,274					3,787	
Estimated casualties among the missing				1,137	...	...						
Aggregate numbers			438,205	14,517	...	49,921	114	14,517	33·0	888,900	86,864	98

* Unsuccessful action.

§ Numbers not ascertained.

Undertaken by	Place	Commenced upon	Duration in days	Result	Besiegers Force	Killed	Wounded	Total	Per 1000 engaged	Est. deaths Total	Est. deaths Per 1000 engaged	Garrison Force	Garrison Casualties Total	Garrison Per 1000 engaged
British	Louisbourg	15 July, 1758	11	Capitulation	13,100	165	354	519	40	217	17·0	2,800	§	§
"	Havana	12 June, 1762	60	Capitulation	13,800	296	650	946	69	392	28·4	§	§	§
"	Monte Neo	28 Jan. 1807	5	Taken by assault	4,000	142	421	563	141	203	50·8	§	§	§
"	Buenos Ayres	5 July, "	2	*Assault repulsed*	7,300	316	674	990	127	416	53·3	§	§	§
"	Flushing	3 Aug. 1809	12	Capitulation	17,000	71	373	444	26	121	7·1	5,800	§	§
British & Allies	Badajoz (1st)	16 May, 1811	11	*Assault repulsed*	16,700	218	1,017	1,235	74	359	21·5	3,700	§	§
"	Ciad Rodrigo (2nd)	8 Jan. 1812	11	Taken by assault	16,600	178	818	996	60	291	17·5	1,764	800	170
"	Badajoz (2nd)	16 Mar, "	21	Taken by assault	25,800	1,035	3,789	4,824	187	1,569	60·8	4,870	*1,600	328
British	Almaraz (Forts)	19 May, "	1	Taken by assault	6,000	33	144	177	30	53	8·8	1,000	§	§
British & Allies	Salamanca (Forts)	17 June, "	10	Capitulation	4,000	99	331	430	108	146	36·5	800	100	125
"	Burgos	19 Sept., "	82	*Assault repulsed*	13,500	509	1,555	2,064	153	731	54·1	2,000	639	320
"	St. Sebastian (1st)	11 July, 1813	14	*Assault repulsed*	11,600	204	771	975	84	312	26·9	...	...	...
"	(2nd)	24 Aug. "	7	Taken by assault	11,000	967	2,478	3,445	313	1,328	120·7	3,200	*1,700	531
British	Bergen-op-Zoom	8 Mar. 1814	1	*Assault repulsed*	3,300	174	726	900	272	276	83·6	2,700	460	170
	Average..		14⅔	Aggregate results...	164,200	4,407	14,101	18,508	113	6,414	39·0	§	§	§
British & Allies	Sebastopol	5 Oct. 1854	338	{ *Brit. assault repulsed* / *French successful* ... }	50,000	1,516	7,445	8,961	179	2,545	54·1	§	§	§
					214,200	5,923	21,546	27,469	131	8,959	42·0	§	§	313
French	Saragossa (1st)	30 June, 1808	41	Siege abandoned	15,570	...	...	3,500	225	§	§	...	3,000	§
"	(2nd)	29 Dec. "	54	Capitulation	43,200	§	§	3,000	69	§	§	31,000	22,800	735
"	Ciudad Rodrigo	15 June, 1810	24	Capitulation	28,100	182	1,048	1,230	44	§	§	5,300	*1,800	340
"	Badajoz	28 Jan. 1811	41	Capitulation	17,000	§	§	1,600	94	§	§	9,000	*2,000	222
"	Tarragona	1 June, "	28	Taken by assault	21,500	§	§	4,209	196	§	§	13,200	*4,000	303
"	Tarifa	22 Dec. "	24	*Assault repulsed*	10,400	§	§	517	50	§	§	2,500	51	20
"	Antwerp	29 Nov. 1832	24	Capitulation	66,500	108	695	803	12	§	§	4,470	491	110
	Average...		33⅔	Aggregate results...	202,270	§	§	14,859	73	§	§	§	34,142	476

* Include losses from sickness.

§ Numbers not ascertained.

vary considerably, being 164 officers to 836 wounded in the former period, and 233 to 767 in the latter.

The battles of Albuera and of New Orleans were attended with the largest losses, and that of Busaco with the smallest loss of modern actions. At Albuera the British loss was 395 per 1000 ; at New Orleans it was 317 per 1000, and at Busaco 22 per 1000.

Mr. Hodge gives the following summaries of the results of battles and sieges :—

Land Battles.—" Table III. .[p. 130] contains the particulars of all the great battles in which British troops have been engaged since the commencement of the present century, excepting those that occurred in India, with respect to which I have not been able to obtain information sufficiently precise to include them in the statement."

Sieges.—"Table IV. [p.131] contains details as to various sieges in which the troops of this country have engaged in the course of the last hundred years, that of Sebastopol being included. I have collected, as far as they were attainable, the particulars of all the English sieges that occurred in that period, excepting such as took place in India, but I have only inserted in the table those with respect to which the information obtained is sufficiently precise to lead to definite conclusions.

" For the purpose of a more complete comparison, I have classified the fortresses captured by both nations under the heads of those that capitulated and those taken by assault, showing the

Average Results of Fourteen successful Sieges.

Places taken by		Number of sieges.	Duration in days.		Aggregate force employed.	Casualties.	
			Total.	AVerage.		Total.	Per 1000.
Capitula- tion.	French armies ...	4	143	85¾	154,800	6,633	43
	English armies...	4	93	23¼	47,900	2,403	50
		8	236	29½	202,700	9,036	44
Assault.	French armies ...	1	28	28	21,500	4,209	196
	English armies...	5	59	11⅘	63,700	11,228	176
		6	87	14½	85,200	15,437	181

" Here we see that, although the places assaulted were taken on an average in half the time required to gain possession of those that capitulated, the ratio of loss suffered by the besiegers before the former was quadruple that before the latter."

Mr. Hodge, in his " Report on the Mortality arising from Naval Operations," states, that " Taking the whole of the casualties in action in the British service during the wars of the French Revo-

lution, the proportion of those returned killed to the whole number
injured in naval engagements was 100 in 398, or rather more than
one in four; while in engagements on land it was 100 in 529, or
rather less than one in five. It may perhaps be thought that, as
a greater proportion of deaths were inflicted in the navy, the injuries suffered by the wounded would also be of a serious character,
but this is not necessarily the case.

"A large proportion of the wounds in naval actions are caused
by round shot; of those in actions on land by musketry. An
injury to a vital organ from a round shot would be more likely to
prove fatal at once than one from a musket-ball; a man mortally
wounded by the latter might linger on for some time, a result less
probable in the former case."

At first sight, there would appear no reason why mortality
arising from disease should be much increased in the navy by
war, as is well known to be the case in the army; but an examination of the facts proves that it was so. It is undoubted that
during the last war the risk of death to persons employed in the
navy, from the accidental destruction of vessels alone, was four or
five times greater than it has been since the peace.

Mr. Hodge adduces the following numbers as in *excess* of
deaths caused by the *war* of twenty and a-half years, between
1793 and 1815 :—

Casualties in action	6,663
Destroyed and wrecked in ships	11,985
From disease on board	44,662
Total	63,310

"The following statement shows that the loss inflicted upon us
in our contests with the navies of different nations, has been generally in proportion to the reputation of their seamen for skill and
discipline, and is an additional proof of the importance of maintaining our superiority in those respects :—

Action.	Enemy's fleet.	Proportion of British loss in killed and wounded.			Number of enemy's ships.	
		To 1000 British engaged.	To 1000 of the enemy engaged.	To each ship taken or destroyed.	Engaged.	Taken or destroyed.
Cape St. Vincent	Spanish.........	32	19	75	25	4
Trafalgar	Franco-Spanish	100	78	94	33	18
Nile	French..........	112	91	82	13	11
Camperdown	Dutch...........	100	115	92	16	9

"The loss sustained in an action is the price of the result obtained by it, and we must compare these elements with each other

before we can arrive at a correct estimate as to either. By the above statement, it is shown, that the casualties of the British in the battle off Cape St. Vincent, were only thirty-two per 1000 engaged, while each of the enemy's ships taken or destroyed cost seventy-five men in killed and wounded. At the battle of the Nile each ship taken or destroyed cost only seven more, or eighty-two men in killed and wounded, although the proportion per 1000 engaged was 112, or between three and four times as many as at Cape St. Vincent. From the general result, it appears, that out of 204 hostile vessels engaged, seventy-three were taken or destroyed by the British, whose total loss, in killed and wounded, was 7349, or a fraction over 100 for each vessel lost to the enemy.

" From the various estimates that have been considered, the following has been drawn out, as the

General Summary of the Mortality in the Royal Navy among an average Force of 110,000 Men during 20$\frac{45}{100}$ Years of Hostilities occurring in and between 1793 and 1815.

Causes of death.	Number of deaths.		Estimated number of deaths that would have occurred from the same causes during peace.	Excess caused by war.	
	Annual Ratio to 1000 mean strength.	Total.		Total.	Proportion to 100,000 deaths.
Casualties in action	3	6,663	......	6,663	10·524
Drowned or destroyed in ships accidentally wrecked or burnt	6	13,621	1,636	11,985	18·931
Estimated to have died from disease or ordinary accidents on board	32	72,102	27,440	44,662	70·545
Total...............	41	92,386	29,076	63,310	100·000

" With reference to every description of armed force, it is of the greatest importance to ascertain what is the average proportion of men unable to attend to their duty from sickness. We have no information of this kind as to the navy. (See Table, p. 136.)

" To facilitate the comparison between the periods of war and peace, the following table has been deduced from the reports on the health of the navy, printed by order of the House of Commons. It contains the results of all the reports yet published, with the exception of those for the East Indian station from 1840 to 1843 : they are omitted on account of the Chinese war, which commenced in 1840.

Table showing the Annual Ratio to 1000 Mean Strength of the Deaths in the Royal Navy (1830 to 1843).

STATION.	1830 to 1836, inclusive.				1837 to 1843, inclusive.					
	Mean strength.	Causes of death.			Mean strength.	Causes of death.				
		Wounds, injuries, and accidents.	Diseases.	From all causes.		Diseases.	Wounds, injuries, and accidents.	Drowned.	Unknown.	From all causes.
South American..	2,465	1·2	7·7	8·9	2,721	6·75	0·83	1·95	0·47	10·00
North American and West Indian..........	3,362	1·5	18·1	19·6	3,645	19·20	1·57	2·57	0·82	24·16
Mediterranean ...	7,958	1·8	9·3	11·1	9,936	10·59	1·91	1·03	0·77	14·30
Cape of Good Hope and West Coast of Africa....	1,513	2·7	22·5	25·2	...	Return	not pub lished.			
East Indian*......	1,849	2·2	15·1	17·3	1,883	14·34	2·48	4·42	0·53	21·77
Various commands........	2,321	3·5	10·3	13·8	...	Return	not pub lished.			
Home.............	3,070	1·9	8·8	10·7	...	Return	not pub lished.			
Average........	22,538	2·0	11·8	13·8	18,185	11·93	1·70	1·68	0·72	16·03

* The deaths in the East Indian command are only taken to the end of 1839, on account of the Chinese war."

From a comparison of the mortality of the army and navy during war, it appears that the man who entered the army, from 1793 to 1815, ran between two and three times, if a private, and between three and four times, if an officer, the risk of injury in battle that was encountered by one who entered the navy, and that the general chance of death in action to the one was double that of the other.

The following Table shows the Mortality in the Navy on the East Indian Station for Fourteen Years ending with 1843.

Years.		Mean strength.	Diseases.	Annual ratio to 1000 mean strength of the deaths arising from				All causes.
				Wounds and injuries.	Accidental drowning.	Unknown causes.		
Peace ...	1830 to 1836.........	1849	15·10	2·20				17·30
	1837, 1838, 1839 ...	1883	14·34	2·48	4·42	0·53		21·77
War ....1840, 1841, 1842 ...		5156	36·78	3·49	4·01	5·95		50·23

PHYSIOLOGICAL OBSERVATIONS, PRELIMINARY TO A CONSIDERATION OF THE PREVENTION OF DISEASE IN TROPICAL CLIMATES.

It is a general opinion among philosophers that the constitution of man is better adapted to bear those changes of temperature, and other circumstances, experienced in migrating from a northern to a tropical region, and *vice versá,* than that of any other animal.   They proudly observe, that this power of accommodating itself to all climates is a distinctive characteristic of the human species, since no other species of animal can endure transplantation with equal impunity.   But it would not be difficult to show that, for this boasted prerogative, man is more indebted to the ingenuity of his mind than to the pliability of his body.   It would appear, in fact, that he and other animals start on very unequal terms in their emigrations.   Man, by the exertion of his mental faculties, can raise up a thousand barriers around him, to obviate the deleterious effects of climate on his constitution ; while the lower animal, tied down by instinct to a few simple modes of life, is quite defenceless.   Nature must do all for the latter; and, in fact, this indulgent mother does compensate in some degree for the want of reason by producing such corporeal changes as are necessary for the animal's subsistence under a foreign sky, in a shorter space of time than is necessary for effecting correspondent changes in man.   The tender sheep, for instance, when transported from the inclemency of the north, to pant under a vertical sun on the equator, will, in a few generations, exchange its warm fleece of wool for a much more suitable coat of hair. " Can the Ethiopian change his hue" in the same period, by shifting from the interior of Africa to the shores of the Baltic? or will it be said that the fair complexion of the European may, in two or three generations, acquire the sable aspect of the inter-tropical natives, by exchanging situations? Assuredly not. Where then is the superior pliancy of the human constitution? The truth is that the tender frame of man is incapable of sustaining that degree of exposure to the whole range of causes and effects incident to, or arising from the vicissitudes of climate, which so speedily operates a change in the structure, or at least the exterior, of unprotected animals.

But it is observed that, of those animals translated from a temperate to a torrid zone, "some die suddenly, others droop, and all degenerate." This is not to be wondered at, considering the disadvantages under which they labour. Man would not fare better, if placed in similar circumstances. Even as it is, the parallel is not far from applying ; for, of those Europeans who arrive on the banks of the Ganges, many fall early victims to the climate, as will be shown hereafter. That others droop, and are forced, ere many years, to seek their native air, is also well known. That the successors of all would gradually and assuredly degenerate, if they remained in the country, cannot be questioned ; for already we know that the third generation of unmixed European is nowhere to be found in Bengal.

" It has been noted that all the races of mankind have their limits of health defined by a rigorous law of climate ; and the most extended experience proves that the white races attain their highest physical and intellectual development, and the most perfect health, with the greatest average duration of life, above 40° in the western, and 45° in the eastern hemisphere. Whenever they emigrate many degrees below these lines, a series of profound physiological changes in the organism commences, and the changes proceed onwards in the ratio of length of residence, and under the conjoined influences of the heat and malaria common to warm climates, and of the altered habits of life incident to emigration to foreign latitudes."

On the other hand, if we look at intertropical natives approaching our own latitudes, the picture is not more cheering. The African children, brought over by the Sierra Leone Company for education, seldom survived the third year in this country. " They bear the first winter," says Dr. Pearson, " tolerably well, but droop during the second, and the third generally proves fatal to them."

The object of these remarks, which at first sight might seem irrelevant, will now appear. Since it is evident that nature does not operate more powerfully in counteracting the ill effects of climate on man than on other animals, it follows that we should not implicitly confide, as too many do, in the spontaneous efforts of the constitution, but, on the contrary, call to its aid all those artificial means of prevention and amelioration which reason may dictate, and experience confirm.   In short, we should study well the climate, and mould our obsequious frames to the nature of the skies under which we sojourn.

The British youth leaves his native shores with vigorous health and buoyant spirits, for a foreign land of promise, where he is to meet with adventures, acquire fame, and realize a fortune. All the happy events, real or ideal, of his future journey through life, are painted by his ardent imagination in prominent characters, on the foreground of the scene ; while reverses, sickness, disappointments, death itself, are all thrown into the shade, or, if suffered to in-trude, only serve as incentives to the pursuit which has been com-menced.

During the short space of existence to which man is doomed on earth, it is a merciful dispensation that youth anticipates no misfortune, and that when the evil day arrives in after life, Hope comes on glittering wing, and gilds the scene even till the last ray of our setting sun is extinguished.

That, so circumstanced, salutary precautions in matters affecting health are too often despised or neglected, need be no matter of surprise ; and a quotation from the writings of a gentleman who resided more than twenty years in India, and whose talent for ob-servation is peculiar, will place the fact beyond a doubt. "Nothing," says Captain Williamson, " can be more preposterous than the sig-nificant sneers of gentlemen on their first arrival in India ; mean-ing thereby to ridicule, or to despise, what they consider effemi-nacy or luxury. Thus several may be seen walking about without chattahs" (umbrellas) "during the greatest heats. They affect to be ashamed of requiring aid, and endeavour to uphold, by such a display of indifference, the great reliance placed on *strength of con-stitution*. This unhappy infatuation rarely exceeds a few days ; at the end of that time, we are too often called upon to attend the funeral of the self-deluded victim."

Before proceeding to the individual disorders which prevail in hot climates, it may be well to allude briefly to some of those gradual and progressive changes in the constitution, and deviations from previous health and habits which, though predisposing and varying towards, yet fall short of actual disease.   These are consequences which, on leaving their native soil, all must expect to feel more or less, and in which all are naturally and directly interested.   For although a few individuals may occasionally return from even a long residence in hot climates, without having suffered any violent illness, or much deterioration of consti-tution, yet the great mass of Europeans will certainly expe-ricuce the effects sketched out under this head, and many other consequences also which will be noticed in different parts of this work. It is, however, by the most scrupulous attention to these *incipient deviations from health*, by early arresting their growth, or at least retarding their progress, that we can at all expect to evade those dangerous diseases to which they inevitably, though often imperceptibly, tend.

PERSPIRATION.

The transition from a climate, the medium temperature of which is 52°, to one where the temperature is from 80° to 100°, or higher, might be supposed, *a priori*, to occasion the most serious consequences. The benevolent Author of our existence has, however, endowed man, as well as other animals, with the power not only of generating heat, and of preserving their warmth in the coldest regions of the earth ;* but has also provided an apparatus for carrying off any superabundance of it that might accumulate where the temperature of the atmosphere approaches to or exceeds that of the body.

" We have seen," says Mr. Erasmus Wilson, " that the temperature of man varies very little in the whole extent of range between the tropics and the pole ; that he can support the intense heat of the former without much elevation of his inward heat ; that he can live where the mercury is a solid mass, like lead, with the most trifling depression of his vital warmth. But it must not be supposed that the constitution of the man is the same in these two opposite conditions ; it is, indeed, widely different ; in the one, he enjoys what may be termed a *summer constitution* : in the other, a *winter constitution* : and we all, without knowing it, have a summer constitution, to harmonize with the warmth of summer, and a winter constitution, to enable us to resist effectually the inclemency of that season.

" The regulation of the temperature of the body is only one of the purposes fulfilled by the perspiration ; another, and an important one, is the removal from the system of a number of compounds noxious to animal life. It was estimated by Lavoisier and Seguin, that eight grains of perspiration were exhaled from the skin in the course of a minute, a quantity which is equivalent to thirty-three ounces in twenty-four hours. Of this quantity, a large proportion is, naturally, water ; but nearly one per cent., according to Anselmino, consists of solid substances, of the latter, one hundred parts contain about twenty-three parts of salts, the remainder being organic matter. An analysis of one hundred parts of the solid matter of perspiration, according to Anselmino, gave the following results :—

* In the polar voyages the thermometer was noted as low as 70° below zero, while throughout Hindostan it rises to 120° Fahrenheit, and upwards.

Osmazome,* combined with common salt . . . . . 48 parts.
Lactic acid salts, with osmazome . . . . . . 29 „
Animal matter, with vitriolic salts . . . . . . 21 „
Calcareous salts . . . . 2 „
                                          ———
                                          100

" To which may be added carbonic acid gas, ammonia, and iron, and, in rare instances, copper. The peculiar odour of perspiration is due to organic matters, and its acid qualities and occasional acid smell to the lactic acid, an organic substance not far removed in composition from distilled vinegar."

The talented author above quoted, adds that, " to obtain an estimate of the length of tube of the perspiratory system of the whole surface of the body, 2800 may be taken as a fair average of the number of pores in the square inch, and 700, consequently, of the number of inches in length. Now, THE NUMBER OF SQUARE INCHES OF SURFACE IN A MAN OF ORDINARY HEIGHT AND BULK IS 2500 ; THE NUMBER OF PORES THEREFORE 7,000,000, AND THE NUMBER OF INCHES OF PERSPIRATORY TUBE 1,750,000, THAT IS 145,833 FEET, or 48,600 YARDS, OR NEARLY TWENTY-EIGHT MILES." Well may the author exclaim, " What, if this *drainage* were obstructed !" This again brings us to the practical conclusion of Moseley, that " *cold* is the cause of almost all the diseases of *hot* climates to which climate alone is accessory." Even in Europe, the summer night affects us with a chill, while the same temperature, a few months later in the winter season, would feel oppressive from its heat. It is during sleep that alternations of heat and cold most seriously affect us.

We are no sooner beneath a vertical sun than we naturally begin to experience the disagreeable sensation of unaccustomed warmth ; and as the temperature of the atmosphere, in the shade, now advances to within ten or twelve degrees of that of the blood, and in the sun actually exceeds it, the heat constantly generated in the body cannot be so rapidly abstracted as hitherto by the surrounding air, and would thus soon accumulate so as to destroy the very functions of life, did not nature immediately open the sluices of the skin, and by a flow of perspiration reduce the temperature of the body to its original standard.

When we contemplate the admirable provision of Nature, against what might appear to us an unforeseen event ; when we survey the resources and expedients which she can command on all emergencies, her power of supplying every waste, and of restraining every aberration of the constitution, we would be almost tempted to conclude that man was calculated for immortality ! But alas !

" Nascentes morimur, finisque ab origine pendet."

---

* The peculiar animal principle which gives flavour to meats and part of the odour of perspiration.—*A Practical Treatise on the Skin*, 1845.

Till at length this wonderful machine, exhausted by its own efforts at preservation, and deserted by its immaterial tenant, sinks, and is resolved into its constituent elements!

But, reverting to the function of the skin: we must not conclude that this refrigerating process, adapted by nature to prevent more serious mischief, is in itself unproductive of any detriment to the constitution, when carried to excess. Far otherwise is the fact; and we may conclude for certain that those Europeans who avoid direct solar exposure, and who are temperate in all ways, but especially in the use of wine, beer, and spirits, will be in enjoyment of health and vigour, and capable to undergo the greatest fatigues, mental and bodily, without injury. One familiar example will illustrate this subject.

We will suppose two gentlemen to be sitting in a room, in the East or West Indies, just before the setting-in of the sea-breeze, both complaining of thirst, their skin hot, and the temperature of their bodies 100°, or two degrees above the natural standard. One of them, pursuant to the instructions of Dr. Currie, who never was in a tropical climate, applies to the negus, beer, or brandy-and-water cup, and, after a draught or two, brings out a copious perspiration, which soon reduces the temperature to 98°. It will not stop here, however, nor will the gentleman, according to the plan proposed; for, instead of putting the bulb of the thermometer under his tongue, to see if the mercury is low enough, feeling his thirst increased by the perspiration, he very naturally prefers a glass or two more of the same stimulating draught " to support the discharge," still, however, "stopping short of intoxication." Now, by these means the temperature is reduced to 97° or 96½°, in which state even the slight and otherwise refreshing chill of the sea-breeze checks more or less the cuticular discharge, and paves the way for future maladies.

Let us now return to the other gentleman, who pursues a different line of conduct. Instead of the more palatable and stimulating drinks, he takes a draught of plain cold water. This is hardly swallowed before the temperature of the body loses, by abstraction alone, one degree at least of its heat. But the external surface of the body, immediately sympathizing with the internal surface of the stomach, relaxes, and a mild perspiration breaks out, which reduces the temperature to its natural standard of 98°. Farther, this simultaneous relaxation of the two surfaces completely removes the disagreeable sensation of thirst; and as the simple " antediluvian beverage" does not possess many Circean charms for modern palates, there will not be the slightest danger of its being abused in quantity, or of the perspiratory process being carried beyond its salutary limits. Nor need we apprehend its being neglected; since from the moment that the skin begins to be constricted, or morbid heat to accumulate, the sympathizing stomach and fauces will not fail again to warn us, by craving the proper remedy.

Taken, therefore, as a general rule, the advantages of the *latter* plan are numerous—the objections few. It possesses *all the requisites of the former* in procuring a just and equable reduction of temperature, without any danger of bringing it below the proper level, or of wasting the strength by the profuseness of the discharge.

During, or subsequent to violent exertion, under a powerful sun, or in any other situation in a tropical climate, when profuse perspiration is rapidly carrying off the animal heat, and especially when fatigue or exhaustion has taken place, or is impending, then cold drink might prove dangerous, on the same principle as would cold externally applied. In persons who have been for some time in the climate, and whose digestive organs are enfeebled, some weak wine and water may not be objectionable; but such indulgence is by no means necessary in the young and vigorous, and it should be reserved for ulterior residence and more advanced periods of life. I may here mention that, during the first Burmese war, while serving as surgeon to the Governor General's body guard of cavalry, I found warm tea, after the most severe marches in the sun, by far the most refreshing beverage.

The habit of Napoleon under great fatigues was as just physiologically, as it evinced the sagacity of that wonderful man. Finding that excessive fatigue constricted the skin, and produced a sensation of cold, he went into a warm bath, and on getting out he took a cup of strong coffee—a sensorial stimulant. He thus became in a few minutes fit for renewed exertions, both mental and physical.

It is hoped that these details may not appear prolix, or unnecessarily minute, to the medical reader; but, considering that this is generally the first erroneous step which Europeans take on entering the tropics, and that the function of the skin, here under consideration, is more intimately connected with other very important ones than is commonly supposed, it has been thought proper to set them right *in limine*. The probability of *future suffering* will rarely deter the European from indulging in *present gratification;* but when stimulating liquids are represented, from high authority, as not only innocent but salutary, it will require some strength of fact, and of argument, to persuade young men to reliuquish their use, or to check the wide-spreading evil.

SYMPATHY OF THE SKIN WITH INTERNAL ORGANS.

In attempting to delineate the influence of tropical climates on the European constitution, although we may endeavour " to chain the events in regular array," yet it must be confessed that nature spurns all such artificial arrangements.

As matter of fact, however, there does exist between different parts of the body a certain connexion or relation, so that when one is affected by special impressions, the other sympathizes, as it were, and takes on an analogous action. Of the sympathies here referred to, none is more universally remarked than that which subsists between the external surface of the body and the internal surface of the alimentary canal. This, indeed, seems more easily comprehended than many others, since the *latter* appears to be a continuation of the *former*, with the exception of the cuticle. I have remarked that, when we first arrive between the tropics, the perspiration and biliary secretion are both increased; and that, as we become habituated to the climate, they both *decrease, pari passu.*

In the first section an instance was given of the skin sympathizing with the stomach, where the cold drink was applied to the latter organ. Had the water been applied to the exterior of the body, on the other hand, the stomach would have sympathized, and the thirst would have been assuaged.

Mr. Erasmus Wilson justly observes, that the sensibility of the skin conveys to the mind a knowledge of the temperature of the body, thus constituting a " thermometer of vital heat, the degrees upon the scale being computed by the expressions *agreeable* and *disagreeable,* in place of the terms of the common thermometer. The value of these expressions to health is not, however, sufficiently estimated; but it is, nevertheless, certain, that a disagreeable impression of temperature in the skin is a warning note of something mischievous to health, acting either within or without the economy." The same author states the rule of health to be, *by food, by raiment, by exercise, and by ablution, to maintain and preserve an agreeable warmth of the skin.* Everything above this is suspicious; everything below noxious and dangerous. For good or for evil, as it may be, the function of the skin is highly important.

It will be found, on experience, that the loss of tone in the extreme vessels of the surface, consequent on excessive or long-continned perspiration, is accompanied, or soon succeeded, by a consentaneous loss of tone in the stomach, and will fairly account for that anorexia, or diminished appetite, which we seldom fail to perceive soon after entering the tropics, or, indeed, during hot weather in England. Now this, though but a link in the chain of effects, seems a most wise precaution of nature to lower and adapt the irritable, plethoric European constitution to a burning climate, by effectually guarding against the dangerous consequences of repletion. This view of the actual subject will set in a clear light the pernicious effects of stimulating liquids, operating on an organ already debilitated, probably for salutary purposes, and goading it thereby to exertions beyond its natural power, producing a temporary plethora and excitement, with a great increase of subsequent atony.

" An important medical law," says Mr. Wilson, " is founded on
the continuity and similarity of structure of the investing and
lining membrane of the body.   This law resolves itself into three
expressions—namely, *that disease affecting a part of a membrane is
liable to spread to the whole; secondly, that disease of the mucous
membrane may spread to the skin, and vice versâ; and thirdly, that
disease of a part of a mucous membrane may become translated to a part
of the skin, and vice versâ.*"   A remark which every person of observation must have made, even in this country, during the summer,
but particularly in equatorial regions, will further elucidate this
subject.   If by walking, for instance, or other bodily exercise in
the heat of the sun, during the forenoon, or near the dinner hour,
the perspiration be much increased, and the extreme vessels relaxed, we find, on sitting down to table, our appetites almost
entirely gone, until we take a glass of wine, or other stimulating
fluid, to excite the energy of the stomach.   Observation and personal feeling have taught that in hot climates, perhaps during hot
weather in all climates, an hour's cool repose before dinner is
highly salutary; and if, on commencing our repast, we find we
cannot eat without *drinking*, we may be assured that it is nature's
caveat to beware of eating at all.   This will be deemed hard doctrine by some, and visionary by others; but it is neither the one
nor the other, and those who neglect or despise it may feel the
bad consequences when it is too late to repair the error.
    There are several other causes also which operate in conjunction
with the above, to impair the appetite; one of which is, the absence of rest at night.   After a disturbed and unrefreshing sleep,
but too common in tropical climates, the whole frame languishes
next day, and the stomach participates in the general relaxation.
The means of obviating and managing these effects will be pointed
out in the prophylactic part of this work.

INFLUENCE OF TROPICAL HEAT ON THE BILIARY FUNCTION.

    The effect of a tropical climate on the function of the liver is
universally allowed to be an *increase* of the biliary secretion.   This
is so evident in our own country, where the summer and autumn
are distinguished by diseases arising from superabundant secretion
of bile, that it would be waste of time to adduce any arguments
in proof.
    Were this a question of mere curiosity, or theoretical specula-
tion, I should pass it by unnoticed; but from long and attentive
observation, as well as from reflection, I believe that I have discovered a connexion between two important functions of the
animal economy, which will let in some light on this subject, and
lead to practical inferences of much importance.   The arguments
and facts adduced in support of this connexion will be found
under the heads Hepatitis and Dysentery, and in other parts of this

work ; and, in the meantime, I shall merely state in a few words the *result* of my observation, leaving the reader to give credit to it, or not, as he may feel inclined.

There exists, then, between the extreme vessels of the *vena portæ* in the liver, and the extreme vessels on the surface of the body—in other words, between the *biliary secretion* and *perspiration*—one of the strongest sympathies in the human frame, although entirely unnoticed hitherto, so far as I am acquainted. That these two functions are regularly, and to all appearances equally increased, or at least influenced by one particular agent, atmospheric heat, from the cradle to the grave, from the pole to the equator, will be readily granted by every observer ; and that this *synchronous action* alone, independent of any other original connexion, should soon grow up into a powerful sympathy, manifesting itself when *either* of these functions came under the influence of *other agents*, is a legitimate conclusion in theory, and what I hope to prove by a fair appeal to facts. This last consideration is the great practical one ; for it is of little consequence whether this sympathy was originally implanted by the hand of nature at our first formation, or sprung up gradually in the manner alluded to, provided we know that it actually exists, and that by directing our operations towards either *one* of the functions in question, we can decisively influence the *other*. That is what I maintain, and what in a future part of the work I hope to prove by facts and cogent arguments.

I shall here offer one practical remark, resulting from this view of the subject, and which will be found deserving of every European's attention on his emigration to southern regions ; namely, that as the state of the perspiratory process is a visible and pretty fair index to that of the biliary, so every precautionary means which keeps in check, or moderates, the profusion of the *former* discharge, will invariable have the same effect on the *latter*, and thus tend to obviate the inconvenience, not to say disorders, arising from redundancy of the hepatic secretion. To this rule I do not know a single exception, consequently its universal application can never lead astray in any instance.

It is well known that if any organ be stimulated to *inordinate* action, one of two things must in general ensue. If the cause applied be constant, and sufficient to keep up this *inordinate* action for any length of time, serious injury is likely to accrue to the organ itself, even to the extent of *structural* alteration. But if the cause be only temporary, or the force not in any great degree, then an occasional torpor or exhaustion of the organ takes place, during which period its *function* falls short of the natural range. To give a familiar example, of which too many of us are quite competent to judge :—thus, if the stomach be goaded to immoderate exertion to-day, by a provocative variety of savoury dishes and stimulating liquors, we all know the atony which will succeed to-morrow, and how incapable it then will be of performing its accustomed office. It is the same with respect to the liver. After great excitement by excessive heat, violent exercise in the sun, &c., a torpor succeeds, which will be more or less according to the degree of previous excitement, and the length of time during which the stimulating causes have been applied.

When Europeans first arrive in tropical climates, the degree of torpor bears so small a proportion to that of preceding excitement in the liver, that it is scarcely noticed; particularly as the debilitated vessels of this organ continue, like the perspiratory vessels on the surface, to secrete an imperfect fluid for some time *after* the exciting cause has ceased; hence the *increase* of the biliary secretion occupies our principal attention. But these periods of torpor, however short at first, gradually and progressively increase, till at length they greatly exceed the periods of excitement; and then a deficiency of the biliary secretion becomes evident. This is not only consonant to experience, but to analogy. Thus, when a man first betakes himself to inebriety, the excitement occasioned by wine or spirits on the stomach and nervous system far exceeds the subsequent atony, and we are astonished to see him go on for some time, apparently without suffering much detriment to his constitution. But the stage of excitement is gradually curtailed, while that of atony increases, which forces him not only to augment the dose, but to repeat it oftener, till the organ and life are destroyed!

It is remarkable that this alternation of redundancy and deficiency, or *irregular* secretion in the biliary organ, should pass unnoticed by writers on hot climates. They, one and all, represent the liver as a colossal apparatus, of the most herculean power, that goes on for years performing prodigies in the secreting way, without ever being exhausted for a moment, or falling *below* the range of ordinary action, till structural derangement, such as scirrhosity or tuberculation, incapacitates it for its duty! A very attentive observation of what passed in my own frame, and those of others, has led me to form a very different conclusion; and the foregoing statement will, I think, be found a true and a natural representation of the case.

Here, then, we have two very opposite states of the liver and its functions;—first, inordinate action, with increased secretion—the periods gradually shortening; and, secondly, torpor of the vessels of the liver, with deficient secretion—the periods progressively lengthening. In both cases the bile itself is *vitiated*. We can readily conceive how this last comes to pass, by comparison with what takes place in the stomach during and subsequent to a debauch. In both instances the chyme passes through the pylorus into the duodenum, in a state less fit for chylification than during a season of temperance and regularity; so, during the increased secretion, and subsequent inactivity in the liver, the bile passes out into the intestines deteriorated in quality, as well as super-abundant, or deficient, in quantity.

In what this vitiation consists it is certainly not easy to say. In high degrees of it with hurried secretion, both the colour and taste are surprisingly altered, since it occasions all the shades between a deep bottle-green and jet black; possessing at one time an acidity that sets the teeth on edge; at other times, and more frequently, an acrimony that seems absolutely to corrode the stomach and fauces, as it passes off by vomiting, and, when directed downwards, can be compared to nothing more appropriate than the sensation which one would expect from boiling lead flowing through the intestines. Many a time have I experienced this, and many a time have my patients expressed themselves in similar language. The slightly disordered state of the hepatic functions, which we are now considering as primary effects of climate, and within the range of health, may be known by the following symptoms :—Irregularity in the bowels, with motions of various colours, and fœtid or insipid odour; general languor of body and mind, slight nausea, especially in the mornings, when we attempt to brush our teeth; a yellowish fur about the back part of the tongue; unpleasant taste in the mouth on getting out of bed; a tinge in the eyes and complexion from absorption of bile; the urine high-coloured, and a slight irritation in passing it; the appetite impaired, and easily turned against fat or oily victuals; irritability of temper; dejection of mind; loss of flesh; disturbed sleep. These are the first effects of increased and irregular secretion of bile, and may appear in all degrees, according as we are less or more cautious in avoiding the numerous causes that give additional force to the influence of climate.

If, for example, I use more than ordinary exercise, expose myself to the heat of the sun, or drink stimulating liquids to-day, an increased and vitiated flow of bile takes place, and to-morrow produces either nausea or sickness of stomach, or a diarrhœa, with gripings and twitchings in the bowels. But a slight degree of inaction or torpor succeeding, both in the liver and intestines, there will probably be no alvine evacuation at all the ensuing day, till a fresh flow of bile sets all in motion once more. These irregularities, although they may continue a long time without producing much inconvenience, especially if they be not aggravated by excesses, yet they should never be despised, since they inevitably, though insensibly, pave the way for serious derangement in the biliary and digestive organs, especially in hot climates, unless counteracted by rigid temperance, and proper prophylactic measures.

LICHEN TROPICUS, OR PRICKLY HEAT.

Few Europeans escape from this the most primary effect of a hot climate, for it can hardly be called a disease.

From mosquitoes, cockroaches, ants, and the numerous other tribes of depredators on our *personal* property, we have some defence by night, and in general a respite by day; but this unwelcome guest assails us at all, and particularly the most unseasonable, hours.

The sensations arising from prickly heat are perfectly indescribable, being compounded of pricking, itching, tingling, and many other feelings for which there is no appropriate appellation. It is usually, but not invariably, accompanied by an eruption of vivid red pimples, not larger in general than a pin's head, which spread over the breast, arms, thighs, neck, and occasionally along the forehead, close to the hair. The eruption often disappears to a certain degree when we are sitting quiet, and the skin is cool; but no sooner do we use any exercise that brings out perspiration, or swallow any warm or stimulating liquid, such as tea, soup, or wine, than the pimples become elevated, so as to be distinctly seen, and but too sensibly felt!

Prickly heat being rather a symptom than a cause of good health, its disappearance has been erroneously accused of producing much mischief; hence some of the early writers on tropical diseases, harping too much on the humoral pathology, speak very seriously of the danger of *repelling*, and of the advantage of "encouraging" the eruption, by taking warm liquors—as tea, coffee, wine, whey, broth, and nourishing meats. Even Dr. Moseley retails the puerile and exaggerated dangers of his predecessor Hillary. "There is great danger," he says, "in repelling prickly heat; therefore cold bathing and washing the body with cold water, at the time it is out, are always to be avoided." Every naval or military surgeon, however, who has been a few months in a hot climate, must have seen hundreds, if not thousands of seamen and soldiers plunging into the water for days and weeks in succession, covered with prickly heat, yet without bad consequences ensuing.

The eruption is seldom repelled by the cold bath, which rather seems to aggravate it and the disagreeable sensations belonging to it, especially during the glow which succeeds the immersion. It certainly disappears suddenly sometimes on the accession of other diseases, but there is no reason to suppose that its disappearance *occasioned* them. At the same time, cold bathing and repellents are not to be recommended in this eruption, even in persons of robust constitutions, recently arrived in the country, and who are in the enjoyment of good health. Where any organ happens to be weak, on the other hand, or any tendency to disease exists, the repulsion of an eruption is by all means to be avoided, and the more so if the sufferer have been long resident in the climate.

Hair-powder, lime-juice, and a variety of external applications have been used for the removal of prickly heat, but with little or no benefit. The truth is, that the only means productive of good effect in mitigating its violence till the constitution becomes assimilated to the climate are—light clothing, temperance in eating and drinking, avoidance of all exercise in the heat of the day, open bowels; and, lastly, the use of the punkah, or large fan, during the night, as is now the ordinary practice in Bengal. The punkah is always safe; and, unlike the thorough-draught or external breeze, it removes the heated air surrounding the body, without exposing it to the dangers arising from sudden night changes in the temperature and humidity of the atmosphere.

NOTA BENE.—In the foregoing sections, as well as in those which follow, from page 165 to page 180, containing special rules respecting dress, food, &c., I have followed Dr. James Johnson, offering occasional additions and illustrations. I have endeavoured to place before the reader a fair abstract of the physiological doctrine—the *cutaneo-hepatic sympathy* of this distinguished author, together with his excellent hygienic rules. His physiological doctrine was propounded by Dr. Johnson in early life, in the East Indies, with a limited range of observation in years, and in the subjects for observation—namely, the crew of a ship of war. But with all these disadvantages, it will, I think, be admitted that, practically considered, in relation to the nature, causes, prevention, and cure of disease, there is much in the theory to "lead to practical inferences of considerable importance;" for it is to the restoring of the lost balance of circulation, of the nervous functions, and of secretion that our main efforts have been, and always must be directed, in the treatment of tropical disease, whether it be fever, dysentery, hepatitis, or cholera.

For all the other articles contained in this work I am individually and exclusively responsible.—J. R. M.

PART II.

THE PREVENTION OF DISEASE.

If it were possible to make men healthy in various ways, it would be best to choose that which is least troublesome, for this is more honest and more scientific, unless one aims at vulgar imposition.—HIPPOCRATES.

In the prevention of disease, as in its cure, we take the same point of departure—namely, etiology; for in the study of causes we shall find in reality the only route to a true prophylaxis.

DESCARTES must have had in view the science of PREVENTION OF DISEASE, or of STATE MEDICINE, when he declared:—" S'il est possible de perfectionner l'espèce humaine, c'est dans la médecine qu'il faut en chercher les moyens." This philosopher felt that whatever tended to improve the physical constitution of man, must promote general happiness and virtue, and thus prevent crime and disease. Health and freedom are two blessings which it is said no man thoroughly appreciates till he has lost them.

Nor did Bacon hold this greatest department of medicine in less estimation; for he exhorts the profession in his time to " exert themselves for the general good, and raise their minds above the sordid considerations of cure; not deriving their honours from the necessities of mankind, but becoming ministers of the Divine power and goodness both in prolonging and restoring the life of man." It would accord with the views of these great men that adequate public provision and arrangement should be made to enable the medical profession to render the services desired; but, in this country, it has, until very recently, been employed by the State individually, and chiefly in its curative or therapeutic capacity only; while it might be employed collectively, in a higher and nobler—namely, in its preventive or prophylactic office.

It is surprising that in so civilized a state of society as ours, we should still be so far behind some of the ancient peoples. Moses imposed sanitary laws upon the Jews; the Greeks and Romans held their officers of health in high consideration. " In the Cyropædia of Xenophon," says Dr. Farr, " the preservation of health is declared a noble art worthy of Cyrus himself;" while in modern England the ruling powers do not yet apprehend the truth, that without the physical care of the people their moral and intellectual improvement is impossible. Wisely said Carew, that "where our prevention ends danger begins."

" In 92 days of the summer quarter, that ended on 30th September, 1857," says Dr. Farr, " 17,653 persons perished untimely in England. What was the cause of this great destruction of life? Evidently the violation of the plain natural laws of life. And the strict observance of these laws must be of the utmost importance to the welfare of the human race, otherwise their violation would not be so terribly punished by the Almighty. Indeed, if the English race could lose strength, beauty, health, and life in the impurities of its dwelling-places with impunity, the imagination of Swift alone could conceive—his pencil depict—the depth of degradation to which the nation might fall.

" The intelligent classes of this country will, however, never acquiesce in the continuance of its present imperfect sanitary condition, and of the resulting diseases which it brings down upon the heads of the population; who often, when they violate the laws of nature, know not what they do."

Let us hope that this humane expectation may be speedily fulfilled.

" England," says Dr. Farr again, " is a great country, and has done great deeds. It has encountered in succession, and at times in combination, all the great powers of Europe; has founded vast colonies in America; and has conquered an empire in Asia. Yet greater victories have to be achieved at home. Within the shores of these islands the twenty-eight millions of people dwell, who have not only supplied her armies, and set her fleets in motion, but have manufactured innumerable products, and are employed in the investigation of scientific truths, and the creation of works of inestimable value to the human race. These people do not live out half their days; *a hundred and forty thousand* of them die every year unnatural deaths; *two hundred and eighty thousand* are constantly suffering from actual diseases which do not prevail in healthy places; their strength is impaired in a thousand ways: their affections and intellects are disturbed, deranged, and diminished by the same agencies. Who will deliver the nation from these terrible enemies? Who will confer on the inhabitants of the United Kingdom the blessings of health and long life? Who will give scope to the improvement of the English race, so that all its fine qualities may be developed to their full extent under favourable circumstances? His conquests would be wrought neither by wrong nor human slaughter; but by the application of the powers of nature to the improvement of mankind."

In the army and navy of England the medical officers have for ages past occupied themselves, spontaneously, and without prospect of reward, in establishing important principles in this great branch of medical science—the prevention of disease;—and the sister science of Medical Statistics may be said to be founded, in this country at least, on the labours of such men as Pringle; Lind, Blanc, Robert Jackson, Trotter, Hennen, and Henry Marshall.*

Dr. Alison, in his " History of Medicine" in the present century, observes that, "Next to the additions which have been made since the end of last century to our knowledge of physiology, we may place the numerous important observations by which our information as to the external causes of disease has been rendered more extensive and more precise.

" These observations and the inferences from them demand the more attention from physicians, that they necessarily involve a kind of evidence essentially different from that on which we proceed in other medical inquiries; and if we durst hope that the progress of human wisdom and virtue would bear any proportion to that of human knowledge, we might expect that the lessons to be drawn from these inquiries would prove of even greater importance to the future happiness of mankind than any which we can gather from the history and treatment of disease.

" These inquiries have in some instances been prosecuted by in-

---

* I take leave here to state that, while serving in the East Indies, in March, 1835, I submitted to the then Governor-General of India, Sir Charles, afterwards, Lord Metcalfe, a systematic and detailed plan for requiring from all competent medical officers throughout our Eastern possessions, reports on Medical Topography and Sanitary Statistics of the districts, stations, or cantonments, whether fixed or temporary, with the localities of which each officer may in the course of service be best acquainted. In the following year, 1837, I placed before the Government of Bengal a detailed "Report on the Medical Topography, Climate, and Diseases of Calcutta," with suggestions for removing the defects, local and structural, which there injuriously affected the health of its inhabitants, European and Native. This report also contained suggestions for the removal of the European troops from the plains to the mountain ranges throughout India. The first measure here mentioned, though it received little or no support from the medical authorities of Bengal, was ordered *by a direct act* of the Governor-General, Sir Charles Metcalfe, to be a standing regulation throughout the three Presidencies of India, and it has stood so ever since. The second proposal for the sanitary improvement of the British Indian capital has for several years been practically carried out under legislative enactments;—the works are still in progress, under an official board, and will continue to their completion. A fever hospital, for the reception and treatment of natives suffering from fever and other acute diseases endemic in Calcutta, formed a supplementary of this my latter plan. This institution is now attached to the Medical College: it was completed in 1853 in all its establishments, and is arranged to accommodate five hundred patients; it is one of the most useful and ornamental buildings in Calcutta, and was erected at the cost of 20,000*l.* Dr. Farr, of the Registrar-General's Office, speaking of the measures above mentioned, says—"We look upon the well-conducted sanitary inquiry, commenced in Bengal, as one of the most important undertakings of the age in India—useful to science, to England, and creditable alike to Mr. Martin, with whom it originated, and to the Government."

Lord Hardinge, referring to the same subject, says—"I am happy to bear testimony to the services you rendered to our Indian empire in originating those valuable measures of sanitary improvement which have so materially contributed to the comfort and prosperity of an immense population. The importance of these benefits will be ever felt; and I am aware, from the interest that, as Governor-General, I took in this subject, that their inestimable results are honourably associated with the active part you took in their first introduction." Thus, although my endeavours were but coldly received by the superannuated members of the Bengal Medical Board, they are approved by persons the most competent to judge of their value, whether scientific or practical.—J. R. M.

dividuals in civil life; but the opportunities of making decisive
observations on some of the causes of disease which occur in the
experience of medical officers of fleets and armies, who are perfectly informed of the whole circumstances of the organized bodies
of men under their observation, and often see these circumstances
suddenly altered, or have even the power of altering them at pleasure, are much superior to those which other practitioners enjoy;
and the peculiar value of such observations has never been so well
understood as during the last war."

The unobtrusive but important services of our brethren in the
army and navy, alluded to by Dr. Alison, are not written in the
rolls of fame, but they will be remembered and appreciated by the
philanthropist and the statesman, for ages after other and more
brilliant services are forgotten. But in public rewards or emolu-
ments our brethren must not as yet expect to share; for " in
medicine alone," according to Marshall Hall, "improvement is
without recompence :"—L'art médicale est la plus noble des professions et le plus triste des métiers.

Referring to " the progress of human wisdom and virtue," it
may reasonably be supposed that by rendering men more healthy
they may become more happy, and that thus the bonds of our common humanity may be drawn the closer, so that the uncertainties,
which are the same to us all, may eventually be regarded as the
true and natural bond of union amongst men.

From what has been stated, it must be obvious that, for the advancement and perfectioning of the science of Prevention of
Disease, we must command the co-operation of the medical pro
fession generally, and, in particular, that of the medical officers of·
the army, the navy, the police, hospitals, dispensaries, lunatic
asylums, parochial unions and workhouses, vaccination establishments, prisons, factories, mines, provident societies, and other
institutions, and public works.

The medical profession has so invariably spurned all selfish
considerations in originating and promoting objects of great sanitary utility, that I would here allude only to the obvious advantages which will result to medicine, and the increased estimation
in which its professors and practitioners will be held, both by the
Government and the country at large, from the realization of the
projects here contemplated. " One of the first steps," says
Heberden, " towards preserving the health of our fellow-creatures,
is to point out the sources from which diseases are apprehended."

It has been well observed, says a great popular writer, that if a
science can be established by its fruits, Sanitary Science may now
take its rank with any of the sciences known to mankind. It no
longer pertains to the class of theories, or inquiries, or specula-
tions. Its laws have been tested by experiment, and are proved
by facts. The object of the new doctrines is an exceedingly simple

one—the improvement of public health, or the prolongation of human life. We know the standard fixed by nature. We can all recollect that the years of man are threescore and ten, and that the age of fourscore is reached only through labour and trouble. So exactly does this estimate fit all generations, that the latest reckoning of our latest calculators produces the very same result.

It has also been observed as very remarkable, that, among all the movements of the working classes, political or social, there is no example of agitation for what would be the greatest boon of all—Sanitary Reform. No workmen ever struck, combined, or agitated for the essentials of a healthy and comfortable existence. No " People's Charter" has ever yet been framed for pure air, pure water, pure food, good drainage, and open spaces for exercise. The classes in question are easily induced to lavish their savings in pursuit of chimerical objects, or to expend the resources of organization upon impracticable ends, but of their lives and health they take little heed. They, however, are the chief sufferers and the earliest victims; and they are the people who should be most anxious for reform.

The Medical Topographer should investigate all the circumstances which tend to deteriorate the human race, and to lower its vigour and vitality; all that relates to the external causes of diseases, their propagation, and their prevention; all plans for improving the physical, and, through it, the moral condition of the people. He should cultivate more extensively the medical topography of the empire; the natural features and peculiarities of every locality which may affect materially the life and health of the inhabitants. Any general system of sanitary inquiry should, therefore, embrace information respecting the surface and elevation of the ground, the stratification and composition of the soil, the supply and quality of the water, the extent of marshes and wet ground, the progress of drainage; the nature and amount of the products of the land; the condition, increase or decrease, and prevalent diseases of the animals maintained thereon; together with periodical reports of the temperature, pressure, humidity, motion, and electricity of the atmosphere. Without a knowledge of these facts it is impossible to draw satisfactory conclusions with respect to the occurrence of epidemic diseases, and variations in the rate of mortality and reproduction.

The result of such inquiries would also, doubtless, show that agriculture is everywhere the most powerful improver of climate, and that its advancement ministers not only to the support of man in the production of his food, but in a greater degree to his health and vigour, by purifying the air he breathes.

The practical connexion, therefore, of agriculture with the nutrition and growth, the sickness and health, the birth and death, of man and of the lower animals, is inseparable from a comprehensive consideration of the public health.

The science of localizing the population, and of constructing towns, cantonments, barracks, and hospitals, is much neglected in this country, and throughout its various intertropical possessions. It is proved over and over again, in the records of the Registrar-General, that, owing to defects in the sites of towns, in the erection of buildings, in the selection of healthy soils and levels, in the supply of pure air and water, in the drainage and cleansing of streets and houses, a mortality of from a fifth to a third part greater occurs in large towns than in small communities and rural districts.

The amount of *sickness* occurring in cities, towns, and villages, and in thinly populated districts, requires a much more careful and extended investigation than it has ever yet received. Evidence should be obtained, on an extended scale, of the moral and physical deterioration of mankind when aggregated in low and crowded towns. "The causes," says the Registrar-General, "that destroy the lives of so many people, degrade the lives of more, and may ultimately, it is feared, have a very unfavourable effect on the energies of a large proportion of the English race. Here is a wide field for salutary and beneficial reform."

Amongst those whose habits and pursuits in life qualify them to be consulted in the objects of State Medicine, the following may be enumerated :—The clergy, the statesmen, colonial authorities, philanthropists, naval and military commanders, the legal profession, the medical profession, quarantine authorities, the landed proprietary and the agricultural body, magistrates, poor-law guardians, actuaries, engineers and architects, shipowners, manufacturers of all classes, the several trades. Professors of State Medicine in foreign countries should be solicited to forward, by their information and experience, the objects in view ; and the various methods which the government of those countries have adopted to investigate and preserve the health of the people, should be ascertained and carefully considered.

It will thus appear that among the more immediate objects of State Medicine, may be enumerated the following :—

1. To direct public attention to the increased security of life and property, which must result from a sustained and organized investigation, by competent persons, of all those agencies and circumstances, moral and physical, which deteriorate, through local or general influences, the public health.

2. To disseminate knowledge amongst all classes of the community, on the most obvious and well-ascertained causes of injury to public health, and as to the most effective and economical measures of sanitary improvement, both in town and country.

It is believed that the union of the medical, clerical, and lay bodies, for the collection of scientific and practical information, for the consideration of sanitary measures within the United Kingdom and its foreign dependencies, and for establishing fixed and determinate principles in sanitary affairs, could not fail to enlarge the sphere of usefulness of the medical profession, for the most extended and beneficent pursuits, and to promote the moral as well as the physical improvement of the population.

"In the science of health," says Dr. Farr, "there are more exact demonstrable truths than in the science of disease ; and the advantages of 'prevention' over 'cure' require no proof." I need, therefore, proceed no further to explain why I here give the priority and the preference to the subject of THE PREVENTION OF DISEASE.

1. The subjects concerning which the State should direct investigation, with a view to establishing settled relations between the science of medicine and the executive, are stated by Mr. Rumsey to be :—

> " A. Statistical.
> B. Topographical.
> C. Jurisprudential.

" 2. In relation to PRACTICAL ARRANGEMENTS for the personal safety and health of the people, requiring for their enforcement either direct legislature enactment, or local institutions or regulations," the same authority divides them into :—

> " A. Preventive, and
> B. Palliative measures.

" 3. In relation to the establishment by law of an ORGANIZED MACHINERY for carrying into effect the aforesaid inquiries, for deliberation and advice on special arrangements and emergencies, and for administration of existing laws, there would be required :—

> " A. The education of medical men, and the qualification of other technical, scientific, and administrative agents.
> B. The institution of official authorities—board and officers —for central and local superintendence and action."

Meanwhile, and pending the ordering of some established regulations for the better care of the health of the national forces by sea and land, there can be no doubt that the first duty of the naval and military surgeon is to preserve the health of the men committed to his charge—a service far higher and more useful than the cure of disease and wounds, however necessary this last function.

" Hygiene," says Cabanis, " teaches the means of preserving health, and forms an important branch of moral as well as of medical science. Ethics, being in fact but the *science of life*, how is it possible for this science to be complete, without a knowledge of the changes which the subject to which it is applied may expericuce, and without a knowledge of the means by which these changes are effected. Hygiene, therefore, and, consequently, some concise notions of anatomy and physiology, should form part of every system of education." The study of nature, he says, is, in general, a study of facts, and not of causes, a knowledge of these last not being necessary. "For studying the healthy and diseased states, for tracing the progress and development of any particular disease, we have no occasion to know the essence of life, or that of the morbific cause. Observation, experience, and reasoning are sufficient for our purposes—we require nothing more."

That the subject of public health has not as yet been taught in our schools is matter of much and general regret, and those of the medical profession who have devoted their time and attention to this branch of medicine, have always done so, in the army and navy at least, gratuitously, and under great disadvantages and difficulties. I can say with truth, that I first became aware of the power of external causes in the production of disease, under circumstances of general and personal suffering of the most painful character, in the marshes of Orissa and Gondwana, and afterwards in those of Rangoon. Our men were dying a miserable, a dismal, a nameless death, by thousands. We lost more men ingloriously than would have made the most bloody campaigns. I have gone through so many storms of febrile suffering, on so many occasions, that I often wonder how I came to survive them. I was young, and inexperienced in the "art of preserving health;" but I laboured hard, and, like others in the public service, I may be supposed to have acquired some knowledge essential to the welfare of the soldiers under my charge.* But suffering, general and personal, was always the school in which I received my instruction.

It was but the other day that the Legislature and Government of this country ordained that a Board for the management of the health-concerns of England should be constituted without any person of the medical profession having a seat in its deliberations. That for this unhappy state of things the medical profession is itself principally to blame is, I think, manifest; for had "the art of preserving health" been taught in our schools of medicine, and been thus placed on its proper footing in the public estimation, no Government, in these days of free discussion, could have resisted the just claims of science. As matters stand at present, there is no remedy;—but the remedy will eventually be found, when medical science shall be represented in the councils of the nation.

I think it necessary here to state my views on this great question, as they have been both misunderstood and misrepresented. Sanitary measures for the good of the army ought, I apprehend, to be explained, advanced, and practised as a part, and the greatest part, of that science which it is the duty of the military surgeon to per-

* "The art of preserving health," says Dr. Farr, "is taught in no regular course of lectures in any of the great schools of medicine in the United Kingdom. Yet the classical sanitary works of Pringle, Lind, Blanc, Robert Jackson, Johnson, and Martin have been framed from observation in the British navy and army."—*Report on the Mortality of Cholera.* London, 1852.

form ; and all this should be done by him, not through subserviency, apology, or solicitation, but as a duty of necessity—as his first duty, in fact. Even Napoleon did not pretend to discover and arrange the sanitary measures necessary to his armies ; these duties he left to those who understood such questions as their proper business, and their recommendations he always carried into effect.

The greatest physician who ever served in the British army invariably treated this subject as a science of the utmost need to the soldier ; and he declared emphatically, over and over again, that to the ignorance of our commanders, and their indisposition to accept and learn from their medical officers what they could not know of themselves, or from any other source, our armies had always been sacrificed. A man of the most rare courage and virtue, and personally of a republican simplicity, he contended that, inasmuch as the medical department of the army shared in the fatigues and dangers of war, so also was it, in right reason, entitled to share in the advantages. In thus acting and writing, Robert Jackson proved himself not only the best friend of the soldier, but, rightly understood, of the officer also.

It is true that this good and great man was in his time assailed and misrepresented by some very unworthy members of his profession, and persecuted by a host of the most vile and corrupt of the army contractors; but he had for his unswerving friends and supporters the Duke of York, Abercromby, Moore, the Adjutant-General, Calvert, and all the best officers of his day, who had known him through fifty years of eminent and honest service. That Jackson was in advance of his time is true, but he was not in advance of our time, and we would do well to follow his useful example.

Had his injunctions, the suggestions of his thoughtful experience, been put in practice, would England have had to lament the disasters and humiliations of Walcheren and of the Crimea ? Let the army surgeon then look well to the science of THE PREVENTION OF DISEASE, as now happily taught at Chatham, and he will serve his country to the best purpose and do much honour to himself. I have all my life urged this on my brother officers of the Indian army, and I venture now to do the same to medical officers of all the services at home. I have served long enough to know the value of a good military officer ; and I have seen, on more than one occasion of active service, how great is the amount of ruin which may be consummated by a bad commander. To honour and obey the first is both natural and necessary ; to conciliate, deprecate, supplicate, and wait upon the pleasure of the latter, in his neglects and wrong-doings, is certainly not the part of an honest or efficient medical officer.

It is true that " the sanitary function has yet to be defined and adjusted" to the wants of the soldier. Let the surgeon, then, advocate its immediate introduction into the army as a measure of absolute necessity—let the STATE MEDICINE OF THE ARMY be modestly but firmly and perseveringly urged, until it shall be regulated and established, " By Order," like the other rules of discipline. It must no longer be said of the army-surgeon that " it depends on his relations with the officers in command whether any suggestions he makes will be listened to ;" in other words, whether the suggestions of science and of experience are to be listened to in order to save the army, or whether the suggestions of the mess-room or the club-house are, without a proved necessity, to be the rule. If " officers in command" do not look to it with more wisdom than heretofore, the House of Commons will some day, not very distant, determine the question in its own way.

Referring to the preservation of the Indian army, it has been said by a great woman, and that woman Florence Nightingale, that " the observance of sanitary laws should be as much part of the future *régime* of India as the holding of military positions or as civil government itself. It would be a noble beginning of the new order of things to use hygiene as the handmaid of civilization." As regards the medical department, it has shed tears of humanity by order to no purpose long enough. It must now stand on its ground of scientific and practical usefulness alone.

Military hygiene now ranks with the State and the public as an accepted science, and we must see well that its results are displayed not only in the economy of military life, but in the expansion of the national resources.

For an exposition of the sanitary necessities of the British army, as now ruled, and of the importance of a well-understood military hygiene, I have but to refer to the health history of the Crimean army as given by Miss Nightingale.

Public opinion is indeed beginning to perceive, in civil life, that the system of calling in the doctor only on the appearance of sickness is radically unsound in itself, quite apart from the question of remuneration. The correct plan, according to the *Standard*, would be to employ the physician's ability and skill for the general and regular superintendence and care of our health and the prevention of disease, and not for applying a remedy to a malady when rendered perceptible, troublesome, or dangerous. " Suppose it were the usage for every family man to set aside a certain sum annually for the regular and confidential attendance of the medical adviser, and let the practice be to prescribe, but never to supply the remedies, we should soon find a change in the entire system of therapeutics and a marvellous diminution of disease."

Hitherto, in place of regarding it as their duty to consult the medical officers of the army, our commanders have proceeded at once, and without any knowledge, to issue their orders in matters affecting the soldiers' health. The results have always been, and ever must be, disastrous. In fact, something like a revolution will be necessary in our armies to gain for military hygiene the attention it deserves.

That men who know nothing of science, general or particular, of war or of administration—men whose knowledge is confined to the very pipeclay of a section, a company, or a battalion, should, as in Chusan in 1840, yet have the power to judge or to order in matters of sanitary science, affecting the very existence of our soldiers, is surely an abuse which cannot much longer be permitted to disgrace our armies.

It is not so much owing to the defects of our ancient sanitary laws, great as these defects confessedly were, as to the utter neglect of their provisions, that matters relating to the public health in this country have been allowed to fall so immeasurably behind the wants, the science and spirit of the age; and it is feared that popular ignorance, national indifference, prejudices, and parsimony will continue yet a while, as of old, to neutralize better measures of sanitary regulation than even now exist! Englishmen, even of classes above the labourer, will agitate and combine for political privileges of no value when secured. They will cry for cheap bread, for holidays, for shorter time of labour, and for higher wages; but they will neither reflect upon, nor combine for, any matters affecting their sanitary improvement. Here, in our cities, as in Paris, the thing must be done for them by an authority which they may not question. The truth I believe to be that, in respect to measures of prevention of disease, medical men have always been ready and capable to direct to good purpose; but society was not, and is not yet, anywhere possessed of sufficient knowledge to co-operate with them. I happen to possess some official as well as professional knowledge on this head; for I was appointed in 1843 member of the Royal Commission ordered by her Majesty "for inquiring into the present State of Large Towns and Populous Districts in England and Wales, with Reference to the Cause of Disease amongst the Inhabitants." As one of the said Commissioners, I examined and reported on the sanitary condition of six of the manufacturing towns of England, and two thousand copies of my reports were printed by order of the Government. The Commission was composed of thirteen gentlemen, including two Cabinet ministers, and its deliberations and inquiries extended over two years. The final "Recommendations" contained in the Report of the Commission to her Majesty, formed the groundwork of the clauses of a Bill, subsequently passed by Parliament, for regulating the health concerns of England and Wales. The Recommendations were, with a very few exceptions, of a permissive character. To this principle I ventured on sundry occasions to object, urging that, on the score of experience, whatever was allowed to be permissive was sure to be neglected; whereas, whatever had been made imperative, like party-walls to prevent the spreading of fire, had surely been obeyed. I urged that Englishmen yield a ready obedience to Acts of Parliament, however stringent, but that to the requisitions of a Sanitary Board they would render neither respect nor obedience.

I think that my anticipations have been amply verified in the workings of the first unhappy " Board of Health," and that its shortcomings have arisen fully as much from defective legislation as from the intrinsic defects of that ill-sorted board. I feel convinced, and I have publicly reported my reasons for this conviction, as member of " The Health of Towns' Commission," that legislation in sanitary affairs, to be effective, must be IMPERATIVE, and based on the principle that no man can be allowed a right to use his property so as to cause injury to the health of his neighbour. In the *Builder* newspaper I find, at the moment of writing, the following common-sense view of this question as regards one out of our many nuisances :—" The total abolition of cesspools must be made compulsory ; landlords *will not* make the necessary outlay *unless compelled* to do so, and the sooner it is done the better." The State does interfere, and has always interfered, in all sorts of ways, in the prevention of crime and on many kindred subjects. Centralization may be carried too far, but so also may respect for local government. " System is not always method, much less progress." Again, and in respect of sanitary matters, it must be confessed that the English people have had full liberty of indiscretion. What heads of families should be made to understand is this—that the general population cannot be making real progress, moral or physical, so long as individual existence on a large scale remains one entire course of sanitary neglect; that in the sum of individual and personal hygiene we shall find the true and general advancement of public health.

The first principles of justice, and the first sentiments of humanity, would seem to be common to all mankind; but who would trust the framing and the administering of a criminal code to local or municipal management? Self-preservation requires that we should stop an evil where we can, if we must stop it somewhere. We cannot give up the right and duty of society to stop crime in the bud ; nor should we hesitate to assert the same right in respect of disease.

The simple circumstance that amongst the destitute poor we must do the cure, and that the cure is very costly and difficult, imposes on us also the duty of prevention. The polite or permissive system of legislating for the public health may do when danger is believed to be suppositious or remote, but in the presence of actual danger it will never answer any good purpose in this or in any other country.

The right to use one's property is one thing, and the right to abuse the privilege is another thing. It is of this last that I complain.

The facts and circumstances here detailed will not be considered irrelevant when the important principle involved in them is taken into account. The establishment of sound principles in sanitary affairs must precede the arrangement of details—a fact

M

not always present to the minds of those who frame sanitary regulations.*

If it be the business of Government to prevent and to punish
crime—to secure the public peace—to enforce industry instead of
rapine, and the settlement of disputes by appeal to reason instead
of by fraud and violence ; if the well-being of the subject be, in
short, the main object of legislation, then would it appear the
special duty of the ruling power to secure the health and the life of
those who, of all others, stand most in need of its protection against
the invasions of individual or corporate caprice, ignorance, or stolid
avarice.   Here we perceive a moral and political duty of necessity.
On this subject it should ever be borne in mind that where there
is disease there also will be found the seat of poverty and crime.
Disease, poverty, and crime, in their worst forms, are constantly
and everywhere found together.   The truth then is, that misery
and crime produce disease, and disease produces misery and crime,
in a circle which revolves, in the same calamitous monotony, from
year to year, of the brief existence of the masses crowded in the
worst quarters of our manufacturing cities.

Whilst men are in the lowest state of physical destitution, surrounded by filth, vermin, privation, and squalor of every conceivable kind—familiar with sickness and death—and strangers to
every comfort—with the mind continually on the rack, or absorbed
in striving against physical necessity—or with the animal spirits
broken down by its pressure ; how is it to be expected that obedience to the laws, that morals, education, or religion should find
a place ?   How can a man whose mind is ruined even more
effectually than his body—the man by whom moral degradation
and physical suffering have done their worst—how can such a man
be expected to give a passing thought even to such matters ?   The
thing is impossible.   But, not to speak of those higher considerations, I should say that the benefits of the surrounding civilization
even are not for the occupants of the lanes, courts, and alleys,
through which I have of late passed.†   Even amongst what are
called the better classes of society we find that, in the false pride of
a *quasi*-science, or of civilization, we continually neglect measures
of precaution known to the rudest people, as if we thought ourselves
not subject to the laws of organization which regulate the functions of the inferior animals.   The nature of brute animals, indeed,

* The Medical Officer of Health, now appointed by the Legislature, is declared by
the "British and Foreign Medical and Surgical Review" to be "a great step in
modern civilization."   The establishment of this sanitary office was exclusively the
result of my persistent advocacy as member of the "Health of Towns' Commission."

† These two last paragraphs are transcribed from my Official Report of 1842, on
the Sanitary Condition of the Labouring Population in our Manufacturing Towns, as
Member of the Health of Towns' Commission.   The observations are believed to be
generally applicable to all persons and places similarly circumstanced ; and they are
here presented in order to show what were then my sentiments on this most important
subject.   The principle I believe to be the same in respect to sanitary regulations for
civil and military communities ; they should be compulsory for both.

we study attentively, and adapt our conduct to their constitution, whilst of our own we continue ignorant and neglectful. " If one-tenth of the persevering attention and labour bestowed to no purpose in rubbing down and currying the skins of horses," says Dr. A. Combe, " were bestowed by the human race in keeping themselves in good condition, and a little attention more paid to diet and clothing, colds, nervous diseases, and stomach complaints would cease to form so large an item in the catalogue of human miseries ;" while another writer declares, with equal truth—" If as much care were bestowed on the breeding of men as upon the breeding of cattle, we should not have books written on the degeneration of the human race."

As regards epidemics, Mr. Cox classifies and enumerates the local causes producing and influencing them. The following table exhibits his views in this respect, being ranged in the order of their presumed importance.

1. *Endemic Atmosphere.*
Produced by—
 a. Human effluvia from lungs and skin ; from over-crowding.
 b. Ditto, from defective ventilation.
 c. Defective house and land drainage.
 d. Personal uncleanliness.

2. *Bad Water Supply.*
Consisting of—
 a. Insufficient supply.
 b. Foul percolation through soil charged with organic matter, &c.

3. *Social Habits.*
a. Drunkenness.
b. Dirt in and around dwellings.
c. Privation of wholesome food.
d. Nature of employment.
e. Neglect of infantile life.

4. *Privation of Solar Light.*

TROPICAL HYGIENE.

Hints for the Preservation of Health in all Hot Climates.

Certain popular means of prevention of disease present themselves to the common sense of most nations to a certain degree, if they would but choose to reflect on their importance and act upon them. But it is with communities as with individuals ; hygienic rules are better known than regarded. They are like the

M 2

vital points in religion and morals;—all men agree in them, yet how easily are they forgotten! In order to think seriously on matters relating to health, most men require to suffer from disease, the lessons derived from such experience being longest remembered.

But there is one circumstance which ought to be impressed everywhere on individuals and communities; and that is, that however useful medicine may be in moderate and judiciously administered doses, under occasional circumstances of change of climate or season, or during the prevalence of certain epidemics, it is yet more on the proper selection of localities, the avoidance of day and night exposure, care in diet, clothing, exercise, &c.; in short, on the adoption of all those well-known measures of avoidance, whether affecting individual habit of life or those more general predisposing causes of disease now so well understood, that the prevention of disease depends, and not on a system of self-quackery with calomel and other mercurial preparations, such as many persons pursue in England, and in India too, to their great injury, for the removal of what they call *"biliousness."*

Many is the robust habit I have seen destroyed by this senseless custom; and I have known several lives lost and others put in jeopardy by the use of saline purgatives during seasons of cholera. In respect of the use of medicines in health, we should hold with the French proverb, that better is the worst enemy of well. It is here that a well-understood personal hygiene will prove of the greatest preservative effect; and it is in seasons of epidemics that its neglect proves most signally destructive.

Another source of great injury to health I must here mention, as it has come frequently under my notice both in India and in England;—I mean the long-continued use of aperient medicines containing the mercurial preparations. Patients frequently obtain from their physicians aperient pills, for instance, containing some blue pill or calomel. They may have been given with a particular view or for a special occasion only, but it often happens that the patient continues for months, or even for years, that which was intended to be used for days or weeks: the results are very lamentable. I have seen persons in a state of nervous irritability bordering on insanity from this cause, with sub-acute inflammation of the mucous digestive membrane and chronic ptyalism—all resulting from long-continued and unconscious use of mercury. A field-officer used blue pill and colocynth for two years and a half, and an American gentleman took the same preparations with ipecacuanha during a voyage from Madras to America, and back to Calcutta. It is quite needless to detail how utterly ruined was the health of both.

"Ingenuity," says Dr. Copland, "cannot possibly devise a more successful method of converting a healthy person into a confirmed invalid, of destroying many of the comforts of existence, and of occasioning hypochondriasis and melancholy, than the practice of prescribing large doses of calomel on every trifling occasion, or when the bowels require gentle assistance; or because the patient erroneously supposes himself to be *bilious*, or is told so by those who should know better." The same distinguished writer ascribes the lapse of occasional indigestion into confirmed stricture of the rectum, and of hæmorrhoidal affections into fistulæ, to the frequent and injudicious use of calomel for the removal of mere occasional derangements of health. The unfortunate word "bilious," as applied to slight disorders, is the scapegoat of the ignorant.

Dr. Paris assures us, that "if the truth were told, a large portion of dyspeptics seek the advice of a physician, not so much for the better adjustment and regulation of their diet as for the means by which they may counteract the ill effects of their indulgences —hence the popularity of those "*antibilious* remedies, which promise to take the sting out of their excesses; and enable the unhappy dupes to fondle and play with vice as with a charmed serpent."

There is, in truth, says James Johnson, and referring to tropical hygiene, no situation where the stranger European may not obviate, in a great measure, the first and most dangerous effects of a tropical climate, by a strict observance of two fundamental rules, TEMPERANCE AND COOLNESS. The latter indeed includes the former; and, simple as it may appear, it is, in reality, the grand principle of intertropical hygiene, so well understood and practised by all classes and descriptions of natives of the East, and which must ever be kept in view, and regulate our measures for the preservation of health.

Common sense, independently of all observation and reasoning on the subject, might, *a priori*, come to this conclusion. From *heat* spring all those effects which originally *predispose* to the reception or operation of other morbific causes; and how can we obviate those effects of *heat*, but by calling in the aid of its antagonist—cold? To the *sudden* application of the *latter*, after the *former* has effected its baneful influence on the human frame, I have traced most of those diseases attributable to climate : nothing, therefore, can be more reasonable than that our great object should be to moderate by all possible means this heat, and to habituate ourselves, from the beginning, to the impressions of cold; so that we may thus bid defiance to the alternations or vicissitudes of both those powerful agents.

This is, in truth, the grand secret of counteracting the influence of tropical climates on European constitutions; and its practical application to the common purposes of life, as well as to particu-. lar exigencies, shall now be rendered easy and intelligible.

DRESS.

When Europeans enter the tropics they must bid adieu to the luxury of linen—if what is uncomfortable, and indeed unsafe in these climates, can be styled a luxury. The natives of the country, from the lowliest to the highest, wear none but cotton clothes, and those of them who can afford luxuries wear them in the largest quantities.

The waterman of Bengal may be taken as an example of a man who works very hard, on wages of from twopence to fourpence per day. His clothing, like his diet, is scanty and precarious in the extreme; the former amounting only to a narrow piece of cloth passed between the thighs, and fastened before and behind to a piece of stout packthread that encircles the waist. Thus unprotected, he exposes his skin to the action of an intense tropical sun—to a deluge of rain, to the dews of the night, and to a cold piercing north-east monsoon—with equal indifference; and with perspiration issuing at every pore, he darts overboard when necessary, and wades through puddles and marshes—this moment under water, and the next in the open air, with rapid evaporation from the whole body. It is true that he, in some degree, supplies the defect of clothing by the assiduous and regular use of oil friction to the entire surface of the body; but, independently of all and every habit, nature has, by race and from birth, done much to secure the hard-working boatman, by forming both the *colour* and the *texture* of his skin in such a manner that the extreme vessels of the surface are neither violently stimulated by the heat, nor easily struck torpid by sudden transitions to cold. Certain it is also, that the action of the perspiratory vessels is different from those of Europeans, the fluid exuded in the native being more oily and tenacious than the sweat of the former.

The dress of the shepherds, again, throughout Bengal, who are much exposed to all weathers, consists of a blanket gathered in at one end, so as to rest on the head, the rest hanging all round like a cloak. This answers the triple purpose of protection from the hottest sun—of a tent in the rainy season to throw off the wet—and of a coat in the cold season to defend the body from the piercing cold. Thus our ridicule of the Portuguese and Spaniards for wearing their long black cloaks in summer, *to keep them cool,* and in winter, *to keep them warm,* is founded on prejudice rather than on correct observation.

But if we look beyond the hardy labouring classes of natives of Hindustan, we observe both Hindu and Mahomedan guarding most cautiously against solar heat as well as cold. The ample turban and khummerbund meet our eye at every step; the former to defend the head from the direct rays of a powerful sun—the latter for the purpose of preserving the important viscera of the abdomen from the deleterious impressions of cold. The khummerbund is certainly a most valuable part of the dress, and one that is extensively imitated throughout India, by Europeans, in the form of a cotton or flannel waistband, worn generally next the skin.

The cotton dress, from its slowness of conducting heat, is admirably adapted for the tropics. It must be recollected that the temperature of the atmosphere, *sub dio*, in the hot seasons, exceeds that of the blood by many degrees, and even in the shade it too often equals, or rises above the heat of the body's *surface*, which is always, during health, some degrees below 97°.

Here then we have a covering which is *cooler* than linen, inasmuch as it conducts more slowly the *excess* of external heat to our bodies; but this, though a great advantage, is not the only one.

When a *vicissitude* takes place, and the atmospheric temperature sinks suddenly far below that of the body, the cotton covering, faithful to its trust, abstracts more slowly the heat *from* it, and thus preserves to the wearer a more and more steady equilibrium. To all these advantages must be added the facility with which the cotton absorbs perspiration. While linen so circumstanced would feel wet and cold under a breeze, and even occasion a shiver, the cotton dress, as stated, would maintain an equable warmth.

That woollen and cotton dresses should be *warmer* than linen, in low temperatures, will be readily granted; but that they should be *cooler* in high temperatures, will, perhaps, be doubted. But let two beds be placed in the same room during the day, when the thermometer stands at 90°; and let one be covered with a pair of blankets, the other with a pair of linen sheets. On removing both coverings in the evening, the bed on which were placed the blankets will be found cool, the other warm: the linen transmitted the heat of the surrounding air to all the parts beneath it, while the woollen covering, as a non-conductor, prevented and obstructed the transmission of heat from without.

From this view of the subject *flannel* might be supposed superior to *cotton*, and indeed at certain seasons, or in particular places where the mercury often takes a wide range in a very short time, the former is a safer covering than the latter, and is adopted by many experienced and seasoned Europeans. But, in general, flannel is inconvenient for three reasons. First, it is too heavy—an insuperable objection;—secondly, where the temperature of the air ranges pretty steadily a little below that of the skin, the flannel is much too slow a conductor of heat *from* the body. Thirdly, the spiculæ of the flannel prove too irritating, and *increase* the action of the perspiratory vessels on the surface of the body, where our great object is to *moderate* the process. From the second and third objections, indeed, even cotton or calico is not quite free, unless of a fine fabric, when its good qualities far counterbalance any inconvenience in the above respects.

The great object of tropical prophylactics being TO MODERATE,

WITHOUT CHECKING THE CUTICULAR DISCHARGE, I would here enter a caution against a too frequent changing of the body linen, a habit confined to newly arrived Europeans principally.   To change morning and evening is enough for all and every purpose, even in the hot and rainy seasons; and to change oftener is simply injurious.   The property which *frequent* change of linen has, of exciting the cuticular secretion, and the effects resulting from the sympathy of the skin with the stomach, liver, and lungs, may account, in a great measure, for the superior health which accompanies cleanliness in our own climate; and, on the contrary, for many of the diseases of the indigent and slovenly, which are so frequently connected with, or dependent on, irregularity or suppression of the cuticular discharge.   But though this is true, by the injudicious, nay, injurious habit of too frequent change of linen in a tropical climate, the fluids on the surface of the body, already in excess, are thus powerfully solicited, and the action of the perspiratory vessels, with all their associations, morbidly increased instead of being restrained.

The necessity which tyrant custom, or perhaps routine, has hitherto imposed on us, of continuing to appear in European dress, particularly in *uniforms*, on almost all public occasions, and in all formal parties, under a burning sky, is not one of the least miseries of a tropical life !

It is true that this ceremony is waived in the more social circles that gather round the dinner-table, where the light, cool vestures of the East supersede the cumbrous garb of northern climates. But it is laughable, or rather pitiable enough, to behold a set of *griffinish* sticklers for decorum, for some time after each fresh importation from Europe, whom no persuasions can induce to cast off their *exuviæ*, even in the most affable company, pinioned in their stiff habiliments, while the streams of perspiration that issue from every pore, and ooze through various angles of their dress, might almost induce us to fear that they were on the point of realizing Hamlet's wish ; and that, in good earnest, their

> " Solid flesh would melt—
> Thaw, and resolve itself into a dew."

To the above observations on dress may be added, that no European should voluntarily expose himself, at any season, to the direct rays of the sun.   If forced to be out of doors, the chatta should never be neglected, if he wish to guard against coup-de-soleil, or some other dangerous consequence of imprudent exposure.

FOOD.

All must agree with Celsus, that *sanis omnia sana*—and with a late eminent physician, that an attention to *quantity* is of infinitely more consequence than the *quality* of our repasts; and

also that an over-fastidious regard to *either* will render us unfit'
for society, and not more healthy after all; yet, when we change
our native climate for the torrid zone, many of us may find,
when it is too late, that we can hardly attend too strictly to
the quantity and quality of our food during the period of being
accommodated to the new climate; and that a due regulation of
this important matter will turn out a powerful engine in the pre-'
servation of health.

It is now well known, from dire experience, that, instead of a
disposition to *debility* and *putrescency*, a congestive, and sometimes
an inflammatory diathesis, with tendency to general or local plethora, characterizes the European and his diseases, for some years
at least after his arrival between the tropics; and, hence, provident nature endeavours to guard against the evil by diminishing
our relish for food. But, alas! how prone are we to spur the
jaded appetite, not only " by dishes tortured from their native
taste," but by more dangerous stimulants of wine and other liquors,
as well as by condiments and spices, which should be reserved for
that general relaxation and debility which unavoidably supervene
during a *protracted residence* in sultry climates. Here is an instance where we cannot *safely* imitate the seasoned European; for
there are no points of hygiene to which the attention of a new-
comer should be more particularly directed, than to the *quantity
and simplicity* of his viands. They are practical points, entirely
within his own command, and a due regulation of them is not at
all calculated to draw on him the observation of others—a very
great advantage.

That vegetable food is, generally speaking, better adapted to a
tropical climate than animal will be admitted, especially in the
instance of the unseasoned European; not that it is quicker or
easier of digestion, for it is slower, but it excites less commotion
in the system during that process, and is not apt to induce plethora
afterwards. These are the considerations which should give preference to vegetable over animal substances in the diet of the unseasoned European, and which should induce him to be at least
sparing in the use of the latter.

Every valetudinarian, and particularly the hectic, knows full
well the *febrile* movement which follows a full meal; and the same
takes place, more or less, in every individual, whatever may be the
state of health at the time. How cautious should we be then of
exasperating those natural paroxysms, when placed in situations
where various *other* febrific causes are constantly impending over,
or even assailing us! The febrile stricture which obtains on the
surface of our bodies, and in the secerning vessels of the liver,
during the *gastric digestion* of our food, as evinced by diminution
of the cutaneous and hepatic secretions, will be proportioned to
the duration and difficulty of that process in the stomach, and
to the quantity of ingesta; and as a corresponding *increase*

of the two secretions succeeds, when the chyme passes into the
intestines, we perceive the propriety of moderating them by abstemiousness, since they are already in *excess* from the heat of the
climate alone, and this excess is one of the first links in the chain
of causes and effects that leads ultimately to various derangements
of function and of structure in important organs, as exemplified in
the fevers and dysenteries, in the hepatitis and cholera of tropical
regions.

The newly-arrived European should content himself with a plain
breakfast of bread-and-butter, with tea or coffee, and avoid indulging in meat, fish, eggs, or buttered toast. The latter alone
often disagrees, and occasions rancidity, with nausea at stomach,
while it increases the secretion of bile, already in excess. A glance
indeed at the *Bawurchee*, buttering our toast with the greasy wing
of a fowl, or an old dirty piece of rag, will have more effect in restraining the consumption of the article than any didactic precept
which can be laid down ; and a picturesque sight of this kind may
be procured any morning by taking a stroll into the purlieus of
the kitchen.

In regard to dinner, were the European master of both time and
circumstance, the early part of the afternoon should be that of his
principal meal ; but the great majority of men of business, whether
official or mercantile, are unable to disengage themselves during
the day, and thus from seven to eight o'clock becomes the settled
hour.

It is true that military men, excepting such as hold staff offices,
may choose their hour of dinner, but fashion and routine rule this
and other habits ; and the mess hour is too late. The naval captain who exclaimed—" Not eat that ! I will make my stomach
submit to anything," represents more persons in every society,
and in every country, than careless observers dream of. Naval
and military men are, beyond all others, devoted to system, and
to a certain extent justly so. But system, like everything in this
world, may be abused so as to degenerate into something even
worse than mere routine. As matter of fact, regiments in general
have luncheon (" tiffin ") on table at one o'clock, with wine and
ale, and a heavy dinner at seven with more wine and ale. Thus
any officer who is so disposed may become the subject of a daily
feverishness, soon to be followed by disease ; and even such as are
temperately disposed commit excesses in eating and drinking, often
without being aware of it.

An old staff officer in Fort William used to say that he had
known more duels, courts martial, and dismissals to result from
the " tiffin " alone than from any other cause ; but what were the
other results, in the olden times, of the tiffin and the dinner, from
year's end to year's end, there is no man alive now-a-days to tell !
Although a great deal that was objectionable in the double meal
has given way to modern improvement in the general habit of

society throughout India, still too much of both tiffin and dinner remains. Both meals are greatly too much after the European fashion; while strong wine and ale are too liberally circulated, at least for health. Claret—" the cup that cheers and not inebriates" —is always to be preferred.

He then who consults his health in the East will beware of late and heavy dinners, particularly during the period of probation, but will rather be satisfied with a light and early repast as the *principal* meal, when tea or coffee at six or seven o'clock will be found a grateful refreshment. After this his rest will be as natural and refreshing as can be expected in such a climate, and he will rise next morning with infinitely more vigour than if he had crowned a sumptuous dinner with a bottle of wine the previous evening.

Let but a trial of one week put these directions to the test, and they will be found to have a more substantial foundation than *theory*.

A limited indulgence in fruits, during the first year, is prudent; and there is little reason to believe that, when ripe and used in the forenoon, they dispose to irritation of the bowels. Particular kinds of fruits have peculiar effects on certain constitutions; thus, mangoes have sometimes a stimulating and heating effect, which not seldom brings out a plentiful crop of pustules, or even boils, on the unseasoned European. The pine-apple, though very delicious, is not the safest fruit to make too free with at any time. The orange is always grateful and wholesome, and good ripe shaddocks are so likewise, owing to their cooling subacid qualities. The banana is wholesome and nutritious, whether undressed or frittered.

The use of spice or condiment, as already stated, should be reserved for those ulterior periods of our residence in hot climates when the tone of the constitution is lowered, and the stomach participates in the general relaxation. They are then safe and salutary, especially during the rainy season.

DRINK.

In a vast empire such as that of India, held by the frail tenure of opinion, and where the current of all the various religious opinions of the natives runs strong against intoxication, it was early found necessary, from motives of policy rather than of health, to discourage the acquisition of habits at once dangerous and disgraceful. Hence the inebriate has always been justly considered as not merely culpable in destroying his individual health, but as deteriorating the European character in the eyes of the natives, whom it is on all accounts desirable to impress with a just sense of our superiority. It is thus that our power may acquire material substance from the gradually improving convictions of the natives

themselves. Happily, what has been promotive of our own interests has been also preservative of our health, as well as conducive
to our happiness; and the general temperance which now characterizes the European circles of society in the East Indies is most
gratifying. We shall no longer hear from medical or lay writers
of "gently stimulating liquids," used during the forenoon "for
supporting perspiration, and for keeping up the tone of the
digestive organs," for all experience has proved such habits to be
actually pernicious. The European who should now take to such
unworthy indulgences would soon find himself excluded from good
society.

It has already been observed that the great physiological rule
for preserving health in hot climates is—TO KEEP THE BODY COOL.
The strong sympathy that subsists between the skin and the several
internal organs, as the stomach, liver, and intestinal canal, has
also been emphatically referred to. The common sense of mankind would seem indeed to point out the propriety of avoiding
heating drinks, for the same reason that we endeavour instinctively
to guard against a high external temperature. But the truth is
that, until men begin to feel the corporeal ill effects of intemperance,
a deaf ear is turned to the most impressive lectures against the
most deplorable of propensities, that which Napoleon declared to
be the least compatible with greatness. With the feeble and
irresolute the magic bowl, which this moment can raise its votaries
into heroes and demigods, will, in a few hours, sink them beneath
the level of the brute creation. Moralists and philosophers have
long descanted on this theme, but with little success, as few will
attempt to prove that water is the simple and salutary beverage
designed by nature for man; seeing that every nation, even the
most refined, has practically repudiated the doctrine. Let the
medical profession, however, do its duty in portraying truthfully
the ill effects of the abuse of drink, in tropical climates especially.
The truth is that, as drunkenness leads, in a moral point of view,
to every crime, so, in a physical point of view, it promotes the
invasion, and retards the cure, of every tropical or other disease.

It may be received as a truth that, during the first two years of
residence at least, the nearer we approach to a perfectly *aqueous*
regimen in drink, so much the better chance have we of avoiding
sickness; and the more slowly and gradually we deviate from this
afterwards, so much the more retentive shall we be of that invaluable blessing—HEALTH.

In speaking of the means of preserving health, which depends
so much on the tone of the digestive organs, we must not omit
the recent luxury—American ice—which has now become an
article of necessity in the East. It would be out of place here to
speak of its uses in the treatment of various diseases, and of fevers
especially, as those of a cerebral and gastric nature. "Nothing,"
says Dolomieu, "is more salutary during the sirocco than iced

beverages; they revive the spirits, strengthen the body, and assist the digestion." Those who have now, during several years past, made use of this real luxury in the East Indies, need no arguments in favour of promoting so remarkable an instance of American enterprise.

I would caution the newly arrived European against a very common and very dangerous mistake, namely, the acting in matters of diet and exercise on the supposition that he may with impunity do as the elder residents; for it is consonant with experience, as with theory, that the *latter* class may indulge in the luxuries of the table with infinitely less risk than the former. To think and act otherwise is to confound all discrimination between very different habits of body which the seasoned and unseasoned possess.

One other circumstance should always be held in recollection, to wit, that when a course of temperance is fully entered on, and the pleasures of temperance fully enjoyed, no consideration should induce us to commit an occasional debauch, especially during our seasoning, for we are at those times in infinitely greater danger of both endemic and epidemic attacks than the habitual bacchanal.

In the last article it has been stated that the subacid fruits are both grateful and wholesome, and so will it be found with moderately acid drinks, such as sherbet. Nature seems to point out the vegetable acids in hot climates, as grateful in allaying drought and diffusing a coolness from the stomach all over the body. To the temperate and the healthy they will generally prove salutary, and I have never seen or heard of any ill effects from their use.

We hear much amongst vulgar habitual topers of the supposed prophylactic influence of spirits and cigars against night exposure, malaria, and contagion; but no medical observer, in any of our numerous colonies, has ever seen reason to believe in any such delusive doctrine, nor is there in reality the smallest foundation for it. All excitement is followed by a corresponding depression of the vital functions, and it is then that the toper is doubly liable to suffer.

I cannot quit the subject of diet without referring to an after-luncheon habit to be met with in India, and one not infrequently imported home by persons in the position of gentlemen; I mean the habit of beer-soaking. This habit may by insensible degrees degenerate into wine and spirit drinking; and then it is unnecessary to mention the very sad consequences.

Surgeons, whether civil or military, can well understand the beneficial actions of wine or of bitter ale, moderately used, in the other sex, after severe confinements, and during protracted wet-nursing, in an exhausting climate. But, unhappily, one sometimes sees lamentable circumstances connected with such indulgences, when they have become habitual; and all I would here insist on is this—that medical officers may never permit themselves, directly or indirectly, to become parties to the initiation or introduction of such abominations into families. To see an English gentlewoman "much bemused with beer," is surely a spectacle the most humiliating.

EXERCISE.

This is one of the luxuries of a northern climate to which we must, in a great measure, bid adieu between the tropics. The principal object and effect of exercise in the *former* situation appear to consist in keeping up a just balance in the circulation, in supporting and maintaining the functions of the skin, and promoting the various secretions. But the perspiration, biliary, and other secretions being already in excess in equatorial regions, a perseverance in our customary European exercises would prove highly injurious, and it often does so, by promoting and aggravating the ill effects of an unnatural climate. As such excess very soon leads to debility, and to *diminishing action* in the functions alluded to, and to a corresponding *inequilibrium* of the blood, so it is necessary to counteract these by such active or passive exercise as the climate will admit *at particular periods of the day or year ;* a discrimination imperiously demanded if we mean to preserve health. When the sun is near the meridian for several hours of the day on the plains of India, not a leaf is seen to move, every animated being retreats under cover, and even the "adjutant," or gigantic crane of Bengal, soars out of reach of the earth's reflected heat, and either perches on the highest pinnacles of lofty buildings, or hovers in the upper regions of the air, a scarcely discernible speck.

At this time the native retires instinctively to the innermost apartment of his humble shed, where both light and heat are excluded. There he sits quietly in the midst of his family, regaling himself with cold water or sherbet, while a gentle perspiration flows from the skin, and contributes naturally and powerfully to his refrigeration. Mr. Twining justly observes that the natives, both Hindoo and Mahomedan, seem to suffer much from the hot season in Bengal. During the latter part of this season those natives whose circumstances enable them to act as they wish, avoid any exertion as much as possible, reducing the quantity of their food, and eating certain fruits which they consider cooling. In the afternoons they drink the fluid contained in the unripe cocoa-nut, or a very simple sherbet, or some sugar and water, deeming the latter especially cooling; and in the mornings they take an infusion of *Nalta Pàt*, or leaf of the *Corchorus Olitorius*, which they say has a cooling effect, at the same time that it acts as a mild tonic, promoting digestion, and preventing lassitude. He adds that the natives, though adapted by nature to bear the climate, take more care to moderate the effects of heat than Europeans, especially in their light clothing, abstemious food, and tranquil habits.

After this example of the salutary habits of all classes of natives of India, it is hardly necessary to urge the injuriousness of every kind of active exercises to Europeans under tropical heats, and especially during the heats of the day; yet hundreds perished annually from this very cause, particularly in the West Indies, upon each influx of European troops during the late war. Happily it may now be said that, owing to the removal of the European troops from the plains to the mountains, the horrors resulting from the climate of Jamaica have been exchanged for health and comfort. This beneficent act is due to the generous and noble nature of the late Lord Metcalfe, when governor of that island.

Who would expect to find *dancing* a prominent amusement in a tropical climate? The natives of the West Indies are exceedingly fond of this exercise; but those of the East are wise men still, for, instead of dancing themselves, they employ Natch girls to dance for them.

Gestation of every kind, whether in palankeens or spring carriages, is a species of passive exercise exceedingly well adapted to a tropical climate. The languid state of the circulation of the blood, in those who have resided long there, is pointedly exhibited in the disposition which they evince to raise the lower extremities on a line with the body when at rest; and this object is completely attained in the palankeen, which indeed renders it a peculiarly agreeable vehicle.

On the same principle we may explain the feeling of satisfaction and the utility of *shampooing*, where the gentle pressure and friction of the soft Asiatic hand over the surface of the body, but particularly over the limbs, invigorate the circulation after fatigue, as well as after long inaction, and thus excite the insensible cuticular secretion. The kecsa, or hair-glove of India, is an admirable means of giving additional effect to the practice of shampooing, a practice which, to the indolent wealthy natives, proves a real and effective substitute for exercise.

The swing might perhaps be rendered useful in the hot and rainy season in the East Indies. In chronic disorders of the viscera it could hardly fail to be grateful and salutary, by its tendency to determine to the surface and relax the subcutaneous vessels, which are generally torpid in those diseases. It might be practised in the early mornings and evenings within doors, whenever the weather or other circumstances do not admit of gestation in the open air.

BATHING.

Moseley's caution to the European residents of his day in the West Indies, may be recorded for the benefit of all who think that, in hot climates, they may do what they please with cold water:—" I DARE not recommend cold bathing; it is death with intemperance, and dangerous where there is any fault in the viscera. It is a luxury denied to *almost all*, except the sober and abstemious females, who well know the delight and advantage of it." The cold bath *is* death, not *during* intemperance, but in the collapse which *follows* a debauch, or indeed any other great fatigue of mind or body. It is also dangerous under every form of visceral disease, but the healthy and temperate of habit may as safely partake of the "delight and advantage" of the cold bath as Dr. Moseley's "sober and abstemious females." The truth is, that the cold bath is a prize due to, and gained by, the temperate. To all else it is eminently unsafe, as any naval and military surgeon of tropical experience can testify. To the European resident in tropical climates whose constitution is sound, and whose habits are temperate, no more efficient means exists of obviating the most unpleasant effects even of the cold season ; for he who reacts well under the cold bath will not be troubled with dry skin, and sense . of internal fulness. To persons of ordinary health, but who are not robust, the cold bath will be found tonic and agreeable from the beginning of March, in India generally, to the end of September. The temperature ranges high in these months, and the determination to the surface is such as to ensure a sufficient reaction. It is a common error to think that, before using the cold bath, we must be *cooled* first, while the very opposite rule is the correct one. To the delicate, indeed, immersion in a *warm* bath for a few minutes is an excellent preliminary, followed at once by *affusion* of some three or four vessels of *cold* water. A glow over the whole surface of the body will immediately follow. This is a safe and excellent mode of bathing to all who shrink from or who feel doubtful of salutary reaction from the use of cold water.

We hear warm and cold bathing recommended without reference to the state of health, to the season, or to regularity of habit, although these circumstances should form essential preliminaries to the choice. It may be concluded for certain that, to persons who have suffered from tropical disease, or who are affected with visceral congestions, or with visceral enlargements especially, the results of fevers or dysenteries, the *warm* bath is the only safe one *at all seasons*. The same rule applies to the dissipated, and to such as are in the habit of keeping late hours. In such persons the balance of circulation is already disturbed, and the effect of cold water is to throw the blood with force on organs already irritated by irregular courses of life, the abdominal viscera especially.

Under such unfavourable circumstances it is not to be expected that the "conservative energies" should be capable of being "roused to successful resistance ;" with the whole external surface parched, and with the digestive mucous surfaces in a state of irritation, how can it be otherwise?

As many persons have but an imperfect knowledge of the relative temperatures of the several baths in ordinary use, the following scale is here presented :—

Cold bath, from	60° to 75°
Tepid bath, from	85° to 92°
Warm bath, from	92° to 98°
Hot bath, from	98° to 112°

By the healthy and temperate European, the use of the *cold* bath should be regularly and daily persevered in, from the moment of his entrance within the tropics ; and when, from long residence there, the functions above referred to begin to be irregular or defective, he may prudently veer round by degrees to the use of the *tepid* bath, which will then be found a most valuable part of tropical hygiene.

The use of the cold bath being a passive operation, unattended by any exercise, it may be used at any period of the day, although the mornings and evenings are generally selected by Europeans in the East ; immediately after leaving their couch, and before dinner. On both occasions the bath is very refreshing, and it powerfully obviates that train of nervous symptoms so generally complained of by our countrymen in hot climates. Before dinner it seems to exert its salutary influence on the surface of the body, and by sympathy, on the stomach, removing the disagreeable sensation of thirst which might otherwise induce a too free use of potation during the repast. It is always imprudent to bathe while the process of digestion in the stomach is going on, as it disturbs that important operation.

SLEEP.

When we bid adieu to the temperate climate of Europe, with its " long nights of revelry," and enter the tropics, we may count on a great falling off in this " solace of our woes." The disturbed repose which we almost always experience there, has a greater eventual influence on our constitutions than is generally supposed, notwithstanding the silence of authors on this subject. Whatever we subtract from the requisite period of our natural sleep will surely be deducted, in the end, from the natural range of our exis- tence, independently of the predisposition to disease which is thus constantly generated. This is a melancholy but a true reflection, and it should induce us to exert our rational faculties in obviating so great an evil.

The great object of the European is to sleep cool, and obtain complete protection from mosquitoes.* Happily both advantages

* Sydney Smith's description of the insects in tropical climates is at least character- istic of the author :— " Insects are the curse of tropical climates. The bête rouge lays the foundation of a tremendous ulcer. In a moment you are covered with ticks. Chigoes bury themselves in your flesh, and hatch a large colony of young chigoes in a few hours. They will not live together ; but every chigo sets up a separate ulcer, and has its own private portion of pus. Flies get entry into your mouth, into your eyes, into your nose ; you eat flies, drink flies, and breathe flies. Lizards, cockroaches, and snakes get into the bed ; ants eat up the books ; scorpions sting you in the feet. Everything bites, stings, or bruises ; every second of your existence you are wounded

may be secured to the temperate by the large mosquito frame and curtain with punkah suspended from the ridge, as now prevalent throughout Bengal. This is not only luxurious but safe, the gentle agitation of the punkah removing the heated air surrounding the body without exposing the person to the dangers arising from sudden night changes in the temperature or humidity of the atmosphere.

The European is thus enabled to procure more and sounder rest than he could possibly do otherwise; and by giving his frame a more thorough and complete respite from the great stimulus of heat, he imparts to it tone and vigour, so necessary to meet the exhaustion of the ensuing day, as well as to repair that of the pre-ceding. Early hours are here indispensable; for the fashionable nocturnal dissipations of Europe would soon cut the thread of our existence within the tropics. The order of nature is never inverted with impunity, even in the most temperate climates; beneath the torrid zone it is certain destruction. The hour of retirement to repose should never be protracted beyond ten o'clock; and at daylight we should start from our couch to enjoy the cool, the fragrant, and salubrious breath of morn.

Without some artificial aid, such as that above mentioned, a great waste of strength—indeed of life—may arise from our inabi-lity to obtain *cool* repose at night. The cold and rainy seasons, heavy dews, or exhalations from contiguous jungles or marshes, often render it impossible with safety to sleep in the *open air ;* a practice, during the *hot season*, fraught with refreshing benefit, where the obstacles mentioned do not prevent its execution.

In Bengal Proper, in the plains of Upper India, and on the Coromandel coast, except during the hot land-winds there, or at the change of the monsoons, Europeans may generally indulge, during the hot and dry season, in the luxury of sleeping in the open *verandahs,* not only with safety, but with infinite advantage. It is an old habit throughout most parts of India, especially of the military classes; and the judicious Captain Williamson says justly that, while it is attended with the greatest refreshment,

by some piece of animal life that nobody has ever seen before, except Swammerdam and Meriam.

"An insect with eleven legs is swimming in your teacup, a nondescript with nine wings is struggling in the small-beer, or a caterpillar with several dozen eyes in his belly is hastening over the bread-and-butter! All nature is alive, and seems to be gathering all her entomological hosts to eat you up as you are standing, out of your coat, waistcoat, and breeches. Such are the tropics. All this reconciles us to our dews, fogs, vapours, and drizzle—to our apothecaries rushing about with gargles and tinc-tures—to our old, British, constitutional coughs, sore-throats, and swelled faces."

After this we may not denounce as extravagant Dr. Clarke's account of the climate of the Crimea :—"If you drink water after eating fruit," he says, "a fever follows. If you eat milk, eggs, or butter, a fever. If, during the scorching heat of the day, you indulge in the most trivial neglect of clothing, a fever. If you venture out to enjoy the delightful breezes of the evening, a fever. In short, such is the dangerous nature of the climate to strangers, that Russia must consider the country a cemetery for the troops which are sent to maintain its possession."

enabling them to rise early, divested of that most distressing lassitude attendant upon sleeping in a close oppressive apartment, communicating a febrile sensation, very few instances could be adduced of any serious indisposition attending it. Healthy and temperate persons, and who are habituated to the use of the cold bath, need be under no. apprehensions, excepting at the places and seasons alluded to, as to transitions from the scorching heat of the day to the serenity of night, for indeed it is gradual and easy.

Those who habitually exclude themselves from the breath of heaven, whether from inclination or necessity, become languid from the *continued* operation of heat and want of repose :—even the slightest aërial vicissitude, or admission of a partial current of cool air, unhinges the tenor of their health, and deranges the functions of important organs. These are they who require the afternoon *siesta*, and to whom indeed it is necessary, on account of the abridged refreshment and sleep of the night; while the others are able to go through the avocations of the day without any such substitute—a manifest and great advantage.

A few words on the incubus, or nightmare—a troublesome visitor to the tropical couch—may properly conclude this section.

From the results of treatment it would appear that the primary cause has its seat in the digestive organs, in whatever way it may act; and that the nightmare originates in defective digestion, producing heartburn, flatulence, griping and eructation, with a train of dyspeptic complaints.

Of all medicines, the carbonate of soda will be found the most efficacious, taken in scruple doses at bedtime, or night and morning, in some aromatic water, such as the peppermint. This medicine not only neutralizes the acids of the stomach, but it promotes the elimination of the bile, and the evacuation of slimy discharges from the bowels.

There are few people with whom particular kinds of food do not disagree, and, being known, these should be avoided. Thus, chestnuts or sour wine will almost always produce incubus in those predisposed to it, as was observed by Hildanus :—" *Qui scire cupit quid sit incubus? Is ante somnum comedat castaneas, et superbibat vinum fæculentum.*" In this country, cucumbers, nuts, apples, and flatulent kinds of food are the articles most likely to bring on nightmare.

THE CONDUCT AND GOVERNMENT OF THE PASSIONS.

Most of the precepts that apply to the regulation and government of the passions in cold climates will be found to apply to them in tropical climates; but it is necessary to correct at once an erroneous impression that there is something peculiar to the tropics which excites certain passions in a higher degree than in temperate regions.

Dr. Moseley says that "there is in the inhabitants of hot climates, unless present sickness has an absolute control over the body, *a promptitude and a bias to pleasure,* and an alienation from serious thought and deep reflection. The brilliancy of the skies and the beauty of the atmosphere conspire to influence the nerves against philosophy and her rigid tenets, and forbid their practice among the children of the sun." However true this description may be in respect of "the children of the sun," it does not accurately exhibit the condition of the stranger European, in whom such a course of relaxation would be very immoral; for such a view would furnish the dissolute libertine with a *physical* excuse for his debaucheries, when the real source might be traced to laxity of religious and moral principle. We would ask Dr. Moseley if the "*promptitude* and bias to pleasure" be increased in hot climates, why the *ability* to pursue or practise it should be lessened? a fact well known to every debauchee.

It has been asked, says Hennen, what has the medical topographer to do with the morals of the natives of a country? and it has been asserted that their immoralities cannot affect the health of troops quartered amongst them, if proper discipline be observed. Such opinions are founded upon a very superficial view of the subject; for the soil and inhabitants, he adds, always react on each other. A sober and industrious race of people will, for example, have a greater desire to improve their country than men of a contrary character, and will also possess greater physical power to carry their desire into execution. Place such a body of men in a district overrun with noxious weeds and timber, and fast degenerating into a morass, and can there exist any rational doubt that they will clear it sooner, and preserve it longer in that improved state than men of a different disposition? Place in a similar situation, or even in a district thus improved, a body of men who are idle and intemperate, and the immediate result will be that the soil will deteriorate for want of proper care, the weeds will reappear, the drains will become obstructed, the edible products of the earth will lessen in quantity, and diminish in their nutritive quality; the inhabitants will become unhealthy from the bad state of their grounds; and the diminution of their physical powers thus produced will disable them progressively more and more from remedying the causes of the evil. Many of these effects will doubtless first be felt in their own persons, but it is undeniable that they must ultimately operate on their visitors. On this obvious principle is founded the axiom in medical topography— " that a slothful, squalid-looking population invariably characterizes an unhealthy country."

Whether the founders of the Hindu faith acted designedly or otherwise, there can be no doubt that, by depressing all the physical energies by a diet purely vegetable, they fastened with a firmer and stronger band the bonds of Brahminical domination on the people of India, until a chain, forged only by superstition, became, in progress of fifty centuries, and through the most powerful of moral and physical agencies, strong as death.

"The use of certain kinds of food and drink," says Cabanis, "may tend to confirm or impair certain moral habits. Sometimes it may operate directly, and by the immediate impressions which it produces; at other times, by the different states of health or disease which it occasions, or by the changes in the fluids and solids which result from it; for all these different alterations in the system soon manifest themselves more or less distinctly in the ordinary dispositions of the will and understanding."

The same great authority in the physiology of climates adds that, "the poor diets prescribed by the legislators of various religions orders, have never had the effect of diminishing the venereal appetite, but have, on the contrary, inflamed these propensities the more, or disordered the imagination in diminishing the physical forces; and thus men have been rendered more feeble, more unhappy, and more easy of domination."

But let us hope that, in respect of the natives of India, the all-powerful benefits of education, and the example of their European governors, may enable them to conquer the influences of climate, and of the depraving religious and political habits of ages. To expect, however, that such changes can be speedily effected were contrary to reason and experience. The caste is of unknown antiquity. "Neither the proselytizing sword of the Mussulman, nor the mild light of Christianity, has had any influence upon it, and the Hindu still worships before the altars of his gods with the same devotion as when Orpheus charmed the wild beasts by the sounds of his lyre, and when Moses ascended Mount Sinai. Religion, manners, customs, costume, civilization, all have remained immovable as the temples hewn out of the granite rocks of Ellora."

After what has been here stated, it cannot be questioned that the habits and character of the people amongst whom we live, during many years, must have a powerful influence on our morals. But to return to the condition of the stranger European. The removal of religious and moral restraint, the temptations to vice, the facility of the means, and the force of example, are the real causes of this bias to pleasure; and in respect to the *effects* of licentious indulgences between the tropics, the reader may be assured that he will find, perhaps when too late, how much more dangerous and destructive they are than in Europe.

The nature of the supposed "propensity" has been explained to him; and as the principal cause resides neither in the air, nor in the "brilliancy of the skies," but in his own breast, he has no excuse for permitting it to grow into the wild luxuries of unbridled excess.

The monotony of life and the apathy of mind so conspicuous in hot climates, together with the obstacles to matrimony, in former times led too often to vicious and immoral connexions with native females, which speedily sapped the foundations of principles imbibed in early youth, and involved a train of consequences not seldom embarrassing, if not embittering every subsequent period of life. It is here that a taste for some of the more refined and elegant species of literature will prove an invaluable acquisition for dispelling *ennui*—the moth of mind and body.

MILITARY HYGIENE, OR PRESERVING OF THE SOLDIER'S HEALTH.

M. Thiers remarks that in ordinary histories of war we see only armies completely formed and ready to enter into action ; but it can scarcely be imagined what efforts it costs to bring the armed man to his post, equipped, fed, trained, and lastly, cured, if he has been sick or wounded. All these difficulties are increased in proportion to the change of climate, or the distance to which the army moves from the point of departure. Most generals and governments, he says, neglect this kind of attentions, and their armies melt away visibly. Those only who practise them with perseverance and skill find means to keep their troops numerous and well-disposed.

Cormenin says truly, that details govern the world ; and Ballyet states as confidently that, in an army, contempt for organization is nothing less than contempt for human life. Both aphorisms have an especial reference to the moral and physical welfare of organized bodies of men, such as fleets and armies. It is different with civil communities, in which the defects of law and of details are to some extent compensated by the moral attitude and conduct of the people. Lord Macaulay expresses this fact when he declares that the Scotch would be well governed without any laws, or under the worst laws, while the Irish would be ill governed under the best laws. But it is not so with an army—an organized and artificial body, in which good regulations and " details" are everything.

It is a beneficent law, also, that all sanitary measures more than repay their costs, and it applies to all such measures, whether in civil or military life. " It is a mean consideration," says the Examiner, " though a true one, that protection against waste mortality arising from neglect of the known laws of nature, leads to a sure saving in money, and that the sanitary physician is the best of recruiting officers."

Of the efforts and difficulties spoken of by M. Thiers, those of the medical officer are not the least ; although nowhere else, if he were fully trusted, could his services be so effective as in the preserving of the soldier's health. As it is, his disadvantages are endless. He is consulted, perhaps on active service, through ignorance or caprice, often when it is too late, but more generally not at all; and thus the soldier always suffers. In the British armies, at home and abroad, the rule is to leave everything, even of a sanitary nature, to the proper authorities, as they are called; and thus much is on all occasions found to be wanting. There is nothing so difficult to deal with, whether in public or private life, as the troubles we create for ourselves. We boast of our " strong towers," in other words, of our stalwart British soldiers; but so careless are we of the sanitary welfare of the matrix whence we derive them, that in the capitals of the three kingdoms there were rejected, of military recruits, between the years 1833 and 1837, nearly fifty per cent. At this rate, were we to require an army of 100,000 men, we must expect that 50,000 would be rejected; for the three capitals are by no means so unhealthy as many of the provincial towns.

Hitherto unhealthiness has been the rule in our armies, and it has often proved but another name for national humiliation and disaster, not to speak of enormous pecuniary sacrifices. In our foreign possessions during peace, and in our foreign enterprises during war, the rule of unhealthiness has been without any exception. We have often got into disasters before we have seen the enemy, and our campaigns have frequently presented the saddest pages in our military history. Our armies have, on more than one occasion, been conquered by their own commanders—conquered and destroyed by the very organization and system of the British army.

When a commander by sea or land is invested with authority, he always desires it to be understood that he is complete master of the situation—that he knows everything, and will do everything. But when such a man knows little, and does less, as too frequently happens, then the results are sure to be disastrous, whether we look to considerations of health or to the completion of warlike enterprises. The truth is that governments may confer material power on governors, admirals, and generals, but if they do not possess moral power, it is as nothing.

Nor are ignorance and neglect of matters affecting the health of the soldier confined, as is supposed in civil life, to blundering and ill-informed lieutenants : far otherwise is the case. When very young, and serving in one of the most pestilential countries known in India, I made a topographic examination of the localities, and reported the result to my commanding officer, suggesting at the same time what I regarded as the most suitable arrangement for encamping the men against the coming rainy season, when it was well known that a great increase of deadly fever would result. The answer was—" I'll be d——d if I do."

Now, here was no blundering lieutenant, but, on the contrary, one of the most able and well-informed field-officers I have ever known ; yet, such was his treatment of a grave matter of duty, and the neglect of which, before the year was over, cost him his life.

Again, on landing at Rangoon, during the first Burmese war, I was credibly informed that the superintending surgeon of the Bengal division there had warned the officer commanding that, without fresh animal food and vegetables, the European soldiers must perish from scurvy. The answer was characteristic, and somewhat more civil than that granted to me. It was this :— " Medical opinions are very good, sir—when they are called for."

Here, also, was no blundering subaltern, but a gray-headed general of reputation, and one who received much honour and profit after his army had perished miserably. How fell is ignorance or weakness when armed with might !

If it be asked how come these things, I answer that it has always been so, and that it always will continue to be so—until it is ordered otherwise. We have hitherto encountered the combined horrors of disease without remedies, and those of climate without protection, and it will so continue with us until persons in command shall be held responsible, in short, for ignorance and neglect of duty. Until this shall be done, it will be in vain to expect that we can in future escape from the administrative collapse of all the departments of the army which so disgraced and ruined us in the Crimea. Mr. J. C. Robertson, late Governor of Agra, remarking on the general question, says—" It may, perhaps, be thought that the duly-qualified subordinate can always supply, by his suggestions, the deficiencies of his superior ; but they know little of the military variety of the genus *homo* who would rely upon such suggestions being frankly made or kindly received. The spirit is nullified, but not extinct, which prompted the reply of a general in the war of 1757 to some wise hint of the youthful Washington. ' Silence, sir; things have come to a pretty pass indeed, when a British general is to be instructed by a Virginia Buckskin !' " I question much whether the old ignorant grudge is in any degree " nullified" which has at all times caused our admirals and generals to eschew common sense as well as science. But the common sense of the country is being made manifest through an influential press, and it becomes more felt in the army and navy every day.

In all our wars, pestilence will everywhere be found to form their most dismal and affecting page ; yet it need not have been so. In none of our most fatal expeditions—in that of Rangoon, for instance—was there any actual necessity for serving decayed rations to our men, or for exposing them through the hot and rainy seasons to excessive fatigue, to the rank air and damp encampment—there to be destroyed without notice and without remembrance.

Governments and communities sympathize readily enough with the soldier's triumphs, but not with his perils and sufferings. Of sympathy with his sufferings from hunger and thirst—from long and forced marches under the burning sun and the heavy dew—

from the cold bivouac—from the long suspense attending field operations; with these, and with his sufferings from inscrutable pestilence, there is but little sympathy; yet they are, after all, the most ordinary as well as the hardest trials of war. For one soldier who is struck down on the field of battle, ten, sometimes twenty, are lost to their country through the unappreciated hardships here briefly recounted. England, often engaged in great wars, is, of all nations, the most slow to learn the real nature of war and of its requirements; and when peace arrives, all the experiences of former wars are forgotten in the pursuits of commerce. When we complain of inhumanity, military errors, and disastrous national failures, political adventurers and sophists are always ready to declare that "we have not suffered more than we have invariably done before on many similar occasions." Such men always have an eye to fair seemings, hollow consistencies, and present conveniences, rather than to truth or humanity.

As a familiar example of the results of mismanagement on the part of governments and commanders, I shall here only notice the hospital arrangements during former wars, and especially the general hospital system. Pringle, writing a hundred years ago, says: "Among the chief causes of sickness and mortality in an army, the reader will little expect that I should rank the hospitals themselves, though intended for its health and preservation, and that on account of the bad air and other inconveniences attending them." Robert Jackson is even more detailed and emphatic in his condemnation of general hospitals, and he quotes the military writer of George the Second's time who characterized this institution as "the destroyer of the army." The truth is that the physical ills they produced, by generating new diseases tending to fatal relapses and counteracting recovery, repressing zeal in the regimental surgeons, and causing delay in early treatment, were not surpassed by their moral ills, which went to destroy the best feelings of the man, and by consequence the highest qualities of the soldier. Here, if anywhere, one would have expected some deference to medical opinion, but the system continued in all its horrors.

The general hospital system, if system it could be called, sprung up afresh for the use of the infantry, and was employed on a large scale in Holland in 1794-95, and the mortality was enormous, ending in "dreadful destruction;" while the cavalry, which "traversed the same fields and lived in the same air," but which carried its own sick and treated them regimentally, had "little or no mortality in the whole course of its service." It was the same with some few corps of infantry that adopted the regimental plan of management. In the parliamentary report of the Military Commission of 1808, the general hospital system is described as "attended with the most destructive consequences to the sick soldiers, and that it has produced expenditure and waste of every kind." Again, we find "the accumulated horrors of ill-arranged hospitals," in other words, the terrible consequences of *hospital miasm*, frequently alluded to during the Peninsular war by the historian Alison. "The military hospitals," he says, "charged sometimes with twenty thousand sick at a time, fostered contagion rather than cured disease;" while the government of England, that lavished its millions on the vain and irregular efforts, prompted by the presumptuous folly of the Spaniards, left their general no funds "to pay for hospital necessaries" for the use and comfort of his sick and wounded soldiers. "The mortality in general hospitals," says Dr. Knox, "after battles, is so terrible to behold, that I feel convinced it would be preferable to tend the wounded in the open field." But, in truth, these general hospitals are establishments to which our soldiers have been consigned, not so much on account of the accidents of war, as through diseases caused by the ignorance and improvidence of our commanders, who have on many occasions proved consummate masters in the art of ruining their own armies. In our military history, how often have the most incompetent commanders proved a fate to the British soldier !

A correspondent writing from the Crimea, in December, 1854, says, "All the officers here concur in describing the general hospital at Balaclava as a perfect pest-house." Thus, from the days of George II., general hospitals have in no way improved on acquaintance; if, indeed, without a previous and complete reformation of our military system, so bad an institution, as formed by us abroad, be capable of improvement.*

---

* "The army, at the census of 1851, consisted of 142,870 officers and men, of whom 66,424 were stationed in the United Kingdom, 2948 on passage out or home, and 73,498 abroad in the colonies and in the East Indies. The annual mortality of men in civil life at home of the corresponding ages is at the rate of 9 in 1000, but the mortality of the troops at home probably exceeds 15 per 1000, and the mortality of the troops abroad, and chiefly in the tropical climates, is such that the mortality of the whole army is said to be at the rate of 30 in 1000 in time of peace. At these rates, 3290 officers and soldiers die abroad annually, of whom about 2193 belong to England, whose names, whatever their connexion with property may be, never appear on the English registers. In the time of war the deaths in the army abroad are raised in two ways; by the augmentation of the forces, and the increased rate of mortality from wounds and from the diseases that have hitherto been incidental to warfare in the field. Thus the mean strength of the British force, officers and men, in the Peninsula, was 66,372 ; the deaths during the forty-one months that ended May 25th, 1814, were 35,525, of which only 9948 happened in battle or as the consequences of wounds : 225 per 1000 of the 61,511 men, were, on an average, upon the sick list, and their annual mortality was at the rate of 161 per 1000.

"To the ordinary deaths of officers and soldiers abroad in 1854 must be added the excess of deaths in the war, which have been caused partly by the extension of the same epidemic of cholera that has prevailed in England, and partly by diarrhœa, dysentery, and other diseases that, like cholera, are made fatal by lying on the ground, by the use of impure water, by dirt and damp, by privation, and by the substitution of salt pork, rum, and biscuits, for the fresh meat, vegetables, bread, fruit, ale, stout, or wine, that officers and men, like the rest of the people, live on at home.

"Sixty-one thousand of the deaths in England, during the year 1854, are referable to the imperfect operation of the sanitary organization of our towns. And the same

When general hospitals must of military necessity be established at the base of operations, even for a short time, their inmates should consist only of such sick and wounded men as cannot be removed to better quarters, and *crowding* ought, above all things, to be carefully avoided; the position, construction, and arrangement being at the same time of the most approved kind; the charge and control being conferred on medical officers of rank and experience, in order that the various abuses, moral, medical, and financial, inherent in the general hospital system, may be guarded against as far as possible. It ought also to be made an understood matter, in the establishment of all field general hospitals, that they should be but temporary, and that they should be abolished at the earliest possible moment.

When the scene of war is in Europe, the sick and wounded should invariably be sent home, where well-arranged and well-administered general hospitals ought to be, and may easily be established in permanence, both for the more systematic treatment of the sick, and for the purposes of schools of professional training to all medical officers, previously to entering on the duties of the army.

So long as the now-existing system of mixed and confused military government holds in England, I see but little hope of our attaining to excellence in general hospital management at or near the scene of field operations abroad. In 1854-55 we were roused by a national clamour, and we effected improvements under violent external pressure. Such pressure is neither safe in itself, nor is it, perhaps, likely to recur. With our command of shipping, this removal of the men from the scene of war may always be done, and there is no just reason for neglecting this duty to the soldier. It is never neglected in the instance of the officer. Our base of operation too, in all our European wars, has been, and must be, the sea.

As illustrative of this subject I may mention that, previously to enlarging the accommodations of the Smallpox Hospital in London, erysipelas, typhus, malignant cynanchy, and other formidable diseases were common; but by spreading the same number of cases over double the extent of surface, these terrible consequences of crowding have been altogether avoided.

causes, exaggerated certainly, with the absence of the comforts and necessaries that are supplied at home, have led to the deplorable destruction of life in the Crimea.

"The deaths, in an average year, among 54,000 in the town and country population of England at the same ages as the men in the army, are 486, or nearly 41 monthly, and about 972 are constantly sick. All the deaths and sickness in excess of these numbers, except the deaths and wounds from battle, are, like the excess of deaths and sickness in our towns, referable to conditions that, in the present state of engineering, chemical and medical science, may be removed to a considerable extent in ordinary climates, even in the field and in the presence of an enemy; for the art of preserving life has, since the Peninsular campaigns, made as much progress as the manufacture of arms, and if skilfully applied, our army will never again endure the mortality from disease that so much impaired its efficiency once in the Peninsula, and again, after the lapse of more than forty years, in the Crimea."—Dr. William Farr; *Reports of the Registrar-General.*

Respecting the ill-regulated general hospitals for seamen and soldiers, the ill-situated and ill-ventilated hospitals of old in our great cities, one might reasonably have asked with Ponteau, " Are hospitals, then, more pernicious than useful to society ?" So much for one item only of neglect, in matters affecting the preservation of the soldier's health.   Those who desire to see further into the health history of the British army will find other numerous sources of disease and death in the land forces, narrated in the famous speech of Earl Grey, delivered in the House of Lords on the 8th of April, 1854.   This noble address went far to inform and confirm public opinion ; and public opinion in this country need rarely be mistrusted if it is but formed on sound knowledge and pronounced with due care ; but the subject is a difficult one.

" The administration of an army," says Audouin, " is sometimes called a trade, but those who understand the subject know that it is a science, and one of so complicated a character that the study of one of its branches might occupy a long life.   To comprehend even the elements of the administration of an army, it is neces- sary to know its origin, progress, and rules ; the various means employed to raise soldiers, organize, arm, equip, pay, and put them in motion ; to subsist them in health and in sickness ; to command them in the field of battle ; to profit by their success ; to remedy their failures ; to reward and to punish them ; and to preserve an account of their fortunate and unfortunate operations."—*Histoire de l'Administration de la Guerre.*

Referring more especially to the preserving of the soldier's health, I would quote the sensible observations of Hennen, who, speaking of the prophylactic value of medicines, says that he does not question their proper use in the cases of reflecting individuals ; " but I don't hesitate to say, first—that they cannot be generally applicable to a whole corps or garrison.   Secondly, that although the soldier may submit in passive obedience, he will invariably make himself amends, as he supposes, for the restriction, by subse- quent excess of one kind or other ; and thirdly, although military officers are sufficiently enamoured of any favourite theory origi- nating with themselves, they view the proposals of medical officers but too often with a jealous eye, especially when the advantages to be derived from them are merely prospective.   We possess the power, by means of the established medical inspections, to meet the approaching disease as early as possible, but I question the prudence, in a military view, of anticipating it before its arrival by a general administration of medicine throughout the garrison; because nearly thirty years' experience has convinced me that no power on earth will reconcile British soldiers to taking physic *en masse*, when they are not sick, nor will they ever view the man who orders it in any other light than that of a speculative experi- mentalist.

" The true preventives to disease are shelter from the heat of the

day, and from the dews and cold of night, avoiding the neighbourhood of marshes and other unhealthy spots in military exercises,
mounting guards at such an hour that the least possible number of
fatigue-parties may be employed in conveying dinners, &c.; timing
duties in such a way that the men may enjoy their natural sleep;
regulating the messes so that the soldier shall always have a due
proportion of vegetables, and especially a comfortable breakfast
before going on morning duties; furnishing every man with flannel
waistcoats and cotton shirts,* enforcing personal cleanliness by
frequent bathing, and by daily washing the feet, &c.; but, above
all, regulating the canteen, so that access can be had to liquor only
in the evening, and then taking every precaution that the bad
spirits and sour wine of the country be rigidly withheld. We may
refine as much as we choose, and we may modify our plans
according to circumstances with critical precision, but these are
the basis on which health is founded, so far as the soldier is individually concerned."

Of all the causes which tend to the premature destruction of the
British soldier in our intertropical possessions, none are so powerful as the neglect in selecting proper localities for camps and cantonments, together with the neglect of suitable structural arrangements in his barracks and hospitals. As compared to these neglects,
the other ills, although great, sink into comparative insignificance.

The dieting of the soldier is another question which greatly
concerns his comfort, health, and efficiency, but which has not yet
received from authority all the attention due to it; and with the
exception that breakfast has been allowed him, I understand that
in most of our colonies the coarse sameness of his food, and the
same inferior cooking of it, remain as in 1793. This subject demands the attentive consideration of competent persons—a complete revision and reform—so that the soldier's food should be
ordered to suit his wants, and changed so as to be adapted to the
various climates in which he serves. He should also be instructed
to dress his food in a palatable, wholesome manner; and these
things can be done with little cost or trouble.

The same indifference is still, after ages of heavy-priced experience, manifested in the ordering of the soldier's clothing and
head-dress throughout our intertropical colonies, no adequate
arrangement being as yet made for climate, for peace or war
service, for the night and day duties.

All the best officers concur in the recommendation of Robert
Jackson, to permit the soldier to do for himself whatever he can do
without injury to his health and discipline; and I feel quite assured

---

* During the hot and rainy season in Bengal the shirt should be changed after exercise, and friction with a dry cloth used at the time of changing; indeed, every soldier
should be supplied with a complete flannel dress, to be worn after the march, or other
fatigue duty, while his clothes are being dried. The bedding should also be daily
exposed to the sun.

that, as regards his food, as one example out of several, there is much truth in the suggestion.

As already stated, I do not believe that there is any one cause so effective to the destruction of the British soldier all over the world, as that of the neglect of fitting positions and other arrangements for the temporary and the permanent encampment of our troops.

In Holland, in 1794; at Walcheren, in 1809-10; on the Guadiana, in 1810; in Varna, in 1854, the same grave errors were committed. To station our soldiers in the plains, at the embouchures of rivers and low harbours in our Eastern and Western intertropical possessions, and in the south of Europe, is to place them where they are sure to die without any necessity. There never can, indeed, exist under any circumstances any reasons of military or political necessity for destroying an army; it is a mere subterfuge and misrepresentation, under which no ignorant or negligent commander should be allowed to shelter himself for a moment. If a disgraceful capitulation is punishable with death, surely some punishment should attach to the wanton sacrifice of an army from causes easy of prevention. Wellington is supposed, by those who know but little of him, to have been considerate towards his men; but his planting of his army in the plains of the Guadiana was a wanton sacrifice, the insalubrity of the country having long been notorious. Sir Charles Napier confirms this view of his character :—" Again, why did he stay in the destructive marshes of the Alemtejo until nearly the whole of the army fell from sickness? It is not easy to comprehend all this, and I have heard no good answer to it." Speaking of Wellington and his generals, he adds—" England has paid dearly in men and money for his education indeed, yet if he has thereby been made a good general, the loss is less. We have very few capable of being made worth a straw, though all the blood and gold of Europe and India were lavishly expended on them." This should seem to be the just estimate of Wellington and his lieutenants :—His hard, narrow intellect and great common sense were slow of being opened and matured : with the others, no amount of sacrifices and experiences could make them "worth a straw."

The extravagant contemporary laudations of Wellington are easily explained. He was a Tory and an aristocrat at a time when Toryism and Aristocracy were rampant.

> "The civil power then snored at ease,
> While soldiers fired to keep the peace."

Abercromby and Moore were only gentlemen, and they bore the sign of the Beast, both of them having been Whigs. Wellington rose far above the sense even of military responsibility, but his great memory will suffer for his neglect of the soldier. Sir William Clinton " considered the Duke of Wellington in most respects an able, but also a very fortunate general—fortunate chiefly in respect of the character of the troops when brought into action, but he also considered him a bad soldier, inasmuch as he neglected the health of his troops and greatly undervalued the medical department. Sir William Clinton mentioned, amongst others, Sir John Moore as being in every sense both a good general and a good soldier—the latter meaning a general who promoted the health and comforts of his troops."

So far back as 1835 I urged on the supreme government of India, as part of a measure sanctioned and carried at my sole instance and recommendation by Sir Charles Metcalfe, then Governor-General of India, for " Collecting Sanitary Reports from all Districts, Stations, and Cantonments in the three Presidencies of India," the following preliminary clause, namely, that

" The topographical reports, when forwarded to each Presidency by the superintending surgeons, shall then be collated by a committee of three medical officers, nominated by the medical boards, and that such as are approved shall be printed and formed into a memoir, a copy of which shall be furnished to all staff-surgeons and officers of the Quartermaster-General's department."

By this clause I intended that information on the all-important question of medical topography should be imparted to the officers of the Quartermaster-General's department;—information which they could not acquire of themselves.

In furtherance of this object, I recommend that a medical topographer, an important OFFICER OF HEALTH, an officer of trust and of rank, be permanently attached to the Quartermaster-General's department, in the British as well as in the Indian army. In time of peace he should inspect and report on the sites of camps, cantonments, and stations, and on the condition of barracks, and hospitals, and transport ships.

In time of war, in addition to the above duties, he should accompany the Quartermaster-General in the field; and, where military reasons do not control, his opinion should be obtained on the sites of encampment, and upon every matter relating to the prevention of disease; all the suggestions of matured sanitary experience being put in requisition for the protection of the soldiers' health.

This great conservative branch of medicine has not even yet been called into sufficient exercise in our fleets and armies; yet it is on the perfection of its civil establishments that the safety and efficiency of our sea and land forces entirely depend.

Had such an officer existed in 1809, the soldiers employed on the expedition to Walcheren would not have been permitted to encamp in a pestilential site, involving as this did the destruction of the army, and the sacrifice of a million sterling per annum in perpetuity; and if Wellington had had such an adviser, he would not perhaps have decimated his army on the Guadiana.

But it is in our intertropical possessions that the chronic waste and destruction of men and money take place; and could we count the hundreds of thousands of British soldiers, and the millions sterling, there lost unnecessarily, even the humanity of commanders and of governments would be shocked.

With a little attention to matters very easy of being understood, and quite as easy of being executed, we may obviate, for the future at least, those dark passages which tarnish the histories of our colonial administration, and of all our wars.

In unhealthy climates especially, and during the prevalence of epidemics in all climates, the medical inspection of the troops should be regular and frequent. This rule tends greatly to the preservation of health, for it is a standing order of all well-regulated troops that every individual soldier be fit for duty in the full sense of the word, or on the sick-list under regimen and medical treatment.

It is a remarkable fact, and one often observed, that in malarious countries especially, and where vicissitudes are great, most diseases have their origin in *night* exposure. "During natural sleep," says Dr. W. F. Edwards, "there is a diminution in the power of producing heat, and this explains why a damp cold air, or a dry and piercing air, which is borne without inconvenience while the individual is awake, even without the aid of exercise, may be hurtful during sleep." Speaking of the yellow fever, William Fergusson says, "It is my belief that malaria can only prevail upon the body during the passive state of sleep; in fact, that to sleep is the danger." It may be remarked, in addition to what is stated at page 45, that the effect of exposure to cold during sleep must necessarily vary according to the power of producing heat. As a means of guarding the system against the effects of atmospheric vicissitudes, I know of none so influential as the cold bath, provided always that the subject be healthy and of temperate habits.

The unnecessary and vexatious restrictions on the soldier's freedom of action, such as we constantly observe in garrisons and cantonments in India, are irksome to his mind, and injurious to his health. In point of fact, they create a profound feeling of discontent—the parent of mutiny. He should be allowed to do for himself whatever he can do without prejudice to health or discipline; and this ought to be made matter of standing regulation, not depending, as now, on the mere will or the uncertain notions of individual commanding officers. "It is easy to conceive," says Pringle, "that the prevention of disease cannot depend on the use of medicines, nor upon anything which a soldier shall have in his power to neglect, but upon such orders as he himself shall not think unreasonable, and such as he must obey."

The flannel shirt was for long a debatable question with military surgeons; and William Fergusson considers it necessary only for the bivouac. As an article of military wear, he says, it is "one of which the healthy, hardy soldier (and there ought to be none others in the army) can never stand in need." This dictum faithfully represents the rough, hardy school of Abercromby, Moore, and Wellington; but we are now satisfied, on the most varied and extended experiences, in many climates, that flannel is a necessary part of the soldier's dress everywhere, and under all circumstances of service. It is best used as under-clothing, for the reason that it readily absorbs moisture from the skin, while, unlike other fabrics, it causes no reduction of the animal heat. With two flannel shirts, sufficiently long to cover the entire trunk of the body, the soldier need not be hampered with cholera-belts; for he will be supplied with enough for warmth and cleanliness. In tropical climates, too, he should have a stout and complete flannel dress to use on coming in from the day's march. Fever, dysentery, and hepatitis follow constantly on remaining for hours in damp or wet clothes. The use of the stout flannel dress gives time also for the drying of the regimental clothing—a most necessary operation after the march, or hard duty of every kind.

The recommendations of Dr. Fergusson are more worthy of attention on another important point—the night-covering and accommodation of the soldier. He urges that, in every part of the British Empire the men should sleep in separate hammocks, which are cool, soft, and elastic, and can be washed like a garment, while they cannot be used without raising the body off the ground, or the hard boards, and they require no aid from flock or straw to make the occupant comfortable, an additional blanket in cold climates being all that is necessary. The hammock-railings have the great advantage of preserving freedom of ventilation, even during the night, and of being altogether out of the way during the day. Wherever a couple of stakes can be driven into the ground, they will serve all the above-mentioned purposes in the bivouac; and the construction of hammock-railings, consisting of uprights, with cross-posts and hooks, would be as simple as economical.

The preservation of the British soldier's health in our various colonies is a matter of paramount importance as regards our political condition, little as the subject has hitherto engaged the attention of the great body of our legislators. "No circumstance," says a popular reviewer, "has so checked the progress of English rule as the maladies peculiar to tropical climates. And it is no exaggeration to affirm, that any means by which this intense mortality could be diminished would more effectually secure our dominion than the most brilliant victories we have ever achieved. Not only does the expense involved in conveying troops to fill the vacancies in the decimated legions fall heavily on the parent country, but another result, more lamentable than any pecuniary loss, invariably follows. A prestige of insalubrity hangs like a cloud over our colonial possessions. The soldier and the emigrant leave home with

o

a melancholy foreboding at the probable speedy termination of their career. Hence the colonies unhappily become too often the resort of the desperate and the reckless. The worst features of English society are there perpetuated, with few of its excellences. This affects the condition of our army to an immense extent."

The rulers of France have not considered this question in its just view, or they never could have conceived it possible to colonize the Algerian provinces under an annual mortality of seven per cent. The result, years ago, has been the sacrifice of a hundred millions sterling, and the loss of a hundred thousand men.

Sir Alexander Tulloch justly observes that military returns, properly organized and properly digested, afford one of the most useful guides to direct the policy of the colonial legislator. Nor is the value of well-ordered numerical returns confined to military questions.

"Whether we wish to appreciate the value of symptoms," says Louis, " to know the progress and duration of diseases, to assign their degree of gravity, their relative frequency, the influence of medical constitutions upon their development, to enlighten ourselves as to the value of therapeutical agents, or the causes of diseases, it is indispensable to count."

The *Tente-d'abri* of the French—the suggestion of necessity in their African campaigns—and used only in provisional encampments, or as a bivouac-cover—is the most useful article yet introduced amongst soldiers. It originated with the French soldier, was amended by him piecemeal, in the accidents of Algerian service, and was perfected there by Marshal Bugeaud. It is three feet high, four and a half long, and is composed of three pieces of canvas, attached by buttons and strings. Two sticks placed at each extremity serve to support it, and it is fixed by pins to the earth. Three minutes suffice to set it up, and two to take it down. Each tent accommodates three men ; each of the three carries a portion of the canvas, and they divide the sticks and pins among them, and so they march. On arrival at their ground, they proceed immediately to fix the tent, and to dig a trench to carry off the water in case of rain. At night they sleep wrapped in blankets, and with their knapsacks for pillows. They are thus preserved from damp and rain.

The *Tente-d'abri* thus proves a protection for health and a guarantee for discipline; it preserves an effective force and assures the duration of the army.

In camps and fleets the officers in command should by every means promote and encourage all kinds of innocent and salutary games and exercises, music, dancing, &c. The monotony of naval and military life, and the varying and sometimes disappointing circumstances of active service, lead to mental despondency and consequent ill health. The fact has often been exemplified ;

so much so, that the *medicina mentis* should ever hold a high place in naval and military prophylaxis.

James Johnson relates, that "His Majesty's ship Russell, 74, sailed from Madras on the 22nd of October, 1806, and arrived at Batavia on the 27th of November; the crew healthy, and their minds highly elated with the sanguine expectations of surprising the Dutch squadron there. Such, however, was their sudden disappointment, and concomitant mental depression on missing the object of their hopes, that they began immediately to fall ill, ten, twelve, or fourteen per day, till nearly two hundred men were laid up with *scurvy*, scorbutic fluxes, and hepatic complaints! Of these, upwards of thirty died before they got back to Bombay, and more than fifty were sent to the hospital there. The Albion did not fare better. The Powerful fared worse: so that in these three ships alone, in the short space of a few months, *full an hundred men died* on board, and double that number were sent to hospitals, many of whom fell victims to the above mentioned diseases, which had been aggravated, and in a great measure engendered, by mental despondency."

With equal truth Sir Gilbert Blane, referring to the converse influences of high spirits, says:—"When the mind is interested and agitated by warm and generous affections, the body forgets its wants and feelings, and is capable of a degree of labour and exertion which it could not undergo in cold blood. The quantity of muscular action expended in fighting a great gun for a single hour, is perhaps greater than what is employed for a whole day in ordinary labour; and though performed in the midst of heat and smoke, and with little bodily refreshment, yet the powers of nature are not exhausted or overstrained—even the smart of wounds is not felt! . . . . It is stated that, when the fleet under Admiral Matthews, in the year 1744, was off Toulon, in the daily expectation of engaging the combined fleets of France and Spain, there was a general suspension of the progress of sickness, particularly of the scurvy, from the influence of that generous flow of spirits with which the prospect of battle inspires British seamen. But if the mere prospect and ardent expectation of battle, without any happy result, could have such a sensible result, what must be the effect of the elevation of mind created by the exultation of VICTORY—a victory in which the naval glory of our country was revived and retrieved, after a series of misfortunes and disgraces, which had well-nigh extinguished the national pride and spirit in every department of the service. The plain and honest, though unthinking seaman is not less affected by this than the more enlightened lover of his country. Even the invalids at the hospital manifested their joy by hoisting shreds of coloured cloth on their crutches."

In accounting for the smallness of the mortality amongst the soldiers in the first month of service at Walcheren, Blane says that " an excited tone of mind, as.well as youth and robust health, had a share in keeping down the mortality at this period ;" and so it was with the health of Hill's division when it surprised that of Gerard at Aroyo de Molinos, in Spain. Dr. Luscombe states that during the week in which this surprise was being executed, the rain was heavy and almost incessant, and the men passed two nights in bivouac without fires; yet the sick in Hill's division, composed principally of Highlanders, was less during that and the subsequent week than in any equal period during that year. Dr. Luscombe, in almost the very words of Blane, assigns as the reason of the immunity of the soldiers from the effects of fatigue and ex- posure to cold and wet, that they were under " exercise and mental excitement."

As an example of the influence of hope in arresting the extension of disease and in repelling it, I may here mention, on the authority of the Statistical Reports, the remarkable fact, that during the epidemic yellow fever of 1822, at Up-Park, Jamaica, among the soldiers of the 91st Regiment, when the order was issued for their removal to another station, the fever ceased ; *and though the corps was unexpectedly detained for three or four days after the order was issued, not one case was admitted into hospital in the whole course of that period."*

Finally, it cannot be too often repeated that on the perfection of the so-called civil establishments—the medical and the com- missariat departments—must depend not only the efficiency, but the very existence of our fleets and armies. I say " so-called," because, in respect to the medical corps at least, it is a complete misnomer, for neither by sea nor on land can there be any absolute protection for the surgeon, during the hour of battle, from the fire of an enemy. The recent calamitous losses in the Crimea have demonstrated another fact, viz., that so long as the departments above-named are dependent and subordinate, and under the management and control of officers holding but an inferior rank, consideration, and power, so long will they remain insufficient to their great purposes. But let them once be ruled and directed by responsible officers of a rank and station adequate to command an instant attention to their respective wants; let such officers be largely and immediately responsible—and then, but not till then, will the two most important establishments of our fleets and armies rise so as to be equal to all requirements, whether during peace or in war.

MEMORANDA ON THE HYGIENE OF CAMPS AND CANTONMENTS IN WARM CLIMATES, WITH A SKETCH OF MEDICAL AR-RANGEMENT FOR FIELD SERVICE.

The first qualification of a soldier is fortitude under fatigue and privation. Courage is only the second; hardship, poverty, and want are the best school of a soldier.—NAPOLEON.

The army is a part of society employed, it is true, in services of a peculiar nature, which require a peculiar organization, but not on that account cut off from the general mass of the community.—COUNT RUMFORD.

Nothing can be so extravagant as to kill good men, who have been trained at such an expense.—LORD HERBERT.

Social science as applied to the army is a very young member of the fraternity of sciences.—CALCUTTA REVIEW.

We have made the discovery that an army may be so constituted as to be in the highest degree efficient against an enemy, and yet obsequious to the civil magistrate.—LORD MACAULAY.

---

1. The moral and material improvement of the British soldier, and the education and training of his officer—two conditions inseparably associated in a true military polity, and whose intimate connexion for good is hardly yet appreciated in this country—are matters with us of such national importance that they can no longer, as of old, be regarded as topics too technical to be understood by the public, or as subjects of indifference to them. Persons of the most ordinary, unmilitary appearance, who have never been seen in public decked out "in scarlet, gold, and cock's feathers"—the feathers "of the male Pullus Domesticus;"—persons who have never been "covered with lace in the course of the ischiatic nerve,"* will now insist on the right to inquire into, and judge of, everything which relates to the soldier; of the "condition-of-the-soldier question," in fact, in all its latitude; "the reason why," and all the rest of it. For the medical officer to be complete master of every circumstance which may tend to secure the welfare, moral and material, of the men committed by the State to his care, is therefore a necessity of his position, if he would maintain it with any credit.

2. Very ordinary-looking, common-place people are now beginning to perceive that, for the conduct of war, the mere gentleman without study and without knowledge, is feeble and inefficient. There must be knowledge, carefully acquired knowledge, before an officer of any rank can deserve the smallest amount of trust or confidence. "By reading," says Sir Charles Napier, "you will be distinguished; without it, abilities are of little use." Of the use and value of the gentleman in the ranks

---

* Sydney Smith, who is here quoted, seems, like Robert Jackson, to have held in special aversion the tailoring endeavours of certain of our commanders—the "sartorial and plumigerous" propensities—and the "clothes-worship."

of our armies, I am deeply and anxiously sensible ; BUT THE OFFICER WE MUST HAVE AT ANY COST : in other words, if the gentleman will not qualify for a duty making certain demands on his time and attention, he must give place to those who are ready for all duties upon all conditions.

3. There are two circumstances in the very nature of our wars which ought to be present to the mind of the medical philosopher ; namely, first, that with us no war can be long carried on against the will of the people ; and, secondly, that war never leaves the country where it found it.   Changes are indeed its necessary consequences.   This truth has not been sufficiently regarded in our country.

4. The public at large is at length beginning to understand that it is HEALTH, and the attentions necessary to secure health, which impart to the soldier " the fortitude under fatigue and privation" which constitutes his " first qualification," and which is so imperiously necessary to him under all the trying and varying circumstances of colonial and of field service.

5. It is further beginning to be understood that the arts of peace must lend their aid to the art of war—that health means efficiency in our fleets and armies—that class interests must be made to cease to injure the public services—and that there ought to be no distinctions amongst our officers by sea or land, but those of merit.   The rusty general who now holds that young officers would fight better on account of their utter ignorance of discipline, tactics, strategy, and all other branches of a regular military education, would have no hearers in any even of our clubs—unless it be the " Senior."

6. " The common sense of the country"—the now alarmed common sense of the country—and the slow teaching of experience, so often invoked, and invoked in vain, in support of the soldier's claims, by Robert Jackson, and the old surgeons of our fleets and armies, have at length forced themselves into this, the soldier's question ; and not too soon, if our forces are to be worthy of our character, traditions, and power.   Formerly, the country was wanting in knowledge ; now, the public has more than enough of that needful qualification.

7. Here, indeed, as in civil life, it will be easy, if we will, to set matters to rights, if only amateurs and monied idlers, of whatever class or degree, be made to take to other pursuits than soldiering. Our ancestors had a wholesome and instinctive dislike of " the fantacied men of warre," and we would do well practically to imitate them in their caution.

8. All this may seem to the superficially informed to be an assuming of a State question ; but what army surgeon does not know it to be vitally a soldier's question !   There is one part of this subject which should never be forgotten, namely, that with our commanders and statesmen it has never been the disaster or

the loss of an army, but always the accusation of having caused it that has disturbed their serenity.

9. But at length, and under a statesman and war minister, singular in the extent of his knowledge and earnest in his purposes, the soldier's treatment, moral and material, has become a system, and been made the great military question of the day. The maxim of Turenne has been practically accepted by Lord Herbert :—" Le bien le plus précieux est le sang du soldat." The principles and the actual reforms which he has introduced into the sanitary arrangements of the army, being of the nature of well-founded institutions, will, it is hoped, ever be felt; for they must go on, under improving knowledge, to more and more improvement.

10. Half a century ago, the people had no information, and in consequence they did not reason on military questions; they took everything as they found it. All this is altered now. The diffusion of knowledge was reprobated by our administrators of old as tending to the subversion of discipline; and ignorance was cultivated on system, as an element of order and of subordination. In no other military power has the influence of the haughty ignorance of routine been so fatally experienced as in this our native country. Seamen and soldiers are presumed to spring from " the vigorous race of undiseased mankind :" we have but to maintain them in their native strength by using the best preservative means with which we are acquainted. Happily, and owing to the sanitary arrangements now in force, this can be done; and it will no longer be permitted to incapacity or routine to annihilate our armies abroad, and decimate them at home.

After these assuring reflections, let us proceed to the more immediate part of our business—the consideration of the comfort, health, contentment, and efficiency of the soldier, and the best means of securing them on active service. Notwithstanding our best efforts in this direction, the " fortitude," which is " the first qualification of a soldier," will be severely tested in the long campaign.

11. It is here held as a principle that in all climates, and under all circumstances of service, the soldier should be encouraged, nay, ordered, to do for himself whatever he can do without injury to his health, morals, and discipline; and further, that he be required to do whatever may be essential to his efficiency and serviceable condition, in the event of failure of the appointed means and appliances. Before the soldier can be held to be completely fitted to undertake his duties to the State, he must be made capable of preparing and ministering everything which may be necessary to his personal care and comfort, in the field and in cantonment.

12. He should be taught certain gymnastic exercises—as running, leaping, wrestling, pitching the bar, the sword exercises, and that of artillery. The swimming bath, where practicable, should be used habitually.

13. Every soldier, or, at all events, a goodly per-centage, should, as a preliminary, be taught to handle the spade or mattock, the axe and saw, the hammer and crowbar—to construct his hut and arrange his tent—to bake his own bread and cook his rations—to mend his clothes and shoes. Instruction of this kind is vitally necessary to our Volunteer Force, if it would act effectively against an invading enemy. Without it our best volunteer battalions would melt away or be nearly destroyed.

14. One of the greatest banes of our military system has always been the permitting our soldiers to take the field and to act as if commanders and departments could everywhere, and on the most remote scenes of operation, be of universal competence and all-sufficient; whereas experience proves that on extended and remote scenes, however great the commander and excellent the departments, very much must be left to the individual exertions of the men, directed by their officers. This may be termed the trained personal hygiene and sanitary skilled labour of the soldier.

15. Nor should the beneficial influences of mental exercises, diversions, cheerful occupations and amusements be neglected. The officers, by habit and example, should encourage all such pursuits, and thus lighten the dreary *tedium* of colonial barrack life and of garrison towns.

16. As the muscles of the body are best exercised in succession rather than all at once, so mental exercises of different kinds ought to be agreeably alternated; thus obviating the tendency of monotony and idleness to degrade both mind and body. In fact, nature seems not to have designed sameness or uniformity of mental pursuit any more than of nutriment for the body: in the one case, the faculties of the mind are rendered sluggish and inane, while, in the other, the very blood is contaminated, and all the functions of the body are thereby enfeebled and depraved. It is with soldiers as with other men—a cheerful and contented mind conducing powerfully to health and morals.

17. The soldier generally enlists so young that we may make of him what we please; and he requires more management to turn him to good account than that of the sergeant and the adjutant. Newly-raised and unpractised corps ought not to be employed on active service, or in the intertropical possessions of the empire; but when such corps must be so employed of necessity, the interior discipline and sanitary economy cannot be too carefully looked to.

18. It is in the earlier years of service—through the sudden change of accustomed habits, the removal from persons and places cherished by them—aided by the influences of change of climate, rapid marches, &c., that the conscripts of the French army suffer the most. General Pelet gives proof of this in the decreasing mortality per 1000 per annum, during the first seven years of service, of from 7 to 2 comparatively.

19. According to Tardieu, the apparent age of full growth in France is twenty years; and the more the rule of nature suggested by that fact is violated in working the recruit, the more the victims of disease are augmented without increasing the real strength of the army. Early enlistment is necessary for the purposes of training; but the soldier should be two-and-twenty years of age before he is called upon to exert his utmost powers, and the age of five-and-twenty would be still better adapted for the hard campaign.

20. Diet.—"Tell me," says Brillat-Savarin, "what a man eats, and I'll tell you what he is:"—so, if we know what the soldier dies of, we can, on some occasions, as at Rangoon and China, in the first wars, and in the Crimea, tell how he has lived. When, for instance, we learn that armies have died of scorbutic dysentery, we know at once and for a certainty that our men have been ill and insufficiently fed, clothed, and housed. The Scotch saying—"He looks like his meat," has a physiological significance in the case of the soldier. In all the Indian examples it was hard to say which was of worst quality, the salt meat or the biscuit. The use of soft bread is strongly urged upon the Government for the use of the French soldiers in Algeria, who regard biscuit, even when good, with an unfavourable eye.

21. The diet of the soldier should vary with the climate, and with the amount of labour required from him. In the field he works as hard as a dockyard labourer, involving, besides the labour, exposure and watching. Under such circumstances of service, the Commissioners of Inquiry into the Supplies for the British Army in the Crimea recommend the following daily ration:—

Soft bread	24 oz.
Fresh Vegetables	8
Rice, or barley	2
Fresh meat	16
Ground or roasted coffee	1
Sugar	2
Total	3 lbs. 5 oz.
Spirits	⅓ pint.

To which it is proposed to add weekly :—

Mustard	½ oz.
Pepper	¼
Salt	½

22. "Assuming this to be the standard ration of troops in the field by which the amount of nutriment is determined, certain equivalents may be substituted for some of the articles whenever economy of transport becomes important; for example, 16oz. of biscuit for 24oz. of soft bread; 2oz. of compressed or preserved

vegetables for 8oz. of fresh vegetables; ½oz. of tea for 1oz. of coffee."—(Report of Crimean Commission.)

23. Dietaries ought never to be estimated by the rough weight of their constituents, without distinct reference to the real nutriment in these, as determined by physiological and chemical inquiry.—(Christison.) An accurate knowledge of equivalents would likewise prove of great value towards securing to our armies a proper system of dieting. Disposed, as our troops are, over every kind of climate from Bengal to Canada, such knowledge is of especial need to us.*

24. The military surgeon should be well acquainted with the economy of food, and with the natural laws of diet, so as to be able to estimate and regulate the labour-value, and the suitableness to the various and contrasted climates of the several dietaries in common use. A scale should be fixed which, as far as can be, may be applicable to all climates and conditions of service.

25. On first arrival in a tropical climate the quantity of animal

---

* For the following valuable information I am indebted to my friend, Dr. Parkes, Professor of Military Hygiene at Chatham :—

PRESENT RATION OF THE SOLDIER AT CHATHAM, SHOWING WHAT IS ISSUED BY THE COMMISSARIAT, AND WHAT IS BOUGHT BY THE SOLDIER.

At Aldershott *everything* is issued by the commissariat, and the same system is to be introduced at Chatham.

The nutritive value has been calculated by Dr. Parkes by a formula which gives the nitrogen in meat and bread lower than Dr. Christison's formula. The carboniferous aliments are divided into fat and carbo-hydrates (starch, sugar, &c.). If the total amount of carboniferous nourishment be required, the fat must be multiplied by 2·4, and the product added to the amount of the carbo-hydrates. The quantity of salts is assumed.

Daily Quantity, Cost, and Nutritive Value of the Soldier's Ration at Chatham (1861).

QUANTITY AND COST.

ARTICLES.	Quantity taken daily in ounces and tenths of ounces.	Price.	To whom paid.
Meat	12 oz.	} 4½d.	Government.
Bread.....................	16		
Bread.....................	8		
Potatoes.................	16		
Other vegetables	8		
Coffee....................	0·33	} 3½	{ Bought in the market.
Tea.......................	0·16		
Salt	0·25		
Sugar	1·33		
Milk	3·25		
Total quantity	65·32 oz.		
Total value	......	8d.	

food should be reduced, during some months at least, allowing compensation in the way of vegetables and fruits. The lighter

NUTRITIVE VALUE IN OUNCES AND TENTHS.

ARTICLES.	Water.	Nitrogenous substances.	Fat.	Carbo-hydrates (starch, sugar,&c.)	Salts.
Meat*.....................	6·75	1·44	0·81		
Bread....................	9·60	1·92	0·36	12·12	
Potatoes...............	11·84	0·24	0·02	3·9	
Other vegetables taken, as cabbage	7·	0·05	0·02	0·52	
Sugar	...	......	...	1·33	
Milk	2·82	0·109	0·12	0·169	
Salts (assumed)	...	......	...	......	1
Total	38·01	3·759	1·33	18·039	1

Total solid nourishment, exclusive of tea, coffee, &c., and 3 ounces for bone................................... 24·128

Water in food .... 38·01

62·138

In addition—

Coffee .... 0·33
Tea .... 0·16
Pepper
Bone .... 3·

3·49

HOSPITAL DIETS.—FORT PITT, FEB. 1861.

Nutritive Value of the Hospital Diets, calculated by Dr. Christison, and communicated by him to Miss Nightingale.

1. TEA.

ARTICLES.	Carboniferous.	Nitrogenous.	Total.
Bread, 8 oz.	4·12	0·84	4·96
Tea, ½ oz.			
Sugar, 3 oz.	3·	0·0	3·
Milk, 6 oz.	0·48	0·27	0·75
	7·60	1·11	8·71

4. MILK.

ARTICLES.	Carboniferous.	Nitrogenous.	Total.
Bread, 14 oz.	7·21	1·44	8·68
Rice, 2 oz.	1·60	0·20	1·80
Milk, 60 oz.	4·80	2·70	7·50
Sugar, ½ oz.	0·50	...	0·50
	14·11	4·37	18·48

* One-quarter has been deducted for bone.

French wines, or the more grateful light wholesome ale, might at first also be beneficially substituted for the rum; and no re-

5. Low.

ARTICLES.	Carboniferous.	Nitrogenous.	Total.
Meat, 8 oz., exclusive of bone......	1·20	1·61	2·81
Bread, 14 oz............................	7·21	1·47	8·68
Sugar, 1½ oz............................	1·50	...	1·50
Milk, 6 oz..............................	0·48	0·27	0·75
Pudding ⎰ Rice, 2 oz.	1·60	0·20	1·80
Milk, 15 oz.	1·20	0·67	1·87
Sugar, 1½ oz.............	0·50	...	0·50
Eggs	0·30	0·40	0·70
	13·99	4·62	18·61

7. Half.

ARTICLES.	Carboniferous.	Nitrogenous.	Total.
Meat, 8 oz., exclusive of bone	1·20	1·62	2·82
Bread, 16 oz............................	8·24	1·68	9·92
Potatoes, 8 oz.	1·96	0·20	2·16
Barley, 1¾ oz.	1·17	0·28	1·45
Sugar, 1¾ oz............................	1·75	...	1·75
Milk, 6 oz..............................	0·48	0·27	0·75
Vegetables, 3 oz.	0·06	0·01	0·07
Butter, 1 oz.	1·00	...	1·00
Flour, ¼ oz.	0·18	0·04	0·22
	16·04	4·10	20·14

10. Entire.

ARTICLES.	Carboniferous.	Nitrogenous.	Total.
Meat, 12 oz.	1·80	2·43	4·23
Bread, 16 oz............................	8·24	1·68	9·92
Potatoes, 16 oz.........................	3·92	0·40	4·32
Barley, 2½ oz.	1·77	0·37	2·14
Sugar, 1¾ oz............................	1·75	...	1·75
Milk, 6 oz.	0·48	0·27	0·75
Vegetables, 4 oz.	0·08	0·02	0·10
Butter, 1 oz.	1·00	...	1·00
Flour, ¼ oz.	0·18	0·04	0·22
	19·22	5·21	24·43

6. Fowl.

Nearly the same as half-diet, with half a fowl or chicken weighing 8 ounces, exclusive of bone, either to be roasted or made into soup, in lieu of the 8 ounces of meat.

8. Fish.

Nearly the same as half-diet, but 8 ounces of white fish in lieu of the 8 ounces of meat.

9. Roast.

Nearly the same as half-diet, but 8 ounces of mutton chops or steak in lieu of the 8 ounces of meat.

cruit should be allowed to use his spirit-ration during the voyage, or yet after landing, until he shall get out of the drill. In hot countries, also, as in Europe, the food-ration should vary with the amount of labour performed by the soldier.

26. A mixed diet will, in all countries, be found the best, and the officers should everywhere see daily to the *freshness and purity* of the rations, both animal and vegetable. Constant attention should also be paid to the cleanly condition of the cooking utensils, and the vessels used in the conveyance of water.

27. The daily ration of the British soldier in the Bombay Fusiliers is detailed by Dr. Arnott to be uniform throughout the year, and to consist of :—

Fresh meat	1 lb.
Bread	1
Vegetables	8 oz.
Rice	4
Salt	2
Sugar	0¾
Firewood	3 lbs.

Spirit ration.

The only alterations ordered in the above dietary consisted in an increase of sugar and a reduction of the salt. Rice is almost discontinued—the men receiving some condiment in exchange. In India, where there is difficulty in procuring leavened bread, the common flour-cake of the country (*chapatee*), warm and fresh from the iron plate, is wholesome and nutritious. Both rice and dhâl are excellent likewise, when well dressed with proper condiments.

28. The fusiliers had breakfast at eight, dinner at noon, and a so-called supper at four—a meal which might advantageously be deferred to six o'clock.

Breakfast consisted in bread with meat, or with fish, eggs, butter, procured by the men at their own cost, with tea or coffee.

Dinner was composed of the meat-ration, with vegetables; while supper consisted of whatever may have remained from the dinner, and of such extras as the soldier may have been able to command. Care was taken that the quality of the ration was good —beef being served out four times, and mutton three times in the week.

29. When salted meat and fish are substituted for fresh meat, they should be carefully soaked before being cooked, and, when practicable, mixed with a certain amount of vegetables.

30. The quality of the soldier's ration is not even now sufficiently regarded at home or abroad. It is too often of so inferior a nature that, if issued singly, it would prove insufficient for his sustenance in barracks even during peace, and while subject to no labour.

31. Condiments in small quantities are good seasoning; in excess they irritate the stomach, and render thirst more difficult

to bear.   Saffron increases the digestibility of rice and flour, and is particularly useful with maize.

32. Food should always be taken before the march.

33. In the " Report of Royal Commission of 1857," of which I was a member, and which was ordered to inquire into " The Regulations affecting the Sanitary Condition of the Army," the Commissioners, in their address to the Queen, express their regret at " the great variety both in the amount and composition of the ration which has been from time to time authorized in the Colonies, the frequent changes in the stoppages, both at home and abroad, at various periods, and the different systems on which the ration has been contracted for and supplied to the troops.

34. " There is no doubt that the frequency of the changes made in the authorized ration since 1813, and the stoppages by which the soldier paid for its value, and the great diversity in the balance of pay to which he has been entitled, according to the station at which he might be quartered, have been sources of suspicion and dissatisfaction to him.

35. " It appears to us, therefore, that all the arguments for a fixed stoppage and full ration in time of war, apply also to a time of peace.   In both cases it is the duty and interest of the government to see that the soldier is provided with such a ration as will keep him in health and efficiency.   In both cases it is advantageous to get rid of a cumbrous and costly system of accounts, by which time and labour are unnecessarily consumed in peace, and which has to be abandoned in war, when the expenditure requires the greatest vigilance.

36. " We are of opinion that no ration can be fixed upon which shall be adhered to in peace and war.   The conditions of life are so different in the two cases, that whatever is suitable for the one must be either too much or too little for the other.   . . . . But the result of the change which we propose will be, that the soldier will receive, whether at home or abroad, in peace or in war, on board ship or in hospital, a uniform net pay and a uniform ration, sufficient both in quantity and quality to provide him with three meals, and to keep him in health and efficiency."

37. DRINK.—No trouble or expense should be spared in securing to the soldier, whether in camp or cantonment, an abundant supply of pure water for drink, cooking, and bathing.   Where the water is of inferior quality, the soldier is sure to compensate himself, as he will call it, by a liberal admixture of ardent spirits.

38. In standing camps and in cantonments water should be carefully conveyed in iron pipes, from a situation beyond reach of contamination.   The French before Sebastopol are stated by Dr. Snow to have laid down iron pipes for conveying water to the army from the hills alone above the camp, whilst the British adopted no such precaution.   In hot climates, ten to twelve gallons of water will prove, on the average per man, a sufficient daily supply for

all purposes, including that required for the barrack attendants and followers. In temperate climates, each man requires about two and a half pints of water daily, as a minimum allowance.

39. The supposition that, in India, tanks which are covered with green weeds therefore contain impure water, is an error—the very opposite being the fact; the weeds, the small fish, and infusoria preserving the water clear and fresh. An English general ordered the "clearing" of one of these tanks; after which operation, carefully performed, the water "soon turned putrid;" but on the return of the duckweed, the water again became drinkable.

40. Water drunk in large quantity is always injurious, even when pure. If, after a fatiguing march, a stream of water is met with, thirst must be sparingly satisfied, and the water reserved for subsequent use. When only a small quantity is procurable, instead of swallowing it, the mouth should be gargled as long as possible, and the water rejected as it becomes warm.

41. When reduced to the necessity of drinking stagnant or impure water, it should, by way of precaution, be strained through cloth, to separate leeches imperceptible from their smallness, and which it is very dangerous to swallow.

42. A mixture of wine and water, brandy and water, or infusion of coffee and water, is always an excellent drink, taken in moderation. It should be mixed at the time of use, and not prepared beforehand, as it then becomes changed, and no longer fulfils its purpose.

43. When troops are fed on salted meat, whether on shore or on board ship, lime-juice, as ordered by the regulations, should never be wanting to the men. It should be served out independently of such fruits and vegetables as may be procurable.

44. Where the spirit-ration is in use, it ought never to be taken in the morning, or before meals : on the contrary, the established rule should be to use it shortly after dinner and supper, diluted with water, and not in its neat state.

45. I have spoken of the "liver-burning" spirit-ration—the "fire-water" of the white man—as being especially injurious to the young soldier on first landing in India; and assuredly it is not beneficial to the old soldier : if he must have it, it should be diluted. Shakspeare was aware of the "liver-burning" action of alcohol; for he says—"Let my liver rather heat with wine."

46. All experience confirms the declaration of Dr. Arnott, of the Bombay Fusiliers, that the advantages which have accrued to the soldier's health and morals from the substitution of sound malt liquor for ardent spirits, are perceptible in the diminution of crime, sickness, and mortality. This excellent and experienced officer suggests the desirableness of prohibiting the issue of the spirit-ration altogether in its undiluted form—porter, ale, wine, and spirits and water affording all the variety that can in reason be desired.

47. But the spirit-ration—another unquestionable form of "regulation poison"—is still regarded by many old officers by sea and land as one of the naval and military institutions; and it may require the intelligence of another generation to get rid of it.

48. Wherever established, the regimental canteens should be spacious and well-ventilated; and whatever else they may contain, they should be abundantly supplied with malt liquors and light wines.

49. When troops are on the march, a cup of warm coffee, or of soup, should be served to every man before quitting the ground; and if some bread or biscuit be added, so much the better. The morning dram was declared by Robert Jackson to be nothing short of "a pernicious bounty."

50. After the most severe fatigues in Burmah, including direct solar exposure during whole days of April and May, and the distress occasioned by volumes of dust, the European officers of the Bengal bodyguard, at the instance of our commanding officer, Major Sneyd, always drank warm tea; and I can answer for the great refreshment derived from this excellent suggestion.

51. I am satisfied that the encouragement to prudence offered by the more general institution of savings' banks, would go far towards promoting the morals and health of the soldier. The arrears of pay due to him, after being long in hospital, constitute another "pernicious bounty." They are notoriously ill-used; often spent in drink, to the injury of health and discipline. In fever, dysentery, and hepatitis, drink is a frequent cause of relapse, and of death consequently.

52. SLEEP.—Whatever may be the opinions of martinets by sea and land, yet is it certain that the refreshment derived from a certain amount of sleep is as necessary to the mental and bodily vigour of seamen and soldiers, as the refreshment derived from a certain amount of food and drink. To the occasional privations of sleep, and to the limited and irregular enjoyment of it at all times, is referred, perhaps with justice, the aged appearance of seamen as compared to soldiers of like ages.

53. Where and how to sleep, are the great considerations in the camp; for on the damp and cold soil, or exposed to malaria, disease comes rapidly and fearfully upon the soldier.

54. Under hard labour, and on the march, the hour of retirement should be early, say, an hour after supper, so that the soldier may enjoy eight hours of sleep. Before Sebastopol, Mr. Woods states that while the French soldiers were "four nights off duty to one on, ours had about ten hours off to twelve on,"—a circumstance which of itself would go far to account for the heavy losses of the British force employed.

55. Sick, wounded, and convalescents should be allowed some additional hours of sleep; and so should soldiers who have undergone hard labour and inordinate exertion.

56. From the circumstance that during sleep the power of gene-rating heat in the system is diminished, much care should be given to the proper covering and clothing of the soldier, as well as to the condition of the soil; for, in tropical climates especially, it is in the night that the danger of contracting malarious disease is greatest.

57. In the West Indian commands, where night duties and night exposure are believed to influence the health of the troops, the British soldier takes his tour of guards or pickets every third or fourth night, " and every six hours stands sentry for two hours at a time." The fact that the mortality of drummers is greatly under the general average among the rest of the troops, in the command referred to, has been ascribed to their comparative exemption from night duties; but it is probable that causes as yet unascertained operate in aid of the freedom from night duty, so as in other ways to favour this class of soldiers.

58. Ordinarily, and in time of peace, European soldiers in the East Indies are much exempted from night duties; but when on garrison employments at the head-quarters of the three Presiden-cies, or when employed at Aden, for instance, the night duties be-come occasionally heavy. Diseases of the liver and hands are stated by Dr. Arthur to have been much increased in Burmah, in the Madras European Fusiliers, by the exposure attendant on night duties. He adds that the men were "on guard about every fourth or fifth day throughout the year."

59. Throughout the British colonies generally, the men, on an average, have from four to five nights of consecutive rest. In the East and West Indies, where soldiers who are natives of those countries are employed largely, the European should not be placed on guard and on sentry duties without a necessity, especially at unhealthy stations, and in unhealthy seasons.

60. COOKING.—That the British soldier, in the field of active service, with its labours and fatigues, should for ages have been left altogether without instruction in the vitally essential matter of cooking his coarse ration, is but another instance of the neglect with which all that related to his comfort and welfare was formerly treated. Let us hope that some general means may speedily be afforded to remedy so great a defect. Every soldier (or at least a goodly proportion per company) should be instructed in the art of cooking his ration of meat and vegetables in a plain and wholesome manner, in making soup and bouillon, and in baking soft bread. These simple matters, so easy of being taught, are essential to the health and comfort of the soldier. It would be a real economy to have a well-trained cook, or even two, in every regiment; and in cantonments and permanent camps, the cooking-places should be spacious and well covered in, so as to afford places of instruction for the soldiers. An instruction-kitchen, in which cooks from every regiment are to be instructed, has been recently established

P

at Aldershott by order of Lord Herbert, and a competent in-
structor in cookery has been appointed.

61. DRESS.—Since the days of the Duke of Cumberland, now
more than one hundred years ago, imitation—that most feeble of
refined flatteries—has been the afflictive principle of the British
army, both in discipline and dress.   It has been injured by a
foreign and unnatural military code, or it has been made to look
ridiculous " by regulation ;" or it has been made to feel cruel discomfort, just as the superior officers—the stage-hero-makers, the
dress-making commanders—as Robert Jackson termed them, may
have been at the time more ignorant or more negligent than
usual.

62. It is, I fear, in vain to talk of such matters as of past and
gone times; for in authenticated publications of August, 1860, in
the Mauritius, Ceylon, and West Indies, our soldiers are spoken
of as dressed in a "red tunic of thick broadcloth lined with serge,
the hard leather stock"—the dog-collar of Colonel Mountain,
condemned half a century ago by Larrey—" that intolerable
shako, precisely the same as at Aldershott."   The dress is said to
be proper perhaps to our northern climate, but cruel in a tropical
region.   The writer then asks—" Is discomfort in dress necessary
to discipline ?"   During the first war in China, the Emperor was
assured by the mandarins that the English soldiers were buttoned
up so tight, that if once down, they could never rise again.

63. In the East Indies a better order of things appears to be
initiated ; but the commanders of Robert Jackson's time have a
wonderful hold on the memories of a certain class of survivors;
and this must always be the case so long as the soldier's dress and
accoutrements are to be regarded as a fashion, and treated from
the officer's point of view only.   The lesson of the life of a great
commander belongs to survivors; but so, unhappily, does that of
a small commander; and this last is sure to be followed in our
country, for a time at least, if he be but a man of a "certain
position."

64. Hitherto, and in our cavalry especially, our imitations have
always been of what is unsuitable, or absolutely bad.   Our
clumsy copyings have been but vulgar compromises in dress—half
German, half Prussian, half French—the poor man remaining an
astonished British soldier all the while.   Cromwell, Claverhouse,
and Marlborough did not spoil their horsemen by foreign imitations.   The system of the Northern military nations has always
been to make soldiers mere machines.   That has never been the
system of the British navy, and it ought never to be the system of
our army.   It required the genius of Cromwell to prove that the
best horse-soldier of the world might be trained in an island.   He
and Marlborough won victories with cavalry.

65. In regard to the equipment of this branch of the service,
Sir Charles Napier says that he could hardly alter it for the worse.

Imitation then is but a poor thing after all; for, with the best men and the best horses in the world, the efficiency of our cavalry is constantly being called in question. The truth of Michael Angelo's apophthegm must here be held in recollection—that he who follows must always be behind.

66. Were I to relate but a tithe of the miseries, sickness, and death described by old officers in India, as resulting from powdered and tallowed heads and queues, polished close helmets, and heat-absorbing heavy black caps, black leather heat-absorbing stocks, heavy tight woollen coats and trousers, leather breeches and jackboots, all worn formerly by our horse and foot-soldiers, under the sun of Bengal, and in the hot and rainy seasons, I should not be credited. But, happily for the European soldier in India, the significant flatteries of imitation are giving place gradually to the suggestions of "the common sense of the country," which is breaking in upon German routine; and our soldiers serving there may at length hope to be reasonably dressed and accoutred; not trussed up and throttled in regulation pillories, as of old.

67. For active field service, the head-dress of the soldier should possess, not the properties of a scalp-lock or ray-trap, but be light, and have small perforations for the escape of the heated and consumed air within. It should, so far as may be, consist of such material as will render it sabre and bullet-proof; and the soldier should be able comfortably to lie down wearing his head-dress.

68. A well-formed, light, and well-adapted helmet, with a good peak in front and rear, would appear to be the best head-dress for both the horse and foot-soldier. For hot climates, it should be constructed on the plan of my friend Mr. Julius Jeffreys, of the Bengal medical corps, as admirably explained in his able work on "The British Army in India, its Preservation," &c.

69. Hitherto the head and body-dress of the British soldier has been the same, whether he served in the humid parts of Guiana or Bengal, or in the winter fogs of Holland; no attempt having been made, until very recently, to adapt clothing to climate; Prussian costume taking precedence of Prussian code, Prussian discipline, and Prussian flogging.

70. But, if we must always be imitating, I would suggest that, in head-dress, we imitate our most unwarlike enemy the Chinese. The helmet represented as worn by the Tartar chiefs appears to unite the best and most graceful exterior quality, with adaptation to all useful purposes. Constructed on Mr. Jeffrey's principle, such a helmet ought to be perfect.

71. Some medical officers, in defect of better means, prefer that in India, the head-dress should consist of a make-shift forage-cap, having a white padded cotton cloth passed round the cap turban-wise, leaving the end of the cloth to fall Templar-like over the nape of the neck.

72. The shirt for Indian service should be of cotton stuff, while the outer dress should consist of the regulation shell-jacket, blue barrack cotton-cloth trousers, stout cotton stockings, and strong high-lows as shoes; the only alteration required for the hot and rainy seasons being the substitution of a white cotton shell-jacket and trousers for those above-mentioned. Such simple dresses, together with a white or coloured cotton stock, are suitable for all seasons in tropical climates, for peace and for war.

73. For marching in all seasons in India Mr. Jeffreys recommends a good flannel dress, as the coolest in itself, and as the best protection against chills; while a comfortably warm and heavier clothing is necessary in the cold weather.

74. The flannel shirt is here of great protective value; and the blanket, which should ever form part of the kit in all climates and seasons, will be in constant use. Where change of body-clothes is not at hand, the men, after the march, may well be covered in their blankets, while their dresses are being dried in the sun.

75. Wet clothes, whenever possible, should be immediately changed—the remaining in wet being powerfully conducive to disease. For the cold season, and for night duties in a warm climate, the great-coat and woollen cloth trousers prove all-sufficient.

76. Changes such as these, much as they are dreaded, because innovations on the Peninsular usages, by some of our older officers, will not be followed either by "a mutiny or a dysentery," as Sydney Smith would have it.

77. The ordinary blue barrack-changes, if made with fixed dyes, are well suited to the soldier's wants, as undress; and the trousers, of whatever stuff, should be made so as to admit of the utmost freedom of movement. The contract system has hitherto proved a failure and an injury to the soldier, both his clothing and foot-gear being far behind the improvements of the day. Country-made boots are best for wear during the hot and cold dry season in India, being soft and light; but the English-made boot is the only one proper to the rainy season.

78. Dr. Cordier, of the Imperial Military School of Medicine and Pharmacy, has carried out some elaborate investigations on the relative values of the various materials for clothing soldiers. The following are the conclusions at which Dr. Cordier has arrived :—

(1.) The colour of the clothing has but little apparent influence on the loss of heat.

(2.) Every fabric is capable of absorbing, in the latent state, a certain quantity of hygrometric water. This quantity is considerable in woollen material, less so in hempen fabric, and still less so in cotton. This absorption occurs without immediate loss of heat to the human body.

(3.) The colour of the fabrics has a great influence upon the absorption of solar heat; and it is sufficient, whatever else may be the nature of the clothing, to modify conveniently the external surface of the clothing, to obtain the advantage by white materials when exposed to the intense heat of the sun.—*Brit. and For. Rev.* Ap. 1858.

(4.) Dr. Cordier's experiments further show that a white cotton cloth placed over a cloth dress lowers the temperature 7° per cent. This is a subject well worthy of a careful investigation.

79. The scarlet woollen cloth of England—that shirt of fire—should never be seen on the plains of India, unless indeed in the northern provinces, and during the cold season. Under any other circumstances the ordinary effect of such a dress amounts to wanton cruelty. The fact is that the dress of our soldiers has yet to be reformed in all ways, so as to secure ease, lightness, and proper texture and colour for different climates and seasons; and, in short, a suitableness to the advanced and advancing scientific and military movements of the day.

80. ACCOUTREMENTS.—" There are five things," says Napoleon, " the soldier should never be without—his firelock, his ammunition, his knapsack, his provisions for at least four days, and his entrenching-tool. His knapsack may be reduced to the smallest possible size, but the soldier should always have it with him." We have here the greatest of all authorities in favour of the soldier's carrying entrenching-tools, such as the axe—an instrument in itself alone immeasurably more useful to him than sword or bayonet: it is of use in forming the camp, in constructing the hut, in entrenching the village, on the retreat, and in many other ways besides.

81. Comfort and ease of movement will to some extent result to the British soldier in India from the introduction of the small pouch on the waist-belt, with the sliding frog for the bayonet, in lieu of the exclusive old heavy chest-constricting shoulder-belt and heavy pouch. By a recent order a shoulder belt, to contain forty rounds, and a waist-belt to contain twenty rounds of ammunition, have been introduced for use in the army of India. This will be some relief, but perhaps not all that might be given. The old shoulder-belt, by throwing the weight of so much ammunition on one shoulder, is injurious; and it is thought by many that two pouches, one in front and the other in rear, changeable when the first is emptied, and attached to the waist-belt, would be better.

82. The knapsack, considered by Napoleon as inseparable from the soldier as his arms and ammunition, is not so in the East Indies, where the heat of the climate precludes the strongest men from carrying so much additional weight. In the East the knapsack is carried for the soldier; and as it gives cover to the "kit," and keeps the men familiar with an old and useful appliance, it is well to have it always at hand. It should be of the description invented by Mr. Berington, and recommended by the Royal Commission of 1857. It is the best that has yet been made in this country .

The knapsack is really a much more important subject than at first appears. To save the soldier's strength he should, even in Europe, be exempted from carrying such a load, when employed on a hard or on a protracted campaign. It must ever be remembered that " force expended is force lost."

83. The knapsack was " permitted" by Lord Raglan to be left on board the transports in Kalamita Bay, on the landing of the British army in the Crimea. The consequences were most disastrous to the health of troops debilitated by previous disease, the result of malarious influences ; and who were now, during six weeks of hardship and exposure, deprived of a change of dress, and of other necessaries.

84. As one error always leads to another, the " permission" to leave behind the knapsack was by the reckless soldier construed into a sanction to throw away his camp-kettles on the march to Balaclava ; and thus began a series of the most astounding blunders and criminal neglects—of military enormities, the very narration of which will interest and shock the feelings of men for ages to come ; a series of cruel ignorances, more ruinous to the soldier and to the military character of England than could have been believed possible of occurrence in the middle of the nineteenth century.

85. BARRACK TENTS.—The tents supplied for the use of the European troops in the Presidency of Bombay, are stated by Dr. Arnott to be in number and quality all that could be desired, being commodious and lofty.* Those supplied for hospital purposes are twenty-four feet by sixteen, having single walls and double flies— the inner fly meeting and lacing to the top of the wall, so as that the outer fly may considerably overhang the wall, giving thus a free and complete escape to rain, along with protection from the sun's rays. The tents for the men on duty in India are generally sufficient.

86. The securing warmth during the night within tents is of the utmost importance to the health of soldiers ; and this is best done by a good layer of straw and a rug to lie on, with camelines, quilts, and the men's great-coats, according to the degree of cold or damp of the nights. Waterproof floorcloths should also be furnished, as being valuable safeguards against exhalations from the ground.

87. When the weather is not rainy or cold, the walls of the tents should be raised or removed on the lee side during the night, and in hot fair weather this should be done on two sides of the tent, so as to secure perfect ventilation. In the daytime the same removal should be made on the shady side of the tent, a gentle removal of the air being thus at all times ensured. The men

* The admirable " Notes on Moving Troops," by Dr. Arnott, of the Bombay European Fusiliers, have often been referred to in this article. They bespeak an officer of much discernment and activity.

should be made to sleep with their heads towards the circumference of the tent, and not to the centre : they thus escape from the consumed air, and breathe a purer atmosphere.

88. In the Crimea, owing to want of marquees, the sick lay in circular tents of the worst and most unsuitable description. Even for men in health, and during the English summer and autumn, they were found insufficient in the camp at Chobham ; yet the same tents were sent for the use of our men in the Bulgarian summer and the Crimean winter. They are stated to have been served in the following proportions :—

Officers of infantry and of cavalry.	Two circular tents to each field officer. One „ „ to each other officer.
To regiments of infantry . . .	One „ „ to every fifteen men. Four „ „ extra for guards.
To regiments of cavalry	One „ „ to every twelve men. Four „ „ extra for guards.

89. Hospital tents and marquees were sent with the original army in sufficient numbers ; but, like the knapsacks, they were "permitted" to be left behind at Varna, and were thus eventually lost to the army, including the sick and wounded, for whose special use they had been furnished.

90. "The circular tent used in the British army, which is estimated to contain fifteen men, is altogether unsuited for an hospital in any climate. It affords very insufficient protection against cold, or rain, or heat. When there is much wind in wet weather, the rain beats through the canvas ; and when it blows upon the door, which is being continually opened for ingress and egress, the rain is driven to all parts of the tent. The pole being in two pieces, for the convenience of carriage, is weak at the joint, and in stormy weather is apt to give way. The side wall is too low to admit of the use of any kind of cot, there being more than two or three men in the tent ; the space is too confined to admit of proper attendance on the patients, even by the medical officer ; and it is impossible, with safety, to use a stove, or other means of warming it. In short, whatever may be the supposed advantages that have led to its adoption as a barrack-tent, it would be difficult to contrive anything much more unfit for the accommodation of the sick." The bell-tent, the worst ever contrived, should never again be seen in our camps.

91. HUTTING.—The soldier should not only be taught to hut himself, but he should likewise hut his cattle of every description. Whenever the systematic or organized means may prove deficient, in short, he should understand that it is his duty so to work for his own benefit, and for that of the army at large. A horse-soldier is worse than useless without his horse ; and on the proper care of the baggage-cattle the safety and efficiency of an army may depend.

92. The huts constructed in England for the use of the Crimean

army, and which arrived too late to save either men or horses, "were framed of the lightest materials that could with safety be used, the boards being about three-quarters of an inch in thickness. They were twenty-eight feet long, sixteen feet wide, and from eleven to twelve feet in height to the ridge-pole, with a gradual slope to about six feet at the side, and calculated to contain from twenty to thirty-five persons, though, under ordinary circumstances, they would scarcely have been considered sufficient for half that number. The men were raised from the ground by sloping floors on each side, of inch plank, leaving an unfloored space of about three feet wide down the centre, in which there was a stove for the purpose of cooking and diffusing warmth. The total weight of each hut, including the iron-work, was about two and a-half tons."

93. EXERCISES AND AMUSEMENTS.—Roger Ascham maintained that " to ride comely ; to run fair at the tilt or ring ; to play at all weapons ; to shoot fair in bow or surely in gun ; to vault lustily ; to run ; to leap ; to wrestle ; to swim ; to dance comely ; to sing and play instruments cunningly ; to hawk ; to play at tennis ; and all pastimes generally which be joined with labour, used in open place, and in the daylight, containing either some fit exercise for war or some pleasant pastime for peace, be not only comely and decent, but also very necessary for a courtly gentleman to use."

94. In modern times, to comprehend so noble a system of moral and physical training, required a Napoleon ; and his management of his armies of Boulogne, and of Poland, in his first Russian war, is a wonderful example in proof. In his great arrangements the Romans could hardly have excelled him.

95. The commentator of Roger Ascham, from whose writings the above is quoted, observes justly :—" But ' the pastimes joined with labour—the vaulting, running, leaping, wrestling, and swimming' —were as necessary for the yeomen, the artisans, and the peasants, as for the gentlemen of England. Such training, ' fit exercise for war,' has won our country's battles, from Agincourt to Alma. Such training, ' pleasant pastime for peace,' has still done something for brotherly kindness amongst degrees of men whom fortune had too much isolated."

96. " To shoot fair in bow or surely in gun," was an accomplishment which made Englishmen for ages the terror of surrounding countries ; and Englishmen are still presumed to possess the precious quality—the coolness in the heat of the fight ascribed to them by Foy. With fair play in the way of exercise, neither Frenchman nor American should be permitted to excel us in the use of the rifle. While, in Robert Jackson's time, one trained British soldier was equal to thirty of the ordinary class, Americans were trained to knock the heads off squirrels with their balls, so as " not to injure the skin."

97. But the life of the British soldier is so exceptional—so arti-

ficial, monotonous, and depressing—that nothing should be left undone which may tend to complete the means for exercise and amusement, wherever he may be cantoned, at home or abroad. According to the men's habits and inclinations, games, amusements, trades, agricultural pursuits, libraries, and theatrical entertainments should be encouraged; and none can encourage practically but the officers.

98. Military labour should always be conducted as a means to advance the social condition, elevate the character, and improve the position of the soldier, both while serving in the ranks and after retiring on the pension-list. The utter helplessness of the mere old soldier, on being discharged, and the miseries he suffers in consequence, are a great reproach to our system. The discharged engineer, on the contrary, finds ample employment and good wages, taking a high position among the working-classes. It is another remarkable deficiency of our system, that, where military instruction is given to the soldier, it is almost entirely confined to the attack.

99. Although much has been done of late years in the East Indies, by Lord Dalhousie very especially, to improve the moral and physical well-being of the British soldier, there are still many things to be accomplished which are necessary to his health and comfort. Of these wants the removal to the hill ranges is the greatest. Here the soldier might be permitted to marry in something like a reasonable proportion per company. Here he might pursue the occupations of trades, of gardening, rearing of domestic animals, &c., so as to prepare him for a return to usefulness in civil life, while, in the meantime, according to all experience, he would be making himself immeasurably a better soldier than the idler and laggard of the barrack-yard.

. 100. It is worthy of remark that while, in all European States, the amusements of the upper and middle classes of society have called into exercise the talents of artists and men of genius of the highest order, those of the lower classes remain confessedly too few, and such as are practised are very ill regulated. As to amusements for soldiers, such things were suggested and written about by the surgeons of our fleets and armies of old; but punishments were the ideas which obtained constant utterance from the mouths of the admirals and generals of those times. In their own persons our naval and military commanders have at all times been ready enough to subscribe to the justice and wisdom of Bacon's observation, that " Perils commonly ask to be paid in pleasures;" but, in the persons of their men, they have, with rare exceptions, forgotten this great and universal truth. In the dreary Sahara of the soldier's life, routine has seldom sought for an oasis in which to refresh or amuse him. The health-giving exercises which elicit the hearty laugh, have never yet been practically offered to our men. Sir John Moore made proposals worthy of him in the West

Indies, and they were disregarded. The imitations of our commanders since his time have been fitful and feeble in the extreme; and thus must such important matters remain, dependent on the freaks of individuals, until they shall be made part of the system and permanent order of our land forces.

101. Robert Jackson, writing in 1791, observes that exercises are no less necessary to the soldier than a knowledge of the use of his arms; and that, in fact, "the essential part of the art of disciplining troops consists in imparting sentiments of heroism and virtue to the minds of the men, in improving the exertions of the limbs, and in acquiring knowledge of the correspondence of their exertions when called into action." He adds, that the subject of exercising soldiers has been but little regarded in the armies of Europe; and that, with us, the ordinary exercises of the soldier "are flat and insipid in their nature—that they occasion no exertions and excite no emulation—that they neither improve the active powers of the body, nor inure the soldier to bear fatigue and hardship."

102. The Romans, who owed more to the discipline of their armies than any other people, were extremely rigorous and persevering in their exercises. They practised their soldiers in every species of service that might occur; so that nothing at any time happened with which they were unacquainted. Actual war was in reality a time of relaxation and amusement to the soldiers of this warlike people, who appear to have been trained for the service of the field, as horses are for hunting or the course. The Romans were not only sensible of the advantages which those habits of exercise procured them in action, but they had also the penetration to discover that they were eminently serviceable in the preservation of health.

103. The exercises now and at all times practised in the British army, so far from exciting emulation, are esteemed, and have always been esteemed by the men themselves, as a mere drudgery; but they might be induced to take an interest in pleasurable exercises, such as fencing, the broad-sword exercises, walking, running, leaping, wrestling, and swimming. Such exercises invigorate the powers of the body and limbs, and thereby impart confidence to the soldier; while indolence is the moth of the mind in all climates.

104. Parades and drills are no exercise; they are generally, in hot climates, and, as now managed, an unhealthy exposure of the men, and nothing more. The march and manœuvre should not take place oftener than three times a week, with the interval of a day of complete rest and refreshment between each.

105. The exercise of marching in the early morning, in light marching order, and with appropriate dress, should be matter of regular regimental order in all tropical climates, and at all seasons, excepting the rainy.

106. The exercise of ball-practice has excitement and emulation in it; and it ought likewise to be made matter of regular order in all climates whatsoever. Robert Jackson, who urges the frequent and liberal recourse to ball-practice, says, that one soldier who is possessed of skill in the use of the musket is equal to thirty or more who have not practised in the careful manner which he recommends; namely, the art of directing fire upon distant, and upon certain given points. No reasonable Englishman will hesitate between parsimony with imperfection and insufficiency, and increase of reputation with expenditure; yet our authorities, until very recently, have always clung to the former.

107. It ought to be for ever in the remembrance of all classes of officers that indolence and sloth are the bane of the soldier in every climate, and that exercise of the mind and body constitute the best preservatives of health and vigour.

108. Soldiers previously trained to handicrafts should be practised in their original trades. The very jollities, competitions, and exhilarations of the workshop would conduce to health; and sheds and huts should be constructed at the public cost to be used as workshops.

109. The use of camps, as opposed to suburban barracks, ought to be—to dispense with all trades, so that the soldier should do for himself everything that may not interfere with health and discipline. The helplessness of the soldier, the forced, or regulation-helplessness, so loudly complained of by Jackson, and which continues to the present day, is very much due to the neglect of such exercises and amusements as are here spoken of.

110. Notwithstanding William Fergusson's declaration that he never knew or heard of a reading army, it is nevertheless true, as he indeed admits, that in hot climates, in which the soldier is necessarily confined to his quarters for many hours of every day, during eight months of every year, reading, writing, the inspection of models and cheap maps, recitation, &c., will prove valuable aids towards dispelling ennui, and preventing recourse to drinking and other vices.

111. Dr. Arnott, of the Bombay Fusiliers, says, that in each European regiment of the Company's army in his Presidency there will be found a savings' bank, a good school, a well-selected library, a printing press, an excellent theatre, and good coffee-shops; while the soldiers are made expert tailors, shoemakers, smiths, farriers, carpenters, bookbinders, watchmakers, &c.; and they meet with support and encouragement in their work. The games are chess, backgammon, cricket, skittles, quoits, long-bullets; with rowing and fishing when opportunity offers.

112. "Under such beneficial operations," says the experienced officer already quoted, "our soldiers are as well behaved in quarters as brave before the enemy; and commensurate with the additions to their comforts has been the improvement of the

habits of the soldier." He adds, that while sobriety is gradually taking place of drunkenness, sickness and mortality are yearly diminishing.

113. In justice to the memory of the Marquis Dalhousie it must be stated that many of the humane measures here described as the results of local arrangement, were systematically and generally ordered in regulations framed during his great administration of India. But those precautions against vice and sickness, those safeguards of discipline, and those sources of contentment and long good service which have been so effective in the East, we should be glad to see extended to the West also—indeed, to all our possessions.

114. Finally, and speaking more physiologically, exercises, by accelerating the respiratory and circulating functions, invigorate the nerve-forces, promote secretion and depuration, purify the blood, and strengthen the muscular system ; not to mention their great influence on the mind of the soldier, in advancing and confirming his moral and military discipline.

115. MARCHING OF TROOPS IN HOT CLIMATES.—The marching qualities of the British soldier have never been so nobly developed and demonstrated as by Sir John Moore—" that model soldier of England"—who taught a lesson which the Peninsular war commemorates, but which the present generation may forget in our home railways. A railway, it is true, will bring the soldier to his post with a speed unknown to our ancestors ; but, if we neglect the march, we shall forget much for which the soldier is brought to his post, and be very little, if at all, the gainers by our mechanical speed.

116. In September, 1812, the Duke of Wellington writes :—" No disorders amongst the old soldiers. Regiments recently arrived from England or the Straits are very unhealthy, and the loss by death is almost confined to them. I am afraid that the soldiers are not sufficiently exercised in marching when at home or in foreign garrisons; and they become sickly as soon as they are obliged to make a march. The non-commissioned officers, and I am afraid the officers, are very bad, and they neglect to attend to the food of the soldiers."

117. The truth is that, as regards health and the results which health may secure to the commander, the march will prove, like other things, exactly what we may make of it. In actual war a march properly conducted leads to vigour, health, and success : a march improperly conducted, ends in exhaustion of mind and body, in disappointment, sickness, and failure.

118. By the more ordinary and unreflecting of the military, the conduct of a march is deemed a matter of trifling routine in itself, and therefore most easy of accomplishment ! If conducted during war, and the march is performed without surprise or loss of baggage ; or, if in peace, and the operation is accomplished without

complaint on the part of the populations along the route, all is presumed to be well; but indeed there are many other circumstances which here demand a very careful consideration.

119. Previously to the march of troops, the regimental surgeon should institute minute and repeated inspections of the men, with the view to prevent weakly and diseased persons from proceeding, and with the purpose also of preserving the means of transport attached to the regiment for the inevitable contingencies only of the march. By such precautionary arrangements disease is prevented, and the slightest cases cured; while the soldiers, knowing that in sickness they incur the risk of being left behind, will use more than usual care against contracting illnesses.

120. Excepting under urgent occasions of service, European troops are not allowed to be moved in India during the hot and rainy seasons; from the beginning of November to the beginning of March being usually regarded as the proper season. A disregard of this appropriate time for movement caused the 78th Highland Regiment, between August, 1844, and March, 1845, to lose 669 men. Even native regiments have suffered most severe losses from similar inattentions to season.

121. The hour of march should be so early as to enable the men to arrive at their ground of encampment before the sun has acquired power;—say, an hour after sun-rise—regard being had to the nature of the country, and of the roads to be traversed by the troops. When conducting the march, care should be taken to place the least effective men in the front—the movement there being necessarily the most free.

122. In hot weather the soldier's neck should be bare upon the march, the head being kept as cool as possible, the face and head being frequently splashed with water. When flushing of countenance or giddiness appears, then the sufferers should be made to halt, and everything done to prevent sunstroke.

123. The pace of the soldier, during the first hour or two of the march, should not exceed the rate of three miles per hour; and the rate ought to have no relation whatever to the walking power of the colonel's horse. At the end of the first hour a halt of five minutes should be ordered, and at the end of the second hour twenty minutes. About half the march being now accomplished, the pace of the men for the remaining half may properly be somewhat accelerated, and a halt of twenty minutes being ordered at the end of the third hour, a march of twelve to fourteen miles may well be performed in four to five hours.

124. In all hot climates the order of march should be open and easy to the men, the close majestic English formation being here something far worse than absurd; unless it be in the very face of an enemy whom we desire to frighten. It is surely enough for discipline and order that, on the line of march, every man may be ready to fall in on the first tap of the drum, as in the French army.

125. In making forced marches, the halt of an hour, in addition to those already recommended, should be ordered at the end of the first twelve miles. Marshal Ney says of the march in Europe :—"If the enemy is far off, there should be a general halt of half an hour after every two hours of march. If it be a forced march, it shall continue four hours, and then a halt of an hour for refreshment."

126. As an example of well-sustained marching, I would adduce that of the heroic Polish commander, Dembinski, in the insurrection of 1831, when he marched five hundred and fifty miles in twenty-five days, surrounded by a host of enemies, bringing his army into Warsaw intact. "The annals of war," says Alison, "do not record a more memorable exploit." The marches performed in our earlier campaigns in India, by Colonel Adams, Coote, and Lake, are very memorable, taking into account the climate in which they were performed.

127. Soldiers in active march, and when the enemy is near, should halt, pile arms, and fall out in their order of march ; so as to unpile, fall in, and march off again at a moment's notice, without disorder or confusion of any kind. A slow rate of march with long halts, on the supposition that the men are thus spared, is a great mistake ; for it implies solar exposure and much distress to the soldier, whether European or Native.

128. Movements in brigade or battalion are never made for the march, excepting in the presence of an enemy—the best mode of marching off being generally by fours ; and when the force is at all considerable, a signal-lantern should be hoisted at the starting rendezvous.

129. It is in devising and arranging the exercises and amusements, and the march of the soldier, that the officer will find himself sure of commanding the personal attachment of his men : it is only by inferior minds that drilling is mistaken for training ;— two things indeed widely distinct and separate. In the language of Marshal Ney, the officer must, without intermission, and with increasing solicitude, attend to the wants of his men, while he insures by the most persevering activity, the execution of his orders.

130. Persons in authority should also hold in careful recollection the caution of this great commander against the too great number of evolutions, invented in time of peace for the soldier's torment, by officers often more systematic than experienced in war.

131. The great French tactician assures us that but "two essential conditions constitute the strength of infantry—that the men be good marchers, inured to fatigue ; that the firing be well executed." He concludes that "victory smiles in general upon those only who know how to command it by good preparations ;" and amongst "good preparations" none assuredly yield better returns to the State than the sanitary arrangements now so well understood :—"Le bien le plus précieux est le sang du soldat."

132. When entering on the Crimean campaign, the following intelligible, common-sense sanitary instructions were issued to the French soldiers :—

" *a*. It is wrong to sleep in immediate contact with the ground. Perfectly dry substances not easily permeated by moisture should be interposed. For this purpose fresh branches of vegetable matters should never be used.

" *b*. When the camp is pitched near a marsh, a tank, pools of stagnant water, or a valley, the chief openings of the tents should be in the opposite direction. In these bivouacs every possible means should be used to exclude the noxious vapours exhaled from such *foci*. At night the openings of the tents, or other coverings, with exception to those necessary for ventilation, should be closed.

" *c*. The greatest care is needed for protection against the freshness of the nights, even when the heat is extreme; it is dangerous to remain clad only with the shirt during the night. At the bivouac and in the tent the soldiers should be very carefully covered.

" *d*. The feet should *not* be washed with cold water, especially when heated after a march.

" *e*. Whenever practicable, the face, and particularly the eyes, should be frequently washed daily, after exposure to the dust of the march.

" *f*. Cleanliness of person, clothes, and dwellings is imperiously required by the nature of the climate.

" *g*. In summer the best protection against sunstrokes, which are often very dangerous, is never to leave shelter without having the head covered.

" *h*. It is necessary to be always so clothed as to be proof against the sudden chills to which one is liable at all seasons, from the abrupt changes of temperature which frequently happen in nearly all parts of this country."

These instructions were explained to the French soldiers.

" *The March.*—*i*. The pace should not on any occasion exceed three and a half miles per hour.

" *j*. One of the junior medical officers, with a native attendant, should always be placed on the march between the column and rear-guard, prepared to administer wine or other stimulant, or order means of carriage for men who may fall out from exhaustion.

" *k*. No man should for any purpose be allowed to fall out without a non-commissioned officer to accompany him, to secure his return to the ranks at the next halt, and to report him immediately to the surgeon, if sick.

" *l*. An excellent suggestion of Dr. Barclay, of the 43rd regiment, is to have all the men who fell out on the march examined by the surgeon immediately on arrival at the encamping ground. He frequently detected disease in this manner which for a time might otherwise have escaped notice.

"*m*. The tents should be pitched as quickly as possible, and they should even be carried on camels or elephants, not carts.

"*n*. European soldiers on a march in India, especially in the hot and rainy seasons, should as much as possible be exempted from duties, and from those of sentries, where any native troops are present.

"*o*. When obliged to go out in the sun, the soldiers should be ordered to place a damp cloth or towel under the forage cap, so as to protect the head.

"*p*. It were a true economy, in the hot and rainy season, to secure the very best description of tents for camp and hospital purposes."

133. TOPOGRAPHICAL PRECAUTIONS—LOCALITIES TO CHOOSE.— When military considerations do not imperatively forbid it, an elevated and dry soil should always be selected for bivouacs, camps, and cantonments, having undulating ground, or the declivity of a hill; the most healthy sites being such as do not, from the natural fall or from the quality of the soil, retain moisture.

a. Where we can obtain the power to choose our ground of encampment, we should give preference to a dry but not hard soil, so that it may quickly imbibe rain, and thus become fit for military operations soon after the heaviest falls. Rapid absorption also saves the troops from the injuries caused by damp.

b. Under great heats, wooded districts, if dry in the soil and subsoil, are good grounds for encampments, the lofty shade affording cool refreshment and a free ventilation.

c. Open downs, so called, are healthy.

d. The elevated banks of rivers that have a sufficient fall either way.

e. Tongues of land, or slender promontories, jutting well into the sea.

f. It is said that wherever pure water is procurable, there the ground is generally fit for encamping or cantoning troops.

g. When marching, to halt, during wet weather, on ground somewhat elevated and sloping, and sheltered from the wind.

h. In such case to increase the number of fires, and to keep them up to the hour of starting.

i. To make the regulated halts where water is good, and to prevent the men from drinking it while heated by the march.

j. In marshy localities the ground of encampment should be on the highest ground procurable.

k. When encamped on a river bank, a station high up the stream should be appointed for drinking and cooking purposes; next below it, the station for watering cattle; and below that the station for washing.

l. When river-water has become muddy, or otherwise unwholesome, wells should be constructed under proper direction—sand or shingle being placed in the bottom of the springs.

m. In all convenient situations the men in health should be marched every morning to the bath, especially during hot weather.

n. Encamped, through necessity, too near a rivulet or river having marshy banks, the extension of ague should be prevented by cleansing and deepening the river-bed, raising the banks, and increasing their inclination, removing the tents to a greater distance from the river bank.

o. Choose a gravelly soil, and if elevated, so much the better— low-lying gravelly soils being less healthy.

p. A chalk formation, with a sufficient inclination, *if poor and barren*, is very healthy, and the air from such soils proves generally dry and bracing; but if the same kind of formation be level, and charged with refuse matters, it will become pestilential.

134. LOCALITIES TO AVOID.—All damp ground, whether sandy or other, to be avoided in all climates; and where the surface may appear parched up and destitute of vegetation, if there yet be moisture underneath, as caused by previous rains or other percolation, it may be charged with the worst exhalations.

a. Lands the woods of which have been recently cut down should be carefully avoided.

b. Half-dried beds of rivers, of canals, tanks, or ditches; narrow gorges. A camp should not be intersected by streams or ditches, nor enclosed by extensive forests.

c. Marshy grounds, and such as are immediately above marshes, and grounds exposed to winds and currents passing over marshes; the near vicinity of canals.

d. Grounds covered with underwood, and the vicinity of such grounds.

e. The low, jungly, or marshy banks of tidal rivers and lakes; especially if the waters be impure.

f. The best ground, if long occupied by masses, becomes contaminated, just as air and water become contaminated by abuse. It is therefore an established sanitary rule in all countries to change the ground of encampment as frequently as may be.

g. Places of proved insalubrity in the estimation of the natives, and places in which troops have suffered on previous occasions of encamping or cantoning, should be carefully avoided. The first of these precautions was neglected, through ignorance, by the British commanders in the valley of the Guadiana and in Bulgaria, and great destruction of life was the result on both occasions.

h. Meadow-lands having vegetation of a marshy nature, combining the presence of amphibious animals, as frogs and tortoises. The presence of the *Rara variabilis* is considered an unerring indication of an unwholesome and marshy locality.*

i. The presence of flies of various kinds, followed by flocks of insect-eating birds, points to an unhealthy locality; and the

* Dr. Aitken's "Climate of Scutari."

nature of the soil, combined with these circumstances, will generally indicate to the careful observer the presence of unhealthy districts.

j. Alluvial grounds at the entrance and at the exit of lakes, especially if there be tracts of slime and mud.

135. TREATMENT OF SOLDIERS ON BOARD SHIP.—The condition of the transport, the state of health of the crew, to be carefully examined. When ships of war are used, a frigate to be preferred to a ship of the line.

a. Old and foul ballasting to be changed, and no fresh or green wood to be allowed in the ship's hold, or any matter capable of ready decomposition.

b. The state of health of the troops to be carefully examined, and cases of contagious disease, or of old or extensive ulcers, to be left behind.

c. The crowding of the men to be especially guarded against, and care taken that berths are secured for the sick and the married : the strictest care to be taken that the aggregate numbers of persons do not exceed the proportion of one person to two tons of measurement, at the least.

d. The men should not be permitted to quit the ship, or to be on deck after sunset, when navigating rivers, or proceeding along level or marshy sea-coasts.

e. Careful and especial examination of the provisions should be made, and it should be seen that the salted meat and biscuit are good and fresh ; the same care being taken in respect of the water, which, when possible, should be taken from springs, and kept in iron tanks. Quicklime should be provided for purifying the water.

f. For distant expeditions there should be hospital ships, well-provided and cleansed, to allow for the proper and immediate separation of the healthy from the sick.

g. Cold and damp in the ship's hold are to be guarded against, and the pumps to be frequently worked, so as to leave but a few inches in the well.

h. Thorough ventilation, and a careful attention to cleanliness, to be promoted by every means ; and in bad weather, when the wind-sails cannot be used, portable stoves or firepots should be carried between decks.

i. In fair weather the men should be much on deck, and they should be made to bathe daily.

j. Moderate exercise, with amusements of every kind, should be encouraged by every means during the voyage ; and a union of kindliness and indulgence with good order and discipline should characterize the conduct of all classes of officers towards their men.

k. It should always be remembered that soldiers who have voyaged in crowded and ill-ventilated ships are peculiarly liable to disease, both endemic and epidemic, on landing in a new country. New-comers are everywhere more prone to disease than residents ; but new-comers who have voyaged in pure air, having ordinary care in other respects, arrive under happy conditions, comparatively. M. Scribe justly observes that such circumstances naturally suggest extra vigilance in the hygienic treatment of newly-arrived troops in foreign countries.

l. The actual loss of British soldiers during the last half-century, reckoned for six months only from their landing in the East and West Indies, and resulting solely from the neglects here briefly stated, would shock the humanity of the present day.

136. BARRACK AND HOSPITAL ACCOMMODATION.—It may be said with truth of all our intertropical possessions, that, next to the injuries to health caused by the ill selection of localities for military stations, temporary and permanent, stand those caused by the ill construction of barracks and hospitals. Of structural errors to avoid we have endless examples throughout the British Empire, at home and abroad; but not one unexceptionable example which might be adopted with advantage in any one of the infinitely various climates of our possessions, temperate or tropical.

137. With a view to settle this most important question on a solid and scientific footing, it was proposed by me, in a memorandum drawn out by desire of Lord Metcalfe, and presented by him to the Colonial Minister in July, 1842 :—

a. That a Commission be assembled in London, composed of medical officers and of engineers, civil and military, to inquire into and determine, on sufficient evidence, the best plans for hospitals and barracks in the various climates in which the soldier serves.

b. That, on a full and careful consideration of the whole subject, a standard plan be prepared suited to the various climates of our possessions, home and foreign.

c. That, provided qualified persons were selected for this duty, the task of arriving at a satisfactory conclusion could not be one of much difficulty; for that much the same kind of barrack and hospital accommodation would be suitable for the East and West Indies, the Cape of Good Hope, Mauritius, Ceylon, and Australia, and also in the Mediterranean stations; while much the same plans would answer for the United Kingdom, and for our North American possessions, and so on.

d. That, until something of this kind is done, the discussions on the subject become nothing more than an useless course of fault-findings and vain disquisitions.

e. Pending the arrival of the proposed settlement, I would beg leave to suggest that barracks and hospitals, situated on the hot and pestilential plains of our hot climates, ought to be raised on arches, and have double roofs, the cubic space within being of the greatest. Here we can make no mistake, for the breathing-space cannot be too large.

138. MEDICAL OFFICER OF HEALTH.—The author also suggests, and he has very long suggested :—

a. That there be attached to the head-quarters of every field force, and specially to the office of quartermaster-general of such force, a highly qualified and selected medical officer in the department of medical topography.

b. That his duties in peace be to examine and report on the proper sites, and on the sanitary condition of military stations and cantonments, convalescent stations and sanatoria;—on the structure and arrangements of barracks and hospitals, and on everything which may relate to the comfort and health of the soldiers.

c. That, in war more especially, such a military-medical officer of health should be attached to the quartermaster-general in the field, and be always in advance in company with that officer, so as to be master of the medical topography of the scene of action.

d. That where military reasons of imperative necessity do not overrule sanitary considerations, the advice of the medical officer of health should be accepted, as to the sites of camps, whether temporary or permanent. Colonel Macdougall, in his excellent work on the " Theory of War," acknowledges what has for more than a hundred years been declared by our army surgeons : he, at length, states distinctly, that " the choice of a healthy site for a camp" is one of those arrangements which is " peculiarly within the province of the medical department."

e. That such an officer, so highly qualified, and possessing rank and station in the army, could not fail to prove of the greatest service, in peace and in war, in all countries ; and that there has not occurred an expedition or a campaign since the reign of William III., not to go further back, in which such an officer of health would not have saved thousands upon thousands of our men, and millions upon millions of our money, not to speak of moral, military, and material savings. To furnish instances in example is altogether unnecessary. Our military history is full of them ; and they will present themselves by the score to every well-informed Englishman.

139. SKETCH OF PERSONAL AND MATERIAL ARRANGEMENT FOR FIELD SERVICE.—(1.) If chemistry and physics, says a modern writer, enable us to commit more havoc among hostile ranks than was possible formerly, surely the advance of medical science ought to enable us to save more of our own troops; or, in the language of the *Times*, " the duties of self-preservation are of primary importance in war, not falling below the art of killing the enemy."

(2.) The naval and military surgeon, under all circumstances of service, and especially during war, should have held out to him all the advantages and encouragements presented to other officers. The difference between officers as combatants and surgeons as non-combatants must cease," says Radetzky, the great Austrian commander in Italy. " I see everywhere military officers and surgeons equally exposed to the fire, and therefore the surgeons shall enjoy advantages and distinctions in every respect equal to those of the officers."

(3.) " Medical officers will not work well," says Guthrie, " without some hope of reward. The promotion on all death and retired vacancies should be granted to those who have worked—not by seniority, but by desert. The medical inspector and the general commanding must judge of their merits; and the Director-General at home should not have a veto."

(4.) For an army to enjoy the advantages of a thoroughly experienced medical staff, it is necessary that a system of rotation of duties be rigorously enforced amongst its members—every military surgeon being employed successively in every department of the service; in the stationary and in the field hospitals—in the field, in the trenches, at the ambulances. Wellington, writing to Sir John Malcolm, from London, in February, 1808, says : " I am employed in this country very much in the same way that I was in India—that is to say, in everything ;" and so ought the army-surgeon to be employed.

(5.) Of the surgeons who accompany an army into the field, those only acquire real surgical knowledge and experience who are detached in charge of the hospitals, and who thus have personal responsibility thrown upon them. Of the surgeons who move with the troops, those only who are attached to the ambulances become familiar with the performance of operations.

(6.) Through a system of rotation the chief of the medical department will readily discover the talents and abilities, and the particular kinds of services for which every officer under his orders may be qualified. Physical qualities with skill in operating will qualify for the field services—such officers being attached to the ambulances; while such as possess peculiar facilities for tending the sick and dressing the wounded should be sent to the hospitals.

(7.) Military qualities will enable the possessor to command, inspect, and superintend, and the mind fitted for organization will find employment in supplying the medical wants of the army and the hospitals, in keeping the registers, accounts, &c.

(8.) The chief must control and direct the *personnel* and *matériel* of his department. The latter was properly designated the " impedimenta " by the Romans ; and our design should be to give to our stores as little of that character as possible.

(9.) After an important action, the surgeons who have attended in the field or at the ambulances, should be sent to the hospital along with the wounded who have been under their care during or immediately after the battle. A surgeon will necessarily take more interest in his own acts than in the results obtained by others, and we ought to employ this tendency for the benefit of the wounded.— *Brit. & For. Med.-Chir. Rev.*, Jan. 1856.

(10.) In 1803, Jackson writes, that in the campaigns and expeditions conducted by Pitt, the " excess" of medical officers over the real wants of the army " was beyond measure great; not less than two-thirds :" in other words, " one-third, or less than one-third, either has performed, or was capable of performing, all the service which has been done in the hospitals during the war."

(11.) He adds, that on the same scenes of action "two-thirds, or more than two-thirds of the medicines ordered for the use of the forces perished in store, before there was an opportunity of applying them to a purpose;" just as our soldiers perished before they beheld their enemy.

(12.) Writing in 1805, the same authority proposes that for a battalion of a thousand men, stationed in Europe in time of peace, one surgeon and one assistant ought to be enough ; having a staff or superior medical officer to each brigade of three battalions. Employed on field service in Europe, or on distant foreign service, then an additional assistant to each regiment is declared necessary.

(13.) Reckoning on the same principle, we should require for service in Europe in time of peace, 231 medical officers for an army of 100,000 men, and 388 medical officers with the same force when employed in the field, or in distant unhealthy climates. But upon Jackson's estimate of what was a fit medical establishment, there was an actual excess over and above the real wants of 100,000 men, of 762 medical officers.

(14.) Jackson estimated the average ordinary sick of his time at one in ten of the effective strength, and at one in five under extraordinary circumstances.

(15.) But a just order with economy had no place in the public arrangements of those times ; and Robert Jackson, to his great honour, was the first and foremost to expose the ruinous consequences. The expedition of 1795 to the Cape of Good Hope consisted of 3000 men, for which 18 hospital staff were appointed, over and above the regimental complement of medical officers.

(16.) The force sent to the Caribbean Islands under Sir Ralph Abercromby numbered 20,000 men ; for which 183 medical officers of all grades and descriptions were appointed.

(17.) The expedition to St. Domingo, calculated at 15,000 men, had 94 medical officers of all grades and descriptions attached to it.

(18.) The total troops employed on these three services, amounting to 38,000 men, had a hospital staff of "two hundred and ninety-five ; or a medical officer for about every hundred and twenty-eight persons, exclusive of the addition of the regimental staff."

(19.) But, including the regimental medical officers, we have "the sum of four hundred and fifty-one medical officers, charged with the care of the health of thirty-eight thousand soldiers ; a high proportion, as affording one medical person for every eighty-eight men." Thus, "had the whole army been all actually sick at one time," the extra provision of hospital staff, not to count the regimental, "was alone sufficient."

(20.) With this "enormous multitude of medical officers," which left "two-thirds of the medical staff idle or but half employed," the sick and wounded suffered "loss in want of medical assistance."

(21.) No wonder that this great authority should declare "a superfluous number of medical officers to be, instead of a benefit, actually an evil in an army;" and that it is the army surgeon who is "choice in quality and important in character" that is wanted, and not a mass of persons "strong only in numbers."

(22.) Dr. Andrew Smith, presenting his views half a century after Jackson, suggested the following personal medical establishment in 1854, for thirty thousand men ordered on service to Turkey, under the command of Lord Raglan:—

Inspector-general of hospitals	1
Deputy-inspectors general	4
Staff surgeons of the first class	12
,, ,, second class	13
Staff assistant-surgeons	48
Chief apothecary	1
Dispensers of medicines	3
Purveyors	3
Purveyors' clerks	6
Medical clerks	2
Cutler	1
Total staff	94

(23.) To every regiment of infantry, averaging 850 men, was, besides, specially allotted one surgeon and three assistant-surgeons. To every two squadrons of cavalry of 250 men one surgeon and one assistant-surgeon. To every troop of horse artillery, one assistant-surgeon; and to every field battery, one assistant-surgeon. For the general duties of the Ordnance Medical Department, one surgeon. Here was personal provision for cure without stint. Had the same amount of care been given by authority to the personal and influential means necessary for the prevention of disease, it is not too much to say that the national calamity of the Crimea would not have occurred.

(24.) The total medical officers allotted to the 30,000 men was two hundred and five. During the Peninsular war it was found that more than one-third, but not quite one-half, of the medical officers of the army were generally ineffective from sickness, &c.; therefore, as an equal amount of sickness might be expected in Turkey, sixty-eight medical officers were constituted a reserve to supply vacancies.

(25.) After providing ample supplies of medical and surgical stores, the Director-General ordered the following material establishment for the conveyance of the sick and wounded:—

Bearers or stretchers 780
Spring-carts on two wheels, Guthrie's 20
Spring waggons on four wheels 20
Flanders waggons 9

(26.) Each waggon was arranged to carry ten men—four severely and six slightly wounded—each having a separate compartment; while the Flanders waggons were intended for the carriage of field-hospital and other stores.

(27.) In addition to a large general material establishment, each corps was provided with a regimental and with a detachment medicine-chest—each such chest being furnished with every requisite medical and surgical means, and also with a box of apparatus for fractures and dislocations.

(28.) Besides the above, the surgeons of each corps had each a full set of capital instruments; the senior assistant a portable set — and the surgeon and the three assistants had each a pocket-case of instruments, with lancets, &c. ; and, for general use, there was likewise a set of cupping instruments and a stomach-pump.

(29.) It is now proper to refer to the scheme of personal and material arrangement proposed by Guthrie, for a force of 12,000 men (twelve. regiments of infantry, and four batteries of artillery), founded on Peninsular experience, on the completion of the war at the battle of Toulouse, when the celebrated author believed that the medical.department of Wellington's army had attained to perfection. This plan, most maturely considered, was submitted for consideration of the Minister for War and the Commander-in-Chief, with reference to the then contemplated expedition to the Crimea. Its purely surgical character is plainly pronounced.

(30.) One surgeon and three assistants to accompany each regiment; one assistant-surgeon to accompany each battery of artillery; and one regimental surgeon to every four batteries. These officers should always remain with their respective corps, except the surgeon of artillery, and go into action with them. At a siege, one assistant-surgeon accompanies each relief into the trenches, and is also exposed like any other person.

(31.) One staff surgeon should be attached to each division, to superintend and regulate its proceedings. He also accompanies the troops into action, but avoids musketry fire and cannon shot, if he can : once an officer loses his regiment at the commencement of an action, it has happened that he could not find it again until it was over, not even if he was a staff officer.

(32.) The staff-surgeon here mentioned, ought to be selected by the general, but should not consider himself permanent. He should form part of the division general's family, and it may be advisable to make him an allowance, as for an aide-de-camp. On this officer mainly depends the efficiency of the division; he should be a young and vigorous person, equal to anything, and when he no longer possesses the confidence of the general, he should be removed.

(33.) The staff surgeon of the division should remain with the wounded as long as he can be spared from the division ; and if the loss be great, one surgeon only should remain with each brigade. Surgeons of artillery should join the general hospital, and also the assistant-surgeons attached to the batteries, whenever their services are required.   One deputy inspector-general should remain at Constantinople, with one staff assistant-surgeon, and one clerk. He should superintend the landing of the troops and the departure of invalids, apportion their supplies, regulate the hospital, and approve the contracts for it.   He should correspond with the inspector-general at head-quarters, and have a separate correspondence on every point relative to the station with the director-general at home, copies of which should be sent to his superior at head-quarters.   He should provide attendance for all sick officers arriving from the army, and report when they become fit for duty. The medical officer here should be of rank, as he will have to transact business with Turkish and other foreign authorities—perhaps even with the ambassador.

(34.) The inspector-general in the field may be of any age, provided he be not subject to back-ache, the gout, chronic cough, or other inconvenient ailment.   "The inspector-general goes with head-quarters.   He is almost entirely a pen-and-ink man." . . . . (Here we have a most remarkable illustration of what had been regarded as perfection in the Peninsula.)   All others will do their duty better if under thirty years of age.   After six campaigns, involving a larger share of practical labour than any one else, and, with one exception, a more responsible duty, I was, at the termination of the war in the Peninsula, twenty-eight years of age. What I could do then any one else can do now.

(35.) Medical officers are not to be computed according to the force employed, but according to the loss likely to be sustained in the first battle.   If a force of 12,000 men should have 1500 wounded, including officers, they would require (Toulouse being taken as an example, and there is no other so good), fifty-two surgeons, besides four apothecaries, or dispensers.   The whole medical force would be thus :—

Inspector-general	1
Deputy inspectors-general	2
Staff surgeons	8
Staff assistant-surgeons	10
Regimental surgeons	12
,, assistant-surgeons	36
Artillery surgeons, four batteries	5
Total	74

(Exclusive of four apothecaries, or dispensers of medicines.)

Deduct inspector-general	1	
Regimental surgeons	12	Always in the field.
Artillery surgeons	4	
Deputy inspector	1	
Staff surgeon	1	At Constantinople.
Assistant-surgeons	2	
Absent, or sick, of the whole	3	
Total	24	

(36.) If 24 be deducted from 74, it will leave 50—being two less than the number required at Toulouse for the first week, to take proper scientific care of 1359 wounded men, and twelve less than were present in the second week.

(37.) If a second battle take place within a few days, there would be only twelve regimental surgeons to depend upon; and if the loss were only half that which occurred in the first battle, all scientific treatment would be at an end. The proposed medical staff is therefore insufficient for the duties required when two battles are fought within a week; yet, in the south of France, three large hospitals were established in less than four weeks—at Tarbes, Orthes, Toulouse, besides some smaller ones. If, in addition to this, any of the diseases common to the country be superadded, the medical officers will be totally unable for the duties—a sad and important consideration.

(38.) If the reports of the inspector-general should, in May or June next, appear to indicate such an evil, twenty assistant-surgeons might with advantage be allowed to volunteer from the regiments at home, some of whom should find themselves promoted to unattached or second-class surgeoncies on their arrival at Constantinople. The general commanding should have authority to require the services of all medical officers from Corfu, Malta, and Gibraltar; and the naval surgeons may, under such circumstances, be able to take charge of the hospital at Constantinople.

(39.) If an addition of 12,000 men be made to the original force of that number, then one deputy inspector-general, eight staff-surgeons, and twelve staff assistant-surgeons should accompany it; volunteers from regiments accompanying them, together with one spring-cart for each regiment, and six for a reserve—in all, eighteen spring-carts; under the belief that 24,000 men will probably suffer more in one action than half their number, if opposed to a superior force.

(40.) The inspector-general should make himself acquainted with the topography, prevailing diseases, and the capabilities of every kind of each place he visits; what it can furnish which the army may require, and the price of each article; so that nothing may be imported from England which can be procured on the spot.

(41.) In the early part of the Peninsular war general hospitals were preferred to regimental and divisional hospitals; but in the latter part, regimental or divisional hospitals were considered the most advantageous. General hospitals should be looked upon as necessary evils, sometimes becoming even pest-houses; and, unless under vigorous management, they very materially impair the efficiency of an army.

(42.) The wounded of each brigade and division should, as much as possible, be placed together, under the assistant-surgeons and hospital establishment of each regiment, the hospital establishments remaining until they can be dispensed with. Regimental surgeons are, in fact, the men for work on such occasions : they understand their business, obey orders, and have an *esprit-de-corps* that carries them through everything. Under a staff-surgeon who knows his duties, and sets the example of them, the regimental surgeons never give in.

(43.) All the accounts of general hospitals, whether on the field or afterwards, should be made up weekly, added together monthly, and finally settled quarterly, by an accountant of repute on the spot, and never reopened : the accountant should not be a person who contracts nor one who pays.

(44.) Contracts should be approved as well as paid by the principal medical officer of each station, who should also examine and approve the weekly account of each separate hospital establishment of the station, whatever be their number. There is little difficulty in doing this, if the principal medical officer have a clerk who understands accounts, and a deputy-purveyor who is willing to do his duty.

(45.) A building should be obtained for a hospital a mile at least out of town, near the place where the troops land. It should be airy, roomy, and capable of containing six hundred sick. It should be walled in, if possible, with a field or garden behind. Supposing 12,000 men to land at Constantinople, there will be some sick, or men unable to march, dependent on the time they may have been on board ship, on the discipline observed, and particularly on the ventilation on board ship during the night.

(46.) The hospital should not only receive all the sick on landing, but all that are left on the advance of the army, and all that return from it as it proceeds. It should be so augmented, from time to time, as always to be ready to admit 200 more, whatever the number present. It may be the depôt for apothecaries' and for all other stores. If the force sent should ultimately amount to 25,000, this establishment must be greatly increased.

(47.) Bedding, less the straw, and all other hospital stores, should go out in the same ships for at least 1500 men. One staff surgeon and one or two of the best staff assistant-surgeons should be allotted to this hospital, with a purveyor and clerk, and two or three hospital serjeants or stewards, if procurable from the pensioners attached to the hospital-conveyance corps.

(48.) There should be a military officer attached to the charge of convalescents, and to repress irregularities. If this officer should not act cordially in concert with the principal medical officer, they should both be removed.

(49.) The first principle of military medical movement in the field is, that wherever a gun can go an hospital-cart should be able to follow and keep up with it. The medical conveyance of an army in the field should be, as far as possible, independent of the commissariat, although receiving assistance from that service on every occasion in which it can be afforded.*

(50.) An hospital-cart should be on two wheels, with shafts and outrigger for two horses, capable of being taken off the springs and easily put on again; having also a light permanent cover and side curtains. It should hold a cot slung high, and a seat for two persons in front, covering a waterproof box for surgical instruments and stores. There should be a similar but narrower seat behind for two persons, affixed to the doors, and everything belonging to the cart should match with similar articles in the artillery, such as wheels, &c. Two horses and two men must be permanently attached to it, and it should carry eight spare horseshoes.

(51.) One of these spring-carts should be attached to each regiment of cavalry, of infantry, and to each battery of artillery not serving with a brigade; while another should be specially attached to the horse artillery, and be capable of accompanying that service everywhere.

(52.) A quartermaster, or two non-commissioned officers, old hospital serjeants, should, if possible, be attached to every twelve carts, the whole being under the orders of the staff surgeon of the division; six of the twelve being in reserve. All the carts should be numbered; and the six attached to regiments should carry nothing but the box aforesaid of medical and surgical stores, and a tent with six bearers, with poles and springs. It should follow the regiment into action at a convenient distance, but near enough, on any movement taking place, to pick up the wounded.

(53.) The reserve carts should carry in addition two hard-pressed packages of ten sets of bedding, each set consisting of one rug, two blankets, three sheets, and one palliasse-case. These carts are to be with the staff surgeon, and as near as possible to the scene of action without incurring much risk.

(54.) Twenty-four carts are thus required for the use of two divisions, and twelve more and a forage-waggon should be attached to the head-quarters of the army; in all, thirty-seven. The forge-waggon should have two blacksmiths and a cutler, a handy man for all hardware work. These carts are intended to replace the defective ones with the divisions, or for particular services. One half should carry the same stores as before mentioned, with the addition of five caoutchouc bed-cases ready for inflation with air,

* In the Indian army of the old Company, the commissariat department, conducted by selected officers from the army at large, has always been the only organ of supply and transport; and it has never been wanting, whether in peace or in war.

while the other six should carry such articles of material for a field hospital as may be immediately required. The inspector-general must take care that every cart should be provided with the best means of carrying water, whether by barrels or skins, &c., as the country will afford, the absence of water having frequently caused much suffering after a battle.

(55.) Thirty-seven two-horse carts will require ninety horses. The non-commissioned officers and men on duty with the carts must walk whenever the carts are required for the use of the wounded; and as servants for the medical staff should be furnished from this corps, one hundred and fifty men will be required in all, although none, perhaps, need be fully efficient for service in the field.

(56.) These carts, &c., should be under direction of the inspector-general for their duties, and under the officer commanding the artillery for their discipline and payment. The great store of materials for general hospitals should be carried on bullock-carts, at a sufficient distance in rear of the army.

(57.) Each regiment should have two bullock-cars for the purposes of the sick only. They should be hired at Constantinople from such persons as can supply twelve for each division, with one superintendent, to be paid for at Constantinople at a fixed price, stipulated rations being granted to each driver and his two bullocks, the commissariat having the power to kill a lame or disabled animal, and to pay for it at a price fixed. The contractor must engage to supply all such casualties at fixed prices, his pay being stopped so long as any carts remain unserviceable. Such a system as this will prevent the irregular pressing found so prejudicial in the Peninsula.

(58.) Return conveyances of every kind, belonging to the commissariat of each brigade or division, should always carry sick to the rear, so as to leave the hospital conveyance as effective as possible for field service.

(59.) Every regimental surgeon should find a horse, mule, or camel out of his allowance, like captains of companies; and two panniers should be furnished by the government for each beast, made with wicker-work, covered by hide with hair on, and having an additional covering or lining made of some waterproof material. A Portuguese field officer's tent should be carried above and between the panniers, the whole being covered by a painted water-deck firmly girded by a rope. The animal thus loaded should never be sent to the rear with the baggage when preparing for action, but should always march in front of the last section of the regiment, if not with the commanding officer at the head of the regiment.

(60.) Each staff surgeon, and each surgeon unattached (absurdly called second class), should have an animal and pack-saddle furnished by the commissariat; panniers, stores, and tent being furnished by the medical department, and the man to take care of the animal being furnished by the hospital conveyance corps, as already indicated. Such, differently arranged and numbered, and with but a few verbal alterations, is the "Sketch of Medical Arrangement" of Mr. Guthrie.

POSTSCRIPT.—I have thought it useful here to record the substance of two intricate and laborious schemes of personal and material arrangement, for forces of but very moderate strength, then about to be employed in Turkey. The perusal will suggest many and varied reflections, according to the characters, opportunities, and experiences of military medical officers; but here I can refer only to one or two particulars. The confusion and collapse of all the departments in the field were, confessedly, amongst the more immediate and powerful of the causes of the loss of our army in the Crimea. "Shining civil qualities," appertaining absolutely to all official military command, according to Napoleon, were here wanting; and thus everything went to destruction.

To take one example out of the two medical schemes of arrangement, we find Mr. Guthrie suggesting that an animal shall be furnished to staff surgeons—the pack-saddle to be supplied by the commissariat, the panniers, stores, and tent to be supplied by the medical department, and the man in charge of the animal to be appointed by the hospital-conveyance department, not to mention the departments required to afford food and cover to man and beast.

In India we have never jumbled our departments. The commissariat there is the great organ of supply and transport. The duties are conducted by commissioned and carefully selected officers. selected under protracted competition and trial. There is not a greater or a more efficient department of an army in the world.

That, after forty years of peace, and of military progress in other countries, the experiences of the campaigns of Wellington had taught us nothing practically useful, whether military or medical, was wofully proved in the Crimea. In India, the beast of burden ordered by Guthrie would have been furnished, with all its own requirements, and the tents by the commissariat; while the medical department would only be charged with the supply of the medical stores and panniers.

With the utmost possible respect and veneration for the great surgical and military experiences and high manly qualities of Guthrie, with whose estimable general qualities I was personally well acquainted, it is most remarkable that in this formal and matured "Sketch of Medical Arrangement," so very little of the first and highest of medical arrangement—the prevention of disease —is to be found.

The perusal of the entire document, formally transmitted by the author to the Secretary of State for War, the Commander-in-Chief, the Commander of the Field Force, the Director-General of the Medical Department, Generals Sir De Lacy Evans and Sir

George Brown, leaves the great blank above mentioned. It is left also in doubt whether the perfections alleged to have been attained at the termination of the Peninsular war of six years, are really worthy of imitation. Sir De Lacy Evans states, in his evidence before the Sebastopol Committee, that "the medical department was quite as inadequate in the Peninsula as in the Crimea," and sundry of the suggestions of Mr. Guthrie, above quoted, proved utter failures in the Russian war.

140. TRANSPORT OF SICK AND WOUNDED IN INDIA.—Whether in the field or in cantonment, access and free immediate communication should be established between the regimental and the staff medical officers, who, being responsible to authority for everything, ought to be invested with independent powers to order and to act for the good of the service, whether in the distribution of medical and surgical stores, means of carriage, dooly-bearers, tents, cattle, &c.

141. During active warfare, or on a long march through a country thinly inhabited, extra cattle and carriage means should be furnished, and there should always be an arrangement for the conveyance of sick officers, who should not, as now, have to depend on such as properly belong to their men.

142. In Bengal, one dooly, or litter, is allowed for every hundred soldiers, and for every ten men in a European regiment. It forms a comfortable bed, and can be taken to pieces so as to admit of dressing the wounded without the removal of the patient, while it affords protection from weather.

143. The comforts of the Indian dooly are so great, not only in sickness but in wounds, that Staff-Surgeon Williamson, in charge of the Museum at Fort Pitt, Chatham, refers to "the large number of cases of gunshot compound fracture of the femur, where patients have recovered with good useful limbs, as compared with the number of thigh-stump cases, and the total by all wounds."

144. "This very satisfactory feature in the classified return of invalided wounded in the Indian mutiny, appears to me not uncommon for Indian wars, but certainly very much so for European wars, as far as records enable me to make the comparison. The difference in favour of the results by Indian wars, I believe to be mainly due to the facilities afforded by the dooly for the successful treatment of this the severest of all forms of compound fracture. Eleven cases recovered, with good useful limbs, out of the total wounded men landed from India—viz., 743, or 1·9 per cent. This is a large proportion compared with the results of the Crimean war—viz., 8 out of 2296, or 0·34 per cent."

145. A field-hospital conveyance has been invented by Sir John Login, an able and experienced surgeon of the Bengal army, of which Sir Charles Napier spoke very highly. The principle of this litter, or *blessière*, is—" to provide such a conveyance for sick and wounded as may render the soldier's removal from it unnecessary until

he can be completely lodged in a depôt hospital. By forming the bearing-poles into shafts to be attached to a light frame on wheels, a single man with leather shoulder-straps can easily run with it at ' the double' on ordinary ground, even while two sick and wounded men are in the litter; the weight of a pair of empty litters, with cover complete, being less than one cot."

146. While surgeons of regiments regulate the disposal and movements of doolies, they must likewise afford the most true and real protection to the hardworking, deserving dooly-bearers, who are otherwise likely to receive rough and injurious treatment on the line of march. Such unworthy treatment ought never to be allowed to pass without the most severe punishment of the offender, for it tends to produce desertion.

147. The regimental surgeon, too, while he looks to the order and care of his sick-carriage, and to the just and considerate treatment of the bearers and cattle, must be watchful of the safe conveyance of the hospital stores and baggage of the sick of his corps, along the line of march. The reverse flank will be found a good position for the tents, hospital stores, and sick-carriage; but, if this may not be, they should proceed in the rear of the reserve ammunition: marching thus in good order, without crowding or confusion, the halting-ground is arrived at without fatigue or damage.

148. FIELD HOSPITALS.—After the application of every means of prevention of disease suggested by reason and experience, the soldier who is wounded or falls sick has still to be cared for in the regimental hospital—there to receive the attention of his surgeon. On the field of battle the field hospital should be placed from four to six hundred yards in rear of the centre, and be distinguished by a flag. Field hospitals for all services, whether near or distant, should be complete in themselves, and have their establishments of officers, hospital attendants and servants, stores, tents, sick-carriage, &c., in readiness, so as to be independent of any occasion to draw upon the regimental establishments.

149. The field and regimental hospitals in India ought always to have a certain number of Peons attached to them, as a native medical police for the services of the camp, where their excellent services will amply repay the costs. A mounted guard should as invariably be allowed for the purposes of protection.

150. To every European regiment in India on active service, one surgeon and three assistant-surgeons will be found absolutely necessary to the proper conduct of duty, while the establishment of well-trained hospital servants should be complete, including even extra hands as security against want in this last essential.

151. Independently of general professional knowledge, the staff and regimental surgeons should be well acquainted with military regulations and organization, and with the aids which may be derived from them towards preserving the soldier's health. No

British commander has yet produced any work approaching to the great and classical treatise of Robert Jackson, on "The Formation, Discipline, and Economy of Armies." Since the days of Marlborough it has been a subject of remark that he who is best acquainted with discipline, and with the character and habits of the soldier, has always the smallest sick-list and the lowest rate of mortality.

I trust that the introduction of the following brief notes, not strictly within the title of this article, may be excused, on account of the interest and importance of the subjects, in a military medical sense :—

152. FURLOUGH, INVALIDING, AND PAY.—Liberal in the extreme as has been the old government of India, in all its general arrangements for men and officers, its furlough and invaliding regulations, as affecting the European soldier in the Company's employment, were until recently peculiarly harsh and ungenerous. When we "have in conquest stretched our arms so far," and felt so nobly secure in our soldiers, we ought sooner to have perceived that to be generous is to be just and wise. The bulk of the nation will not fight in person, and all our ministers of all parties shrink from the ballot.

153. Good service pay, and pension, with permission to come home for the recovery of lost health, must be generally conceded to the European soldier of the army in India; and even ordinary furlough must be granted to non-commissioned officers, and to selected soldiers also. It will not do to adhere any longer to traditional systems.

154. India, it must not for a moment be forgotten, is a country in which the military service is, according to Wellington, "of a severity unexampled in any army that is or that ever was in the world."

155. "Every means should be taken," says Napoleon, "to attach the soldier to his colours. This is best accomplished by showing consideration and respect to the old soldier. His pay likewise should increase with the length of service. It is the height of injustice to give a veteran no greater advantage than a recruit." If this be true of the French soldier of the first empire, what shall we say of the claims of the British soldier in India, under the conditions described by Wellington?

156. To the British of the old Company's European regiments there was no good-conduct pension—no sick furlough to England with right to return, excepting under the rare circumstance of recovery during the voyage home. Regulations such as these, so mistaken and illiberal, increased the mortality greatly—the poor fellows preferring the risks of death in India to the horrors of being thrown to starve in the streets of provincial towns in their native country.

157. "I have no doubt whatever," says Dr. Arnott of the Bom-

R

bay army, whose reports are here so often referred to, "but that the illiberality of the invaliding regulations greatly augments the mortality of the Company's army." Setting aside the question of humanity, this officer justly considers that a large gain in ready-made soldiers might be made by the indulgence of sick furloughs, retaining the absent men on the musters while regaining their health in England.

158. Furlough to Europe should be granted to all such British soldiers as, during a certain number of years, have exhibited good conduct : the extension of so reasonable and just an indulgence would render service in India popular in the United Kingdom, and ensure the enlistment of the best class of recruits; it would hold forth an object to the soldier, and he would thus become frugal, temperate, and healthy, comparatively : the canteen would be less frequented, drunkenness would be less frequent, disease would diminish greatly, and crime would become rare.

159. The soldiers of her Majesty's army serving in India enjoyed, through the improvements introduced by Lord Howick and Sir Henry Hardinge, many advantages which, until recently, were unknown to the European troops of the Company. These last, until within the last few years, enjoyed no increase of pension for good conduct; and when incapacitated by sickness, they were for ever discharged and cast adrift. To this rule the only exception was in the instances of men who recovered on the homeward voyage. They were sent back to their colours in India; while their less fortunate comrades, who were longer in recovering their health, re-enlisted into their old regiments, to which they were much devoted. These national errors ought not to be overlooked or forgotten; for they were common to the Home and Indian administrations alike. Here the English administration happened to take the lead.

160. To preserve to his armies their vigorous temperament, their warlike manners, and to destroy their remembrance of their native soil, Napoleon, though ruling an empire placed in a very temperate climate, always fixed the residence of a large portion of his armies in Northern Germany; while England, possessed of rich but pestilential tropical colonies, sent her soldiers there to perish miserably in vast numbers, the survivors, languishing for years in unwholesome stations and worse barracks, becoming enfeebled and enervated in body, and fearfully depressed in mind, and rendered thus unfit for the hardships of military service in Europe. It may reasonably be inferred that the sagacity of the incomparable statesman and commander would have suggested to the French Emperor, had he possessed tropical continents and islands, the necessity for recovering his soldiers, by frequent reliefs, into neighbouring cool and healthy mountain ranges, without waiting for suggestions to this effect from the superior medical officers of his armies.

161. Napoleon judged wisely in his disposal of the French

armies. Because the greatest of his Continental enemies were of northern climate and race, he cantoned his Frenchmen in large proportions in the higher northern latitudes; and for this distribution of his forces he assigned moral and physical reasons of unquestionable truth. But for the army of the British Empire, occupying her varied and extensive foreign possessions, the policy of frequent removal and consequent change of climate, ought to become a State necessity, and must constitute ere long a fixed principle of military arrangement, as regards the soldiers of the line—the foreign service and principal offensive force of the empire. It is quite different with the militia and volunteer force—the home-service and principal defensive force of the United Kingdom; this must be comparatively stationary, ruled on a different principle, and by a different class of officers.

162. The first part of these brief and necessarily imperfect memoranda having now been brought to a close, in so far as they relate to the personal medical wants of troops employed on the march, we may here with advantage take a glance at the character and capabilities of the object of all this care—the British soldier; a subject in the treatment of which our naval and military surgeons have at all times and in all places been masters. I say " naval," because seamen are but soldiers on the waters, and because human nature is in the main the same in all situations and under all circumstances and conditions of military service.

163. Miss Nightingale, who, with the highest powers of discernment, was at much pains to observe and appreciate the character of the man, says—" I have never been able to join in the popular cry about the recklessness, sensuality, and helplessness of the soldier. I should say (and, perhaps, few have seen more of the manufacturing and agricultural classes of England than I have before I came out here), that I have never seen so teachable and helpful a class as the army generally. Give them opportunity promptly and securely to send money home, and they will use it. Give them schools and teachers, and they will come to them. Give them books and games and amusements, and they will leave off drinking. Give them work, and they will do it. Give them suffering, and they will bear it. I would rather have to do with the army than with any other class I have ever attempted to serve; and when I compare them with . . . . . I am struck with the soldier's superiority as a moral, and even as an intellectual being." Again, she says—" I speak from experience of two things, viz., that unmurmuring as the soldier is, a more forlorn being does not exist than he, separated from his comrades in a general hospital, nor one who feels more the thought and care of his country, if, in such a situation, he is provided for by her in an hospital with the comforts of home. And such will always be the case with the Anglo-Saxon." ·

164. The Duke of Wellington, who condemned alike our military

system, borrowed from the Prussians, and the soldiers it produced, but who never improved the one or the other, or mitigated, until forced to do so by public opinion, " the barbarity of the English military code," declared that our soldiers " were detestable for everything but fighting, and that the officers were as culpable as the men. . . . . We are an excellent army on parade, an excellent one to fight, but we are worse than an enemy in a country ; and, take my word for it, that either a defeat or success would dissolve us."

It was said, on the other hand, of Gustavus Adolphus, that " the carriage of his army made him to be beloved of the enemy themselves ;" but Wellington was not beloved by his own men even, who regarded him always with a cold respect only. "In war, as in literature," says Napoleon, "each man has his own style." Wellington's style of making war was generally good, but, regarding his men without any feeling of sympathy, we can readily perceive how he came to do so little for them.

165. The historian Napier, commenting on these sweeping condemnations of our men by their Peninsular commander, says, most justly,—" There were thousands of true and noble soldiers and zealous worthy officers who served their country honestly, and merited no reproaches. It is enough," he adds, " that they have since been neglected" (Wellington being then all-powerful) " exactly in proportion to their want of that corrupt aristocratic influence which produced the evils complained of."

166. It is unnecessary now-a-days to criticise these several judgments, the general voice of the country having determined both what is just and generous and what is absolutely true. "The Duke" did not know, he did not care to know, the real sentiments and character of the soldier. Being removed above him, he had no sympathy with him or with the class whence he sprung ; and he knew nothing of him but as a great instrument for battle. It was very different with Cromwell and Napoleon, and, I rather think, with Marlborough. From the narrow and unjust point of view whence Wellington regarded his men, it resulted that he knew neither how to improve or to reward them.

167. In the astounding declarations of the Duke of Wellington against granting a war medal to the Peninsular soldiers, that they had already received so many votes of thanks from Parliament, we discover the most astonishing absence of knowledge, not to speak of want of sympathy with the feelings and longings of both officers and men ; and all this while we find that the mere representations of his own medals and decorations are sufficient to fill a goodly volume ! Could the soldiers who had fought so nobly under him for six years feel, wear on their persons, or hand to their wives or children so many parliamentary votes ? Did " the Duke" rest satisfied in his own person with republican rewards ? No ;—he

claimed and he obtained the most ostentatious and the most substantive rewards, and he used both to his own purposes.

168. The character of the commander, as stated over and over again in course of this work, is matter of primary consideration and importance, as relating to the physical and moral welfare of the soldier; it is therefore a question everywhere proper to the medical topographer; and on this score alone, as one of absolute duty, is the subject here noticed.

It is, indeed, on all accounts more grateful task to recal attention to the conduct of the great naval and military surgeons of the Revolutionary War—of officers who not only deeply knew their men, and warmly sympathized with them, but who went forth to advocate great moral and physical reforms with the true portrait of the British seaman and soldier in their hands.

It was on the ground of superior knowledge and experience of the hardest and severest kind—of a knowledge far in advance of that of all persons of their time—that Robert Jackson, Trotter, Blane, McGrigor, William Fergusson, Hennen, and Henry Marshall became naval and military reformers when reform was feared, and therefore unknown to and unheard of by our naval and military commanders.

That the reward of Jackson, the most able, the most bold, and the most persevering friend of the soldier, should have been an unremitting, unsparing official persecution, throughout a long life, is nothing more than might have been expected from the times in which he lived. For any man, wearing the British uniform, to write and act as Jackson did from 1791 to 1805, was to incur the constant risk of being degraded and ruined in his prospects; and nothing but a moral courage quite equal to that rare physical courage which he had so often displayed in battle, could have sustained him in his conflicts against the most powerful and corrupt influences. At the head of Jackson's enemies was always to be found "the successful apothecary of Weymouth"—the approved of George III., Sir Lucas Pepys—who would have treated the great army physician as Muir and Palmer had been treated, if any law could have been perverted and corrupted to his purpose.

169. "The boldness and enterprise of medical officers," says Sydney Smith, "is quite as striking as the courage displayed in battle, and evinces how much the power of encountering danger depends upon habit." If by "habit" is here meant a peculiar education and training—a familiarity from early life with every kind of danger—a knowledge everywhere acquired and matured under the hardest and most severe circumstances occurring in civil life, and of the experiences of military service the most trying —then the term "habit" has a real application to our course of life. Our naval and military surgeons were of the true caste. They possessed, besides their native courage, that moral courage

which is engendered by liability to varied responsibility, and by constant exposure to all kinds of dangers by sea and land.

170. Towards the close of the last, but principally in the beginning of the present century, certain of the army-surgeons, and Robert Jackson, the foremost of them, denounced the British military code as foreign, un-English, barbarous, and cruel, while the discipline, they said, cramped and crippled the man, soul and body. Jackson, with an invincible courage, moral rectitude, and power of knowledge peculiar to himself, urged that, instead of the rule of the lash, the soldier should be treated as a reasoning being—that he should be free to do for himself whatever he could do without injury to his health, morals, or discipline. But the commanders of his day heeded him not; so the government of the lash—of the lash in one hand and the rum-ration in the other, as Henry Marshall describes it—went on to the complete satisfaction of the generals for another half century. At length, the public press, backed by the " common sense of the country," decided the matter; in exact accordance, of course, with the humane demands of our army and navy surgeons.

SANITARY PRECAUTIONS NECESSARY IN CAMPS, BARRACKS, AND HOSPITALS.

1. CAMPS.*—The greater part of the diseases of camps, and the mortality resulting from them, are due in all countries mainly to zymotic affections, as fevers, dysentery, diarrhœa, and cholera. Soldiers just arrived in a new country are peculiarly liable to suffer from zymotic diseases; and no given amount of reinforcements will compensate for the loss of the same number of the original force; and hence the necessity for effective sanitary precautions, and the discovery of immediate and effective means for treating the earlier stages of disease.

2. But, besides the morbid peculiarities connected with general climate, and the powerful influences of locality; making allowance also for the influences of the nature of the duties, the diet, and clothing, the prevalence of zymotic diseases will obviously be connected with the results of military discipline and hard military service, as well as with such local favouring causes as are continually observed in civil life, as—

The prevalence of damp.

Impure air.

Impure water.

3. Attacks of zymotic disease will be found to occur in connexion with the three following sources of dampness :—a wet soil—a retentive surface-soil—a confined locality ; and of these three

---

* "The Report of the Crimean Sanitary Commission" is here followed, with certain alterations and transpositions.

conditions, a wet subsoil will, as in the Crimea, occasion the largest amount of sickness.

4. One of the worst sites for a camp is that in which a thin but porous material rests upon an impervious bed, retentive of the water, and which keeps the subsoil charged with it, while the surface may afford little or no indication of the fact. The evils of such a site have often been experienced by British armies; and Holland, Walcheren, Portugal, Spain, and the Crimea are familiar examples.

5. Unhealthy sites of this kind are frequently marked by a greener and more vigorous vegetation than that of the surrounding district, or by water-springs coming to the surface, or by evening fogs settling over them sooner than over the country around.

6. Before fixing upon the position for a camp upon unknown ground, it will be found advisable to dig trial-holes a few feet deep, to ascertain the condition of the subsoil drainage, so as not to risk the health of troops by encamping them on ground in which the trial-holes show the presence of water near the surface.

7. Where reasons of military necessity require the occupation of a position having a wet subsoil, the whole should as speedily as possible be thoroughly drained by deep trenches; and if there be a hill-side or water-shed above the ground, the surface-water from it should be turned aside from the site of encampment by deep catch-water drains, as in the Crimea.

8. If the position be such that deep trenching and draining cannot be executed, it is more than probable that such ground, if held long, will seriously affect the health of the troops.

9. Wet clays, from the retentive character of their surface-soils, keep the air near the ground damp and cold, so as injuriously to affect the atmosphere of tents and huts. Such localities proved very injurious in the Crimea. Where such positions are occupied of necessity, there should, besides the general drains, be hut and tent trenches.

10. Dampness of the air, arising from the confined nature of the locality, as from valleys, and especially from such as contain lakes, proceeds from certain local peculiarities readily appreciated by the medical topographer. The resulting dampness, stagnation, and impurity constitute powerful causes of disease.

11. It was observed in the Crimea that in certain hollows and valleys occupied by the troops, white damp mists settled down, and were followed by epidemic diseases, especially by cholera. Surface-water, stagnant lakes, trees, and brushwood, favour the formation and retention of such injurious collections of vapour; and troops in occupation of such positions have often no escape from the consequent sickness, except by their abandonment.

12. The evils resulting from these local causes are not unfrequently aggravated by the careless manner of erecting huts and

pitching tents, the sites and the ground around being left undrained and uncleared.

13. Deep trenching round the tent-site is the best remedy, and, in the case of huts, the site should be isolated from the surrounding ground, and the area to be occupied by the hut, drained by a trench dug around it of at least a foot below the level of the floor.

14. If it be not practicable to drain the subsoil, and if the position must be held, adequate provision should be made with every material at hand for raising the beds of the men above the ground.

15. Huts should never be banked up with earth against the wood; Crimean experience having shown the danger of the practice as causing fevers. An interior lining, even of paper, affords a far better protection, being sufficient against draughts.

16. The flooring of the tents should be occasionally raised, the surface of the ground being cleaned, and strewed with quicklime and charcoal.

17. Various sources of atmospheric impurity are apt to accumulate unless carefully guarded against; and of these the most frequent are:—manure-heaps and picketing-grounds, cattle-depôts and slaughtering-places; latrines having too large a surface, and that are kept too long open ; graveyards. When an army can shift its ground at will, dangers from such causes may always be avoided by doing so.

18. Filth of every kind is readily washed into the ground by the rains, and trodden into it by the steps of men and animals. To avoid such injurious consequences, the most scrupulous cleanliness is necessary all over and about the camp, all refuse matter being at once swept away and removed to a distance; refuse blood and bones should be buried.

19. Manure-heaps and stable-litter should always be opened, to admit of being dried by the air to expedite their combustion—a process which should never be neglected.

20. All offal and carcases of animals should be buried at least three feet below the surface. If charcoal or quicklime be not procurable, the burned stable-litter should be thrown over the tainted ground.

21. The latrines should be made deep and narrow, earth being daily thrown into them, until they become filled up within two feet of the surface. They should then be closed over with earth, and others dug, and treated in the same manner.

22. When an army is to occupy the same ground for many months, it becomes unsafe to bury refuse matters, as thus the ground would become saturated with organic substances dangerous to health. In such case the construction of furnaces is a necessity towards the destruction and rapid removal of all organic products.

23. With a view to obviate overcrowding, and promote the

necessary ventilation of tents, the number of men sleeping in them ought to be diminished as much as may be practicable; but, considering the limited means at the disposal of commanders in the field, the evils of overcrowding may be greatly obviated by a free general ventilation, such as that of Mr. Mackinnell, and by the introduction, under all circumstances of service, of a free means of escape of consumed air around the top of the tent-poles. In the case of huts wanting Mackinnell's appliance, ridge-ventilation will prove tolerably efficient.

24. The usual practice of striking tents and shifting the ground, will prove an excellent means of avoiding the effects of saturation of the earth by refuse matters, and the emanations resulting from occupancy.

25. Lime-washing of huts inside, especially of hospital huts, purifies the air, and should never be neglected. The same process applied outside the huts cools them, and protects them in some degree from the intense sun's rays.

26. All engineering works for the water-supply of camps should comprehend :—

a. The selection of the purest obtainable source.

b. The water on delivery to be as pure as at its source.

c. When the pound is necessary, the tank should be covered.

d. When practicable, water should never be drawn by dipping, as it is thus liable to become muddy.

e. Where a water source of sufficient purity cannot be obtained, the water should be filtered; and a good filter may be made with sorted gravel, clean sand, and charcoal.

f. All troughs for the water-supply of horses should have separate inlets and overflows.

27. BARRACKS AND HOSPITALS.—On taking military possession of a town, if troops are to be stationed there for any length of time— but, above all, if it is to be made the base of operations—a powerful sanitary police should at once be established, the duties to be clearly defined and vigilantly exercised, in the following order :—

a. To make a thorough sanitary examination of the whole town and neighbourhood, and to report thereon.

b. To organize immediate measures for a thorough cleansing and removal of nuisances; all offensive matters should be removed to a safe distance from the outskirts of the town, or burnt if inflammable, or buried.

c. To provide for the daily cleansing of all streets, lanes, courts, alleys, and open spaces, as well as of back-yards, stables, cattle-sheds, &c., and for the safe disposal of refuse matters.

d. In situations where the surface of the streets or roads is so defective as to retain and accumulate foul waters, and to interfere with surface cleansings, the defects should be repaired, and proper channels formed for carrying off such refuse liquids.

e. In clearing out foul ditches, care should be taken not to throw the mud over the surface, and thus expose it to the action of the sun. The work is best done in the coolest period of the day, or under rain ; quicklime or charcoal being freely used under the operation.

f. All buildings to be occupied by troops as barracks or hospitals should be treated as already mentioned, by a complete system of house drainage, ventilation, and cleanliness.

g. All wells and sources of water should be carefully examined and guarded, to prevent pollution or waste, whether through design or neglect.

h. Wet and unwholesome grounds may be rendered less injurious by effective trenchings, and by covering them over with fresh earth ; but, besides such measures, additional precautions are requisite to prevent the evils resulting from the occupation itself.

i. A sufficient number of latrines should be provided immediately, and regulations established for their management.

j. Stable manure, offal, and carcases of animals should be daily removed, and buried or burned, which latter is best.

k. The dead should be buried far from the habitations of the living.

l. Refuse charcoal-dust may be used with advantage for deodorizing latrines, and the filth which it may not be safe to remove. Quicklime prevents decomposition ; but sand and fresh earth are very useful when used in large quantities.

m. Deodorizing agents should never be used as substitutes for the removal of organic matters to a distance, or for their destruction by fire.

28. That the impure air of barracks and hospitals, arising from defective ventilation and drainage, is sufficient to account for a large proportion of sickness, always existing under such defects, has been proved in all camps and cities. To obviate such occurrences in buildings to be occupied as barracks or hospitals, it is requisite that the following circumstances be attended to :—

a. The local position of the building must be carefully examined, to ascertain the sanitary topography of the site, with a view to the removal of every noxious element from within and from without.

b. All buildings situated in low, confined, and malarious positions, or where the ground cannot be easily drained, or where there is a damp, relaxing local atmosphere, having a depressing influence on health, should be carefully avoided.

c. The sanitary condition in and around every building occupied by men and officers should be examined, with a view to the immediate removal of every nuisance.

d. It is especially necessary to examine most carefully the state of the drainage and sewerage ; for, however spacious and suitable a building a barrack or hospital may appear, when viewed externally and superficially, it may nevertheless have germs of disease concealed beneath it to such an extent as to render it little better than a pest-house in certain states of weather and directions of wind.

e. Drains and sewers built of rough rubble stones, with a square section, or without proper attention to the fall, or too large for the volume of water to be carried away, are liable to accumulate foul deposits, and to generate poisonous gases. If, on examination, deposits be actually found within sewers, it is quite certain that such sewers may at any time become dangerous to the health of the occupants of the building, especially if they pass under or near an inhabited apartment, so that the air of the room become infected with the exhalations escaping through their sides. Deaths from fever and cholera occurred within the barrack-hospital at Scutari directly traceable to this cause.

f. Still more dangerous do sewers become when there is a direct communication between them and the interior of the buildings, by means of untrapped privies or sinks. In this way the air becomes tainted to a much greater degree, and may alone, or in combination with other sanitary defects, give rise to disastrous consequences.

g. To prevent such occurrences, it is always necessary, before putting men, whether well or sick, into buildings, to cleanse thoroughly the whole drainage, to provide a suitable apparatus, with water for flushing the sewers, to prevent accumulation in them, to trap the outfall of the sewer, to prevent the wind or tide, as the case may be, from driving foul air up inside the building, and to provide ventilating openings for sewers, in such positions that the offensive effluvia cannot reach the interior of the building.

h. It may be necessary to destroy and relay sewers, giving them a better form and inclination. When made of stone or brick, the section should be as nearly oval as possible; but whenever pipes of sufficient sectional area can be obtained, they form the safest and best drainage for buildings.

i. The experiences of all the hospitals around Constantinople, during the war, go to show that it is not only possible, but highly advantageous for the salubrity of any military hospital, to substitute the pan-closets for any arrangement whatever of open privies, and that, with ordinary care on the part of the attendants, those closets act perfectly.

j. Wherever practicable, water-closets should be under a separate roof, and in all cases they should have a ventilation distinct from and independent of that of the main building. Box latrines, with flushing apparatus, may be used with advantage for barracks. They save water, but they require for their proper care a daily and strict attention.

k. The state of existing ventilation, as well as the capabilities for ventilation, of every building to be occupied as a barrack or hospital, should be very carefully examined.

l. It may be received as a principle that a building in which a number of persons, whether sick or well, are to be congregated for any length of time, should never depend for its ventilation solely on doors and windows. Doors and windows may be placed in wrong positions for ventilation; they are liable to be opened and closed irregularly; and they are generally closed during the night, when the air is pure and cool, and when the ventilation is more necessary for barracks and hospitals than in the daytime.

m. Wherever there is want of freshness in the air of a barrack-room or hospital-ward, it may be concluded that there danger to health exists, and no means of ventilation ought to be accepted as sufficient which does not remove the evil.

n. In carrying out an independent plan of ventilation for a barrack-room or hospital-ward, it is of primary necessity to afford a free and constant exit to the warm foul atmosphere, and this as near as possible to the ceiling of the apartment. Ventilating openings of sufficient size, whether through the walls into the external air, or by ventilating tubes through the ceilings and roof, are well adapted for the purpose.

o. The size of the openings must depend on the number of inmates, and they should be somewhat larger for a barrack-room than for a sick-ward, on account of the greater numbers inhabiting the former.

p. But, while providing carefully for the removal of the consumed air, it is necessary to introduce means for the constant admission of fresh air; and this can be best effected by the removal of a sufficient number of panes of glass, or else by making openings through the walls near the level of the floors.

q. In most cases it is necessary to moderate the current of air admitted, especially in the instance of sick wards, by substituting for the glass removed, or opened on hinges, panes of perforated zinc, or of wire gauze, or by narrow, overlapping louvre-boards, which may be made of wood, or by nailing over the apertures pieces of open canvas, coarse gauze, or bunting. These means must be modified according to the season and weather; but, in hot climates, the free perflation of the entire building, by opening both doors and windows, is most necessary. Such arrangement does not by any means obviate the necessity for other and permanent means, such as have already been mentioned.

r. The cubic contents of any room or ward in which men are to be placed should be accurately ascertained beforehand; and the number of inmates should not be apportioned solely on the basis of the cubic contents. Barrack-rooms and wards of hospitals may be very lofty, but if the beds be placed too near to each other, on the assumption that there is cubic space enough, the men may still suffer from all the evils of overcrowding.

s. In large stone buildings to be occupied as barracks, or for hospital purposes, beds should never be placed nearer to each other than six feet, measured from centre to centre; and the cubic space allowed for each man should never be less than a thousand cubic feet.

t. The cubic space required for healthy men occupying stone buildings, depends on the climate and season, but above all on the presence or absence of an epidemic constitution of the air, indicated by a tendency to zymotic diseases. A smaller amount of cubic space may be allowable in a colder than in a warmer climate, in a winter than in a summer season. It is unsafe, with a good constitution even, and in a temperate climate, to allow of less than five hundred cubic feet for an adult man in health; and much more should be given in seasons of epidemics. In Turkey, as in all countries, cholera broke out in the barrack hospital when the allowance was between 250 and 350 cubic feet per man.

u. When the atmosphere is polluted with the foul emanations from sewers, or through defective ventilation, a small amount of cubic space is of course far more likely to dispose to disease than if these additional elements were not present. The only safe rule of practice, therefore, is, to attend strictly to cleanliness within and without the buildings, to correct defects in sewerage and ventilation, and to spread the troops as much as the accommodation will allow.

29. It is far safer to encamp, or even to bivouac troops than to overcrowd them in barracks or hospitals; for overcrowding and defective ventilation have at all times and in all countries been followed, in the British army, by disease and consequent danger to the efficiency of the forces, and the success of the military undertaking.

30. During seasons of epidemics especially, one or other of the above-mentioned evil conditions, or the two conjoined, will be certain to lead to immediate loss, and during ordinary seasons this loss is but protracted by being spread over a wider extent of time.

31. Should cholera break out under the ill conditions contemplated, the troops should at once be removed from the buildings, and put under medical inspection, with a view to the immediate discovery and treatment of the precursory diarrhœa. The encampment of the troops on an elevated, dry, and healthy position, and spreading over a wide area, constitute the best securities.

32. It is always hazardous to quarter troops in unwholesome localities, or in houses obviously overcrowded with inhabitants. Regiments, while on the march even, when quartered in filthy overcrowded towns or villages, especially during seasons of epidemics, have, from the mere circumstance of this very temporary and intermitting exposure to overcrowding, become affected with fevers and cholera; and have left these diseases in nearly every town and village through which they have passed.

33. The walls and ceilings of all apartments are liable to become

saturated with organic matters, absorbed from emanations proceeding from the bodies and breath of persons inhabiting them. This is one of the most ordinary and most overlooked of the consequences of filth, overcrowding, and defective ventilation, and it is a common predisposing cause of epidemic diseases.

34. It follows therefore that all buildings about to be occupied by troops, whether as barracks or hospitals, should have their walls and ceilings scraped and thoroughly cleansed, and then washed with several coats of fresh quicklime-wash to make them white throughout, and this last process should be frequently repeated. This simple proceeding has in numerous well-known instances been found to arrest and to avert the progress of zymotic diseases, when nothing else appeared to be of use. The tools and the materials required are easily obtained, and every labouring man can be instructed to do the work effectually.

35. It is hardly necessary to specify that everything likely to give off injurious emanations, whether it be foul linen, the remains of food, or the excreta of the occupants, should be at once removed outside the apartments, whether of barracks or hospitals.

36. Ships, unless specially fitted up, and moored in healthy places, are not adapted for hospital purposes, and should not be used either for sick or convalescents, if suitable accommodation can be obtained on shore.

37. It may be mentioned, in respect of barracks and hospital huts, that an interior lining of boards, or building a rough rubble-stone wall outside, as done in many of the regimental hospitals in the Crimea, affords a good protection from the severity of weather and from external heat.

38. The result, lastly, of all experience goes to prove that the neglect of military hygiene, whether as regards the soldier's person, or the sanitary condition of stations, camps, barracks, and hospitals, has hitherto, in all climates and seasons, and in our various possessions, at home and abroad, been the cause of an enormous amount of sickness and mortality in our armies; and the whole subject, as closely connected with the moral advancement and physical efficiency of the British forces, demands for the future a thoroughly practical development, commensurate with its importance to the general welfare.

39. "A man," says Lord Bacon, "owes a duty to his profession." Had our commanders by sea and land held this simple truth in recollection, by assuring, as was their first duty, the welfare of their men, our statesmen and the legislature of the country would have been spared many unseemly and humiliating investigations. But want of knowledge in officers, and until recently, in the public at large, has been the parent of endless calamities. "Our army," says Lord Herbert, "is, perhaps, at present, the least professional of all our professions. The education for the

army, and the examination previous to admission, has been as yet but very superficially military."

40. The army, as a profession, having thus been behind all other professions, it resulted that the soldier was for ages made to inhabit pestilential stations, cantonments, camps, barracks, and hospitals; that he was made to observe a most injurious sameness in diet, while the quality of his food was often deficient in nutriment; that he was ordered to wear clothing which in one country was insufficient, and in another country burthensome and injurious; that he was exposed to night duties under very unfavourable circumstances, as to climate, season, and protection; that his employments were insufficient, and that such as he had were monotonous and wearisome; that he was subjected to a foreign, barbarous, and cruel military code; and that, owing to all these unhappy and unnatural circumstances, he became the reckless, intemperate, and unmanageable man whom the Duke of Wellington described to us.

41. Peace is the time for perfecting the military system, and the military institutions of the country. Little indeed can be done in this way during the hurry of war; for how can a man think in a mill? The great and progressive prosperity of England has been but slow in reaching the soldier, whose fate has been the sport of commanders, and, until quite recently, of departments, negligent and ignorant of his requirements, and regardless of his value and deserts. Time, which, according to Shakspeare, gallops with some men, has moved sluggishly for the soldier's advancement; but, if we would guard against arousing the most dangerous spirit, we should lose no more of it. We would seem, in our military policy, for ages to have trusted very much to chance, and to the native "pluck" of our soldiers; but such chance-medley will no longer answer our purpose. "We must confess," says Napoleon, "that fate, which sports with man, makes merry work with the affairs of this world."

NOTE ON THE VENTILATION OF BARRACKS AND HOSPITALS.

The following, amongst other memoranda, was, with some slight corrections, presented by the author, as member of the Royal Commission of 1857, appointed to inquire into "The Regulations affecting the Sanitary Condition of the Army:"—"The suggestions respecting ventilation draw important but confounded distinctions, and which, I feel assured, have not presented themselves to the minds of those who have advocated before this Commission certain favourite plans. A practically approved ventilation is the real question to be compared and determined. It is not the mere size of the barrack-room or hospital-ward which determines the excellence or the evil, but its good or bad construction in promoting or impeding a just plan of ventilation. A large ward, constructed like those which so long existed at Fort Pitt, Chatham, for instance, will be impure and unhealthy, while a large ward, with suitable appliances for natural ventilation, will be both pure and wholesome. There can, in short, be no just comparison between a separate and detached room, having separate and independent ventilation, with no thorough draught, exposed to, and with openings into, the external air, and other rooms forming portions of an extended mass of building having one common continuous roof. In commending without discriminating small huts, or hospital-huts, again, it is forgotten how great the number of doors and windows these last contain comparatively to their space, and that they are separate and detached, each having a separate and detached roof; but it is these united circumstances, and not the circumstance of their being small, which constitute the real advantages of small huts and hospitals.

But, in a sanitary point of view, it is not possible to obtain a gradual and equable natural ventilation, or an equable temperature in a small room or hut. It must have the thorough draught which, though it kills a few, is better for the health of the many than the defective ventilation of ill-constructed large apartments, which injures all. Again, the defective ventilation of large rooms and wards is altogether of our own creation. It need not be. With the due proportion and dimension of doors and windows for summer ventilation, and with the ordinary ventilating apertures for use in cold months, a large room or ward will be as pure, while it will be more healthful, because more equably warmed and ventilated than a small barrack-room or ward.

No system of ventilation can prove, in reality and upon fair trial, successful, which does not work through an ascertained natural law or laws of aërial currents.

Those who advocate the use of small rooms and wards do not appear to be aware either of their advantages or their disadvantages, because they are unacquainted with the causes of both. Nor do they comprehend the real advantages of large apartments over the smaller, both in adaptation for ventilation and for the regulation of temperature.

HABITS OF THE BRITISH SOLDIERY AND
THEIR INFLUENCE ON HEALTH.

THE helpless, listless condition of organized bodies of men, as compared to the active, independent condition—the free agency, competitions, and private enterprise of civil communities, is a subject which, with its moral and physical results, has not yet been appreciated either by official bodies, or by the public, which pays for all the labour of naval and military organization. Well may the British grenadier exclaim with Antony,—

"Ten thousand harms, more than the ills I know,
My idleness doth hatch."

In civil life, men are very much masters of their actions and of their habits of life; while in the army and navy a man is neither master of his diet, exercise, clothing, fuel, hours of rest, nor of anything else, in short. The government that employs the seaman and soldier is the sole arbiter of their habits and customs, and of everything that relates to their condition. In all this the governing power incurs an obvious responsibility; and it would prove a mournful as well as unprofitable labour to trace, since the days of Charles the Second, how this responsibility has been used for the soldier's and seaman's moral and physical welfare. There was doubtless much in the former habits of the officers which provoked the very neglects of duty in the British soldier which all military men must condemn; but much may be done, under modern improvements in the habits of the officers, towards raising the moral standard, and giving a hopeful occupation and excitement to their men.

The barrack-life of the British soldier in India, imprisoned as he is by the sun—what a world of wretchedness and misery, moral and physical, does that term bring to the memories of all who have witnessed it in our tropical possessions! Here we find men at the mean age of twenty-six, "at the healthiest period of life, and selected from the healthiest of the population," yet "fallen below the health level of their native country, where all the chances are in their favour;" and this, in part at least, owing "to the reckless dissipation incident to all military bodies," as we have managed them. The soldier, according to a British war minister, was to be found, a few years previous to 1856, either in the parade-ground or in the canteen. He would nowhere else be received.

The sad sameness of the barrack-life and the dull routine of duties, in India and in all our colonies, have led, by a physiological

S

law of necessity, to irregularities in the habits of life and in the conduct of the soldier. If not looked to in time, this want of attention to the healthy mental life of the men must end in some very serious events. In the barrack the British soldier has found until very recently no home—no employment for mind or body— no amusement—no varied society. Here he is still very much cut off from all industry and enjoyment—he has no solace when ill. Mr. Wilson, in his excellent work on malaria, says that when young soldiers thus circumstanced are exposed to the causes of epidemics, or to the intense malaria, it is no wonder they should " die off like flies."

At home, and in many of our colonies, the soldier finds companionship in civil life ; but in India, if he would have his associates out of the barrack, he must fall into the snares of the vilest and worst class of natives, whose business is to plunder and minister to his worst vices. Much consideration is due to the soldier on this score. The barbarous restrictions on his marriage must ere long give way to a more just and humane system. This question, as regarded by Sir Charles Napier, " affects the health, morality, and strength of our army in various ways, such as desertion, population, and other points."

The late Inspector-General of Hospitals, William Fergusson, says :—" I never saw a barrack that was not too crowded, or in other words, where, if the men had been lodged in separate cottages, or even in hovels, they would not have been healthier.

" Of the soldiers' life within these barracks there is much to be said, and much to be amended. To take his guards, to cleanse his arms, and attend parade seems to comprehend the sum total of his existence ; amusement, instruction, beyond the drill, military labour, and extension of exercises, would appear, until very recently, to be unthought of ; as it is impossible that the above duties can fully occupy his time, the irksomeness of idleness, that most intolerable of all miseries, must soon overtake him, and he will be driven to the canteen or the gin-shop for relief.

" Labour in every shape seems to have been strictly interdicted to the soldier, as water for his drink. All, or nearly all, must have been bred to some trade or other before they became soldiers, but they are to work at them no longer. Labour, the labour of field works and fortifications, strengthens the limbs and hardens the constitution, but that is never thought of in our military life at home ; so thought not the ancient Romans, whose military high- ways still exist, and who never permitted their soldiers to grow enervated in idleness during peace. Better, surely, would it be that every one should work at his own craft, or be employed on the public works, in regulated wholesome labour, than thus to spend his time in sloth and drunkenness.

" But his exercises, without even going beyond the barrack pre- mises, may be made manifold ;—running, wrestling, gymnastic

games of every kind, swimming, leaping, pitching the bar, the
sword exercise, that of the artillery, all that hardens the muscles
and strengthens the limbs, should be encouraged; and when the
weather forbids out-door pastimes, the healthier exercise of single-
stick, in giving balance and power to the body, quickness to the
eye, and vigour to the arm, may properly be taken as a substitute
for the drill, which, after the soldier has been perfected in his
exercise, is always felt to be a punishment. So is the unmeaning
evening parade, and perpetual roll-calling.

"Surely, if the soldier present himself once every morning, correctly equipped and in order, the most teasing martinet ought to
be satisfied, and then no more should be required than to see that
the men are all in their quarters on the beating of the tattoo.
Surely the use of the sword has been too much frowned down, as
if it had been a forbidden thing. In the night attack, the musket
is worse than useless, its fire leading to every kind of confusion;
and at the breach it is little better, for it can only be presented
against stone walls and ramparts that conceal the defenders; but
it would cover the swordsman advancing to the breach, and a couple
of chests of ship's cutlasses furnished to every regiment as regimental baggage—a single horse-load—provided the men had been
taught to use them, would generally supply all that could be wanted
for the exigency of the service.

"Let any one reflect on the fearful expenditure of life at the
breaches at Badajos and St. Sebastian, and say if some means
should not, if possible, be devised to render it less costly hereafter.
One is almost tempted to regret the times ' when,' according to
the old song, ' our leaders marched with fuzees, and we with hand-
grenades:' and could the good grenadier have carried a sword by
his side, to use after he had tossed the ball, he would, I believe,
have done much more execution than with a musket and bayonet:
and why should the artillery be to him a closed book, as if in the
course of his service he was never destined to handle or to suffer
from it? A couple of guns, even if wooden ones, in every barrack-
yard, with an old invalid bombardier to teach the use of the
rammer, and the sponge, and the match, would fill up many a vacant
dreary hour, and open his mind to a most useful professional lesson.

"The lesson, moreover, would be as useful to the infantry officers
as to the privates. He would then, should he ever prove the captor
of a prize gun, at least know what it was, and be able to turn upon
the enemy the engine that had just been used for the purpose of
destroying himself. Every sailor, even on board a merchant ship,
where there are no idlers, must become more or less an artilleryman,
and why should not the too often idle soldier?

"Foot-racing, too, the art of running, so little practised, and so
supremely useful, should be held amongst the qualities that constitute military excellence. It was so held at the Isthmian games
of ancient Greece, and deserves a better place than has hitherto

been assigned to it in the military pastimes of modern Britain. In our school books we are told that the youth of ancient Persia were taught to launch the javelin, to ride the war-horse, and to speak the truth. Let the young British warrior be taught to use his limbs, to fire ball-cartridge, to cook his provisions, and to *drink water*. The tuition may be less classical, but it will stand him in far better stead during every service, whether at home or abroad.

"Barracks, from time to time, should be evacuated for purification. The evils and dangers of accumulation will otherwise beset them, inducing disease; and to obviate this, it would be well, whenever practicable, to march out their inhabitants, in the summer season, to the nearest heath or common—always, however, without tents—and there make them hut themselves. No military lesson could be more useful than this. Every man so hutted would be advanced in soldiering to the full instruction of the campaign. The change, breaking the monotony of barrack-life—the novelty, would animate; he would be taught how to live in a camp, how to cook and to forage, to use the mattock, the shovel, and the axe.

"Tents, when the soldier lies upon the cold ground, with a crowd of comrades enclosed within a superficially heated atmosphere, loaded with animal exhalations, can only be considered hot-beds for the generation of dysentery. On their return to barracks, they will find everything healthy and refreshed, and they will know that they have been made better soldiers.

"Some have strenuously recommended barrack libraries; and surely, when we think of the dismal monotony that hangs over the soldier in barrack-life, no one with good feelings could object to them. Still, I must confess that I never knew or heard of a reading army. The military exercises and pastimes would seem better adapted to the soldier's character; and I acknowledge I would rather see him a cook than a student, for on that art his very existence may depend; but if he feel disposed to read, let him have every advantage and opportunity that the rules of the service can admit.

"Music would seem far better adapted than even books to fire the soldier's mind, for when played in national airs, it awakens a chord which has often electrified armies; and amongst all nations, at some period or other of their history, it has been the accompaniment and incentive to war. The highly civilized English soldier now fights, and can fight, without it; but if taught to feel its powers, would he not fight better with it? To the Irish and the Scotch soldier it still speaks the language of the heart, and the Highlander, when he hears the gathering of his clan blown from the mountain war-pipe, becomes elevated and transported beyond himself; he will then encounter anything in human shape, unappalled by all the forms of death that the engines of war can inflict." This admirable military physician concludes:—" Regular bodily pleasurable exercise has been said to be worth a host of physicians for preserving military health ; and occupation without distress or fatigue is happiness. The philosopher can make no more of it; and every idle hour is an hour of irksomeness, and every idle man is, and must be, a vicious man, and to a certain extent an unhealthy one ; for the mind preys upon the body, and either deranges its functions in a direct manner, or drives the possessor to seek resources incompatible with health."

Thus spoke William Fergusson, after an experience of actual war of twenty years, and thus had spoken before him Robert Jackson ; but in everything relating to the soldiers' welfare, Jackson, Fergusson, Hennen, Henry Marshall, and Ballingall will be found to have been half a century or more in advance of all opinion, and especially in advance of military authority. That the warnings of such men should for so long have been unheeded is but another instance out of many of the utter disregard of the subject by the authorities of the state, both civil and military, who for ages regarded the soldier as but a red-coated pariah. In France it is well understood that "the degree of perfection of military medical science is the true measure of the importance attached to the preservation of the soldier."

It was with a rare sagacity and penetration of the subject in all its bearings, belonging only to an officer of the highest order of talent, that Sir John Moore—"that model soldier of England"— the intimate personal friend of Robert Jackson—declared, in addressing Sir Ralph Abercromby, that "a Roman army would have gone through their military exercises in the West Indies and have been healthy." The same distinguished commander added :— "The troops, I observe, which have been most active, are the most healthy ; a proof that the sun is not the cause of sickness. But in general the greater part of the sickness proceeds from want of interior discipline and economy in regiments. Great attention should be paid in this country to the cleanliness and even neatness of the soldier's person and the regularity of his diet, an addition to the eating part of his ration instead of rum ; sea or river bathing, constant activity, and movement. In short, General (excuse the pedantry of the expression), but with a Roman instead of a modern exercise and discipline, the troops in the West Indies might, I am convinced, be kept healthy. A parade twice a day, consisting merely of an inspection and exercise of arms, is easy for officers ; it leaves them what they call more time, but it leaves the soldier also to lounge the whole day in barracks, where the air cannot be good, and where, from indolence, his body becomes enervated and liable to disorder." How much that is preventive of disease do these short sentences enjoin, and how applicable is the entire reasoning to the condition of the European soldier in the East Indies as well as in the West. No wonder that, living in the miserable manner here described, condemned formerly to a re.

sidence of twenty years in the East Indies—moving from bad stations to worse—hope should have shed but a feeble influence over
the soldier's enjoyment or future prospect, and that he should thus
yield, as he still does, to the temptation of momentary gratification.

The description of the soldier's life given by Colonel Lindsay of
the Guards, while it relates to his condition in the middle of the
nineteenth century, might quite as justly have been given of the
men of George the Second's time :—" Perhaps no living individual
suffers more than he from *ennui*. He has no employment save his
drill and his duties. These are of a most monotonous and unin-
teresting description; so much so that you cannot increase their
amount without wearying and disgusting him. All he has to do
is under restraint : he is not like a working man or an artisan.
A working man digs, and his mind is his own ; an artisan is interested in the work on which he is engaged ; but a soldier has to
give you all his attention, and he has nothing to show for the work
done. He gets up at six. There is no drill before breakfast ; he
makes up his bed and cleans his things ; he gets his breakfast at
seven. He turns out for drill at half-past seven or eight ; his drill
may last an hour and a half. If it be a guard day there is no drill,
except for defaulters. The men for duty are paraded at ten o'clock ;
that finishes his day's drill altogether. There is evening parade,
which takes half-an-hour ; and then his time is his own till tattoo,
which is at nine in winter and ten in summer. This is the day of
a soldier not on guard, or not belonging to the company which is
out for Minié practice."

Dr. Julius Jeffreys, writing in 1858 of the condition of the
British soldier in India, says :—" If any one would see a picture .
of the gnome *Ennui* reigning absolute, not even the descriptive
power of the poet Spenser will so well supply it as the scenes
within a barrack compound in India, surrounded or not by the hot
and dull mud wall. There is life there truly, for there is respiration and perspiration enough ; but life a blank ! Eyes looking
upon nothing—minds caring for little and hoping less—thoughts
of home long suppressed."

Robert Jackson states, that " Planters, who may be said to work
hard, experience good health comparatively ; even soldiers are
healthy when actively employed ; they suffer when they remain
immured in barracks in ease and apathy." Again :—" The writer
ventures to say, by fair induction from fact, that if the soldier in
the West Indies, instead of being restricted from labour, were
permitted to do for himself whatever he is capable of doing, his
health would suffer less than it now does; the mind would be
occupied, there would be satisfaction, and fewer of those causes of
temptation which in idleness lead him into error."

The most complete army of modern times—in health, discipline,
and equipment, was that mustered by Napoleon in 1805, on the
shores opposite to England, and which a popular historian declares

to have "acquired a degree of perfection, in point of discipline, organization, and military habits, unprecedented since the days of the Roman Legions."

This great army amounted to one hundred and fourteen thousand combatants; and it is highly deserving of remark, that its exemption from disease was ascribed by its incomparable leader to habitual light and cheerful occupation of mind and body, short of fatigue.

"Constant employment," says one of his Generals, "was the true secret both of their good health and docile habits; neither officers nor soldiers were ever allowed to remain any time idle; when not employed in military evolutions, they were constantly engaged either in raising or strengthening field-works, or in levelling down eminences, draining marshes, or filling up hollows, to form agreeable esplanades in front of their habitations, and where their exercises were performed." The same army, according to Tardieu, marched from the sea-coast without halt to the field of Austerlitz, over nearly 400 French leagues, leaving hardly any sick behind; but then it was an army of matured and seasoned soldiers, the youngest man in it being twenty-two years of age.

We have seen how the French soldier is made healthy and happy, and no one who knows him can doubt that the British soldier is quite as capable of both attributes as his gallant neighbour. Activity is the moral and physical type of the French soldier; he is taught that while a certain amount of rest is good, too much of it produces weakness and disease; that exercise is its contrast, its antidote.

What "the interior discipline and economy" of Marlborough— England's greatest commander—may have been, I have no means of knowing; but there must have been something notable in that order which, according to one who served under him, made his camp resemble "a well-governed city. Cursing and swearing were seldom heard among the officers; a sot and a drunkard were the object of scorn; and the poor soldiers, many of them the refuse and dregs of the nation, became, at the close of one or two campaigns, tractable, civil, sensible, and clean, and had an air and spirit above the vulgar." Such results were worthy "the head of European captains," as Napoleon termed him; but how melancholy to look on the reverse of this picture, and to reflect that, in the middle of the nineteenth century, so much should remain to be done to render the British soldier healthy and happy. On the abuse of ardent spirits in our various colonies it were almost in vain to speak. Before that terrible vice can be overcome, something far more powerful than medical reasoning on facts, or the warnings of experience founded on them, must be brought into active operation. Discipline must still further alter its direction;— in place of being active only to punish wrong, it ought and must be exerted further and further in the encouragement to good conduct.

Henry Marshall, speaking of the British soldier in the East Indies in his day, says :—"By the daily custom of imbibing spirituous potations, a new want is created, intemperance is established as a habit, and frequent intoxication is the consequence. The wretched drunkard must now have a large supply of liquor in the morning to recover him from the effects of the quantity drunk on the previous night. He perhaps has neither money nor credit, and his clothes are then sold at a small portion of their value. Some do not stop here; for, after having sold all their clothes, they will rob their comrades, and with the proceeds of their dishonesty, provide the means of intoxication. Confinement follows upon confinement, court-martial upon court-martial, and punishment upon punishment, until the worn-out wretch dies in hospital of the 'HORRORS,' fever, or dysentery; or if he should for a time resist the fatal effects of disease, his constitution becomes broken down by the combined influence of the poison of spirits, an exhausting climate, and repeated attacks of illness, so that in a few years he is found unfit for further service in India, and he is sent home to be invalided.

"Death is the last, but perhaps not the worst consequence of intemperance. This description of the life of a British soldier in India is by no means highly-coloured. But the evil does not fall on the heads of the unfortunate sufferers; military discipline in all its branches becomes deeply affected by habits of intemperance. To the generally prevailing vice of drinking are to be attributed almost every misdemeanor and crime committed by British soldiers in India.

"The catalogue of these, unhappily, is not a scanty one, for, by rapid steps, first from petty, and then more serious neglects and inattentions, slovenliness at and absence from parades, follow disobedience of orders, riots, and quarrels in barracks, absence from guards and other duties, affrays with the natives, theft, and selling of their own and their comrades' necessaries, robberies, abusive language, and violence to non-commissioned officers, and last of all, desertion, mutiny, and murder may be traced to this source. This frightful picture is not exaggerated. I have seen thirty-two punished men in a regimental hospital at one time, perhaps not a single individual of that number suffered for a crime which was not a direct consequence of the immoderate use of spirits.

"I recollect attending to the punishment of seven men of the same regiment, who received among them four thousand two hundred lashes. They had been all tried for crimes arising from habits of intemperance. Since the institution of the Recorder's and Supreme Court at Madras, no less than thirty-four British soldiers have forfeited their lives for murders, and most of them were committed in their intoxicated moments."

Such were the ferocious punishments which disgraced our armies in former days ; punishments to be matched only in an American merchant ship, or among the barbarities of a Virginian plantation.

That these are not altogether tales of bygone days is but too apparent. In General Orders of the Commander-in-Chief in India, addressed to the soldiers of Her Majesty's army, and dated 2nd August, 1844, 25th May, 1847, and 14th August, 1852, the frequency of "violence to their superiors" is noticed in the most cogent and emphatic terms. These outrages, so disgraceful to the character of the army, and so subversive of its subordination and discipline, are stated, in some instances, to have been prompted by "a desire to get transported to the penal colonies." His Excellency adds, "The acts of which many of these men have been convicted rendered them liable to a sentence of DEATH ; and the Commander-in-Chief, therefore, deems it necessary to call the attention of all concerned to the remarks contained in the General Order of the 2nd of August, 1844."

That much has been done, at home and abroad, to improve the condition of the soldier, all must admit ; but to account for depravity and insubordination such as this, we must refer again to the barrack life, and to the long and dismal catalogue of moral and physical defects and neglects which still remain unredressed. As to the difference in the treatment of military offenders in India, it consists only, according to Dr. Jeffreys, in the less severe corporal punishment now inflicted, and the greater frequency of transportation.

On these and other points it is as sure as Holy Writ, that "our neglects will find us out," and that the evil consequences can only be staved off for a time. There must come a day of reckoning with the soldier, as with other creditors.

How, it may be asked, can courts-martial and officers in command altogether reject the excuse of intemperance, so long as a soldier has it in his power to command the means of depriving himself of his reason ? Beccaria is of opinion that the punishment of crime cânnot be just, or, in other words, necessary, if the laws have not endeavoured to prevent that crime, by the best means which times and circumstances would allow.

We used to instil the moral and physical poison with one hand, and hold out the lash with the other, as the antidote against indulgence. Coercive measures have at all times been found very ineffectual for preventing the evils arising from intemperate habits, partly because the soldiers do not generally regard drunkenness as an ignominious vice. Where punishment has no influence in checking a man from repeating a breach of discipline, or in preventing others from committing a like offence, it is worse than useless.

These truths should be repeated by us until the odious, foreign, and unnatural punishment of the lash shall be abolished from our armies.

On the uses of libraries, my friend, Dr. Julius Jeffreys, offers some just and discriminating remarks. "Enlisted as a soldier, there are, during times of peace, both an end of the labourer's toil and an improvement in his diet in India; but a hereditary organization cannot be changed in a day. So given to muscular action had he been by nature, that, at the end of a long day of toil, as a labourer in England, you might have seen him of an evening, *by way of relaxation*, lying at his length and reading a book! No, but playing at bowls, skittles, or even cricket! When you shut him up in a barrack in India, and give him books, treat him however kindly you may, he chafes from inaction. He would be happy to have to make the paper of your books, to print them, press them, bind them, pack them, carry them, and *do anything* but read them. Exceptions of course there are; men whose brains would not generate toil-energy alone, but were apter for intellectual. Some of these have sought the greater leisure of military life. Invite more of such minds by promising them full play, and your ranks will be greatly improved, and will supply you with mighty commanders, if you will love war." But to return to our more immediate subject.

Where endemic fevers prevail, the temperate, it is true, are attacked as well as the intemperate; but it is universally admitted by medical men, that the former have a much better prospect of recovery than the latter. Desgenettes, in his medical history of the French army in Egypt, observes that daily experience demonstrates that all the soldiers who indulge in intemperate habits, and that are attacked with fevers, die; nay, we may go still further and say, that they have been more liable to an attack of disease. Sir James McGrigor repeats the same observations even more emphatically.

The obvious purport of Henry Marshall's able report is, to recommend the withdrawal of ardent spirits from the canteen, and the abolition in the East Indies, and everywhere, of the indiscriminate and uniform issue of spirit rations to the troops, with a view of abating the extent of crime, of lessening the proportion of sick, of reducing the rate of mortality, diminishing the numbers discharged on account of disabilities, and of promoting the welfare, efficiency, and discipline of corps.

But there is another habit respecting which I shall venture to say a few words, because it is both a bad one, and a comparatively new one,—I mean the immoderate use of tobacco—a habit brought amongst us from the continent of Europe, on the cessation of the French revolutionary war. Young military men are apt to regard the habit as a manly one, until severe dyspepsia, giddiness, shattered nerves, sallow complexion, disturbed action of the heart, and other symptoms show themselves, and then it is frequently too late to stop. "The sallow complexions, black, broken and unsound teeth" of the Germans are matters of notoriety to all travellers. "You may," says one of them, "smell a German in any part of the room, or scent him at a quarter of a mile's distance in the open air, if the wind be favourable."

Much is talked of the good effects of tobacco-smoking in damp and malarious localities, by persons who, in defiance of geographical differences, carry the habit wherever they go—from the marshes of Burmah to the arid plains of Hindustan, forgetting that, meanwhile, in the language of Cassio, " they put an enemy in their mouths to steal away their brains;" but I think there is good reason to question the benefits of this habit of smoking even in the fatherland of fog and damp, or that tobacco ever acts as a preventive to any disease, and least of all to fever.

The truth is, that many persons puff themselves into the good graces of snobs and spoonies like themselves, and use cigars by the score now, as Lord Chesterfield drank and smoked in his time, notwithstanding his aversion to wine and tobacco—" because he thought such practices very *genteel,* and made him look like a man." How his lordship may have looked under the united influence of wine and tobacco, his biographers have failed to relate; but we all know how our modern " spoonies" and " snobs" in our thoroughfares look, after a course of cigar-smoking alone.

Damp and cold climates may confer a greater tolerance of, or partial immunity from, the evil effects of the drug, but this is perhaps all that can justly be admitted.   Dr. A. T. Thomson, speaking of the medicinal effects of tobacco, says:—"Its narcotic power, when it is employed in excess, weakens the digestive organs, obtunds the nervous sensibility, and depresses the whole vital energy."   Of the empyreumatic oil of tobacco, which is produced in minute quantities in the ordinary process of smoking, the same author says that, when introduced into a wound, "it causes instant death."   Of the other active principle, the nicotina, he states that it is a direct sedative; and that, medicinally, under all circumstances, tobacco must be employed with the utmost caution.

If such checks and cautions are necessarily put on the use of this powerful drug, in the hands of the physician, what need be added on the continuous and unlimited use of it by the reckless and ignorant soldier.

Of hookah-smoking I need say nothing, as happily its day is nearly gone; but I have seen many cases of severe constitutional and cardiac disturbance from its abuse, with perfect recovery of health on the discontinuance of the habit; the digestive functions, those of the heart and nerves, having been seriously affected in the most inveterate smokers.   Of the miseries, mental and bodily, which I have witnessed in the persons of young officers, from the abuse of cigars, I will only say that they very far exceed those detailed in the " Confessions of an Opium-eater."

Many persons flatter themselves that by long use such habits become a harmless second nature—the truth being that they can never become a second nature, *for they have nothing to do with the first,* as has been said of graver matters.

Lallemand has reported, on an extensive personal observation, that the use of tobacco deadens the generative functions. " I am convinced," he says, " that this must be much more frequent than is generally believed, if I may judge by the torpor into which the organs of generation fall, as soon as the narcotic action of the tobacco is experienced, and by the habitual indifference evinced by confirmed smokers for the society of women."

Professor Lizars of Edinburgh, after enumerating the modes in which syphilitic ulcerations of the lips, mouth, and throat are propagated by the short pipe and cigar, and how carcinomatous ulceration of those parts is produced by the same cause, states that the constitutional effects of tobacco are numerous and varied, and occasionally truly deplorable. Amongst these he enumerates dyspepsia, vitiated taste, a loose condition of the bowels, congestion of the brain, loss of memory, amaurosis, deafness, nervousness, palsy, emasculation, and cowardice, or want of moral courage.

" The physiological operation of nicotine," says Van Praag, " is at first stimulant, and at last depressing, not only to the circulation and respiration, but also to the nervous system. Accelerated circulation, increase of respiratory movements, and excessive irritation of the muscular system are the phenomena observed first ; the concluding symptoms are those of general depression, both of animal and organic life."

There can be no question, I think, as to the injuries inflicted on health by the protracted or excessive use of tobacco in any of its forms. It may assuredly be classified amongst those substances which produce chronic poisoning.

Mr. Solly, of St. Thomas's Hospital, regards smoking as the curse of the present age. " Amongst the various insidious causes of general paralysis, smoking is one. He knows of no *single* vice which does so much harm as smoking: it is a snare and a delusion ; it soothes the excited nervous system at the time, to render it more irritable and more feeble ultimately."

That the habitual abuse of tobacco leads certainly to mental and physical degradation is becoming daily a fixed impression in both France and England. In the Ecole Polytechnique and other public schools of France it has been proved that the youths who smoke fall behind in their studies, and that their healths are injured.

" A hundred pounds of tobacco-leaf," says Professor Johnstone, "yields about seven pounds of nicotine. In smoking a hundred grains of tobacco, therefore—say a quarter of an ounce—there may be drawn into the mouth two grains or more of the most subtle of all poisons ; and this dose, frequently repeated, cannot fail to injure the strongest constitution." This authority adds that, besides this poison, many other hurtful agents and gases are carried into the mouth and lungs, in the act of smoking tobacco.

Dr. Prout states that " tobacco disorders the assimilating functions in general, but more particularly, as I believe, the assimilation of the saccharine principle. I have never, indeed, been able to trace the development of oxalic acid to the use of tobacco; but that some analogous and equally poisonous principle, probably of an acid nature, is generated in certain individuals by its abuse, is evident from their cachectic looks, and from the dark and often greenish-yellow tint of their blood. The severe and peculiar dyspeptic symptoms sometimes produced by inveterate snuff-taking are well known; and I have more than once seen such cases terminate fatally with malignant disease of the stomach and liver. Great smokers also, especially those who employ short pipes and cigars, are said to be liable to cancerous affections of the lips." Dr. J. P. Murphy states most truly that there is nothing more injurious to a flaccid heart than smoking, many cases being traceable to this cause alone.

Were I to relate but a small portion of the results of my personal observation, as to the effects of the abuse of tobacco, I might be suspected of exaggeration, I therefore prefer to place before the reader the results of other men's observations.

It must not be supposed from what is here stated that I would place the stout British soldier on a diet of vegetables, treacle, and tea: far from it; I would take nothing from him which constitutes a liberal, nutritious, and wholesome diet; not even a moderate spirit-ration to the seasoned soldier—especially when in work or in full exercise. Cooped up in barracks, however, the present plan of dieting in the East Indies is too uniform and unvarying, and much too highly stimulating; and the spirit-ration, whether in or out of the canteen, constitutes "a pernicious bounty" to the men. The whole of the dieting of the army requires revision and regulation, so as to adapt it to the wants of the soldier under the various climates in which he is called upon to serve.

"Exercises which might inure the body to hardships," says Robert Jackson in 1791, "have not been sufficiently enforced; and such sorts of diet, and such modes of life as might obviate the danger of diseases, have been little attended to."

William Fergusson justly observes, that a great physiological principle seems always to have been overlooked, and that is, the natural appetite for change and variety. "It is ever the same, and no man, even if he will, can be satisfied with this. His stomach and digestive organs will be heard in their own cause; and if they be not attended to, their owner will fly to *alcohol* in solace of his disappointment. There is a mistake here; for if we wish to wean the soldier from drunkenness, we should be careful to place within his reach more wholesome indulgencies, of which a diet suited to his taste (and it cannot be suited without variety) must ever be the first. Were he allowed to cater for his own mess (always, however, under due superintendence), there can be little doubt of his better relish for his meal, besides learning that most useful of all lessons, the art of subsisting himself. In the case of the soldier, to cook is to live ; for if he cannot prepare his food, he will be poorly fed, even with flocks and herds at his command. In all this the soldier ought to have been trained and supported by the wisdom of the country. But has it been so ?"*

These most excellent because practical suggestions, if they evince less learning than some chemical rules of diet which I have seen, nevertheless contain more knowledge. They are also highly important and interesting in another sense, as showing how far the author was in advance of what is called professional opinion. While naval and military men, scouting and scorning all opinion but their own unauthorized dicta, and asking the old worn-out question—"not being a naval or military man, what can he know of naval or military affairs?" we have here a most eminent and experienced army surgeon calling upon "the wisdom of the country" to "train and support" the soldier. The miseries and horrors of the Crimea, with their disastrous results, have at length roused the people to a sense of the national danger ; and the common sense of the country, guided by the common interests of self-preservation—in other words, "the wisdom of the country" is brought to bear on naval and military organization—not, however, before it had become an urgent state necessity.

Referring, in conclusion, to the more especial subject of this article, we find that Dr. William Fergusson, whose "Notes and Recollections of Professional Life" were published in 1846, says : —"The exceeding vulgarity of the prejudice that ardent spirits impart strength and vigour to the human frame, is disgraceful to educated men ; yet true it is that many of our most experienced commanders of the army and navy still attempt to justify and continue the practice."

ON THE SELECTION AND IMPROVEMENT OF LOCALITIES FOR THE EUROPEAN TROOPS IN OUR INTERTROPICAL POSSESSIONS.

It has been justly observed by an able military surgeon of old—a survivor of climate and English club-house generalship—that "where the hygiene of an army is judiciously regulated, the soldier may be kept in health and vigour ; but allow an ignorant general to encamp on a marsh, let filth stagnate, fatigue excessively the men, crowd them in low damp rooms, and, despite of

---

* Neglect in the use of fruits and vegetables has at all times proved a source of injury to the health of our soldiers in India ; and the subject of an ample supply of these requisites has not, even in our own day, received the attention from authority which, from its importance, it deserves.

drugs, they will fall as unripe and blasted fruit, not by the sword, but by the fever."

Sufferings and sacrifices such as these have at all times been regarded by the army and navy surgeons with sympathy and sorrow; nor have they ever been slow to offer cautions against their causes, nor to censure the criminal neglect of their cautions. Robert Jackson, writing in 1791 of the expeditions to, and occupations of Carthagena, the Havannah, Martinique, Guadaloupe, St. Lucia, St. Juan, and even Jamaica, declares that much of the destruction of life arose " from the inexperience or ignorant inattention of those who conducted the expeditions. We have many instances of expeditions apparently well concerted which have failed from the excessive sickness of the troops; and too many proofs of this sickness proceeding from a neglect of such precautions as might have contributed to the preservation of health." From the days of the occupation of Carthagena and the Havannah, to those of the occupation of Varna and the Crimea, the sacrifice has been consummated with all the cruelty of ignorance and mismanagement. Truly has our great military historian, Napier, declared of the British soldier, that he " conquered under the cold shade of aristocracy : no honours awaited his daring, no despatch gave his name to the applauses of his countrymen; his life of danger was uncheered by hope, his death unnoticed."

From the utter ignorance of our commanders of what is necessary for the preservation of the health of their men, they frequently propose to stay an evil by increasing it. Our surgeons, on the contrary, have at all times been quite unmilitary in the efficiency and completeness of the sanitary measures they have proposed.

Frederick of Prussia has stated that fever cost him as many men as seven battles; so that, between the fever and the battles together, it must have fared badly with " the tyrant's counters" in his day. It were well if we could be assured that in our own time the external causes of fever have become less rife in our camps, and that our commanders by sea and land have become more vigilant and better informed as to the means of preventing them; but I fear that neither can be affirmed with any confidence. As to commanders, we would appear to cling, as of old, to men ignorant of, and disinclined from learning the most simple rules affecting health : we hug our mismanagements.

When shall we have done with the times when, according to Hughes's "History of England," " British troops were led to slaughter by generals scarcely fit to conduct a review?" When shall we have done with commanders wanting in strategic power, in administrative capacity, and in knowledge of, and willingness to apply, the means of saving their men. The experience of all our wars shows that the worst economy is not to be prepared, and that it costs more than double to make up for a bad beginning. The truth again is, that, under an inefficient commander, every kind of disaster is not only possible but very practicable.

We have lost an army in every quarter of the globe, and precedent has consoled us: it has always been so in our campaigns, and in our colonies. We have often appointed unproved men, and men of proved insufficiency; and we have retained them in their places, because it has always been so with us. Our principle has been "that nothing bad should be mended." But a better order of things is at hand: in truth, matters could not continue much longer as they have been.

To the neglect of healthy localities for camps, cantonments, and stations—to the absence of proper structural arrangements in barracks and hospitals—to inattention to the suitable feeding and clothing of the men—the neglect in promoting and cultivating better habits of life—the absence of instruction in cooking, hutting, exercising, and bathing—to the neglect of change of air and of climate in the remote stages of the diseases of seamen and soldiers;—to these neglects, which it must at all times rest with governments and commanders to remedy, we must refer the constant and terrible losses of the British army in our intertropical possessions.

I venture to say that, from the causes here briefly enumerated, we have in every score of years, during the last century and upwards, lost unnecessarily, in our fleets and armies, more men than have fallen in our battles from the landing of Julius Cæsar to the present time.

Sir A. Tulloch has stated to me, as the result of his investigations in the War-office, that amongst British officers and soldiers of the Queen's and Company's armies, serving in the East Indies alone, there occurred, from 1815 to 1855 inclusive, exclusive of casualties, a total mortality of about one hundred thousand men, "the greater portion of whose lives might have been saved, had better localities been selected for military occupation in that country." Estimating each soldier at the minimum value of 100l., we here arrive at a loss in money of 10,000,000l.*

Nor are the causes of such destruction of life difficult of being discovered and prevented. Robert Jackson says that, "There are instances where the sick-list in armies amounts to one-third of the total force, and others, where it does not exceed one-fiftieth, even one-hundredth part. The causes of such difference are sometimes visible and obvious. To discover their sources, and to prevent their operations, is important; and it is frequently a work of no great difficulty."

Samuel Johnson, in his " Political Tracts, 1771," referring to the contests of his time with France and Spain, states, that " The wars

---

* It was my intention, in the present edition, to have quoted largely from the valuable and admirably prepared works of Dr. Norman CheVers, on "The Means of Preserving the Health of European Soldiers in India," and of Dr. Ewart, on . " The Vital Statistics of the European and Native Armies of India ;" but I was reminded that I had already exceeded the limits prescribed for my Volume, and thus, much to my regret, my purpose was frustrated. Both works do much honour to their authors, and to the medical corps of the Indian army.

of civilized nations make very slow changes in the system of empire. The people perceive scarcely any alteration but in an increase of debt; and the few individuals who are benefited are not supposed to have the clearest right to their advantages.

"The life of a British soldier," he adds, "is ill represented by heroic fiction. War has means of destruction more formidable than the cannon and the sword. Of the thousands and tens of thousands that perished in our late contests with France and Spain, a very small part ever felt the stroke of an enemy; the rest languished in tents and ships, amidst damps and putrefactions, pale, torpid, spiritless, and helpless; gasping and groaning, unpitied among men, made obdurate by long continuance of helpless misery; and were at last whelmed in pits or heaved into the ocean, without notice and without remembrance.

"By incommodious encampments and unwholesome stations, where courage is useless and enterprise impracticable, fleets are silently dispeopled, and armies sluggishly melted away. Thus is a people gradually exhausted, for the most part with little effect. In the last war Havanna was taken; and at what expense is too well remembered. May my country be never cursed with such another conquest."

The attack on Carthagena is yet remembered, where "the Spaniards from their ramparts saw their invaders destroyed by the hostility of the elements, poisoned by the air and crippled by the dews; where every hour swept away battalions, and in the three days that passed between the descent and re-embarkation half an army perished."

Nor can these events be regarded as matters of a bygone history, for Walcheren, the Peninsula, Arakan, Rangoon, China, Sindh, Varna, and Sebastopol have brought them back to our very doors; and they have occurred always from the same causes. The maxim that what cannot be remedied ought to be forgotten, does not apply to the conduct of war. On the contrary, all our errors should be treasured in our memories, with a view to their avoidance for the future. The masses must learn wisdom from retrospection; they are of the very few who possess prospective wisdom. Although the past cannot be redeemed, the experiences of the past ought to suggest lessons and cautions for the future. The ancients held the prudent maxim never to pardon the second blunder in the conduct of war. Let us hope that England may eventually learn this necessary lesson. In the Crimea it should seem as if all the bunglers of the British army had been assembled, each in his respective line, to try what mismanagement could do—how far mismanagement could be carried—how far, in short, the forbearance of the country could be made to extend. "It is passing easy," says the *Examiner*, "to talk of putting the saddle on the right horse, but here the saddle is one and indivisible, and the horses to be saddled are many."

Sir Gilbert Blane, speaking of the neglect of the seaman's health in his earlier experience, says :—" In former times they had not the attention paid to them which would have been due even to inanimate machines of equal utility ; for there seemed to be much more anxiety about preserving arms from rusting and cordage from rotting, than about maintaining men in an effective state of health."

The naval commanders here referred to were not men of the school of Lord Metcalfe, who always urged his maxim—" Economy in the department of stores is ruinous. We ought to be lavish of the contents of our arsenals, and saving of the lives of our men." A soldier lost in India costs at the least 120*l.*, so that the necessary reinforcements to keep an army of 100,000 men, which some think necessary, will cost 1,200,000*l.* per annum.

We have, in the instances cited, witnessed our armies scourged and wasted away as of old, through the ignorances and incapacities of authorities at home and abroad; but a higher order of intelligence is dawning upon us, having its origin in the sanitary investigation of our naval and military surgeons. " The wisdom of the country," too, invoked to her soldiers' aid by men like Robert Jackson, William Fergusson, and Henry Marshall, is being manifested through a free press and a Parliamentary inquiry ;— sharpened, perhaps, by a sense of the common danger resulting from abuses and ignorances without end. We are said to have acted hitherto as if armies had been made for generals, and not generals for armies; but let us hope that the time is not distant when soldiers and seamen shall cease to perish without necessity, and without results.

Let us hope also that Englishmen may not again witness, as in the instance of Walcheren, the degradation of the sovereign's grant of " approbation" for " perseverance and celerity—for the promptitude with which he had commenced, and the vigour with which he conducted " and consummated the destruction of an army. One such humiliation—one such shameless laudation of a commander who ought in justice to have been cashiered by sentence of a court-martial—ought to be enough for one century.* The practical working of the British military system in the Crimea was regarded by the public with alternate indignation and sarcasm ; and of Walcheren we have all heard how—

> " The Earl of Chatham, with his broadsword drawn,
> Stood waiting for Sir Richard Strahan ;
> Sir Richard, anxious to be at 'em,
> Was only waiting for the Earl of Chatham."

---

* The expectations here hazarded have not as yet been fulfilled, commanders of the most lordly degrees of ignorance having been rewarded and decorated for similar services to those of Lord Chatham—the destruction of their men.

There is no country in the world in which the responsibility of public servants is so little felt as in England ; and so long as this state of things holds, great public calamities may be looked upon as certain of occurrence.

The pestilential island of Walcheren received the largest expedition which had ever, up to that time, left the shores of England, amounting in seamen and soldiers to seventy thousand men.

The climate into which this most powerful and admirably disciplined force was thrust—*during the months of its utmost insalubrity*, those of summer and autumn—was such that the Scotch regiment in the Dutch service had been known to bury their whole numbers in three years; a climate in which the French army lost annually one-third of those employed, or 33 per cent.; and in which a Dutch corps, which on arrival, three years previously to the British landing, amounted to 800 strong, numbered but eighty-five men on this occasion. Such was the country and such the climate—all within sixty hours' easy sail of us—in which our ministers and commanders proceeded to make war.

The climate and its diseases had been accurately described by Sir John Pringle so long ago as 1764; yet nothing was known to our ministers, who sent the imbecile toilet-loving Chatham in command of the finest army that England had possessed since the days of Cromwell. How often have folly and factious ignorance paved the way for the death of the British soldier! With us, when a question was raised in Parliament on the subject of the soldier's wants, the stereotyped reply used to be—"it is under consideration"—and there it was allowed to remain.

The conduct of our enemy, on the occasion of our very characteristic expedition to Walcheren, was characteristic of his surpassing genius: "Only keep them in check," said Napoleon, "and the bad air and fevers peculiar to the country will soon destroy their army."

The forces sailed on the 28th July, and were landed on the 31st July and 1st August; and by the 10th October, 587 per thousand of the strength had fallen sick, while there died 142 per thousand. Such inquiries as these ought certainly to "contribute greatly to direct us to the best means of promoting the welfare, improving the efficiency, and preserving the health of the soldiers," as stated by Henry Marshall; but, somehow or other, governments and commanders are peculiarly slow of deriving lessons from experience.

Marshall concludes with the following quotation from the "Edinburgh Review:"—"*The expedition to Walcheren, planned and conducted as it was, was the fruit of statistical ignorance in every one, everywhere, from the Prime Minister to the Commander-in-chief, and from him to the surgeon's mate. That ignorance which every Middleburghian and Dutchman could have enlightened or dispelled, cost us ten thousand brave men, not a little money, and not a little credit, and not a few tears and inconveniences to those whom statesmen never consider.*" This miserably conducted expedition cost the country twenty millions sterling, and imposed a burthen of one million of annual taxes.

Its other consequences, in the language of a popular historian,

T 2

were ignominious retreat, pestilence, and destruction—because, according to custom, the worst possible general was selected to command the finest of armies. Again, we have the expedition to St. Domingo, in which, according to Dr. Maclean, the British force was reduced in three months to 1100 men, from an original army of 10,000; and all this "without striking a blow or seeing an enemy."

In round numbers, there were treated in the Peninsular and other hospitals, according to Sir James M'Grigor, for disease and wounds, from the 21st December, 1811, to 24th June, 1816—346,108 men, of whom 232,553 were discharged cured. Of these last, so-called cured, how many thousands were harassed and distressed, during the whole course of the war, by the habitual recurrence of the fevers of Walcheren and the Guadiana, so as to weaken them and render them frequently unfit for duty? How many, in after years, in our various colonies, suffered cruelly and perished miserably and prematurely, from sicknesses resulting from the same original ills?

Thus, death is the last but not the only result of "incommodious encampments and unwholesome stations, where courage is useless and enterprise impracticable."

It had long been a subject of complaint and remonstrance on the part of Robert Jackson and other military surgeons, that, in the West Indies, facilities of accommodation for trade—the polar star of British policy—had condemned the soldier to the scourge of disease without a necessity; and whoever looks at the distribution of the European military force in the East Indies will come to the conclusion that the soldiers have been exposed to disease there on grounds even less justifiable than have held sway with the authorities in the West.

"It is positively true," says Robert Jackson, "proved to a demonstration, in numerous instances, but proved by accident, not by avowed experiment, that European troops may be so stationed in the islands of the West Indies as to retain health nearly as well as they could be expected to retain it in their native country. The air of the interior and mountainous parts of the larger of the intertropical islands is comparatively cool and pleasant, and not unfriendly to the European constitution.

"The expense of filling up the military ranks, thinned by sicknesses which arise from bad position and badly constructed quarters, actually amounts, in course of a few years, to a greater sum of money than would be required to erect barracks of the best form of construction at the most eligible sites in the country, even at the extravagant price of government contract."

The truth of what was here many years ago advanced, Jackson proved in a statistical summary of the "Inspection Reports of Military Positions, Barracks, and Hospitals," submitted to the Commander of the Forces on the West India station. His representations, though so true and so easy of comprehension, met with no attention whatever; and after a public life of the highest honour and of the most noble labour and usefulness, extending over half a century, every day of which, during peace and during three great wars, was devoted to the moral and physical good of the soldier, Jackson concludes with a pathetic appeal to "the legislative branch of the government;" there being "a presumption amounting almost to proof that it has no chance of obtaining attention from the executive;" that is, from military or naval authority;* and after the lapse of another half-century of terrible experiences, the watchword with our commanders is still, "As you were." With the ordinary run of commanders by sea and land it must be so: they are but servile formalists.

Referring to the fact that in England "much opposition was raised by the subordinate authorities" to his suggestions for compiling statistical reports on the sickness, mortality, and invaliding among the troops in the colonies, Henry Marshall adds that "ignorance of the principles of military hygiene, and an inveterate

---

* I have already suggested that if, by the usages of war, the punishment of death be applicable to a disgraceful capitulation on the part of a commander, some heavy punishment ought in justice to await the man who, through wilful neglect, and a wanton ignorance, causes his army to perish. It was once a rule of English and French history that "responsibility meant death."

But in these days of canting speculative or pseudo-philanthropy and dreamy sentimentality, death must not be so much as mentioned for the holocaust even of an entire army. Yet death has been awarded, and suffered too, for very minor crimes comparatively. Certain am I, that the very first Sir Michael or Sir Peregrine who shall be made to suffer the mild sentence of cashiering for such a crime, under the award of a court-martial composed of medical and military officers in equal numbers, will prove the last of his class who will venture on the same course of shameful neglect in time to come. From the day that this act of common justice shall be done, we may hope never thenceforth to hear again of armies being planted in marshes, there to die, while the surgeons had for fifty years urged their removal to the hills, where they would have lived well and happily; of soldiers being thrust into barracks and hospitals unfit for the reception of convicts. Let this be done, and we shall no more be told by a statesman in Parliament that "nearly one half of the lives that used to be sacrificed in the West Indies was sacrificed through neglect," and that "this mortality might have been prevented by the most ordinary precautions;" that "while the soldiers, who were unstained by crime, were condemned to five days' salt provisions weekly, the convicts were allowed five days' fresh meat; and that while the troops were suffering, the convicts were in good health." I say, let the right judgment be brought to bear on the right man, and we shall hear no more of such atrocities.

Commanders, in short, must be rewarded or punished in like manner as other public servants; and as they always receive the highest rewards, so they should be made responsible in the highest degree. They accept the advantages with the disadvantages. It should be remembered, also, that the sacrifice of a fleet or an army might prove the ruin of the empire. For such crimes excuses and soft names must no longer be found. I have long been strongly impressed with the conviction that, of all the responsible servants of the public, the responsibility of those who undertake the management and command of fleets and armies should be made the most direct and immediate. "Where there can be no responsibility below, there should be double responsibility above," says Lord Macaulay. Hitherto they have been the most irresponsible of public servants. There was hardly a chief or a subordinate actor in the Crimean tragedy of horrors who did not receive some reward or honorary distinction from the Crown. They have each and all been, in fact, rewarded in proportion to the injury they have done to their country. "*Dat veniam corvis, vexat censura columbas.*" The culprits were rewarded first, and tried by a sham commission afterwards, which was assembled and indeed designed only to whitewash them.

prejudice in favour of former usages, seemed to be the leading cause of the opposition to the measures recommended, the adoption of which has proved so singularly beneficial."

Very different was the conduct of the generals of Napoleon. On the landing of the British forces on Walcheren, and on the capture of Flushing, there was found a Memoir by the French commander, General Monnet, on the preservation of the soldier's health. It was a document full of interest, and of much scientific and practical value.

But, referring to our subject, the removal of the British troops from the pestilential plains to the healthy mountain regions of Jamaica was at length ordered by a man who united the most active and enlarged benevolence to the most invincible firmness and resolution in carrying out every measure that was right—Lord Metcalfe. And, strange to say, the result has been to the very letter as Jackson foretold; the British soldiery now retaining their health in the mountains " nearly as well as could be expected in their native country."

The result as regards the mortality of British troops is, in simple figures, as follows :—From 1803 to 1816, and for how long before we do not know, the soldiers perished in Jamaica at the rate of 130 per thousand per annum, while by the simple and easily arranged measure ordered by Lord Metcalfe, the mortality has, since 1842, been reduced to 35 per thousand per annum.

This beneficent act, so becoming the generous and noble nature of the Governor of Jamaica, was " characteristic of Metcalfe. He made the first movement on his own responsibility, and offered himself to pay the expense. He saw that the troops under his command were being sacrificed to ignorance, negligence, and false economy ; and he exerted himself, not without success, to establish a new order of things, by locating on the high healthy grounds of the island the European regiments which perished miserably on the plains."*

Detachments of British troops were stationed at Maroon Town at different and uncertain times between 1795 and 1839, by direction of Lord Grey and others ; but nothing fixed or determinate was arranged until Lord Metcalfe gave the final order. When will any of our great foreign possessions fall under the charge of such another governor?

Robert Jackson speaks also of the value of military labour in securing military health—a subject not yet sufficiently taken into consideration by our authorities. Fort King George, he says, in 1803, stood in lee of a swamp, and the exhalations from it being considered by Colonel Macdonald, commanding the Royal Scots Regiment, to be injurious to the health of his men, he ordered them to drain it. "The planters lent the tools, the soldiers of the Royals drained the bog ;" and Fort King George, which formerly

* Kaye's " Life of Lord Metcalfe."

stood noted for unhealthiness, is now "one of the healthiest quarters in the Windward and Leeward Islands Station, as appears by a comparative view of the sick returns of the army."

In Jackson's various writings there are numerous instances of similar results from the gratuitous labour of the soldier ; and, what is very important also, this most eminent military physician always concludes by declaring that " the thing was done—with obvious effect upon health, morals, and happiness, while the work was under execution."

With reference to the purposes for which British soldiers are sent to the East Indies, and to the efficient exercise of their powers when called into action, it has always surprised me that so large a portion of the European army has been retained in the plains of Hindustan. It is justly observed by Drs. Hooker and Thomson, that India presents more contrasts and varieties in climate than any other area of equal extent in the world. Holding this fact in view, we must take advantage of the irregularities of surface, and varieties of soil, to found healthy stations. With urgent political reasons or state necessities I do not pretend to deal; but if these do not exist, I know of no defence that can be set up, on the score of humanity or of expense, in plea of the cruel and unnecessary sickness and mortality—of " the serious loss in the balance of national accounts," consequent on the loss of men. "The case is important, and the sovereign power will be false to its own interests, if it do not apply a remedy when furnished with proof that a remedy is attainable, and particularly when informed that it is not difficult of attainment."

Independently of the revenues of British India, England, possessing property to the amount of nearly ten thousand millions of pounds sterling, and an annual produce therefrom of about four hundred millions, need surely not descend to haggling about the money-value of the soldier, nor yet about the cost of means necessary to his health and efficiency. Dr. Julius Jeffreys observes justly that, " costly to India as a large British force must necessarily be, it is the most profitable investment she has ever made, and it is not at present quite costly enough to satisfy the demands of justice and sound policy." And now that extensive lines of railway are about to be laid down throughout the length and breadth of Hindustan, the time, I trust, is at hand when the British soldier may have the advantage of recourse to the mountain ranges and solitary mountains scattered over the several provinces of India, not only as sanitary stations, but as places of permanent residence.

But the evils resulting from neglect in choosing proper sites for our colonial emporiums do not end here. The choice of such sites having, as stated, reference to trade only, and not to health, the sickness which is ever present is not referred to its true cause, the inherent unhealthiness of the place, but to the arrival of some trading vessel from some other equally insalubrious locality; and hence quarantine, with all its evils.

Sickness is always prevalent in such places, ships are always arriving; and people always dislike to believe that they are living in a pestilential locality; so, disease is readily ascribed to importation. With the unreasoning many, the suppositious foreign ill is always more dreaded than the real home-bred pest.

In the East, as in the West Indies, the loss of military life from endemic and epidemic diseases has always been unnecessarily great—sometimes enormous. " If the subject be viewed correctly and without prepossession, the loss sustained will be found to have been principally owing to mistake, that is, to inattention to truths furnished by experience for the choice of healthy positions."

These just and manly sentiments are quoted from the celebrated work of Robert Jackson on the " FORMATION, DISCIPLINE, AND ECONOMY OF ARMIES," and especially from that portion of it which is devoted to a " General View of Service in Tropical Climates;" wherein, though he speaks in special reference to the West Indian colonies, there is necessarily much which applies with equal justice to all hot countries. This admirable work, which I had the pleasure to get republished, ought to be in the hands of every officer, whether military or medical.*

I may here mention that I prepared, by desire of the late Lord Metcalfe, without previous notice, a memorandum relating to arrangements for constructing barracks and hospitals, and which he handed to Lieutenant-General Sir George Murray at a meeting, held by desire of Lord Stanley at the Colonial Office, on the 16th of July, 1842. This note was of a purely suggestive character, no time having been allowed me for entering into details; and the following quotations are here presented :—

" 1. The author of this note has satisfied himself, from an extensive range of observation in the East Indies, that great loss of

---

* The great military work of Robert Jackson is not sufficiently known to the British or to the Indian army; and as I am desirous that military men should have a better warrant for its excellence than my opinion, I subjoin that of one of the highest and brightest of military critics—that of Sir John Moore :—

" My DEAR JACKSON,—I have perused your military book, with which I am much delighted. There are none of us, even the most experienced, who may not derive instruction from it; and I only regret that you, who possess a soldier's mind, had not been a soldier by profession."

Although no royal honours awaited Jackson in his time, honours have been freely awarded to his memory by his countrymen, of which scores of club-house generals— those slayers of their men—may indeed be envious. In his professional career in the British army he was exposed to continual slight and persecution at the hands of his professional superiors; and a personage, designated by Ballingall "a successful apothecary at Weymouth, who had made himself acceptable to George III."—Sir Lucas Pepys—was placed over him as head of the medical department of the army. This was the person who refused to proceed to Walcheren, declaring as his excuse that " he knew nothing of camp or contagious diseases but what he had learned from Sir John Pringle's book." Cobbett observed on this occasion that the old apothecary had only one other declaration to make, "that he was unable to draw his pay." Thus was the royal choice justified in the person of this miserable favourite.

life, injury to health, and sacrifice of the public money have resulted from the present modes of locating and constructing barracks and hospitals for the European troops there; and his information, derived from printed and other sources, leads him to conclude that similarly injurious results are also produced in various of her Majesty's colonies, from similar causes. . . .

" 4. To obviate for the future such extensive waste of life and money, and with a view likewise to improve such existing buildings as may admit of amendment, it is proposed that standard or model plans be prepared for barrack and hospital accommodation, in scale proportioned to certain given numbers of men, and suited to the various and contrasted climates occupied by British troops. The most cursory observation will satisfy us that, of certain given plans, one only will prove excellent; whereas now, all over the British Possessions, we find in existence every conceivable plan, ending in no approved or fixed plan whatever; so that, in fact, that which ought to be settled, and is very easily capable of being settled by regulation is, up to this day left, as I have stated, to the fancy of individuals.

" 5. It is not apprehended that either difficulty or the expenditure of much time would be encountered in carrying out the proposed plan, provided it were undertaken by persons competent to the task; for the same plan of barrack and hospital accommodation would suit the climates of the East and West Indies, the Cape of Good Hope, Mauritius, Ceylon, China, and Australia—the stations of Gibraltar, Malta, and the Ionian Isles—while plans for the other colonies would be easy of settlement.

" 6. To arrange and complete so desirable an object, it is respectfully suggested that a committee of engineers and medical officers be assembled in London, and that power be given, in furtherance of the purposes in view, to call in evidence such persons as may be supposed to possess experience and a knowledge of the subject."

Sir George Ballingall, in the last edition of his admirable " Outlines of Military Surgery," says of the memorandum just quoted: —" This excellent suggestion has not been as yet acted upon, and consequently no established plan has been adopted for the construction of barracks and hospitals either at home or abroad."

It is impossible to overrate the influence of structural arrangements, of an abundant supply of pure air and water, whether in military or civil communities. That sickness and mortality increase in proportion as the population increases in density, has been established so as to demonstrate a strict relation between these elements. The Registrar-General has found that where the mortality was 15, 16, and 17 in 1000 living, the average number of persons on 100 acres was respectively 9, 17, and 22. Again, in certain town districts the ratio of mortality ranged from 28 to 36 in 1000 living; the numbers of persons on 100 acres in these districts being respectively 279 and 693.

Miss Nightingale, speaking of the utter neglect of ventilation in the treatment of our soldiers, says :—" With regard to overcrowding, both for barracks and hospitals, the regulation of our service is overcrowding. But even the regulation-space was not adhered to."

"The population of England," says Dr. Farr, "is, there is reason to believe, collectively healthier than any equal amount of population in any other kingdom; but the rapid increase in the proportion of the town population—in which the mortality is 27 per cent. higher than it is in the country, and the sickness, the suffering, the debility, the physical degeneracy of race, are in an equal excess—makes this question of the health of towns and the fertilization of the surrounding fields one of the great questions of the day, demanding immediate solution. It is difficult for the imagination to conceive all the beneficent effects that would flow from the possible diminution of the mortality which the above figures express.

"The population of large towns," says the same authority, "was 6,838,069 in 1841, and 8,247,017 in 1851. The question of the health of towns is therefore a question of the strength of England." . . " National health is national wealth."

The practical question may now be asked—Have we not within our Eastern possessions, almost everywhere, mountain tracts and solitary mountains conveniently situated, wherein the European soldier might live in health and vigour through the advantages of a cool and a better climate, and the proper application of his own labour ; and, if so, why are they not made use of? That such favourable localities abound throughout India, no one can doubt ; and I am disposed to hope that the calling the attention of authority to their sanitary advantages, for the benefit of all classes, civil and military, will prove one out of the many valuable results which may accrue from the detailed and systematic plan of requiring, from military surgeons serving in India, "Reports on the Medical Topography of the Country generally, and of its Districts, Stations, and Cantonments in particular."*

Such courses of investigation can hardly fail of important sanitary results ; and they should be carefully and systematically conducted, so as to ensure success, for hitherto the selection of hill stations has had too much of caprice or of chance in it to command the benefits that might otherwise have been obtained. It is probable that some of the lower ranges of hills, and solitary hills, may prove

---

* The plan here referred to was a measure submitted by the author, on the 26th of March, 1835, to the Governor-General of India, Sir Charles Metcalfe, Bart., and sanctioned and ordered by him for the three Presidencies of India and the Dependencies to the Eastward. The order bears date 23rd November, 1835, and was a *direct* act of the Government—the medical authorities of Bengal having afforded the measure a very equivocal support, or rather no support at all.

This great question is now in the hands of a highly-intelligent body of medical officers ;—the field is almost untouched before them, and we must not doubt the eventual results, whatever obstruction may be offered by the *vis inertiæ* of old men.

available for military stations, and that medium degrees of elevation may be found which, while not so lofty as to cause bowel and
other disorders, may yet prove of sufficient height to place the
soldier above fever-level.   This would be a most important topographical discovery.   Maroon Town, Jamaica, is elevated but little
more than two thousand feet above the level of the sea, yet this
has proved a sufficient protection against the deadly fevers of the
country; and even against the yellow fever, a rise of 2500 feet is
everywhere found to be a sufficient protection.   The same security is obtained in Constantinople and in Cairo, in the instance
of plague, by the elevation of Alem-Daghe in the former, and of
the citadel in the latter.

Looking to the serious character of the great Sepoy mutiny of 1857,
and perceiving that in all future time the main prop of our Indian empire must consist in a well-ordered British force, I presented, on the
12th Aug., 1857, to the Chairman of the Court of Directors of the East
India Company, " Suggestions for Promoting the Health and Efficiency of the British Troops serving in the East Indies."   Here, and
in a subsequent report, the necessity of investigating, in a manner
the most deliberate and scientific, the various mountain climates
throughout India was insisted on, and the details of investigation
were at the same time furnished; beginning with the examination
of the " medium elevations of from 2000 to 4000 feet," and ending
with the examination of those " of from 4000 to 8000 feet."

The proposed course of investigation, immediately approved and
ordered by the Home Government of India, will open out and demonstrate the whole subject of mountain climates, and establish for the
lasting good of our armies the national importance of this subject.
In India, beyond any other of our possessions, every individual
soldier becomes of importance; and it is only in the mountain
ranges that his health can be preserved.   Hitherto our trials of the
elevated climates of the East have been exclusively confined to the
higher ranges, and those bordering on the hot and pestilential
plains, where the air is cold and extremely humid, to the neglect
of those elevated slopes bordering on the snowy ranges, where the
atmosphere is buoyant, comparatively dry, and bracing.   As to the
medium elevations, their climates have been altogether overlooked
by us in the East, although they have proved of the greatest
sanitary value to our troops in the West Indies.

Nor are the moral influences of the mountain climates to be
disregarded by the medical philosopher.   Montesquieu and Malte-
Brun have assigned topographical reasons why the inhabitants of
the plains should of necessity be weak, effeminate, idle, and timid,
while the elevated and cold regions are inhabited by their conquerors;—regions wherein the severer forms of fever are unknown.
It would seem, indeed, that the diseases of tropical climates, like
certain vegetable productions, are restricted to certain altitudes
and particular degrees of temperature.

"If British colonies," says Horace Wilson, "be ever formed in the East, with a chance of preserving the moral and physical energies of the parent country, it is to the vales and mountains of the Indian Alps that we must look for their existence." The removal of troops even to short distances from their stations and encampments has, I am happy to learn, been acted on systematically in various of our colonies since the publication of the "Army Medical Statistics," and in every instance with a most satisfactory result. I trust this important subject will continue to be present to the minds of both military and medical authority, and that no narrow contracted notions of economy will anywhere be allowed to stand in the way of a duty imposed alike by considerations of humanity, and of the best interests of the State.

I had continually to treat the ailments of men of business in Calcutta, which I often found to be of an anomalous and perplexing nature, affecting both mind and body. In such cases mere medical treatment very often proved vain, until the sufferer was released from the cares of official duty, by change of air, a trip to sea (which I always preferred), or by a removal to the Upper Provinces :—indeed, where the circumstances of the patient admit of it, this last resource of medicine should never be neglected. It acts as a general tonic, invigorating the whole frame, improving the quality of the blood, and stimulating every organ to a more healthy performance of its office.

Of the advantages of an apparently trivial change of position on health we have a very interesting example in the instance of Augusta in the southern division of the United States. Prior to 1829 this arsenal was situated on the Savannah, and fever prevailed to such an extent that, in the third quarter of 1825, all the garrison except two men suffered from it ; while, by a removal to Sand Hills, three miles from Augusta and two from the Savannah River, where the soil was hard, dry, and sandy, with no marshes in the vicinity, the ratio of cases of intermittent fever was reduced to 150, and of remittent fever to 156 per 1000 annually.—*Brit. and For. Med. Rev.*, July, 1843.

The selections of localities for barracks and hospitals are very generally faulty throughout the East Indies, while the cost of their erection has sometimes been enormous. "The different erections of the Company for the accommodation of their troops," says Tennant, "have cost several millions, and may be regarded as splendid instances of their economical principles giving way to the comfort of their army. The sums thus expended, laid out at the compound interest of this country, would, at a determinate period not very remote, have equalled the national debt."

The buildings for the European troops at Berhampore in Bengal, lately abandoned on account of the unhealthiness of the station, are stated to have cost, including capital and interest, the enormous sum of 16,891,206*l.* The details are from the office of the Accountant-General, and that of the Military Board, Calcutta.*

Happy the condition of the European soldier in the East as in the West Indies, had a tithe of the sums wasted in erecting barracks and hospitals in low and marshy sites, been applied to purposes of preparing less costly but yet suitable accommodation in positions of ascertained salubrity ; but, instead of that, we have everywhere throughout our intertropical possessions, buildings occasionally of good construction, erected at enormous cost, which are eventually abandoned because, from their improper positions and proved insalubrity, their inmates are found to die in a proportion to shock even the humanity of Governments.

Dr. William Maclean, of the Madras army, says of India generally, in 1854 :—" Barracks have been built, and costly repairs wasted on others that for half a century have been mere pest-houses. Our cantonments, for the most part, are to this day in a most disgraceful condition, well-known causes of disease being rife and abounding on every hand ; and all for want of some person, or body of persons, who can speak out on the subject so as to compel a respectful attention."

By a table furnished me by the late Inspector-General Macleod, the average annual admissions into hospital during thirteen years, at Berhampore, was 2196 per 1000; while the deaths averaged 106 per 1000 per annum.   The proportion of deaths to cases treated in hospital was, during five years, as follows :—

In fever, one in . . . . . . 21 and a fraction.
dysentery, one in 10
hepatitis, one in , . . . 9

Secunderabad, Madras Presidency, now also in course of abandonment, has long been noted for its bad locality—bad barracks and hospitals—all which have long operated destructively on the health of British soldiers : yet it is surrounded by stations which are noted for their healthiness.   The barracks are described by the late Inspector-General Burke as " composed of two squares enclosing one another, so as to make assurance doubly sure against the possibility of perfect ventilation ;" and added to all this we have defective drainage and sewerage.

Dr. Burke is worthy of being heard on another important question arising out of this subject—namely, that of finance :—" It has

* The military buildings of Berhampore were estimated, in the
year 1757, at 302,278l., or rupees 3,823,657 14 8
Compound interest on this sum for 77 years at 5 per cent . 163,702,404 0 0
Average annual charges for repairs, &c., during 77 years, at
the annual average of rupees 18,000 . . . .   1,386,000 0 0
Total . . . . Rs. 168,912,061 14 8
Total (sterling) . . £16,891,206 3 10
Exchange at 2s. per rupee.

been stated that every European soldier landed in India costs the state 100*l*. sterling; calculating from which the intrinsic loss of 117 European soldiers by Secunderabad in four and three quarter years, is 11,700*l*. sterling; but as these 117 men have to be replaced, the doing so will cost also 11,700*l*., to which must be added the loss in acclimatizing these latter, amounting, on the lowest calculation, to one-eighth, or 1462*l*., giving a sum total of 24,862*l*. as the actual loss sustained in four and three quarter years, or probably three lacs of rupees in five years. But as Secunderabad would appear to have been a station for European troops for at least thirty years, the cost to the State for that period may be estimated at twelve lacs at least," or about 150,000*l*.

Man is a dear article in England; and with whatever little care we have hitherto treated him, the old seaman and soldier have at all times been most difficult to replace : but human labour for battle must be paid for as for other national works. The whole of this subject, as affecting troops, is of the highest importance. It was owing to ignorance of military and medical topography that so much suffering and death attended the several attempts against Ava during the first war with that state, and that every object aimed at by the Government of India, in sending a force to Rangoon and Arakan, failed for so long ; and it was a neglect in commissariat arrangement, and of medical topography, that caused the destruction of both the Rangoon and Arakan armies. But to return to our more immediate subject :—

In no station in the south of India, the old abandoned one of Masulipatam excepted, has the mortality been so great as at Secunderabad; and it is produced, as might be anticipated, by fevers and dysenteries of formidable character, principally : in short, it would be difficult to determine which is most to be lamented in this unhappy station, the defects of nature or those of art. There died there, between 1804 and 1835, the large number of 2620 men and officers, women and children, inhabiting the bad locality and buildings described.

According to a return made by the Madras Medical Board, the average annual deaths amounted to 84·89 per 1000 of strength, or 96·89, according to other corrections. These are melancholy reckonings; but they will continue to be the rule of the British army, "until," according to Robert Jackson, "physicians have the place in the councils of military commanders that is due to science. The health history of the late wars in Europe is demonstrative in proof of the important fact that military life has been sacrificed in an enormous proportion to ignorance; that is, to the unwillingness of commanders to be advised on subjects which they could not themselves be supposed to know."

So serious a charge as this against the commanders of his country, by one so far-seeing, so just, so learned and experienced, so humane and virtuous as Robert Jackson, is deserving the most serious consideration. The declaration of this celebrated army physician was not only true when it was made, some fifty years ago, but it remains emphatically true to the present hour, notwithstanding the unremitting labours of such men as Jackson, Blane, Hennen, Trotter, Fergusson, Ballingall, and Henry Marshall, and their endeavours to bring about a more enlightened, just, and humane treatment.

While all the horrors related by Earl Grey, in his celebrated speech in the House of Lords on the Administration of the Army, 8th April, 1854, were in full and destructive existence, the Duke of Wellington was all-powerful in this country; he was Master-General of the Ordnance, Commander-in-Chief, Prime Minister, &c.; but if he had held no official station during the forty years of peace—the time for perfecting military institutions, as well as improving the condition of the soldier—his power to ameliorate (had he been so minded) was without limit. That he did not move more actively in the cause of improvement, or cause others to do so, must always be a subject of regret to those who best appreciate the Duke of Wellington's military services in actual war.

During the period of his active field career in India and in Europe, he rendered vast services to his country; but in the forty long years of peace which followed, and when the military institutions of the empire, as well as the locating, housing, clothing, feeding, and arming of the soldier, might have been leisurely and most appropriately perfected, "the Duke" did not sufficiently consider those easy, obvious, and incumbent duties, for the discharge of which his previous course of life and experience might at least have been supposed to qualify and prepare him. During this long peace his conduct in civil affairs, and in relation to the military administration of the country, was marked by a narrow and obstructive spirit, injurious to the best interests of the army. In politics he is said, by those who knew him best, to have had no other wisdom than to see when he was beaten.

In place of pursuing a course becoming his military experiences, and one apparently so natural, his Grace took to politics, which he did not understand, and in which he could not succeed. He not only did nothing, or but very little, so far as I can discover, to improve the moral and physical condition of the soldier, to whom he owed so much, but he is said to have opposed many vitally important suggestions for the improvement of our military organization and administration. Here we perceive, for the hundredth time, how much that relates to the soldier's welfare—how much for good or for evil—depends on the character of the commander.

But the Duke of Wellington did take an active part on one occasion of sanitary importance, and it went to curtail the already scanty breathing space allowed to the soldier in barracks—to take from him all indulgence in the way of more air. In 1827 his Grace wrote a letter to commanders on foreign stations, since embodied in the regulations of the army, to the effect "That officers and troops must not at any station have more accommodation than the regulations allow them ; that the use of single iron bedsteads having diminished in almost every barrack, *which the same space would have accommodated under other circumstances,* it will not answer still further to diminish the numbers accommodated, after the diminution already caused by the arrangement." Well may the *Westminster Review* characterize a regulation such as this as "simply absurd."

If our commanders will not be instructed betimes—if they cannot be made to look before them and pay a just regard to the warnings of the medical staff of the army—it is quite within the range of possibility that the soldier may some day be induced to take the question into his own hands—for this is essentially a soldier's question—and thus bring it to a summary conclusion. One month's arrest of the voluntary enlistment, and matters would arrive at a most unpleasant issue. But another difficulty may arise from the circumstance that, for the future, the extent to which a fleet and an army can be maintained in peace must depend entirely on the strength of the good opinion the public may have of the way in which they are managed and administered. After a peace we always find ourselves unprepared for war—not because money has been unwisely saved, but because it has been unwisely spent. Another war of mismanagement might prove too much for popular patience, and cause short work to be made with some of our institutions.

If we would look well to our recruiting, and to the maintenance of our old superiority by sea and land, we must bring this sanitary question to "an immediate solution."

The disasters of the Crimea have at length opened wide the eyes of the public to some of the necessities of the case. "The worst waste of all," says a popular writer, "the waste that can least be afforded—the waste the most extravagant—is the waste of the soldier's life ; and no means which can contribute to keep him in health and condition should be spared. The best economy now is to make the most of our men, and to furnish freely whatever will contribute to their health, their strength, and their efficiency. For this they will not fail to make a return in action which must conduce to the restoration of peace."

The greatest of all commanders was most careful of military health ; and being Emperor as well as General, he ordered so that all the arrangements of the military hospitals were excellent throughout the armies of France ; the historian Napier declares that Napoleon "furnished his hospitals with all things requisite, even with luxuries."

He also knew how to appreciate and reward the difficult and dangerous services of the military surgeon : he acted on the principle urged by Robert Jackson, that as " the medical staff shares the fatigues and dangers of war, in just reason it is entitled to a share of advantages."

Napoleon designed that there should be rewards for every rank —from the common soldier to the field marshal; and he bestowed the highest grade of the Legion of Honour on the field of battle, on Barons Larrey, Desgenettes, and Percy. The commanders of the French army considered that the Legion of Honour derived lustre and renown from the enrolment of such names in its ranks; while, in the British army and navy, neither mental sympathy nor material aid has ever come from our admirals or generals—always excepting the honoured names of Abercromby and Moore, the friends of Robert Jackson, and of Sir Howard Douglas and Sir De Lacy Evans, in our own day. The Austrian commander in Italy seized the right and justice of the question when he said, "The difference between officers as combatants and surgeons as non-combatants must cease. I see everywhere military officers and surgeons equally exposed to the fire, and therefore the surgeons shall enjoy advantages and distinctions in every respect equal to those of the officers." In free commercial England we have not yet arrived at this stage of enlightened fair play. Decorations are the gifts of governments, and they are not generally granted in this country to men who have honestly earned them. After more than a century of good service, the medical department is still subjected to a systematic depression.

It would seem to have resulted as a matter of course that, from the former systematic neglects of the army and navy, the friends of the seaman and the soldier—the Trotters and Jacksons of our fleets and armies—should also have met with ill-usage:—persecution was the constant lot of Jackson, while the equally long and meritorious services of Trotter, on his element, were treated with a cruel neglect. It was not thus with their contemporary Larrey, whose memory has recently received in France the highest honours.*

* MILITARY SURGEONS IN FRANCE.—"In the *Lancet* we have some details touching the inauguration of the statue erected in honour of Baron Larrey in the great entrance court of the Val de Grâce, in Paris. We subjoin the speech of M. Dupin, President of the National Assembly. The President spoke as follows, in a very impressive tone of voice:—

" ' I have the honour of addressing the military surgeons of the French army, and I tell you—if any one were bold enough still to dispute your right to proportionate rank in the army, proudly answer by pointing to this statue, and by citing the life of the man it represents—the life of the worthy Larrey.

" ' I have said it elsewhere, and I will repeat it whenever an opportunity offers—the military surgeon, fearless in epidemics, fearless in the field of battle, possesses all kinds of courage. He has military courage, because he faces death offered on all sides by fire and sword; and another courage, far superior to this, for he preserves his calm coolness and presence of mind when his life is in the greatest peril. The blow which is aimed at him, and which he sees threatening, cannot, and even were he able, would not, be returned by him. He knows his hazardous situation, and does not hesitate to fulfil his dangerous duties.

" ' Kneeling by the side of the disabled, with as firm a hand as when he is studying nature in the anatomical rooms, he dresses their wounds. But with these two kinds of courage he reaps two kinds of glory; and Larrey, who has shown his courage

U

If in France "the degree of perfection of military medical science is held to be the true measure of the importance attached to the preservation of the soldier," so, in England, the neglect by the authorities of the science of military medicine, and of those who, under such great discouragements, so ably and so disinterestedly professed and cultivated it, may be taken as the true measure of the disregard shown in this country, until very recently, for the soldier's health and comfort.   Such it has been for ages with us : our soldiers have, on too many occasions, been condemned to the worst miseries of defeat in the very midst of their triumphs and glories.   In the olden times it was "famine and the ague;" at Rangoon, in China, and the Crimea it was scorbutic dysentery—a term which ought to be expunged from the registers of our fleets and armies.

But let us hope that a better order of things is at hand; that the soldier is about to receive the cares and attentions that are due to him, and that harshness may not in future be the reward of the army surgeon.

Harshness, says the historian Napier, is the essence of the aristocratic principle of government; and he might have added, with a great statesman, that of all tyrannies the worst is that which works with the machinery of freedom.   But, whatever may be the essence of the aristocratic principle of government, the influence of aristocracy on our military institutions and discipline has not been beneficial.   It may be reckoned, in fact, as only so much more of that amateur element which has so often saddened our experiences.   It cannot be denied, also, that we owe some of our blue blood to the aristocracy borne on our musters; a goodly portion, too, of our white feathers being furnished by that class. For the proof we need not so much as examine our cavalry, or go so far back as the battle of Minden.   The opposite notion is indeed founded on popular error.

The *Examiner*, remarking upon Lord Raglan's most unjust censure of two medical officers, says :—" We should be glad to see some praise as well as blame, and that the meritorious services of medical officers do not escape notice more than their faults.   Was

equally in both, now deserves to be honoured with double glory. He has proved, when twice wounded, that the dangers which the military surgeon runs are not imaginary. He was wounded once in Egypt, in times of glorious memory, and another time at Waterloo, on that mournful day for France.

" ' You heard, from those who addressed you before me, what the life of Larrey has been, and what services he has rendered to science! It is not for me to enter into the details of this noble career. I am, besides, not prepared for it ; I speak, carried away by momentary impulses, and by the admirable speeches which have just been uttered. I judge this learned man—this defender of mankind—by considering as a whole his useful life, marked by the most enlightened and noble services, and I bow before this statue which so worthily represents him. Yes, I greet Larrey ! the virtuous, devoted man whose self-denial and devotion triumphed even over the elements, and who has been among us as an incarnation of genius and humane feelings. He deserves the thanks of science, the army, France, and the whole civilized world !'

" What would they have said in France to the memory of ' that hero of the morrow of. Alma'—the Surgeon Thomson ? "

a word of honour given to the memory of Dr. Thomson for a noble example, who volunteered the charge of 700 wounded Russians on the field of the Alma, assisted only by a single servant as devoted to duty as himself? This hero in the cause of humanity died of cholera, immediately referrible to his exertions and exposure among putrefying bodies. Had he lived, would he have obtained the praise which is bestowed on a staff officer for galloping with a message on the field of battle, or for helping the Commander-in-Chief in doing nothing in a soldier's battle and victory? The smallest services of the men with names and positions are overweeningly prized—the noblest services of the unconnected and humble are unnoticed and unhonoured." Thus, while the ignorance, prejudices, and inert obstinacy of the great bulk of our admirals and generals long effectually resisted the just claims of the naval and military surgeon, the first of all commanders—the greatest master of the art of war—thought and acted on directly opposite principles. He did not reward his naval and military commanders for fatal services.

Napoleon, on the other hand, in a manner for ever memorable, and while in the agonies of a disease which he knew to be incurable, remembered with kindness the surgeons of the Grand Army. He bequeathed "To Baron Larrey, Surgeon-in-Chief, one hundred thousand francs. He is the most virtuous man I have known." Again, he bequeathed "To Surgeon Emery, one hundred thousand francs." Nor should the conduct of this illustrious patient to Dr. Archibald Arnott, of His Majesty's 20th Regiment, be forgotten. "The Emperor, on his death-bed, desired that a valuable gold snuffbox might be brought to him; and having, with his dying hand, and last effort of departing strength, engraved upon its lid with a penknife the letter ' N,' he presented it to his kind and valued friend as a parting memorial of his deep esteem and heartfelt gratitude." Not satisfied with this mark of personal kindness and regard, the dying Emperor bequeathed to Dr. Arnott a sum of money also. It is only with those of the highest natures that the gentler and warmer feelings survive the practical acquaintance with the world. From the coarser and more rude minds such acquaintance carries away with it all the sympathies of our nature, leaving men cold, callous, and selfish. But such was not the case with the great Napoleon; his heart warmed to the last towards the old soldier, the honest public servant, the man of merit and of science.

The treatment of the army surgeon by this incomparable commander and statesman is not only important and interesting in itself, but also on account of the memorable reasons which he urged in support of his conduct—reasons which ought to be known to, and appreciated by, the medical profession.

Napoleon deemed the honours conferred on such men to be called for alike by justice and necessity, in any plan which should pretend to give "consistence to the system of recompences" granted by the State to its servants. He considered their exclusion from honorary distinctions as founded on the "injustice of feudalism." In the awarding of honorary distinctions he acted promptly, and upon the standard of true merit :—"Returned to Paris, Napoleon gave the gold cross he had worn through the Russian campaign to his physician Corvisart." With him the cross of the Legion of Honour was but a symbol which expressed the gratitude of the country—the outward sign by which the State recognised equality of merit.

In the Council of State held to frame the laws and regulations of the Legion of Honour, it was proposed by Count Mathieu Dumas, that the several divisions of the Order should be conferred only on military men.

"Such ideas," said Napoleon, "might be well adapted to the feudal ages, when the chevaliers combated each other man to man, and the bulk of the nation was in a state of slavery; but when the military system changed, masses of infantry and phalanxes, constructed after the Macedonian model, were introduced, and after that, it was not individual prowess, but science and skill, which determined the fate of nations. . . What is it now which constitutes a great general? It is not the mere strength of a man of six feet high, but the *coup-d'œil*, the habit of foresight, the power of thought and calculation; in a word, pacific qualities, not such as we find in a lawyer, but such as are founded on a knowledge of human nature, and are suited to the government of armies. The general who can now achieve great things, is he who is possessed of shining civil qualities; it is the perception of the strength of his talents which makes the soldiers obey him. . . We must not reason from ages of barbarity to these times. France consists of 30,000,000 of men, united by intelligence, property, and commerce. Three or four hundred thousand soldiers are nothing in such a mass; not only does the general preserve his ascendancy over his soldiers by civil qualities, but when his command ceases, he becomes merely a private individual. The soldiers themselves are but the children of citizens. The tendency of military men is to carry everything by force; the enlightened civilian, on the other hand, elevates his views to a perception of the general good. The first would rule only by despotic authority, the last subject everything to the test of discussion, truth, and reason. I have no hesitation, therefore, in saying, that if a preference were to be awarded to one or the other, it belongs to the civilian. If you divide society into soldiers and citizens, you establish two orders in what should be one nation. If you confine honours to military men, you do what is still worse, for you sink the people into nothing." Elsewhere, this wonderful commander said, "Justice is one only in France—the citizen precedes the soldier."

"Moved by these profound observations, the Council agreed

that the proposed honours should be extended indiscriminately to civil and military distinctions;"*—while in our country such men as Chatham and Whitelock, Sackville, fourth-class politicians, such as Mr. V. Smith, and a host of generals not worth mentioning, have been deemed more deserving of honours than public benefactors like Pringle, Blane, Trotter, Robert Jackson, M'Grigor, Henry Marshall, James Johnson, Wm. Fergusson, Ballingall, Hennen, Guthrie, and a host of distinguished medical officers who have bravely encountered every kind of danger in all climates and situations, and who have conferred incalculable benefits on the fleets and armies of England, as well as on mankind at large. The great surgeons of our fleets and armies, in the far greater proportion, have received no honours but those which no man could give or take away.

After a digression which, to the military surgeon, may not, I trust, appear irrelevant, but rather as excused by the occasion, I return to the concluding subject of this article :—

Rigaud de Lisle, with Drs. Aiton and Parkin, have accepted the following as some of the ascertained laws of malaria :—

1. The malarious poison, although not confined to such situations, is extricated in greatest abundance in low, marshy, and alluvial soils.

2. Malaria is extricated from all wet lands, the muddy surface of marshes, and the slimy banks of lakes and rivers during what has been termed the drying process.

3. Malaria is never extricated from the surface of water, under any condition whatever, so long as the particles of the latter fluid hold together.

4. Malaria becomes innocuous at a certain distance from the source whence it is given out.

5. The specific gravity of malaria is greater than that of atmospheric air; but winds of a higher temperature enable the heavy malarious gas to ascend to higher elevations than under ordinary circumstances.

6. The interposition of a forest, a mountain, a wall, or even a mere cloth, is sometimes sufficient to preserve an individual, or individuals, from the pernicious effects of the miasmata given out on the opposite side.

In reference to these laws, it may be concluded that above a certain height all situations are free from endemic fever, not only in temperate but in tropical climates, although "the line of perpetual health" will be higher in the latter than in the former.

To conclude the subject of this article :—Were it desirable even, which it is not, to dispense with a Native Indian army, it is financially impossible, with the revenues of England and of India united, to maintain in Hindustan an European force independently adequate to the support of the British rule there.

* Alison's " History of Europe."

"Our force," says Lord Metcalfe, "does not operate so much by its actual strength as by the impression which it produces, and that impression is the opinion by which we hold India." If, again, the declaration of Colonel Sutherland be correct, that the groundwork of our power in India consists in our substantial British soldiers, then are they deserving our most serious care, in everything which relates to their moral and material welfare.

Their highest qualities may at any moment be subjected to the severest trials; and it behoves the ruling power to see that these men are at all times and places maintained in the most complete readiness for action.

ON THE TERM OF EFFICIENT SERVICE IN INDIA.

DURING a long and varied course of service in India, I had extended opportunities of observing the effects of climate, as well on the moral as on the physical nature of Europeans—"the slow blight of the constitutional power"—but especially amongst the military classes; and the result, so far as I can judge from an unusually wide range of observation at home as well as in India, is, that the term of thirty years of actual residence in the East is the very utmost during which persons under ordinary health, and of an average constitution, may be expected to retain their British vigour of thought and action. Thirty years constitute, in fact, a good average working portion of life in any climate, although, in Europe, a man may work long and well beyond that term.

Lord Metcalfe gives the following reasons for employing young men :—" In contending that the employment of young men is no necessary part of the Delhi system, I wish to guard against the impression that I am opposed to the employment of young men. Under control, they may be employed with advantage in any situation. There is a zeal, an energy, an activity of virtue in young men which often more than compensates for mere age and even experience, too often accompanied by apathy, lethargy, and inertness, the consequences of disease caused by a climate, the fiery ordeal of which few constitutions can stand unimpaired for a number of years. In rejecting the services of men when young, in situations in which they can be efficiently controlled, we may lose the best aid that they can ever bring to the public interests. But while the young of all the services, especially of the military branches, ought thus to be encouraged and promoted, let us not be deprived of the advantages to be derived from the maturer experiences of our civil officers. Burke complained eighty years ago that India never saw the gray head of an Englishman."

Of the precocity described by Doctors Moseley and Ainslie, I have never seen any evidence : they would seem to have found in every other British youth within the tropics a second Grotius :— *Reliqui viri tandem fuere ;* GROTIUS *vir natus est.* Cabanis speaks of but one form of precocity in hot countries—that of old age (*vie-illesse precoce*)—and I fear this last is, with the majority, nearer the truth ; for, if the age of forty-eight be the stage of highest intel· lectual power in Europe, that period would appear to be anticipated in tropical climates ; and, after the maximum has been attained there, the decline of the mental and corporeal powers is both silent and rapid. Of hot climates and their effects we may say in an especial degree what Napoleon said of the political career :—" We may stop when we are rising, but never when we are going downwards."

Certainly, of my profession, and I think I may say of the Indian public services generally, all who have attained to eminence in the East, have done so long *before* the term of thirty years' service ; and few indeed have retained much of it long *after* that term.

We are glad to see in general society occasional exceptions to this melancholy rule ; but how rarely ?   One may, perchance, see the veteran of forty years' service, in all the mental freshness of youth, and beside him the officer of thirty years' service, superannuated and enfeebled in all respects ; but the first is the exception ; the last is the rule that must ever govern the mass, or, more properly speaking, the average of Europeans.

In India we are too much attached to the absolute rule of seniority in military promotion, a rule which does not work well for command.   It may serve the interested purposes of individuals, but it ill serves the interests of the State.   It is but a perverse adhesion to the old maxim of " age before honesty or honour."

The disposition to rise by the rule of the muster-roll, rather than by the exercise of knowledge, diligence, and discernment, is injurions in many ways :—it brings men who never were fit to command into the list of generals ; while it causes others, who were once efficient, to linger in the army, and to look to the rewards which seniority may bring them—after their energies have faded. Any system, therefore, which should induce young officers to look to the acquisition of rank rather than rupees, would prove an advantage to themselves and to the service.   The Marquis Wellesley said, forty years ago :—" The army in India rested too much on the footing of profit, without reference to honours at home ;" and this owing to circumstances over which the army had no control : its officers " were not held forward to public view as much as other officers in other parts of the world"—persons whose " services were not more meritorious or important than their own."   But if the authorities of the India House and Board of Control, with their uninformed and impeding subordinates, were unjustly slow to advance and reward merit in the Indian services, there never has been, on the other hand, any power in the East which could step in between misconduct and neglect of duty and the visitation of justice—between the wrong-doer, the criminally negligent, and his punishment. In England, on the contrary, we see men placed on the staff of the army, promoted twice, and decorated for so-called services in the Crimea and elsewhere, who in India would have been cashiered for dis-service and criminal neglect of duty. In India punishment comes quickly and certainly, while reward comes slowly and with uncertainty, or not at all. The manner in which rewards are often bestowed at home, again, deprives them of all semblance of merit; while in France, although the numbers decorated are large, the decoration being honestly deserved, the honour is highly desired and much prized.

Rank has been withheld from the officers of the Indian army until too late in life to be of use to the recipient, or to the State. Nor can education and experience united counterbalance the deteriorating influences of age. The officers of the Indian army are, as a body, remarkably well educated. Lord de Ros, in his work for the guidance of young officers, states that the superior education of the officers of the Indian army has become an object of remark during the late campaigns in India, where the talent and services of many of the younger ranks have frequently attracted the notice and praise of the most distinguished authorities.

Here, again, we perceive that it is in "the younger ranks" that the benefits of education produce the most efficient results; while Brigadier Hodgson, of the Bengal army, assures us that the "average age of the major-generals of the Indian army is somewhat above sixty-five years, and the average length of service alone of the lieutenant-general is about sixty years. This is altogether a state of affairs most unjust to the Indian army, and politically criminal as regards the great national interests at stake, and which are indeed perilled by a great standing army being kept in so palpably inefficient a state with respect to its senior grades, the members of which are already unfit from physical decrepitude to exercise energetic command in the field."

It is evident, from all that is here set forth, that a superannuation list has become a necessity to the Indian army.

The promotion by absolute rule of seniority—so injurious in so many ways—often causes our older Indian officers to be superseded in command; and thus their experience even is made to give way, and is set at nought, under an arrangement grounded on a hard necessity.

Nor is this important subject to be regarded as foreign to medical investigation; for the moral qualities, age, and physical capabilities of the commander do not involve military and political considerations and results only, but also the moral and physical welfare of the army under his orders—its health, comfort, and efficiency;—everything, in short, depends on the character of the commander.

Governments may confer material power on a general, but if he do not wield moral power, he is as nothing. When the great Lord Chatham read over the list of British generals, with a view to their employment in the first American war, he observed:—" I know not what effect the reading of those names may have upon the enemy, but for my own part, I confess it makes me tremble." Seniority had at that time done its worst for our commanders.

" The arguments in favour of purchase," says the *Times*, " all assume as their basis the pre-existence of a system of seniority, and derive their force from the necessity of remedying the intolerable abuses to which the unmitigated system of seniority, as we have it in the artillery and engineer corps, gives rise. Seniority has in it a certain degree of fairness, since it is the fate of all men, noble or plebeian, rich or poor, to grow old, but it buys this single advantage at the expense of every other defect to which a criterion of promotion can be liable.

" For the first twenty years of military service, increased age may be some indication of increased efficiency, but after that period, this congruity gradually ceases, till every year that is added to the age of the officer detracts from his utility, and seniority declares him fit for the highest command just when the inexorable hand of time has stripped him of his last qualification for any. Moreover, seniority, by annexing the highest rewards to the longest service, strengthens the inducement to continue in the army after health, strength, and faculties have failed, thus keeping down rising merit, and applying the strongest incentives to old men to undertake duties which they cannot fulfil.

" It is a vivid perception of these enormous evils which has induced mankind to betake themselves to the system of purchase, as involving, with all its absurdity and injustice, a less practical mischief than seniority ; and certainly, if the alternative lies wholly between the two, we shall not be disposed to doubt the wisdom of the selection. . . . . We believe that the assumption that there is no alternative between purchase and seniority is fallacious ; and that in war with much ease, and in peace without insurmountable difficulties, a system of promotion by merit might be devised which would supersede both the one and the other."

Mill, the historian, says :—" It cannot be too often repeated, that in a country like India everything depends upon the personal qualities and capacities of the agents of government. This truth is the cardinal principle of Indian administration.

" The safety of the country," he continues, " is that those by whom it is administered are sent out in youth, as candidates only, to begin at the bottom of the ladder, and to ascend higher or not, as, after a proper interval, they are proved qualified." Should India be handed over to place-hunters from St. James's-street—to men knowing and caring nothing about the country, and anxious only to seek their own gains, and return home speedily, the end of our rule there cannot be far off.

In the French army I believe the system of promotion consists in giving one-third to seniority, one-third at the recommendation of the officer in command, and the remaining third under direction of the Minister-of-War. This system gives satisfaction to all classes; and it gives to the armies of France Commanders-in-Chief of the age of five-and-forty.

The retiring pensions of public servants in India have been ordered as follows :—

For the Civil Service, pension on 22 years actual service.
```
 ,,   Military    ,,   ,,    22    ,,    ,,
 ,,   Medical     ,,   ,,    17    ,,    ,,
 ,,   Clerical    ,,   ,,    15    ,,    ,,
```

In reference to the respective ages on entering the several public services, this scale must be admitted to be fairly fixed : but all the annuity funds, whether civil or military, are founded on the general expectation of a longer course of service than that which earns the government pension; and such expectation is verified in the result—but few indeed being in a position to retire on completion of the government term. It therefore would seem as if some term—intermediate between twenty-five and thirty years' service, had been in contemplation both of the government and of the founders of the annuity funds, in respect of the civil and military servants at least; and such an idea is justified by the actual influence of the climate of India on the European constitution.

This article formed part of a Report on the Medical Topography of Calcutta, presented by me to the government of Bengal, and published by its order at the public cost in Calcutta, in 1839. I am now gratified in the support afforded to the opinions I have so long entertained, by so eminent a public functionary as Mr. Welby Jackson, of the Bengal Civil Service, who, in a Memoir submitted to the Government of India, states as follows :—

" In appointing persons to offices of high trust and responsibility, though no positive and distinct reservation be made as to the time they are to hold the appointments, it is tacitly understood that they are not to occupy them longer than they are able to discharge the duty efficiently.

" This is evidently a part of the contract between the State and the nominee ; and where public opinion exists, and can make itself heard through the press, or the delegates to a national assembly, the condition is sufficiently enforced. No one, under such circumstances, can long continue to hold an office for which he has become unfit by reason of old age, or other fortuitous circumstance incapacitating him, or impairing in a material degree his ability to perform the duty. In India there is no public voice. The people, as a body, know little or nothing of the administration of

the government; they take no part in it, either directly or by de-
putation. It is therefore incumbent on the government, and more
especially on the Honourable Court of Directors (who in some
measure supply the place of the public by acting as a check on the
Executive), to frame and adopt such rules as may prevent incapable
and inefficient persons from continuing to occupy offices of public
trust.

"In regard to the chief offices in India, the principle is fully acknowledged and acted upon. The appointments to the offices of
Governor-General, of Governor, of Member of Council, as well as
of Brigadier, and General of Division in the army, are made for a
limited period of five years. There is no rule against a second appointment, though it is of rare occurrence. Apparently, it is considered probable that at the age when these dignities are conferred,
the efficiency of the nominee will not last much longer; and,
further, it is perhaps thought advisable to have periodical opportunities of correcting any error of judgment which may have taken
place in the selection.

"The principle is applicable to all offices, of every description,
high or low, ministerial, judicial, fiscal, or representative; but
more particularly to offices held by an exclusive service, the members of which rise by seniority, and become eligible to promotion
as they grow older. It is true that the government which appoints
has always the authority to dismiss; but, in practice, this has been
found insufficient, and hence the custom of appointing for a definite
period to the high offices above mentioned. There is one standing
reason why the period should be defined; it is quite certain that,
in every instance, official capacity is impaired after a certain time
of life; the period may vary with individuals, but an average may
be fixed, beyond which the services of very few would be worth
retaining."

"The Civil Service Annuity Fund is framed on the principle,
and with the expectation that civil servants will, one with another,
remain twenty-five years in the country; this includes three years
passed on furlough. It is expected that by that time their means
will permit their retirement, and that their physical and mental
powers will require it. I believe that the period is very properly
fixed; but there can, at all events, be little doubt that, after
thirty years' service in India, the proportion of civil servants who
are worth keeping is very small indeed. I will assume, therefore,
thirty years as the average efficient portion of a man's life in
India."

The truth and justice of what is here so ably set forth cannot be
gainsaid; yet, happily, the evils of the seniority system do not
press with such severity on the civil service as might, *a priori*, be
expected—safety being found in selection for all the higher offices
throughout the country.

But the unmitigated application of the absolute rule of seniority promotion, staff and regimental, to a scientific corps, like the medical department of the army of Bengal, was until lately, as might be anticipated, attended with the worst and most disastrous results of all—the necessary detention of the whole administrative staff till altogether worn out in mind and body; till long after the term of efficient service in India has passed away.

The three senior members of the medical service of Bengal formed what was called the medical board of that presidency, and numbered between them about 120 years of service, or an average of forty-two years each; while the next ten officers on the list, constituting the administrative staff of the service, were not far behind in this groove of seniority.

To speak of such a system as this is to waste time; for a board so constituted must be superannuated by science as much as by years—the ebb of opinion having everywhere left this pernicious rule of seniority high and dry on the drift of old custom. An institution which was not respected had lost its salt. A slavish adherence to the principle of seniority is, in truth, only a pretence for avoiding a modern reality.

Henry Marshall observes that—" Under certain circumstances, competition is as necessary to promote intellectual exertion as it is to effect mechanical production. Where persons are remunerated by time, instead of according to the beneficial results of application, or where there is a uniformity of reward without reference to that which is produced, competition may take a wrong course, and he who labours least thinks he has gained the prize. Establishments in which the enrolment and advancement in rank are chiefly awarded in accordance with length of service, or where the advantages are professedly administered on that principle, involve a spirit of COMMUNISM which is very unfavourable to zealous intellectual industry beyond those routine duties which cannot be evaded; and without the energetic exertions of individuals, we are not warranted in expecting much progress towards the cultivation of science and the diffusion of information; a result which rarely occurs except from competition, honestly, impartially, and widely administered."

Robert Jackson, speaking on this subject, says, that " If reward or emolument be the portion of a man borne so many years on the muster-roll, rather than of a character distinguished for activity, diligence, and discernment, the purpose of bounty is mistaken."

The sedative effect of a fixed situation, with a fixed salary, was nowhere so thoroughly exemplified as in the Bengal medical service; it surpassed the hop-pillow in its results.

The subject of this article, I repeat, is proper for the consideration of the medical officer, and it has not been sufficiently placed before authority; but it demands the most serious attention, so long as we may be expected to hold India by what, in Europe, is termed the power of opinion. There is no country in the world where so much depends on the PERSONS of the functionaries, and on the spirit which animates them, as in India, and consequently, where the RIGHT SELECTION OF PERSONS is of so much importance. Asiatics always look to the persons, and never to the departments. The Sepoy, for instance, whose own "idea of loyalty," according to Lord Metcalfe, " his loyalty to his ' salt,' a sense of what is due to the hand that feeds him," knows right well who and what his colonel is—who the general of division, and who the commander-in-chief; but he has only a very vague notion of what our departments are—his own views being always personal.

Thirlwall observes, that "the character of every people is more or less closely connected with that of its land ;" and we should take but a limited view of the effects of climate, and especially of localities abounding in marsh poison, if we considered only the more familiar effects of those agents on the European constitution, such as the various forms of fever, anæmia, &c. The states of the air affect the mental energies and moral feelings of many individuals, to a degree inconceivable to those who have not thus been subject to their influences, or who have not watched their varied effects. Even in Europe, the long application of such causes, as in Tuscany and Switzerland, affects the mind to very idiocy ; and I have seen a complete, but temporary prostration of the mental powers result from a residence in our taräis and jungly districts in India, as in Gondwana and Aracan, but especially after the fevers of such districts.

Finally, and independently of the influences of climate, I believe with Lord Macaulay, that official aptitude is everywhere acquired at the expense of the general powers, and that in all countries a fixed limit in years should be ordered, beyond which public service should not extend.

ON THE

MORTALITY AND PHYSICAL MANAGEMENT OF EUROPEAN CHILDREN IN BENGAL.

FOR children of strumous habit, or for the offspring of parents that are what is termed weak-chested, the climate of Bengal, and of India generally, is favourable. Under ordinary precautions, they may be freely exposed to the open air at all seasons, during the early morning and evening, without risk of being chilled; an inestimable advantage, and one for the absence of which hardly any other circumstance will compensate.

The diseases of childhood run their course also very mildly in Bengal ; and, upon the whole, it cannot be said that under proper management of diet, and with precautions against extremes of temperature, the climate of Bengal is unfavourable to European infant life, up to the age of five or six years, when they begin to exhibit the necessity for change of climate by emaciating, and by out-growing their strength.

The climate of Italy has in like manner been found beneficial in the instances of weakly children, who in England suffered from swellings of the lymphatic glands, gastric irritation and catarrhs; and there can be no doubt that at the tender age here spoken of, and also at the more advanced age of puberty, the removal for a few winters to the south of Europe would tend powerfully to the prevention of pulmonary diseases in weakly children, and those in whom a hereditary disposition to them is suspected.

Of accurate or statistical record, bearing on this interesting question, we have as yet little in India; but I believe that the results of a close observation would afford corresponding facts to those obtained in England and France, as to the greater mortality among infants under the extremes of temperature—the very cold and the hotter months. The winter and spring seasons have been observed at the Military Asylum, Chelsea, to be very productive of tuberculous disease in the children born in the East and West Indies especially.

Dr. Duncan Stewart, of Calcutta, states, that amongst the European inhabitants of that city, the ratio of mortality of adults is greater than that of infants in the proportion of five to one; while, with the poor degenerate Portuguese, the mortality of children exceeds that of adults in the proportion of four to one. The late Inspector-General Burke states Fort William, Calcutta, to be " one of the worst, if not the very worst, of the military stations in India for children," the average annual mortality per cent. being 16·29. Here we perceive the difference in the fate of the British soldier's child in the garrison of Fort William, and that of the better classes of his countrymen, residing within half-a-mile of him.

In the excellent reports on the health of the Bombay European Fusiliers, by Dr. Arnott, we find the mortality of the women was nearly six per cent., while that of the children was nearly seven per cent. The order, discipline, and general sanitary condition of this corps have during many years been highly creditable to all its officers, military and medical; but the barrack accommodation for the married men is stated to be very defective. Mr. Clark states that in Sierra Leone the difficulty of rearing European children is great, especially about the stage of teething. At this time they are frequently harassed with intermittent fevers, followed by enlargement of the spleen and cachexia. Unless they be speedily removed from the climate, they sink into an early grave.

From tables recently obtained by the government of India, the following annual rates of mortality for the children of European soldiers are deduced by Dr. Chevers, in his admirable " Review of the Means of Preserving the Health of European Soldiers in India :"—

Bengal	. . .	1850-51 to 1853-54	. . . .	84·2 per 1000.
Madras.	. .	1850-51 to 1853-54	. . . .	39·8 ,,
Bombay	. .	1852-53 to 1854-55	. . . .	70·7 ,,

From this record it appears that as for the British soldiers and their wives, so for their children also, the Presidency of Bengal is by far the most unhealthy of the three. The ages and sexes of the children are not here given ; nor are the European children distinguished, in the Bengal and Madras reports, from the Indo-British, amongst whom, in Bombay, the mortality is somewhat lower than that of the Europeans.

The observations of Dr. Edwards on the differences of constitution at different periods of life are of the highest importance as relating to children ; and if more generally understood, and more carefully put in practice, they would considerably reduce one of the greatest sources of mortality. The power of generating heat is so feeble in the infant system, probably from a smaller consumption of oxygen in proportion to the bulk, that it is impossible to be too guarded in the important article of clothing during the cold season in Bengal, where scarcely a year passed in which I had not occasion to witness the most serious, and sometimes fatal results from the exposure of infants, imperfectly clothed, to the piercing N.E. wind. It may be concluded that the younger the infant, the more necessary does caution become on this head.

But where the opposite system is adopted, or that of *hardening* by means of half-clothing, or the equally unreasonable system of *strengthening* by means of a double diet, the results are even more speedily destructive than in Europe, and they are brought about by the supervention of gastric fever, with cerebral determination— severe diarrhœa, or the more slow process of mesenteric fever. In respect of the management of infant health, and referring to the theories and empiricisms brought to bear on it, I have every-where observed, that even the fatal results of mismanagement but rarely cure the mother of her theory or her quackery—so much stronger are ignorance and prejudice than death.

It may be said that, under ordinary care in diet and clothing, the operation of the teething process proceeds kindly in the climate of India ; and speaking from my personal experience, I should say that severe teething irritation is seldom a primary affection, but that, on the contrary, it generally follows upon previously existing gastric, intestinal, or febrile disorder ; and it is not too much to say that, in eighteen cases out of twenty, these last are but the results of mismanagement in diet and clothing— errors of ignorance and weakness more common to the most civilized than to the most barbarous communities. To read some books, and to hear some people talk, one might be led to suppose

that the teething process of infancy is a *morbid* one from beginning to end.

I believe that the seasons in which the greatest mortality occurs
amongst European children in Calcutta are—the cold season of
December and January—April and May of the hot season.   In
the former, congestive and catarrhal fevers prevail, and in the
latter, remittent fever, occasionally of an ardent character, and
diarrhœa.   Altogether the deaths are not numerous as compared
to the births ; and this circumstance is mainly due to the generally
rational plan of rearing the children of the better classes, where
the wet-nursing, the aliment, clothing, cleanliness, air, and exercise
are carefully attended to.

I did not see one case of smallpox amongst the children of the
better classes of Europeans during my residence in India ;—a fact
which speaks powerfully in favour of the protecting influence of
vaccination ; for not a year passed that smallpox did not prevail
in the native portion of the city.

It is stated by Lind that " European women in general enjoy a
much better state of health than the men ;" but that " child-bearing is peculiarly fatal to them in Calcutta ; on which account it
would be advisable for them to retire to a more healthy situation
at the approach of their delivery.   Dr. Clark observes that, on the
coast of Coromandel, parturition " is not attended with such great
danger as in Bengal ; neither is the puerperal fever of such a
putrid nature."

From whatever cause it arise, the very contrary of the above holds
at present, parturition being unattended with even so much risk as
in Europe.   Puerperal fever I never saw in Calcutta ; and during
sixteen years in which I was familiar with the state of health among
the better class of Europeans there, I heard of but one death connected with child-bearing, independently of previous disease ; and
I remember but very few instances of children being born dead.
Some three or four instances of remittent fever or of dysentery,
inducing premature delivery and death, I have heard of during the
time specified ; and that was all.   I would therefore ascribe the
fatality spoken of by Drs. Lind and Clark to the circumstance
that, in the olden times, the management of parturition was left to
ignorant native nurses ; indeed, in *Hickey's Journal*, published in
Calcutta in 1780, the public is frequently warned against permitting what the editor terms, the *improper* interference of European
physicians !

It has been asserted by careful observers at home that for every
year below twenty-one at which marriage is contracted, the
female constitution sustains a proportionate damage.   The early
marriages so common amongst English females in India must
prove injurious both to mothers and to their offspring.

On the subject of rearing children in India I would observe that
all experience is against it—that it is altogether a cruel and an

impracticable endeavour—and that I have seen several deaths result from the unnecessary attempt to wage war with the climate. Dr. Kenneth Mackinnon observes justly of the children of European soldiers in Bengal, that we have proof of the effect of climate in their early drooping and decay. " Even when there is no tangible disease, nutrition and oxygenation do not appear to go on favourably ; the skin is pale, the muscles wanting in substance and in tone ; the joyous spirits of children are wanting—the body is inert, the mind listless."*

The late Mr. Twining states that, after much and careful inquiry, he was not able anywhere to find a sample of the third generation from unmixed European stock. I believe that such is scarcely to be found in any part of our Eastern possessions, and least of all in Bengal Proper :—so much for the question of European colonization in India, respecting which much has been said and written— regardless of the fact that Nature has set her ban—a blighting interdict—upon it. The European has not been made for the climate, and the climate is not made for him. The Principal of the Lawrence Asylum says that the children of soldiers in the plains die so early that only about one in five is found surviving the fifth year of Indian sojourn, while in the mountains they flourish like children in healthy country districts in England.

Volney, the eloquent historian of Egypt, states " that neither the Mamelooks, who were a *Caucasian* race, nor the Turks, who are Mongolians, unless they married native women, which the Mamelooks never did, could continue their race in Egypt ;—all their offspring perishing in the first or second generation."

Without an accurate census and correct tables of mortality, returns such as the following can be of little use ; but I could obtain no better information on the spot :—

Burials in Calcutta of Protestant Children.

Years.	Adults.	Children under 5 years.	Total.
1820	239	43	282
1821	196	50	246
1822	275	47	322
1823	215	55	270
1824	209	63	272
1825	240	54	294
1826	234	36	270
1827	190	45	235
1828	157	77	234
1829	128	32	160
1830	180	28	208

* The " Treatise on the Public Health, Climate, and Hygiene of Bengal," by this able and experienced officer, is one well worthy of perusal by all military medical officers who may have to serve in the East.

PART III.

ACUTE TROPICAL DISEASES AND THEIR CURE.

THE REMITTENT FEVER OF BENGAL.

THIS fever has been long known to, and carefully described by, British writers on the diseases of the East. Some of the older observers termed it Putrid Intestinal Remitting, and Putrid Remitting Marsh Fever; perhaps without being sufficiently aware that in those days, owing to the salt diet, crowding, and other sanitary neglects in their then long voyages, a general scorbutic taint existed, amongst the newly-arrived Europeans especially. Since then, and under the various designations of Jungle, Hill, Tarái, Bilious Remittent, Marsh Remittent, or Malarious Fever, it has been described by more modern writers. In reference to all these designations it must be remembered that the surface and soil of Hindustan present more contrasts, and give rise to more varieties of climate, than any other country of equal extent in the world.

Robert Jackson terms it Gastric, or Bilious Remittent, and describes it as a fever belonging to all countries; but as endemic in the West Indies at all seasons of the year. Though common to all countries, and observed occasionally at all seasons of the year, he justly adds that it prevails more generally in warm countries, on extensive alluvial plains, and in the autumnal season.

Remittent fevers will be found almost everywhere throughout the East Indies, varying in their intensities and in their complications, as they may occur in the Deltas, along the marshy banks, or in the embouchures of rivers; in the plains extending from the bases of mountain ranges, termed "Taràis;" in partially inundated or irrigated lands, or in such as are traversed by percolating streams, or by canals; in wooded districts, termed jungles; or in certain hill districts. The seaboard, especially where there is jungle or salt marsh, and the adjacent islands, when of a jungly or marshy nature, are peculiarly pestilential; and so are often found the drying-up marshes, and the drying-up beds of rivers. Of the various obstacles which bar the colonization of the white man in tropical climates, and of the many causes which reduce the strength of our armies there, remittent fever is the principal.

The British army has often been fever-stricken, and occasionally destroyed, in low, dry-looking, sandy plains, such as those of Rosendaal ard of Walcheren; on the elevated, rocky, and dry-looking countries, and in the half-dried water-courses of Portugal; on the plains of Spain, along the course of the Guadiana; but everywhere, in the latter-named localities, there was "water to within a few inches of the surface;" the ravines were always "half-dried," and the Guadiana itself consisted of but "lines of detached pools."

Whether on the coast of Kent, about Dungeness, "during the hot summer and autumn of 1807," or in the West India Islands, the same topographical conditions were found to exist by William Fergusson;—"there was generally the presence of actual marsh, or damp; and always the antecedents of heavy rain, or of "flooding in the rainy season." "The fevers of Cadiz, Carthagena, Gibraltar, and Zeeland," says James Johnson, "may compete, in respect to virulence and fatality, with those of Batavia, Bengal, St. Domingo, and Philadelphia."

Varying somewhat in type and in complication, each depending on locality, on constitution, and on habit of life, the essential characters of the remittent fever are still everywhere very much the same; and whether as cause or effect, this disease has much to do with almost all the derangements of health of the European in the East. It is also by far the most prevalent of Indian endemic diseases; and on the right understanding of its movements, peculiar nature, complications, and just treatment, will always greatly depend the usefulness of the Indian medical officer.

According to a table furnished to me by Sir Alexander Tulloch, out of an aggregate European force of 25,431 men, of her Majesty's army, serving in periods of eight and ten years respectively, between 1823 and 1836, in the stations of Calcutta, Chinsurah, and Berhampore, all in Bengal Proper, 13,596 cases of fever, remittent, intermittent, and continued, occurred;—whereas, out of the same aggregate force, 8499 cases of dysentery and diarrhœa occurred— thus establishing the far greater prevalence of the more strictly malarious fevers over diseases of the bowels.

My friend, the late Dr. Kenneth Mackinnon, of Bengal, an excellent officer, says that fever is wonderfully prevalent in the plains of the Ganges; and adds that out of an average European force of 8700 men, there occurred in Bengal Proper, during seven years, 4772 cases of fever; and that even in the healthier Upper Provinces, out of an average force of 23,731 men, there occurred in the same seven years, 14,159 fever cases.

Mr. Waring, of Madras, states that fever in all its forms constitutes fully one-half of the admissions into Indian military hospitals; and in Bombay, among persons of all classes, castes, and climes, forms about forty per cent. of the total deaths.

In the history of the remittent fever of Bengal, during the last hundred years, the first observation that presents itself is—the great difference as to its intensity in the present as compared to former times; and secondly, the causes of this difference.

The earliest account we possess of the state of public health, and of the season of greatest mortality in Calcutta is that of Capt. Hamilton (1688—1723), wherein he mentions 460 burials out of 1200 British inhabitants, from August to the ensuing January.

Of Major Kilpatrick's detachment of 240 men, mostly Europeans, stationed at Fultah, Ives tells us, that "not thirty of the whole were left alive between August and December, 1756, by one of these epidemics." He adds that, "the number of men buried in Bengal amounted to more than half of all who died in the several hospitals in India, during the whole term of Admiral Watson's command, a period of three years and one month." Dr. Bogue, who also served in Watson's fleet, says that, "out of three ships of the line and a twenty-gun ship, and those not fully manned, we lost in six months upwards of two hundred men, most of whom died of these fevers."

Dr. James Lind was surgeon of the *Drake* Indiaman, and writes of the fever "which raged in Bengal, in the year 1762," and which he terms putrid and remitting marsh fever. This fever "raged more or less in different places, according as the soil was more or less swampy;" and "became so violent," during the rainy season especially, "as to end in death during the third fit, which is generally the case." Others, he says, "were exposed to the danger of dying at every fit;" and "when the disorder continned for any time, without a change, it generally ended in death; while the weather grew better it sometimes, in the space of a few days, from a common fever became an intermittent one, and the patient recovered, unless his liver, which was sometimes the case, happened to be affected."

Stavorinus, the Dutch naval commander, speaking of "the sort of sickness or fever" which prevailed amongst the European inhabitants of Calcutta, during his visit to that city in 1766-1771, says that "it generally sweeps away those who are attacked by it in the space of three days."

Dr. John Clark, who visited Calcutta between 1768 and 1771, says that "the fever and flux" were very fatal in the former year. Of the fever, he states that "it frequently carries off the patient in twelve hours." . . . "During the sickly season in Bengal, the uncertainty of life is so great that it frequently happens that one may leave a friend at night in perfect health who shall not survive the following day. There have been several melancholy instances of persons who have returned home in a state of perfect health, from performing the last duties to a deceased friend, and have next day been numbered with the dead."

The same authority records that out of 189 cases of fever treated in ships trading to the various ports in the East, "105 recovered, and 84 died." Again, "out of 876, the complement of men belonging to eight ships, 78 died in Bengal, and 55 at sea, or nearly *one* in *six*. Both the fever and flux, if obstinate, have an equal tendency to terminate in abdominal obstructions, particularly in fatal swellings and suppurations of the liver." From this truthful record, and looking to the sanitary condition of the sufferers, and to the results of the exclusive treatment by bark, we are constrained to infer that the ultimate recoveries must have been but few, out of all who were the subjects of the fever or the flux.

Mr. Magennis states that in 1784, out of the crew of his ship, the *Valentine*, and six others stationed at Khidgeree, there died of fever and dysentery, 170 men, the usual period of their stay in the Hooghly being from August to January. Curtis writes that about the same time, out of two companies of the 98th and 100th regiments embarked in England for India, there died during a " suffering and tedious passage of exactly eleven months, 75 men, 40 of them being from fever, 18 from dysentery, and the remainder from scurvy and cachexy." It was on this occasion that the 2nd battalion of the 42nd regiment alone suffered a loss, by the time it landed in Calcutta, of five officers and 116 men, all from fevers, bowel complaints, " and the scurvy." It would appear that the unfortunate companies referred to by Curtis, had " some occasional fillings up from the other ships as the numbers decreased ;" but, making allowance for this circumstance, the loss of life was horrible —especially when we reflect that each ship in a fleet shared a like mortality.

The ships were, in the language of Clive, " crammed with soldiers ;" so that, along with salt rations, there was crowding, and consequent filth and want of ventilation—making altogether a combination of the most unfavourable circumstances to the soldier's health.

That a scorbutic taint was very general in these times may, I think, be admitted ; and this circumstance will account for the general term " putrid," as applied by the older writers to the endemic fevers and dysenteries : this unfavourable complication will go far also to account for the enormous mortality. Curtis states, that in the open well-ventilated Naval Hospital at Madras, containing from four to five hundred men, " the great bulk of the cases were *ulcers ;*" indeed he constantly refers to the scorbutic taint as prevalent amongst both soldiers and seamen, a fact almost entirely overlooked by modern writers when treating of the earlier results of treatment in tropical diseases. Dr. Lind, in his excellent " Treatise on the Putrid and Remitting Marsh Fever of Bengal in 1762," refers expressly to the prevalence of scurvy amongst the crews of all the ships off Calcutta.

That there also prevailed a certain amount of scorbutic taint on shore, even among the better classes of Indian society, may be reasonably inferred from the observations of Tennant and others. Tennant, writing from Cawnpore in 1798, says :—" The mode of living in this part of India has, within the last ten or fifteen years, undergone a very great alteration. Before that period the civil and military servants of the company of the first rank were lodged in bungalows worse than those of a subaltern of the present day : as the practice of feeding beef, mutton, pork, and poultry was not then introduced, their tables were poorly supplied ; even vegetables were not to be had, though an article indispensably necessary in this climate. These inconveniences were aggravated by a constant routine of irregularity. After dinner it was the usual custom to go to sleep in the hottest time of the day ; from this every party was awakened in the evening to partake of supper, which protracted a drunken sederunt till a late hour of the next morning. Amidst continued repletion, and frequent irregularity, the climate operated with fatal influence ; for trying as Bengal still is to almost every European constitution, there was a time when it was deemed far more hostile."

"A reformation highly commendable has been effected, partly from necessity ; but more by the example of a late Governor-General" (Lord Cornwallis, it is presumed), " whose elevated rank and noble birth gave him in a great measure the guidance of fashion. Regular hours and sobriety of conduct became as decidedly the test of a man of fashion as they were formerly of irregularity. Thousands owe their lives, and many more their health, to this change, which had neither been reckoned upon, nor even foreseen by those who introduced it."

" One species of dissipation often led to others ; the late hours and hard drinking induced gaming, which prevailed to a degree ruinous to many individuals : the same nobleman, by giving this practice a decided disapprobation, and by promoting such as refrained from it, has in a great degree lessened the habit, by bringing it into disgrace. Much dissipation, however, still remains."

How the condition of the blood, of nutrition and innervation, and of the secreting functions, must have been depraved by such a course of life, and with what deadly results the jungle fevers of those days must have operated on constitutions thus depraved, we need hardly stop to inquire. So recently indeed as the beginning of the present century, James Johnson states that, in the small portion of the river running between Calcutta and Khidgeree, full three hundred European seamen, or more than a fourth of the ships' crews, fell annual victims to the ravages of remittent fever ; many of the cases, even within so recent a period, having doubtless been complicated with scurvy.

But happily we have no longer to record any such fearful ravages by endemic diseases in the capital of the East ; neither do such sweeping epidemics as that recorded by Clark in 1770, with its *cold stage of twelve hours*, occur, carrying off 80,000 natives and 1500 Europeans. Such pestilences seem to have gone from us ; and we find that here, as in the Western hemisphere, the malignant fevers of former days, if they have not disappeared, are at least mitigated. Even in Jamaica, although severe epidemic fevers sometimes recur, they do not now, as formerly, destroy " to the amount of the whole number of its white inhabitants once in five years."

A just and useful comparison between former and recent times can scarcely, therefore, be instituted, so far as relates to the means of cure and the results. But this much may be conceded in favour of the position of modern Indian medical officers ; that owing to the better sanitary condition of their patients, to the better understanding of the value of depletory means, of a cooling regimen, and of the power of improved antiperiodic means, we not only save many more lives, but we have far fewer of the sequelæ to fevers and dysenteries than of old. For instance, out of 284 Europeans treated by Dr. Paisley in the Military Hospital at Madras in 1782, 182 men suffered from some form of " visceral obstruction"—the assured evidence of an exclusive treatment ; in other words, from organic disease of the liver or spleen, or of both, rendering death more or less speedy a necessary result.

The object of these remarks is, principally, to excite the attention of the younger members of the profession in the East to the superior efficacy of measures of prevention to those of cure of disease ; however much may be due to the careful consideration of this latter subject by the conscientious physician. In the first-named department of our profession, although a new science, the progress has already been immense ; whereas in the last, although a science of some two thousand years, or more, the results are by no means so signally useful comparatively, whether as regards the benefits to the individual, or to the community.

With all the advantages of modern medical science, no one could, even in our day, pretend to any very great success in the cure of Europeans suffering at once from the united influences of the most concentrated malaria and of scorbutus. We know, in fact, that in the olden times, owing to the joint influences of the marsh poison, and of the blood depraved beforehand by a salt diet, and by crowding in ships and barracks, the seaman and soldier were destroyed by fever and dysentery within a few hours of their admission into hospital. Such men were in truth almost beyond any, and all, medical means of cure :—no amount of cinchona could have cured them ; but very easily devised, and very obvious means of prevention MIGHT HAVE PRESERVED THEM IN HEALTH.

The causes of the present comparative improvement in public health must be of the highest interest and importance, especially to communities living within the tropics ; and, with all just confidence in modern medicine, guided by the lights of an improved physiology, and those also of pathology, I cannot yet agree with those who would ascribe the *whole* of the difference here spoken of to superior modes of medical treatment, great as these confessedly are. It is not through modern improvements in the treatment of disease, as contrasted with the older modes, that public health has been so much amended, as through the great measures of prevention of disease, consequent on the progress of improvement of localities, institutions of police, &c. It is to the preservative power of knowledge, to the reciprocal actions of the social state and of political events upon each other and upon medical science; to the perfection of the arts of civilization, in short, that the advancement of public health is most indebted, and so it will continue to be, although these circumstances are not sufficiently weighed by some of us when, in our hurry to praise ourselves, we forget what is due to our predecessors of old, and that those last had frequently to treat a violent and complicated form of disease which we have never seen, and with whose fatal severity we are consequently unacquainted.

It is justly observed by a popular writer, that there never were any specifics discovered against the plague, the sweating sickness, or the leprosy; and yet the leprosy, the sweating sickness, and the plague are now among the things unknown to us. They disappeared, not before any marvels of medicine, or any perfection of chemical science, but before the gradual amelioration of our condition through sanitary improvements.

PREDISPOSING CAUSES.

The predisposing causes of fever will be found in all those conditions of the body, and in all those habits of life, which tend to spoil the blood, and which lower the tone of the nervous system. The depressing passions of the mind also tend greatly to the advent of fever, whether endemic or contagious; and here we are carried back to the voyages of thirteen months to Bengal, to the crowding of soldiers and seamen, to the mental despondencies, to the scurvies, to the mortal "putrid remitting marsh fevers" of Europeans on landing in India, in the days of Clive and Hastings. The endemic causes of fevers, remittent and intermittent, are believed to be common to both, the poison being supposed more active or more concentrated in the former disease. The two fevers occur in the same stations and districts, and they frequently take the place of each other—the remittent fever more generally constituting the first illness of the European, to be followed immediately and temporarily, or sometimes for years together, according to local and constitutional influences, by intermittents more or less regular in type.

Extremes of every kind—extremes of supply and deficiency, of repletion and of privation;—excesses of every kind, especially in the use of spirituous liquors, wine, fermented drinks, and of tobacco, each and all of them dispose to fever; and so does exposure to extremes of heat and of cold, to heavy dews and fogs, to night air, to changes of season and other influences. Amongst seamen and soldiers proceeding to our various intertropical possessions, the salt rations and the spirits served to the men during the voyage used to be to a great extent, and are still to some degree, very injurious to health, and very predisposing to fevers, dysenteries, and hepatic diseases.

Excessive labour and the consequent fatigue, whether from the operations of sieges, or from long marches, powerfully dispose to fevers amongst soldiers ; and when to labour and fatigue we add the absence of proper diet, the want of necessary cover from tents, want of sufficient clothing, and want of sleep, we shall be at no loss to account for the ravages of disease in camps—especially when to all the above causes we superadd the abuse of stimulating liquors, and the malarious influences. Mr. Waring states that the temperate men—they who neither totally abstain nor who too freely indulge in alcoholic drinks—present the smallest number of admissions into hospital from fever, and likewise the lowest rate of mortality when attacked.

After the brief sketch here offered of the history and causes of the remittent fever of Bengal, the reader will be prepared to enter on a consideration of its symptoms, pathology, and treatment as they are presented to us in our day.

SYMPTOMS AND PROGRESS.

In no other morbid state is the physiognomy of disease so marked with general distress as in the severer forms of tropical fevers; for whether we behold the sufferer in the stage of rigor, reaction, or that tending to collapse, the countenance and manner are expressive of anguish, varying only in degree according to the stages.

The attack of the Bengal remittent fever is usually sudden, though occasionally the patient may complain for a day or more of weakness and lassitude, headache, nausea, and general uneasiness, accompanied by mental depression or subdued anguish. The countenance is pale and shrunk—the conjunctivæ clear, and of a dull whiteness. During this precursory stage of malaise the pulse is small, contracted, and frequent, with a slight increase of the temperature of the surface, especially over the forehead and præcordia, and a diminished action of the intestinal and urinary organs, as well as of the skin.

The actual invasion of fever is ushered in by debility of the mind and body—a hebetude indicative of diminished power of the nervous system ; by shivering or horror, the sensation of cold recurring in paroxysms, not being continuous. The headache now becomes intense and darting, with sense of tension across the forehead as if with a tight-drawn cord, and with pain in the back and loins, or on moving the eyeballs. The eyes now look muddy, or are tinged yellow, being void of lustre and expression; or else they have the appearance of deep-seated inflammation; occasionally, they are protruded, giving a wild and passionate expression to a countenance already flushed and anxious. At other times the countenance is bloated and torpid, expressive of general congestion, of epigastric distress, or of what the patient terms *inward suffering*. There is frequently a distressing giddiness, which occasionally proceeds to delirium. When this last symptom appears early, and runs high, we may anticipate a dangerous form of fever.

The tongue is red at the tip and edges, loaded, clammy, and moist; at other times, with a bitter or bad taste, the organ is but little changed from the healthy appearance. The thirst is usually most distressingly urgent, and the previous nausea is now increased to actual and severe bilious vomiting, accompanied by distressing sense of oppression and burning pain of the præcordia.

On examining the surface of the body, we find the skin thick, dry, and corrugated, giving to the hand a rough unpleasant sensation of pungent, deep-seated, and intense heat, as if derived from the blood: occasionally, in severe complicated cases, the skin is of a deep yellow. In the fevers of the rainy season, especially in persons in a state of anæmia, or of a phlegmatic habit and large abdomen, the skin is moist, clammy, and cadaverous, indicative of prostration of the nervous and vascular functions.

The abdomen generally, but more particularly the epigastric region, will be found tender on pressure, tumid and inelastic; this condition is accompanied by great anguish and oppression, caused by sanguineous congestion around the nervous centres. The secreting and excreting functions are all seriously disturbed, the bowels being usually constipated; but occasionally there are copious biliary evacuations; at other times, they are acrid and watery, while the urinary excretion is always scanty and depraved, though occasionally it also is copious, limpid, or tinged with bile.

The blood-current, previously oppressed, becomes now hard and quick, ranging from 110 to 120 pulsations in the minute; and the force and frequency of circulation through the brain, superadded to the already disturbed condition of the nervous functions, gives rise to confusion of ideas and loss of mental command, amounting occasionally to actual delirium.

The respiration is hurried and irregular, sometimes interrupted by deep sighing, the act seeming as if performed with over-heated air, and causing a feeling of heat in the lips and nostrils during expiration; and with all these accumulated distresses, there is not a point on the entire sentient surface of the body on which the patient can recline for a moment with comfort. No posture affords ease or rest, the sufferer being harassed with a restlessness which nothing can appease, characteristic at once of gastric irritation and oppression, with much general disturbance of the great central nervous functions of life. In a brief space the sufferer goes through a terrible storm of diseased action, his throes of anguish, mental and corporeal, being truly distressing to behold.

After a time, this general distress of body and mind, so diffi-cult, if not impossible to describe, begins to subside ; and, with a relaxation of all the symptoms, comes a state more or less ap-proaching to regularity of function, termed remission, more or less complete, according as the fever is mild or severe in its cha-racter.

These symptoms rise and fall in daily succeeding paroxysms, until they advance perceptibly into a condition of returning health, or recede and become aggravated and complicated into a state of imminent danger—the paroxysms running imperceptibly into each other, so as hardly to leave the least interval from suffer-ing, during the brief but retrograde process that now remains to be gone through.

It sometimes happens that the paroxysms prove erratic, a double paroxysm occurring within the twenty-four hours—a circumstance to be carefully ascertained, lest the physician's visits and his appli-cation of active remedies, and especially of bleeding and purging, should be mistimed ; that is, used at the wrong time of remission, instead of the right time, or that of the accession of fever.

The favourable stage of abatement again, or that of remission, is indicated by a general perspiration, a reduced temperature, a soft and expanded pulse, diminished in frequency to about 90 in the minute—a full, free, and regular respiration, and a more abun-dant action of the secreting and excreting functions. In the rainy season and in dissipated and unhealthy subjects, as well as in the worst of our fevers, the stage of remission is the period of greatest danger—the relaxation proceeding too far, as shown by profuse sweats, coldness of the extremities, great anxiety, and sink-ing of the vital powers ; in short, there is no stage of this fever that does not require careful observation and anxious watching ; for each succeeding event has strict relation to its antecedent, and all of them vary in degree of intensity according to the locality and season—according to the age, constitution, and previous habits of life of the patient. The night is a time of increased distress to the sufferer from fever. Malaria is notoriously more influential at night ; and it has been noticed besides that the electricity of the atmo-sphere is at its daily minimum at about three A.M., while atmo-spheric pressure is at one of its daily minima about four A.M.

In the ordinary forms of remittent fever, the first stage, or that of cold, is but short, while that of reaction, or of heat, varies from two to eight hours' duration ; and this again is followed by relaxa-tion or remission, which is more or less complete, of longer or shorter duration, proportioned to the severity and duration of the previous stages. In its more concentrated forms, on the other hand, the remission of symptoms is so trifling as to require a close observation for its detection; and unless the progress of disease can be early arrested by art, paroxysm follows paroxysm with increasing rapidity and severity, until life is destroyed.

In the milder or less dangerous forms of this fever, under the influence of proper treatment, the daily paroxysms steadily decline in force and frequency; and towards the fifth or seventh day, or earlier, convalescence may be completely established, and a return to health ensured. But however mild the fever may appear, the inexperienced practitioner should be on his guard against evil. In fact, he who has to watch the progress of this fever should be always expecting the unexpected; so suddenly and insidiously may unfavourable symptoms set in. He must be on the watch for the sudden accession of symptoms at once dangerous, unlooked for, and rapid in their progress, if allowed to go on unchecked. Changes also take place suddenly in the constitutional powers of the patient; especially in persons of weakly condition, in such as have suffered from previous disease, or from great bodily fatigue, from privation, or from mental distress.

The previous detail of symptoms will have shown how greatly the nervous and vascular functions have been disturbed, even in the course of one paroxysm, and how much the cerebral and abdominal organs have been oppressed; it is then to these two regions that the attention of the medical observer must be principally directed; for what serious results may he not anticipate from many such paroxysms, if unrestrained and unmitigated! The truth is, that, in respect of changes within the two cavities named, our circumspection cannot be too keen; for congestion, more or less severe, to end perhaps in inflammation and effusion, and consequent destruction of some organ essential to life, may be the result of carelessness, or of inattention. The most serious, rapid, and unexpected changes will be found to occur within the cerebral cavity; but indeed this latter, as well as the abdominal viscera, should be regarded throughout every stage of the fever with the most anxious attention. Here, to be forewarned will go some way to render us forearmed. The true wisdom, as regards fever, is the faculty which anticipates dangers, and which prevents their occurrence. We are all wise after the event, but true wisdom should endeavour to obtain a fore view of ulterior consequences.

Such is a detail of the symptoms and progress of the remittent fever of Bengal, the average duration of which may be estimated at from six to eight days. In no instance, perhaps, will each and all the above-mentioned symptoms be presented, for the fever varies with the locality and season; but so many of the symptoms described will be found in every case as to leave no doubt whatever as to the real nature of the disease.

A consideration, however transient, of the outline here given, must satisfy any one that the disease under consideration is one which involves the safety or the destruction of the most important organs of the body. It is likewise, though varying in degree, the most prevalent form of disease known to the world, and that by which it is supposed the greater portion of the human race is prematurely destroyed; it therefore claims a paramount attention on the part of the tropical physician, as on his intimate acquaintance with its nature and treatment will mainly depend his character for usefulness. The dangers which more immediately affect life in the remittent fever, arise from liability to collapse of the vital actions; the more remote dangers are connected with visceral enlargements —the sequelæ to fevers, remittent and intermittent, and their results.

In placing before the reader a detail of the symptoms of the Bengal remittent fever, I have confined myself to the mention of such as are present in the ordinary and severer forms of that disease, omitting all notice of the minor forms and degrees, as these last may appear at different seasons of the year, in persons of peculiar temperaments, habits of life, or in persons of different ages and sexes.

I have done this with a view to avoid confusion and the entanglement which results from over-minute descriptions of symptoms which vary only in degree; believing too that he who can appreciate the circumstances of danger in the graver forms of fever, so as to overcome them, will be at no loss when called to treat such as are mild and almost free from danger to life. After having been familiar with the mastering of great dangers, it is easy to bring one's mind down to considerations for the removal of the smaller ills. There is, in short, nothing in the nature or progress of disease which can disturb or embarrass the man who has been habituated successfully to encounter the storms of tropical fevers.

PATHOLOGY.

A consideration of the phenomena constituting a paroxysm of remittent fever, in a person previously healthy, and the fact that the violence of succeeding paroxysms has, during life, fallen with augmenting morbid force on the organs within the abdominal and cerebral cavities, will prepare the pathologist to find that, after death, the results of congestion, or of inflammatory action, are manifested in the peritonæum, stomach, liver, and bowels in the one case, while the membranes, the cavities, or the substance of the brain suffer injury in the other case; and so it is in fact. Another circumstance deserves a preliminary and special notice, namely, the almost universal application to the fevers of the East of the significant term BILIOUS. That it has not been in the olden time, any more than in our own day, an accidental or a misapplied term is evident, for modern statistics fully attest to its pathological accuracy in the most extended and unquestionable manner. We are thus, in India, continually thrown back on the just observation of Clark, that, of all the organs of the human body, the liver is the most liable to disease.

The great majority of the complications in the fevers of Bengal are abdominal, whether these consist of mere irritation, of simple congestion, or of congestion proceeding onwards to inflammation ; and this would appear to be the principal cause of the prostration, with tendency to collapse, so common, especially during the rainy season ; for, even within a few hours, there occasionally exists here an oppression of the vital functions alarming to the stranger physician.

The depression caused by a violent blow on the abdomen more nearly resembles the febrile collapse than any other morbid condition with which I am acquainted ; and both probably depend on a disturbance of the functions of the organic nervous system—the powerful though silent source of many symptoms known to us only by their effects.

The proximate cause of fever has been referred by various pathologists, German and British, to congestion around the central nervous ganglia with consequent alteration or diminution of the organic nervous influence—a perversion of innervation in short, together with a depravation of the blood through the entrance of a morbific cause, the nature of which is unknown. This prostration of the organic and cerebro-spinal nervous functions, produced by the immediate application of malaria, comes on with a speed and violence proportioned to the dose of the poison. We have at first the universal sense of cold, then the accession of a great and universal heat—the acceleration of pulse—the racking pains—the restlessness and burning thirst—the suppression of the secretions—all referable to injury done to the nervous centres. Essentially and specially we have, in fact, a paresis of the great sympathetic and cerebro-spinal nerves, with dilatation of the arteries, resulting in congestions and inflammations in those organs which derive their nerves from the sympathetic. The beneficial effects of venesection, practised at the accession of the stage of reaction, have indeed been supposed to result, in part at least, from the removal of so much of the mass of heated blood which disturbed and excited the heart's action.

Dr. Handfield Jones states that—1. The sympathetic plexuses are distributed on the arteries of the abdominal, the thoracic, and the cerebral organs. 2. Paralysis of these plexuses dilates the arteries they accompany, and increases heat and tissue-change in the localities where they are distributed ; it establishes active hyperæmia, which, in states of debility, may pass into inflammation. 3. The action of malarious poison is sometimes paralysing, at others irritating. Neuralgic pain, rigors, or convulsions must be regarded as signs of irritation; numbness, coma, or loss of muscular power, as signs of paralysing influence. These two effects may be produced at the same time in different nervous structures of the same body.—*Brit. Med. Journal*, October, 1857.

The condition of the several organs as to vital power is, as stated by our author, much concerned in determining the occurrence of inflammation after hyperæmia has been set up; and the more we regard also jaundice with free flow of bile, and other secretion-fluxes—the dysenteries, the hepatic and splenic tumour—as the results of the same poisonous influence which produces palsy of the solar plexus and fever, the more we shall approach to a true pathology. This is an old doctrine, in fact; "the difference of constitutions," according to Huxham, "thus altering the face and nature of the disease."

It must be held in recollection that what are termed congestions, subacute and acute inflammations, tend, firstly, to destroy life speedily; and secondly, in their remoter results, they found organic diseases which have the same eventually fatal effects. In either case they form conditions of the utmost importance; for, in the first instance, the immediate cure is involved, so as to save life—in the second, the prevention of disease more or less remote and deadly.

The oppressive fulness, tenderness, and anguish of the epigastric region, with nausea, vomiting, or retching, forming so urgent a feature in the symptoms during life, are followed, in fatal cases, by alterations of structure in the mucous digestive surfaces, more or less extensive and destructive according to the intensity or the duration of the previous fever.

These lesions will be found in the stomach, duodenum, and mesocolon principally, and they are generally of a congestive or inflammatory nature, as evidenced by a turgid or dirty-red condition of the inner surfaces, and by interstitial effusions; in very severe or protracted cases the results of congestions, or of inflammatory actions, as redness, ecchymosis, or even ulceration, will extend to the mucous surfaces of the small and large intestines, while the liver, spleen, omentum, and mesentery exhibit various degrees of vascular engorgement. A severe disturbance of the hepatic function is almost universal in the progress of the remittent fevers of the East, and the evidences of congestion, sometimes of inflammatory actions, in the liver, gall-bladder, and ducts, will very generally be found after death. The spleen is not so frequently the seat of morbid changes; and when they do exist in persons previously healthy, the conditions are those of simple enlargement, or of softening of the organ. The case of Captain F——r (referred to at p. 372) exhibits the great violence and the enormous extent of abdominal inflammation sometimes resulting from · severe malarious fevers, and impresses a lesson how to treat them. The neglect of antiphlogistic remedies led here to the destruction of a powerful constitution, and to premature death.

Nor are the evidences of congestion, or of inflammatory action within the cerebral cavity, of a less prominent or declared character. In general these results consist in effused serum, sudden and dangerous in its occurrence, and such as we should most anxiously guard against by a prompt and effective treatment; for when effusion occurs within the head, the fatal termination is too often close at hand. As already stated, however, the greater proportion of the complications, in the remittent fevers of Bengal, are abdominal, and, though hardly of less danger to the patient, they are not so sudden in their invasion, nor so immediately dangerous to life, as those which are cerebral. But it is well to remember that against the one or the other, or against both together, the tropical practitioner must be unceasingly and carefully on his guard.

The evidence that serous effusion is threatened, or taking place within the cerebral cavity, will be found in mental incoherence and a wandering indifference to objects of former interest, ending in stupor more or less complete, if the disease advances. To questions relating to his condition of health, the patient replies that he is " very well." This insensibility to, or unacquaintance with, his actually dangerous state, indicates imminent peril; and the sufferer, when not relieved by timely and proper treatment, first " sinks in bed," under the laws of gravitation, and afterwards with dilated pupils, flushed cheeks, cold extremities, and increasing stupor, he sinks in death.

The effusion of serum within the abdominal cavity is accompanied by increased præcordial anxiety, and increased tendency to collapse; the abdomen feels full and inelastic on examination, and sometimes there is tenderness on pressure. The tendency in the remittent fevers of Bengal to found visceral disease within the abdomen is so great that we should be on the careful watch against such complications, from the first hour of treatment until convalescence shall be established and matured.

Death from remittent fever being usually an event of speedy occurrence, there can seldom exist time for emaciation of the body; but the surface generally exhibits a sallow or greenish-yellow appearance. Where jaundice occurs in the course of this fever, and especially where it is associated with cerebral disturbance, such as drowsiness, the danger is again imminent. The collapse here has a double source—a cerebral as well as an abdominal origin; and the surface of the body after death exhibits a deeper tinge of sallowness, with livor of the face and neck.

A presentiment of death is a very unfavourable circumstance in the progress of remittent fever, and one that is too often verified by the result. A soldier will say: "You have been very kind to

me, sir, but this time I shall not get over it." There may exist
in the poor fellow's case nothing that has the appearance of absolute or immediate danger at this time—yet the man generally dies,
and that in the course of a few paroxysms. The fatal impression
is instinctive, and is not at first shared by the medical attendant, who is seldom able to trace the pathological source.

In July, 1840, the height of the rainy season, when, as stated,
the fevers are more than usually severe in type, I passed a gentleman, the head of a mercantile firm, while driving through the
streets of Calcutta. He remarked to a friend on my healthy appearance, and on the amount of labour I appeared to undergo with
impunity. At 2 p.m. of that day he was seized with the remittent
fever ; and at 4 p.m. he was informed that, although the younger
and stouter of the two, my life was despaired of by my professional
friends. His countenance speedily assumed a very grave expression, and after some days he refused to use any means of cure,
truly declaring himself to be a dying man. On examination after
death a purulent collection was found under the descending colon,
a condition not suspected during life.

THE SELECTION AND APPLICATION OF THE MEANS OF CURE.

In every form and variety of fever,—in every climate, and in every
season of the year—one of the most important circumstances to observe, is, the nature of the prevailing disease, whether endemic or
epidemic; for not only do fevers differ in their nature in different
localities and seasons, but so also do their complications, whether
congestive or inflammatory, so as to require a different and carefully proportionate treatment. It should likewise be impressed
on medical officers that too much attention cannot be paid to the
type of every fever, endemic and epidemic—to its general character, as well as to each individual case. " In inflammations,
in fevers, in fluxes, in hæmorrhages," justly observes Dr. Handfield Jones, " we see the existence of the same types of morbid
action ; the asthenic where arterial paralysis, through vaso-motor
nerves, dominates ; and the sthenic where tissue excitement and
irritation come to play the more prominent part. Nearly the
same therapeutic proceedings are appropriate in each of the four
sets—the character of the type being the all-important circumstance."

We are told by Sir James M'Grigor, in his admirable history
of the diseases of the Peninsular army, that not only had fever
very different forms in different seasons, and in different quarters
of the same seasons, but they required very different, nay, opposite
kinds of treatment: the knowledge of this, he adds, strongly impresses on us the necessity of becoming acquainted with every attending circumstance, before we venture to censure any particular
practice. These circumstances should be for ever present to the

mind of the physician.   And here I would remark on the serious
disadvantages under which the tropical practitioner undertakes
the cure of fever, as compared to his more fortunate brethren of
temperate climates.   The former has, in a large proportion of
instances, to treat a fever violent, concentrated, and rapid in its
nature and tendencies :—he has but a few days, and sometimes but
a few hours, between the invasion of disease and the recovery or
death of the sufferer.   The means of cure, too, while they require
the most cool, measured, and careful judgment, must be prompt,
direct, and powerful to a degree not known, and therefore not
required elsewhere.   All this involves a most grave responsibility.
In Europe, on the other hand, owing to the comparatively subdued
and protracted character of the fevers generally, we can afford to
watch the slow progress of events, so as cautiously and indirectly
to treat symptoms, and thus aid nature in her endeavours to free
herself from disease.   By him who would conduct his patient with
safety through the troubles and distresses of a tropical remittent
fever, two preliminary conditions must be settled :—he must first
select his means of cure with judgment, and apportion them carefully ; and having done this, he must apply them promptly.   In
fever, above all diseases, we must ever admit with Trophilus that
—" he who is able to distinguish what can be done, and what
cannot be done, is the true physician ;" but how great and difficult
his task !   He must measure his means to the wants of nature,—
doing neither too much nor too little—carefully avoiding what
ought *not* to be done.

Before proceeding to the cure of this formidable disease it is
always necessary carefully to observe the age, length of residence in
India, and the constitution, whether plethoric, bilious, or anæmic ;
for on these conditions must rest much that concerns the nature,
amount, and persistence of our remedies.   The physician must
likewise inquire minutely and carefully into the duration and
actual stage of the fever ; — that is, whether it be of some
hours' or some days' duration, and whether the actually existing
paroxysm be at its accession, or its decline.   These are the first
and more immediate points for consideration ; for, by the daily
recurrence of these paroxysms, changes take place in the relative
balance of power in the several functions, nervous and vascular,
which render a proportionate modification in our more active
means of cure necessary to successful treatment.   The means
which would be salutary within the first few days cannot be used
later with the same effect, or to the same amount ; and so again the
means to arrest fever and save life, if applied at the accession of
the paroxysm, would induce a dangerous collapse, or even destroy
life, if applied at the stage of its decline, or towards its termination.   After these preliminary cautions the reader will be prepared
to enter into the general details of remedies in their usual order of
application—into a consideration of their respective physiological

actions—into the preferences to be given to some of them, and their application to particular cases.

It is of great importance to arrange such means as are primary, so as to separate them from such as are but secondary, or of minor consequence to the cure. For this purpose I have marked, under their respective heads, the various means in use for the treatment of remittent fever, very nearly in the order of their importance; and I would here observe that whoever pretends to encounter remittent fever with a mind unprepared, incurs a fearful responsibility:—the suitable education and training cannot here be postponed till the emergency arises.

EMETICS.

Certain authors in various countries have recommended that, in the treatment of fevers, we should begin with the exhibition of an emetic, and each has had his favourite—sulphate of zinc, antimonial preparations, or ipecacuanha—the latter being by most persons believed to be the safest. Certainly, when a patient seized with fever is found with a stomach loaded with food and drink, the sooner he is vomited the better; but the coincidence cannot be a frequent one anywhere, and within the tropics the practice of early vomiting in fever has not obtained or held ground. In the treatment of Europeans, suffering from the periodic fevers of India, I have very seldom exhibited emetics; but I am bound to say that, in the treatment of natives of all classes, civil and military, I ever found a combination of compound jalap powder with a few grains of calomel, and one or two grains of emetic tartar, to act in a manner frequently to cut short the progress of fever—the patients very generally requiring neither bark nor arsenic, the free action of both stomach and bowels, having proved curative of the fever.

In the instances in which emetics have proved of real service to European patients, I was disposed to refer the benefit generally to the sudorific and sedative effects, and not to the action of vomiting— a severe and distressing symptom already present in almost every violent case of remittent fever. There exists, in the East at least, a prejudice against the use of emetics; but I apprehend that the just application of this powerful means has not yet been arrived at, through a careful course of observation and experience. All that seems to be really known is, that there are cases of fever in which emetics may act beneficially, and others in which they prove injurious.

Robert Jackson says that, in periodic fever, particularly in the bilious remittent of the autumnal season, the emetic is often the first remedy prescribed; and, in certain cases, its operation is not unfrequently beneficial, so beneficial indeed in many instances that the disease is arrested, or a condition induced by its action under which it is easily arrested by other applications. This celebrated physician adds, however, that emetics do no good, but even do harm, " where the habit is full, the arterial action high, the pulse hard and tense, or small, deep, and concentrated—the skin thick and torpid, or where the functions of important organs, viz., the head, lungs, or liver, are oppressed by sanguineous congestion."

Mr. Wade, of Chunar, published a book, in 1791, in which he detailed the results of treatment by means of a solution of Epsom salts and emetic tartar, with a success " unbroken, except by two cases of unfortunate termination, in the treatment of about four hundred cases of fever and dysentery." That the fevers and dysenteries amongst the old hard-drinking European pensioners forming the garrison of Chunar in 1791—men whose ambition was limited to possessing abundance of cheap grog—could not have been of a very formidable character, is sufficiently apparent. Mr. Wade invites " the medical world to draw their own comments ;" and the medical world has done so long ago. Meanwhile, this same plan of treating every disease alike was copied by and attempted to be practised at the General hospital of Calcutta, under the influence of bayonets, by a late medical officer of that institution; but it had no better success with " the medical world." As to the patients in this latter instance, no power could induce the Europeans to submit, either to the continued nausea, the frequent vomitings, or the incessant purgings which resulted. There was, in fact, no power at that time in the government of British India sufficient to enforce the emetic-cathartic treatment.

This is the kind of *case-book* that is calculated to do so much harm with the inexperienced and the inattentive, who are averse from the trouble of learning their duties, except by the shortest and easiest of ways.

THE WARM BATH—TEPID AND COLD AFFUSIONS— COLD DRINKS.

Robert Jackson began his treatment of the congestive fevers of the West Indies by a warm bath and active frictions to the whole surface of the body. While thus immersed, with the sensibility of the skin " augmented by the heat of the bath and by friction," and with the fluids powerfully derived to the surface, he abstracted blood from the arm. That such means are powerful, and require the hand of a master, no one can doubt; but, in point of fact, neither the warm bath nor the tepid and cold affusions have had, any more than the emetics, any systematic or sustained support from the practitioners of the East. Perhaps the great tendency to collapse in the fevers of Bengal may have at all times deterred us from the very liberal use of means which tend powerfully to affect the balance of circulation.

I remember the instance of an European who was employed on the deadly island of Sagor, and whose case interested me greatly at the time. His fever was in its seventh day when I saw him, and the native boatmen, to prevent his leaping overboard, had tied him in his delirium to the benches, in which state he was exposed, bareheaded and half naked, to the direct rays of a March sun during the two days of his passage up the river to Calcutta. The whole surface of the body was of a lurid lead-and-brick hue, as were the eyes. His delirium was subsiding into stupor, no coherent reply being obtained from him; his restlessness was of the most distressing kind, for he tossed and changed his posture violently in every few seconds of time; his tongue was black and dry, and his pulse was extinguished by the weight of my fore-finger :— the case looked hopeless. I seized, however, on what appeared to me the most urgent feature of this poor fellow's case, namely, the most excessively pungent and unpleasant heat of skin I had ever felt by means of the touch; and I ordered him at once, and under my inspection, to be dashed with cold water over head and trunk, from a few feet of height. Some six or eight earthen pitchers of water were thus poured on the patient, after which he was well rubbed and put in bed. The fearful restlessness at once subsided, and in half an hour he was in a gentle perspiration and sound sleep. I have never seen such a case, or such a result, before or since. A few mercurial purgatives concluded this man's cure, and I did not see him until two years subsequently. But it now became apparent how severe had been his fever, for the faculties of the mind never regained their former power, and he was eventually sent to his friends in England. The unusual nature and amount of heat in this case induced me at once to apply the cold bath; and I was of opinion at the time that, had I adopted any other course of treatment, the patient must have died. But it is only fair to state that Robert Jackson, the originator of this plan of treating fevers (and not Dr. Currie, of Liverpool), and who had had more experience of its effects than any other person since his time, declares that the salutary action of cold affusion, in febrile diseases, is not necessarily and indispensably connected with the presence of increased heat. His caution that cold affusion is "ineffectual or dangerous where deep congestion or strong inflammation exists in any of the interior organs," may constitute another reason why this means has not been more generally had recourse to in the fevers of the East Indies. Measures difficult of application and sometimes doubtful of result—excepting when used with an extraordinary tact, like Robert Jackson's—will not be generally adopted or employed by ordinary medical practitioners. This great military physician appears to be the most original of modern medical writers, partly for the reason that he practised longer, read more, and remembered more, than any of our modern physicians, some of whom, with a complete absence of fitness, aim at a feeble and false originality; but Jackson was, in fact, a most acute observer, and a most original thinker and practitioner.

The topical use of cold and tepid water is much practised in

India, and that with signal benefit when applied to the scalp, forehead, and temples, where cerebral determinations occur with severity, as in the ardent fever of the hot season.

Warm baths have been limited, in my own practice, to the latter
stages of fever, dysentery, and hepatitis, and when convalescence
was approaching. They will then be found both grateful and
beneficial.

Nature prompts the free use of cold drinks in all forms of fever,
and the extinction of thirst is everywhere esteemed a powerful
means of cure; so much so that certain mild forms of fever are
curable by cold water alone. The abundant introduction of
American ice into the three capitals of India has proved of great
service in the treatment of the fevers of those cities. The ice is
useful not only as a local and general refrigerant, but as a powerful means also for allaying the distressing irritability of stomach
so common to our fevers.

BLOOD-LETTING.

I come now to consider blood-letting, — the most powerful
remedy, the most difficult of just application, but the most needful
of any we possess, if we would cure the congestion or inflammatory sthenic remittent fever of Bengal, and save the patient from
subsequent visceral disease. The question of blood-letting in
disease is almost the most important which can engage the attention of the practical physician. I am aware that a kind of fashion
is at present moving against the practice, almost to the desire for
its total exclusion; but those who are acquainted with the history
of medicine, and who have seen and understood the nature of
acute inflammatory and congestive tropical disease, will take
fashion here at its proper value, and at no more.

In temperate climates general blood-letting is demanded in
acute inflammations of internal parenchymatous organs, and of
the serous membranes and coverings; nor has fashion as yet superseded this rule of practice, in the instances of persons of unimpaired constitutions. But if a man be so enthralled by routine,
says Mr. Cumming, that he must either bleed every case, or not
bleed at all, he had certainly better not bleed in any case; otherwise, while he may save ten cases of sthenic inflammation he will
destroy ten cases of asthenic inflammation, and injure the remaining eighty of a mild character. The scientific Virchow
speaks deliberately of general blood-letting as " *a revulsive means
which prepares the system for other modes of restoring its equilibrium.*
It is in the latter way that it has most value in sthenic and
hypersthenic inflammations: *it places the patient in a favourable
condition for the regulation of inflammatory disturbances.*" In other
words, it prepares the patient for the actions of those secondary
but necessary remedies which conduce so materially to the completion of the cure.

" It may be very well," says a Dublin critic, " to refrain from blood-letting in the treatment of feeble and unsound patients in large cities, but what will our provincial friends say to the whole-sale interdiction of the lancet? That we do not now bleed as we formerly did is obvious enough; but do we err in the opposite extreme? We have ourselves ' a theory,' that it might be better at once to diminish the quantity of the circulating fluid than to render it unfit to support life or repair injury, by slops and physic. By the way, if it is so bad a practice to bleed, how does it happen that we have so much leeching and cupping, especially in private practice? These questions are worthy of consideration, both in a pathological and medico-ethical point of view." Certainly, these questions *are* worthy of consideration; and, to borrow their own language, how long will medical critics persist in thinking that if any given proceeding be wrong, its directly opposite must necessarily be right;—that if profuse and indiscriminate bleeding and mercurialization, for instance, be wrong, the not bleeding and the not giving calomel in any case must be right?

One very important circumstance should be impressed on the attention of all young naval and military surgeons, viz., that when, upon careful consideration, general blood-letting is deemed neces-sary in the severer forms of tropical fevers,—when there is violent tumult of arterial action, or an oppressive venous congestion,—conditions alike dangerous to life—the general blood-letting, to be effective, should be practised as early as possible, and be sufficient in amount to make an impression on the febrile movement; to relieve the stress, morbid energy, and force of the circulation. A small bleeding, or repeated small bleedings, may moderate a mild, but can never arrest a violent tropical fever.

Balfour, writing in Bengal in 1789, says :—" The loss of blood, both general and local, is very effectual in removing these partial affections"—complications described as virulently and obstinately inflammatory. " Even when it fails, it prepares the way for a free exhibition of opium to alleviate the pain, and of bark to sup-press the fever; by the violence of which these partial affections are often supported and aggravated, more than by any topical cause."

In the practice of Robert Jackson, in the West Indies, the largest bleedings were made from young and plethoric soldiers, chiefly in the ardent and inflammatory cerebral fevers, and occa-sionally in the congestive abdominal complications common to the West as to the East Indies. Of the complications referable to the abdomen and cerebrum, the latter are the more ardent, and the more immediately dangerous to life. It is but proper to add, that " this apparently revolting practice," as Jackson terms it, was of such effect in his hands, " that the greater number of persons who were treated in this manner returned to their duty within a fortnight." A sthenic condition of the vital functions, with a morbid state of the nervous system, must have been present when depletions to the amount of "ten pounds in twenty-four hours" were made with signal relief; for the same amount of reducing means would in the present day sink the patient. As here stated, the rule of depletion that applies to an acute or ardent fever, applies with equal force to the same means of cure in the more difficult and formidable form of congestive fever; and there is not in the whole range of practice of medicine any question of a more nice discrimination than that of the measure here referred to; and next in importance comes that of the proper time and manner of using blood-letting. To render this important operation "the more certain, and the more perfect," Jackson urges :—

" 1. That it be made within six hours from the invasion of continued fever, or before the paroxysm of the periodic fever of violent excitement has attained its acmé.

" 2. The simple act of abstracting blood from the circulating system is often decisively effectual in arresting the course of fever, where it is resorted to at an early period, and where the process is properly conducted.

" 3. It is still salutary, but of less decisive effect, where the course is more advanced, that is, beyond the third day. It is not of dependence, but is not prohibited, and it is occasionally useful even at late periods. It is thus not safe to carry it to the extent of effecting precipitate arrest; it is safe, as well managed, to alleviate impending dangers, and often to facilitate the development of regular crisis :" thus he conceives that guarded blood-letting favours the tendency of fevers to subside under the law of periodic action.

" 4. If employed thus, it obviates or removes congestion, and thereby prevents effusion into internal cavities, and into the substance of internal organs. '

" 5. Abstraction of blood is, moreover, safe, and its effect is often important, at the first moments of relapse.

" 6. Prescribed with consideration, and applied with management in execution, blood-letting is both a safe and powerful remedy, either decisive of cure by its own power, or preparatory of the curative powers of others. It is the main engine of successful practice; it is not the sole remedy.

" 7. But though I say this in truth, I do not say that bleeding in a large, even in any quantity, is uniformly proper, or uniformly safe.

" 8. Though the abstraction of blood is generally beneficial, it is only so conditionally, and under management. If the effect produced by it be not seconded by well-considered means of stimulation, or conservative of auxiliary power, general or local, adapted to the circumstances of the case, the chances are that the harm will be greater than the good. But while blood-letting is a remedy of nice management in cases of relapse, it is to be avoided, as well as other remedies of strong operation, where there exist appearances of approaching a favourable crisis. On the contrary, where the critical power labours, and the critical effect is marred through internal impediment, the abstraction of blood in a given quantity is often followed by signal benefit; it gives facility to the course of the salutary process artificially obstructed.

" 9. If there be no prohibitory circumstance in the case, one bleeding is preferable to repeated small bleedings.

" 10. But though I regard the abstraction of blood as a remedy of the first importance, for the abrupt and successful cure of fever, either primarily or secondarily, I am yet free to own that its good effect depends principally on the manner of adjusting the subtraction to the condition.

" 11. It often fails, and even sometimes does harm where, employed as principal, its real place is only that of auxiliary; and *per contra*, where employed as auxiliary, its real place is that of principal."

12. The increased relative tolerance of blood-letting in inflammatory affections with fever has been tabulated by Dr. Marshall Hall; and Dr. C. Williams apprehends that the explanation of the fact will be found in the increased excitability of the heart's action and tonicity of the arteries, which maintain a sufficient force and tension to preserve the circulation, especially through the brain, even when much blood is abstracted. The quantity of the blood in the system, and a more stimulating quality of it, may contribute to the same result.

Not to speak of the practical importance of the rules here laid down by our greatest military physician—a man of the most rare powers of observation and truthfulness—and numbered by me the more to mark their separate import, they are of extreme interest in the history of tropical fevers, and of their treatment; and it is principally on this latter account, and not as rules of practice in India, that they are here presented to the reader's consideration. Such histories I conceive to be of great importance, as from their attentive consideration and comparison we learn, generally after a lapse of years, to deduce a just balance in the use of all the known means of cure, old as well as new. In the principles involved in the rules above quoted from the writings of Robert Jackson, he will, I think, be found just, although the degree and extent to which he carried blood-letting will not apply to the fevers of our day, in the East Indies at least. The rational and the timely employment of blood-letting are the two great points for consideration and determination by the tropical physician.

It has been well observed that the most distinguished physicians of all ages, who have treated of fever, coincide entirely in the feeling that with regard to this important class of disease it is impossible, in the short life allotted to the most aged, to do anything more than add a little knowledge to the common stock. If this be true, and who that knows anything of medicine can doubt it, we should study with care the history of fever, and learn from it not to boast of our success, or blame those who have gone before us; for in truth we are too often only able to see the defects of the older writers by the lights which they have placed before us. The accurate observer Tennant, speaking of the treatment of the fevers of his time in Bengal, 1796, says that it was "simple and decisive, and more efficacious than that of any sort of diseases equally malignant in Britain."

Jackson, by the most active depletion, designed to produce immediate curative result by cutting short the progress of fever, and so did the older medical officers in our tropical possessions by "throwing in the bark." In the circle of varying opinion, doctrine, and practice, we come again, after the round of a century, to the same exclusive treatment last mentioned, in heroic doses of quinine. This plan of arresting fever has been of late had recourse to in the continued types of Europe, and in the formidable paroxysmal malarious fevers of tropical regions, but as yet without any determinate results. The treatment by Peruvian bark, and by bark chiefly, was long and faithfully practised in former times, and an enormous amount of visceral disease—the infarctions of the older writers—was the result; and it is to be feared that, in hot climates at least, such will again be the result, whether we employ, after an exclusive manner, the disulphate of quina, or the more galenical preparations of the bark. All experience points, in fact, to the union of the depletory and refrigerant with the antiperiodic means in the cure of tropical fevers, remittent and intermittent, thus blending all the safe and effective means of cure, not limiting ourselves to one exclusively. Robert Jackson wisely and candidly observes of cutting short the course of fever, by any or by every means, that all attempts to cure on this plan, as they must be at random, so they cannot be adopted without danger : in other words, fevers cannot be cut short by any one means, although their violence may be reduced and their duration shortened by the consecutive and conjoint actions of various medicinal agencies.

In the treatment of fevers, as of other acute diseases, we must be content with what *can* be done with safety and efficiency—in the language of Pitcairn, we must be content, in the great majority of instances, to " guide" the fever. As matter of theory, or even of reasonable endeavour, it seems sound in principle to cut short a fever in its career, however difficult the execution ; for, as in military affairs, what can be done most speedily is done most effectively, and we should bring into action all our forces as soon as possible. As yet, however, we have nowhere succeeded in absolutely cutting fever short by *coup-de-main*, either by blood-letting or by Peruvian bark ; yet the two means constitute beyond doubt our heroic remedies. Robert Jackson was supposed to have come nearer the desired result, through blood-letting principally, than any physician with whose practice we are acquainted; but it is admitted also that, in hands less skilled than his, the practice of large and repeated bleedings was not always safe. In the East Indies they have never been used, nor would they there be justifiable as a general rule. No tropical practitioner can peruse the works of Jackson, however, without great benefit; but it is to those practising in the West Indies that, with a certain reservation, they will prove of more special interest.

Dr. Graves, of Dublin, says of bleeding in typhus, within the first ten or twelve hours of seizure, that by its means the patient, if plethoric, has " a very good chance of escaping the disease ;" but he adds, that " it is only during this stage that you have a chance of extinguishing the fever at once by abstraction of blood from the system." After all, this great practical question must be determined by the known character and course of the disease—by a just observation of every individual case, and by experience. On mere theory we may be led to use or disuse this most powerful means, and in either case erroneously.

All circumstances considered, I give a very decided preference to general over local blood-letting, in all cases of acute sthenic, flagrant, tropical disease, whether it be the remittent fever, dysentery, or hepatitis. When the medical attendant bleeds from the arm he sees and knows what he is doing; he measures his means, and adapts them to the circumstances of the case, and he sees carefully, and at once, that it is not carried too far; whereas, by the application of leeches, no one knows the exact amount of blood abstracted in the first instance, and the amount of subsequent oozing, in the absence of the medical attendant, is even more uncertain, and in remittent fever even more dangerous when, as occasionally happens, this oozing takes place during the night, and in the declining stage of remission. This much is certain, however, that so much blood does occasionally ooze from leech-bites as to cause an immediate prostration of the powers of life amounting to dangerous collapse, with a subsequent anæmia very difficult of cure. Of these facts various emphatic examples are daily presented to me in the instances of invalids returning from India, and the proofs will be furnished in a subsequent portion of this work. From the recorded histories of the cases it is often evident that, where the medical attendant in India intended to abstract the amount of twenty ounces, sixty ounces have been lost, or three times as much as was intended. Now, no medical officer of ordinary education, however young, could look on venesection, and see his patient approach to a sunken condition without immediately tying up the arm; but where leeches have been applied I see very lamentable results from neglect and oozing, the patients being at the time under the general care of very able and experienced medical officers.*   The application of leeches is too often left to relatives and to servants, a contingency which cannot in the nature of things happen in venesection. Besides these considerations, we must remember that leeching cannot produce the same kind of beneficial result on visceral congestions and inflammations as the general abstraction of blood. It is different with external inflammations in which leeches prove supremely beneficial.

When I ordered the application of leeches in the fevers of Bengal, I invariably sent a native dresser to apply the requisite number, with directions to dress the leech-bites so as to preclude any oozing. I would strongly recommend, therefore, that whenever it is proposed to abstract by leeches so much blood as twelve ounces or more, the operation be performed by the lancet instead.

Fevers, idiopathic and symptomatic, are traced by Dr. Billing "to a loss of the functions of the nervous centres, and subsequently of the organs depending on them." Fever, he says, results "from injury to the centres of the nervous system, which arises either from peripheral injury propagated to them, or through lesion by miasm, which, by the route of the circulation, directly poisons them—most probably by chemical combination or alteration— instantaneously lowering their power or energy." I have shown throughout, that the immediate effect of the lowering of the power and energy of the nerves or the nervous system is inflammation, or congestion of the capillaries, the first degree of inflammation. Referring to the treatment, he says:—" If we can relieve his debility of body and mind, the patient will recover from his fever ; that debility we have shown to be caused by an overloaded state of the nervous centres. We uniformly see that the only successful means of relieving them consist in diminishing the injecting force when the pulse is strong, increasing at the same time the contracting action of the capillaries by antimony, mercury, salines, bark, &c. &c., or even when the pulse is not strong, we find bleeding sometimes necessary to diminish the actual quantity of the load, as the constringents alone may not be sufficient to produce contraction, so that, with reference to the indication of bleeding, we have much more to consider the state of plethora of the internal vessels than the state of the pulse or *vis a tergo*.   And though emetic substances have an influence similar to that of bleeding in lowering the *vis a tergo*, they are, nevertheless, of most essential advantage when the pulse is even almost gone, by their immediate constringent effect on the internal capillaries : hence it is evident that the pulse, which was so long considered as the indication for the use of bleeding or sedative medicines, is often no guide at all ; in which cases the necessary practice of sedatives, from having been hitherto unex-

---

* Some surgeons are in the habit of placing cupping-glasses over leech-bites applied on the trunk—a plan which has the effect of abstracting the quantity required rapidly, and of preventing any subsequent oozing.

plained, has always been called indirect practice." This distinguished physician adds, " I do not admit this term, and never practise indirectly ; my indications are always founded upon physiology, as I have explained them up to this point." The doctrines here propounded appear to have anticipated that of Virchow, who refers the primary phenomena of fever to "loss of power in the nerves ;" and likewise that of Traube, who ascribes many of the symptoms of fever to " a weakened, more or less paralytic condition of the vagus." Dr. Handfield Jones has brought much ability and power of observation to bear on this question, in his admirable essays on the operation of malaria.

It has been observed that blood-letting is well borne where the organs of the abdominal cavity are involved in congestion or in- flammation, as compared to the toleration of loss of blood when the lungs are similarly affected. Large quantities of blood are lost by the bowels in typhoid fevers without any sensible depression of the patient; and such persons as suffer from intestinal hæmor- rhage generally recover from this disease.

In the recent controversies respecting the physiological effects and the efficacy of blood-letting, much stress has been placed on the relief afforded by venesection to the oppressed and congested condition of the heart, which is presumed to arise as a consequence of internal inflammation. On such a subject I would not here offer an opinion; but, in reference to tropical diseases generally, and to tropical fevers especially, it is with oppressive congestion of the nervous centres—with malarious poisoning of the foci of organic influence—that we have first to deal. These morbid conditions once overcome, the great abdominal viscera are saved.

PURGATIVES.

When we reflect on the intimate pathological connexion which exists between the stomach, small intestines, and liver, and on the facility with which morbid irritations of the former organs are con- veyed to the latter, when to these circumstances we add the fre- queney with which the liver is congested or inflamed in the course of the febrile movement, we shall be at no loss to perceive how it is that purgatives have at all times been held of high repute in the treatment of the remittent fevers of Bengal. When we regard the intimate nervous and vascular inter-communications of every organ within the abdomen, the one with the other, and that each and all of them are disturbed in their functions during this fever, while some of the organs are more liable than others to become con- gested or inflamed during its progress, we shall be prepared to find that purgatives rank as powerful means in aid of the cure, and such they have always very justly been held to be.

Given in their uncombined forms, and with reference to their special and peculiar actions, they remove retained or vitiated matters from the bowels, thus carrying out of the system sources of contamination, while they promote a more free arterial and venous circulation ; they excite the secreting and excreting functions of the bowels, and by these several actions they produce a sedative effect, while they derive from the head, so as to relieve that cavity, as well as the abdomen, from an oppressive load of congestion. Combined with mercurials they act as cholagogues, and thus relieve the portal circulation from stagnation, and the liver from consequent disease. They rouse the dormant sensibilities of the bowels, and aid in restoring the balance of the general circulation, especially when blood-letting has preceded their administration so as to remove congestions, and thus afford a renewed activity to the functions of secretion. When we consider the certain action of purgative medicines, and that their influence is exerted on the most extensive secreting surface of the human body, we shall at once perceive how powerful must be their effects. By previous depletion, the system is, in fact, prepared for the more free and effective action of this class of remedies, whether exhibited in their simple or combined forms. M. Pierre Campet, Surgeon-in-Chief of the Military Hospital in French Guiana, more than a hundred years ago, observes on this subject, in reference to the dangerous fevers of that colony :—" Toutes ces maladies ne cèdent point d'abord aux purgatifs ; mais elles deviennent plus traitables, lorsqu'on commence par la saignée,"

The compound extract of colocynth, with calomel and James's powder, followed in a few hours by infusion of senna with sulphate of magnesia, or by the compound powder of jalap, is a favourite mode of purgation in this fever. It is usual also to add the sulphate of quina to purging mixtures, so that the tonic and antiperiodic may thus be applied to the whole mucous digestive surface. I found this last an excellent remedy, both in hospital and private practice. Where, in the latter stages of fever, the bowels are torpid and the hypochondria inflated, Robert Jackson recommends a tincture composed of aloes and myrrh, and also the oil of turpentine. He is partial to the use of the tincture ; but the oil of turpentine, he says, while purgative, stimulates the whole alimentary system to the proper exercise of its functions.

DIAPHORETICS.

If the main cure of fever, as stated by Robert Jackson, consists "in turning the tide of circulation to the exterior, in maintaining it there, and thereby disembarrassing the interior organs," the contra-stimulant value of diaphoretics must be great. In the very mild forms of fever a few doses of purgative medicine, with or without mercurials, followed by sudorifics, given so that their action shall be maintained, and by diluents, will cure the disease; but in the more grave cases here under consideration, blood-letting and purging must precede and give effect to the sedative action of diaphoretics by their relaxing effects on the system, and by their reduction of its unnatural heat. As in the instance of purgatives, so with sudorifics—the system must be prepared for their full effects by other and more powerful means.

Minute and repeated doses of tartar emetic have always appeared to me to constitute the best diaphoretics, given simply; but when mercury in any form was added, I then used James's powder in preference.

"All the metallic salts," says Dr. Billing, "have, more or less, an astringent effect on the capillaries ; and to this influence I attribute the universal efficacy of antimony as an antiphlogistic remedy, it being doubly valuable in acute cases from its sedative effects on the heart and pulse, combined with its locally tonic or astringent effects on the capillaries of inflamed or congested·parts, as well as on those of all the secreting structures. Hence, too, its efficacy, in small repeated doses, in cases where there is great depression of the system, by its relieving the relaxation of the capillaries by which the depression is caused. Nay more, we can manage to insure its full antiphlogistic effects without the inconvenience of nausea, by combining it with a little opiate and aromatic."

MERCURY.

Second generally in time of application, and only second in importance as a cholagogue and depurative, and as a means of preparation for other and final measures of cure, comes the action of calomel. When blood-letting shall have produced its results on the circulation, the febrile movement, though subdued, being still in serious progress, we have recourse to this mineral. When properly administered, it is at once the best aid to the abstraction of blood, and the best preparation for the effective action of antiperiodics, such as quinine, arsenic, &c., through its active operation on all the depurative functions. Robert Jackson, though no favourer of mercurial treatment, admits that in fevers complicated with abdominal congestion, calomel is a remedy of the first importance. He says that it repairs mischiefs which no other means with which we are acquainted are capable of touching. This is the simple truth, and it constitutes the reason why this remedy has at all times held so high a place with the practitioners in our worst climates.

As it is better to repeat than to leave an important subject in any doubt, I here beg leave to transcribe from my article on "Hepatitis" a summary of the actions of mercury, and especially of those of calomel:—It is for the very reason that calomel assists powerfully, both in "drawing off" accumulations, and in promoting "*increased secretion*" that it proves of such value in aid of blood-letting. It is, in fact, by this very double action of purging and increasing secretion at the same time, that calomel relieves the loaded and inactive vessels of the diseased gland; not to speak of the other acknowledged physiological influences of this mineral—such as its increase of *all* the secretions and excretions of the body—its influence on the capillary circulation —its febrifuge effect—the peculiar specific power ascribed to it by Gooch and others as an antagonist to inflammations, whether general or local—its stimulant power over the absorbent function —its power of unloading, at the same time that it gives a new im‧pulse to the vascular system—its peculiar power in removing viscid and tenacious intestinal secretions—its alterative, solvent, and antiplastic effects on the blood;—these are the actions and uses ascribed to mercury by the ablest of our physicians and surgeons, and they are such as to place this remedy second only in order and in importance to blood-letting, in all the more acute hepatic affections of India. That mercury enters into intimate union with the elements of the blood is now an ascertained fact. It must, therefore, "modify its plasticity, and influence all the organic functions to which it is subservient." I have only to add here that the above summary is quoted from the former edi‑tion of this work, with commendation, by Dr. Copland, in his article on "Diseases of the Liver."

Dr. Billing, speaking of the treatment of disease by "calomel and opium," says justly, that though powerful allies to the anti‑phlogistic treatment, they have often failed from being employed without being supported by bleeding, or purgative, or emetic, or diaphoretic medicines. This is equally true of tropical diseases, and I have seen enormous quantities of calomel given with no‑thing but evil effect, because its action was not solicited and sup‑ported by previous depletory means.

In the most acute and rapidly fatal of infantile diseases, croup, Dr. West states that, "after the severity of the disease has been subdued by antimony, the time has come for the administration of calomel. From the very commencement of the attack, mercurial inunction may be had recourse to every two or three hours : but the action of mercurials is far too slow to overtake a disease which tends so rapidly to a fatal issue. At this period, however, calomel seems to have a twofold utility ; it counteracts the tendency to the formation of false membrane in the air-passages, and prevents or subdues that inflammation of the lungs which is so frequent and so fatal a complication of this disease."

That the preparation of the subject by previous abstraction of blood is indispensable to the success of mercury and of quinine in the more concentrated fevers of tropical climates, is admitted by all the best practitioners of all times.

It is thus, by regarding each means of cure as constituting a part only of a whole, that we shall best avoid the errors and dangers of relying upon exclusive means in the treatment of dangerous and complicated diseases, and that we shall learn to apportion to each remedy its just value.

At the end of the last and beginning of the present century, calomel was greatly abused in the treatment of tropical diseases; but I think it may be said with truth that, for several years past, this mineral has been used in India sparingly, as a truly remedial agent, and in a scientific manner.

BARK.

Sir James Annesley observes, that visceral disease is the necessary result of the neglect of depletory means, including mercurial purgatives; and that congestions often lead to inflammatory action, especially if bark or arsenic have been freely administered during the stage of congestion, and of disturbed and impeded secretion; and this is in accordance with general experience. Here again we perceive that quina, like other powerful remedies, may not only prove of no effect, but may be administered so as actually to be injurious. The extreme of right, says an ancient maxim, is often the extreme of wrong; and quina may do signal good, or even prove hurtful, according as the patient may or may not have been prepared for the action of the bark.

"The too hasty use of bark," was condemned by Huxham in his day. He prepared the system for its best effects by previous bleeding, purging, vomiting, and the use of attenuants. "Never be too hasty in giving bark, or chalybeates, where the patient hath *a yellow cast of countenance, a tense abdomen,* and a very costive habit of body." And these just views have continually been urged by the best writers and practitioners of tropical climates, down to our own day. Dr. Kenneth Mackinnon, speaking of the exclusive treatment by heroic doses of quinine, says that we have no proof that the formidable fevers of India can be safely or successfully treated without blood-letting, purgatives, and other antiphlogistic means. Nor can this be proved until it be shown first that the endemic fevers of the country have changed their types and complications; and then, of course, treatment must conform to the altered circumstances of the disease. Meanwhile, and until a remedy of equal or of superior power shall be found, we may safely affirm that, properly applied, the cure of severe malarious fever, always difficult with quinine, is indeed imposssible without it.

To apportion the dose and determine the right time for exhibiting it, so as to secure the full tonic and antiperiodic influences of the quina, we must appreciate accurately the circumstances in each individual case, the stage of the fever, and the effect of the previous antiphlogistic means. The stage of remission or of abatement of fever is naturally chosen for the exhibition of tonics and antiperiodics, because of the then diminished force of diseased action, and of the nearer approach to a natural condition of the functions. Generally speaking, the quinine is exhibited throughout India in accordance with the judicious rules propounded by Cullen.   The random exhibition of quina by timid, careless, reckless, or inex- perienced practitioners does infinite harm; and, in former times, when bark alone was relied upon for the cure of all tropical fevers, the results were deplorable.   The exclusive and all but uniform success claimed for bark by Balfour, Clark, and others among the older writers, is only another instance out of many of the laxity in classification, in manner of recording, and in narration, in their times.

Where, with a state of general plethora, visceral congestions remain unsubdued, or only partially removed, the secretions being scanty and depraved, with the pulse full and hard, and the skin constricted, dry, and hot, the time for the exhibition of bark has not yet arrived.   Robert Jackson says that bark is not to be re- lied on for the precipitate arrest of remittent fever, either in the West Indies or in other countries.   Bark and the disulphate of quina are efficacious in arresting the remittent fever of Bengal when venous congestions have been overcome by previous deple- tory means, when the pulse has been reduced in force and fre- quency, when the secretions are in free action, and the skin re- laxed; when these preparatory results have been obtained, we may then be sure of establishing the antiperiodic influence of quina with the best effect, and without risk of producing any injury. It then becomes a sovereign remedy; and the nearer the patient can be brought to the state of remission, the surer will be the operation of the antiperiodic.   It must now be given in full doses, so as speedily to establish its influence.   The amount of dose, and the frequency with which it is to be repeated, will depend on the nature of the fever;—where paroxysms are violent, or where the sufferer is in a malarious locality, the doses should be large, and often repeated.   It is better to exhibit the quinine in five- grain doses, often repeated, than to give scruple doses as recom- mended by some writers; for by the former plan we have the ad- vantage of observing the effects as we proceed, and we can with- hold excessive doses.

"Quinine," says Dr. Bence Jones, "acts in weakening the pulse in a similar way to arsenic, hydrocyanic acid, opium, and other narcotics, antimony, and nitre."

Quoting the general conclusions of M. Briquet, he adds :—

" (1.) That the maximum diminution of the pulse is rarely twenty to twenty-five pulsations a minute, even in typhoid fever.

" (2.) That the diminution is always in direct relation to the previous frequency of the pulse.

" (3.) That the reduction is never below forty beats a minute.

" (4.) That much fibrin in the blood, or active inflammation, prevents the depression.

" (5.) That large doses of quinine produce so serious a perturbation of the economy that they should not be given unless the
illness, as regards length, seriousness, and accidents, is sufficiently
important."

With regard to the pathological action of quinine, M. Briquet
considers :—

" (1.) That it does not act directly on the marsh poison.

" (2.) That it does not act on the general state of the organs, or
on the blood; but it has especial action on the nervous system—
C'est la médecine du quitte au double, celle que les militaires em-
ploient quand pour couper la fièvre ils avalent une double ration
d'eau de vie chaude mêlé de poudre à canon.

" (3.) It does not act by increasing the vital forces or by sustaining them.

" (4.) It is not by a tonic action, or an astringent action, or a
stimulant action, but by a sedative stupifiant action that it acts on
the marsh poison.

" Lastly. The absorption of quinine by a sound skin is very
doubtful."

In the administration of arsenic for the cure of lepra, and in the
uses of the same mineral and of quina in the cure of intermittents,
" we can trace no known relation between the physiological effects
of the remedies and their therapeutic influences :" we know the
ultimate facts, and the general facility of the cure. But the
exhibition of quina in exaggerated doses, as recommended by some
writers, implies, besides other errors, no reference or application to
peculiarity of habit and constitution, in certain states of which such
inordinate doses of a powerful nervine tonic produce stimulant and
irritant effects, disturbing the functions of the stomach, causing
disorders of the alimentary canal, as shown by thirst, constipation, or purging; disorders also of the cerebro-spinal system, as
evinced by throbbing headache, giddiness, deafness, &c.

That the quinic intoxication, whether acute or chronic, is not a
harmless result of overdosing, is a fact that has frequently come
under my observation. Several officers who had been treated in
India with half-drachm doses of quinine, often repeated, have not
recovered at home from the resulting cerebral and general nervous
disturbance until a residence of two years there. In New Orleans
" blindness, deafness, and insanity," frequently followed what the
doctors there termed "*the abortive treatment* of yellow fever by
enormous doses of quinine." We must hold, therefore, in repect
of quinine as of any other remedy, that the dose (homely as the
doctrine may appear), should be so much as shall cure the disease,
and no more. To administer more is surely unphilosophical and
unpractical, all authorities condemning the large and long-continued use of powerful remedies. But it is to be feared that until
the medical profession shall become more generally well-informed
as to the real nature of diseased action, and as to the physiological

influences of medicine upon it, feebleness, timidity, and foolhardiness will continue alternately to disfigure the practice of our art.

In the use of Peruvian bark and its preparations we have seen that of old, as now, some tropical practitioners proceeded so as to afford their patients too much of a good thing—too much even of quina—to which, then as now, men of limited and exclusive means betook themselves, after the fashion of the one-remedy-man. Here, as in other instances, we find, in fact, that the exaggeration of an acknowledged truth may cause as much harm as the practice of an acknowledged error.

Campet, writing of the fevers of French Guiana, says that cinchona is the best known febrifuge; but that experience has abundantly made known certain evils which the remedy is capable of producing, when exhibited à contre-tems; that is, when given to arrest fever before the patient has been freely evacuated. In such circumstances he states that it arrests the secretions, produces visceral obstructions, and at length dropsies. His conclusion, as applicable to-day as it was in 1754, may prove worthy the attention of certain persons in the Eastern as in the Western Hemisphere: " Eh! quel remède ne devient pas dangereux administré par de certaines mains."

Quinine, the great febrifuge, justly administered, acts purely as a nerve-tonic to the cerebro-spinal and visceral sympathetic systems: exhibited in extravagant doses, it is toxical and not therapeutic. Its free use, indeed, should be guardedly considered before exhibition, and carefully watched in its effects afterwards. " Given in large doses," says Dr. Hughes Bennett, " quinine produces very inconvenient effects, cephalalgia, vertigo, tinnitus aurium, deafness, and other symptoms, which, should any cerebral complication exist, would render it fatal;" and death in this manner he witnessed at La Pitié, from "acute meningitis, with exudation of lymph on the membranes."

The exhibition of quinine in liberal doses, suited to the urgency of the occasion, was no uncommon circumstance in my own practice in Calcutta; and one instance out of many I will here relate. My late distinguished friend, Mr. John Turner, of the Bengal army, at the time surgeon to Lord William Bentinck, was seized with severe remittent fever. On the morning of the fifth day, finding himself in a state of dangerous collapse, accompanied by the most violent hiccup I ever witnessed, he despaired of recovery and refused all medicine, believing that a fatal termination was at hand. This fearful condition increased up to eight p.m., when the countenance and expression were quite cadaveric, his limbs cold and soddened, the pulse in the extremities extinct, and the hiccup terrible to behold. He was now at length induced, by the urgent entreaty of friends, to use the quinine solution, which I had early in the morning prepared. He took it every two hours through the night, and by five o'clock the following morning he had . taken a drachm of the drug. The hiccup had entirely ceased, circulation and warmth were restored to the extremities, and he rapidly recovered. This occurred in Calcutta in 1833.

The advocates of the exclusive treatment of remittent fever by enormous doses of quina, in their eagerness to effect an immediate cure, overleap their object, and overlook the visceral disease which so often takes the place of the fancied cure. A wise man cele-brated by Bacon was wont to caution those who were in too great haste to come to a conclusion, by saying—" Stay a little, that we may make an end the sooner;" and so it is with those who remove visceral engorgements before having recourse to antiperiodics— they, in reality, are those who stay a little, in order to make an end the sooner, and the surer.

ARSENIC.

This mineral acts as a powerful nerve-tonic and antiperiodic, ranking in these qualities next to the cinchona. But its most signal benefits are experienced in the sequel to remittents and intermittents; cases of an asthenic nature, where the patient suffers from irregular forms of fever. Arsenic has been used from time immemorial in Hindustan by the native doctors; and I saw at the Native Hospital of Calcutta daily examples of permanent injury to the circulating system, and to the mucous digestive organs, from the abuse of this mineral by the Bazar practitioners in their endeavours to cure fevers, rheumatisms, and venereal diseases. "Arsenic," says Dr. Billing, "often acts as equivalent to a union of bark and mercury; for arsenic, besides its tonic effect on the nervous system, increases the secretion of bile, and otherwise acts on the liver; it possesses also the power, like mercury, of curing chronic inflammations; and even further resembles it in occasionally producing the inconvenience of salivation."

We should commence the use of this mineral in small doses, and not persist many days in its exhibition; in fever not beyond eight or ten days. If, besides its tonic and antiperiodic effects, it acts "on the liver as much as mercury," according to the last-named authority, we should hold this remedy in more regard in India than we now do. It is one that may safely be administered during the paroxysm of fever; and the number of days stated is sufficient to test its virtues. In the practice of the medical officers in the East Indies, in so far as the fevers of the country are con-cerned, the exhibition of the arsenical preparations is almost ex-clusively confined by them to the intermittent forms; and, even in these, arsenic is far from being in general use.

Mr. John Turner, of the Bombay army, has since 1841 exhibited the Fowler's solution in fevers, remittent and intermittent, in doses every two hours, of from twelve to thirteen minims. This is done during the apyrexy, as we are assured in official reports, with unusually successful effect.

M. Frémy gives an account of 316 cases of ague treated at the Military Hospital, Roule, near Paris. Of these 106 were cured by arsenic, not having been subjected to prior treatment; and 158 after quinine had failed. The following are the conclusions he draws:—

1. The use of arsenic in ague is of very ancient date; but it was in the seventeenth century that its employment became, so to say, popular in Germany, England, and India. At the present day it is habitually used as a preservative of health by the inhabitants of the Tyrol and the southern provinces of China, where tobacco is always mixed with it. Moreover, most of the mineral waters of high repute, especially those of Vichy, Mont d'Or, Neris, Plombières, &c., contain very notable quantities of arsenic. Thus, when administered with care, it should not be regarded as a hurtful or poisonous substance.

2. Arsenious acid will cure intermittent fever, its influence not only being exerted on the return of the paroxysms, but also on the hypertrophy of the spleen, which it rapidly and certainly reduces to its normal size.

3. The arsenic should be given in doses of twenty-five milligrammes (a millig. is one-seventieth gr.), dissolved in weak white wine and water, or it may be given in doses of from 40 to 80 millig. in glysters. Fowler's solution produces the same effects.

4. Not the slightest symptom of poisoning has been met with; and several patients have borne the increase of the dose to fifty-five millig., or to 250 in lavements, without inconvenience.

5. The statistics here produced were derived from observations made in the hospital between June and October, 1855, and corroborate the results of prior observation.

6. It is an error to say that arsenic should be preferred to quinine. It will completely cure cases that have resisted quinine; but it is only preferable to this substance from its great cheapness, which is a point for consideration in country practice, where the poverty of his patients disarms the practitioner. It is well, however, to note that quinine sometimes gives rise to serious symptoms, so that several patients prefer bearing the fever rather than go on taking it.

7. The fevers here treated were all old cases, the majority being instances of relapse.

8. The patients who took arsenic soon acquired flesh, and a considerable appetite. They became active, and the skin assumed a rose-colour, and a peculiar freshness of appearance.

9. Arsenious acid seems to have the advantage over quinine, in rendering relapses less frequent and more delayed.—*Moniteur des Hôp.* No. 20.

I find myself during the last ten or twelve years continually prescribing arsenic; not that I have a preference for it over quinine, but that invalids say—" I hope, sir, that you are not going to order quinine for me; it is of no use. I have taken so much of it that it has ceased to stop my fever, while it produces indescribable distress." Thus, through over-dosing—by the abuse of a really superior remedy, and by the consequent intoxication and disgust of the patient, I am often driven to prescribe arsenic, and find it indeed a noble remedy.

WINE.

In the treatment of the ordinary remittent fevers of Bengal wine has little to do; for unless a tendency to collapse occur, with profuse sweats, an anxious countenance, a laborious respiration, a cold damp skin, and sunken pulse, we have not to exhibit spirituous or vinous stimulants. On the occurrence of collapse, however, diffusible stimulants are invaluable, and they are always resorted to. In cases where the cure is delayed for many days, either from neglect of early treatment, or from constitutional peculiarity, wine is occasionally requisite. But whether in recent or in protracted cases, the tendency to sinking is the event to be carefully watched; and then the wine should be given, with or without soup or farinaceous food, according to circumstances, and with quina in the intervals. Wine and spirits must be regarded as simple stimulants; they do not change the course of events in periodic fevers. This is so much the case that, after the use of wine, we may in the next coming paroxysms have to use antiphlogistic means:—such are some of the difficulties to be encountered in the management of this formidable disease.

In some forms of continued fever, and in certain malignant periodic fevers, Robert Jackson admits of the use of wine; but he says that the application must be nicely adjusted. Champagne he considers a good wine for the occasion; and porter, he adds, is relished by the British soldier.

OPIUM.

Opium is a means for much good or for serious evil, just as we may apply it. Its physiological actions are of great value as repressive of nervous irritability, and consequently of vascular action; while morphia is held by many to possess antiphlogistic power. Used in stimulating doses I have seen opium prove of great value, under two circumstances not uncommon in the progress of remittent fever. The first is, the disposition to faintness or to profuse perspiration after blood-letting. Here half a grain or more of opium with calomel, or tincture of opium with chloric ether, given with the calomel, will relieve from vascular and nervous depression, and rouse and restore the patient. The other occasion is when, after the use of depletory means, the hard-living patient, or the man habituated to the free use of various stimulants, begins to feel the depressing effects of fever, and of active treatment, and of the absence of the accustomed exciting beverages;—then it is that symptoms of nervous exhaustion come to be complicated with the existing fever, so as frequently to constitute a masked or subdued delirium tremens.   There is here great danger, in the hands of the inexperienced or the inattentive.   Depletory measures would now destroy the patient; whereas opium, applied in a moderate dose, at the right time, calms while it restores the sunken nervous functions, and the patient is saved.   The calming influence of opium on the cerebro-spinal system, and on the sympathetic and vaso-motor nerves, must not be forgotten.   Given in the manner proposed, and for the occasion only, conjoined with calomel in mild doses, the opium imparts its influence to the nervous system, without locking up the secretions—an important reserve in the case before us.

COLCHICUM.

This powerful drug is valuable in itself, on account of its purgative and eliminant qualities.   It assists the cholagogue and diuretic action of calomel, rendering, by these actions, the dose of the mineral less than might otherwise be necessary.   The power of colchicum in reducing articular inflammation is such that it must be regarded as a valuable aid in all sthenic affections, whether febrile or inflammatory.

BLISTERS.

Blisters are of much service in the middle and later stages of severe remittent fevers.   Used subsequently to measures of general and local depletion, they relieve cerebral and abdominal complications, and help the cure of the sequelæ to acute congestive and inflammatory affections within those cavities.   Employed with judgment, they exercise a powerful derivation, and abate morbid, while they rouse defective sensibility.   Robert Jackson applied blisters largely—often to the shaved scalp.

THE DIET.

While fever runs high, with or without complication, there can hardly be any question as to the diet—nature demanding the use of cooling diluents, which are all that the case requires.   But, as the fever advances, and the powers of life retrograde—especially where collapse threatens—then farinaceous articles and thin broths become necessary, in aid of stimulants, tonics, and antiperiodics. Such aids from diet will be more particularly demanded where the patient is anæmic, reduced in his constitutional powers, or of long residence in India.   The careful practitioner will be on his guard against the advent of exhaustion, and he will not delay the use of such restorative means till he sees his patient sinking. All that is here suggested in respect of diet in fever applies with equal, if not greater force to that proper to low types of dysentery.

Finally.—Let the young medical officer consult with his superiors early in the progress of remittent fever. Whenever obscure or doubtful symptoms may appear, let the ablest of his brethren be consulted *at once*. Such a course of open, honourable, and humane conduct will bring with it external indications of esteem and respect, while to the young surgeon it will impart internal comfort and peace. To defer consultation until stupor, abdominal tumidity, and induration have occurred, is to incur a fearful responsibility, if not disgrace. Such a deferred consultation may gratify the fancy and caprice of female relatives, but it cannot rescue the young medical officer from the severest blame.

Let it be said of the young surgeon as of Edmund Burke— that he read everything, saw everything, and foresaw everything. In the medical profession, indeed, no man is deserving the public confidence who is not a hard student and a careful practitioner every day of his life; and to this rule I have never known an exception. We none of us know how much of our actual knowledge we owe to study—how much to our own observation; for, without previous study and training, what would be the value of the observation and experience of the best of us; and, generally, the obtrusive pretender to originality in writing and practising will be found but very ill or very partially informed both in the science and practice of medicine—an original blunderer, in fact.* This is especially true of everything which relates to the great subject of fever; a subject so difficult that "it is remarkable how entirely the most distinguished physicians of all ages who have treated of this subject, coincide in the feeling that, with regard to this important class of disease, it is impossible, in the short life allotted to the most aged, to do anything more than add a little to the common stock." Let the best of us but try to separate, with a singleness and truth of purpose, what amount of knowledge he has acquired from others from what he has learned for himself, and the result will certainly not be a pretension to originalities, novelties, or discoveries. To attain a just estimate and balance of doctrine and of practice is what now constitutes a good physician.

The greatest histories must in great part consist in compilation; and all medical writing, to be worthy, must consist in the history of what is known from one age to another.

---

* "What you don't know, sir, would fill a large book," is especially applicable to such discoverers.

APPLICATION OF REMEDIAL MEANS TO THE INDIVIDUAL CASE.

After the general view of the various therapeutic agents employed in the treatment of fever, and of their effects, we come to consider their joint and several applications to the individual patient suffering from the remittent fever of Bengal ; and here we find, on experience, that the first and most immediate object is to reduce the force and frequency of arterial action during the paroxysm, which, if allowed to go on unrestrained, would, in the severer examples, injure or destroy some organ essential to life.

If the patient be seen in the forenoon, on the accession of the first, second, or third paroxysm of ordinary remittent fever, if he is of a sound constitution and not beyond middle life, blood-letting from the arm, while the patient is in the recumbent posture, should be practised to the extent of relieving the sufferer from præcordial oppression, from visceral fulness and congestion, or from the intensity of headache, whichever may predominate. If along with reduced force and frequency of the blood-current, and reduction of the morbid temperature, we obtain from the operation a gentle relaxation of the skin, we have the best evidence of relief from visceral congestion, whether the operation be performed for the cure of fever, dysentery, or hepatitis ; the quantity of blood abstracted being regulated by the effect, and not by an arbitrary measure in ounces. It will sometimes happen, however, from peculiarity of habit or other causes, and notwithstanding the utmost circumspection, that the relaxation of the skin will proceed to sweating, with symptoms of depression of the vital powers ; then from half a grain to a grain of opium, or from fifteen to twenty minims of laudanum, with as many of chloric ether, should be administered. This will impart tone to the heart's action, and soothe the nervous excitement, while it will allay gastric and intestinal irritation. It is only in cases of depression, however, such as this, that opium is to be recommended in the very early treatment of fever ; but, when requisite, it will be found to calm both mind and body. Let the physiology of the disease, and the habit and condition of the patient guide the application of remedies, and we shall approach as nearly to the correct measure of means of cure as human endeavour can compass.

Unless the fever assume a severe form, one general blood-letting, practised as stated, in the recumbent posture, and under the studied observation of just time and of effect will, on the average, be found sufficient to relieve the patient from abdominal or cerebral oppression. Blood-letting, used as here directed, will be found to simplify the application of all the subsequent means of cure ; and where the fever is not of the most concentrated form, one sufficient abstraction of blood is much to be preferred to repetitions of the operation—a practice depressing to the constitution, and occasionally perversive of the type of the existing fever. Within an hour after the bleeding, a dose of calomel, with compound extract of colocynth and James's powder, should be exhibited, followed in two hours by a powerful cathartic, such as infusion of senna with sulphate of magnesia. After the free action of these remedies we shall obtain in the afternoon some degree of remission; and the patient should be directed to take, at bedtime, from six to ten grains of calomel, with four of James's powder, if the skin be dry. Here, within eight or ten hours of first seeing the patient, we perceive that, of the means above generally described, blood-letting, mercury, a sudorific, and a purgative have been used, while the patient has been allowed free recourse to cooling diluents.

On the early morning visit of the following day the patient will probably be found in a more complete state of remission, when the sulphate of quina alone, or in combination with the purging mixture, should be freely and repeatedly administered;—given in this latter manner the quina applies itself to the whole extent of the mucous digestive surface, so as to give full effect to its tonic and antiperiodic influences; and a larger dose of it can thus be borne in the early stage of fever than if given without the purgative. This is an important consideration; for the quina rightly administered will arrest the progress of a mild fever, and save the life of the patient in a severe one, by mitigating the fever and its morbid associations.

By the forenoon the paroxysm may recur in a milder degree, though to such an extent as to demand the application of leeches to the epigastric region, if any oppression or fulness exist there, or behind the ears if there be headache; while a mixture composed of antimonial wine with the acetate and nitrate of potash should be given every two hours, so as to soften the skin and determine increased action of the kidneys. Robert Jackson, in treating the remittent fevers of Jamaica, exhibited a combination of nitre, camphor, emetic tartar, and opium, and he speaks of it as a means to the efficacy of which he can bear testimony. But I think that, in general, diuretics of the class of *renal depurants* are to be preferred, such as the acetates, citrates, and tartrates of soda and potass. These remedies not only increase the volume of water excreted by the kidneys, but they are believed likewise, by a direct chemical action, to increase the metamorphosis of tissue.

It is usual, in the remittent fevers of Bengal, to give from five to ten grains of calomel, with or without antimonial powder, at bedtime, followed in the early morning by an active purge, and when the last is under operation, quinine in solution is given freely. This is a good practice, and a sufficient means in itself to cure some of the milder forms of the fever under consideration:—preceded by an adequate abstraction of blood, this practice will even cure a severe fever. ·Thus, under the favourable circumstances contemplated, we witness the daily decline of the disease, and the daily diminishing occasion, therefore, for the use of active measures of cure, until towards the third, fifth, seventh, or ninth day, convalescence is completely established.

In treating the more ordinary remittent fever we have thus, very much in the order of detail previously described, to use—blood-letting at the forenoon accession ; cold, affusive, or tepid sponging, when proper to the case; cooling diluent drinks ; saline diaphoretics, refrigerants, and diuretics, during the mid-day and afternoon exacerbation; calomel with antimony, at bedtime, or with opium, as the particular case may require ; a powerful purgative in the very early morning, followed immediately by, or taken along with, the quinine ;—all intended to subdue morbid actions, to assuage and anticipate the coming paroxysm ; wine and diffusible stimulants when collapse approaches or occurs. Such are the means, and such the proper order of their administration. The whole subject must be earnestly weighed and determined : whatever the surgeon does must be in earnest, even where he is most cheerfully confident. Earnestness is the soul of enterprise and of success in this as in all human affairs.

If remittent fever has existed unrestrained, however, for several days, and the patient is not seen till the accession of the third or fourth paroxysm, or even later, provided the general powers of the constitution remain uninjured, a general blood-letting is still the principal means to save life, followed by calomel, purgatives, antimonials and refrigerants, and quinine, in the manner previously indicated. But if, on the other hand, the duration of the disease being as above, the paroxysms have become indistinct, running into each other with but brief or ill-defined intervals, while abdominal or cerebral complications arise, as indicated by epigastric fulness with anguish, or by approaching stupor or delirium, congestion now wearing the aspect of inflammation ; then the time and manner of applying our more active means demand the nicest care to insure, not only their just effects, but their safety. Blood-letting may even now constitute the principal means to save life, but the blood must be guardedly abstracted, whether generally or locally; and calomel becomes indeed a remedy of necessity, as Robert Jackson would rather refuse to call it, in the treatment of the fevers of the West. To save the patient from impending dangers, in the case of unrestrained fever here contemplated, the medical officer must be neither rash nor supine : sinking would result from the rash application of means, and effusion into one or both cavities involved in those fevers would be the result of timidity or indecision. Generally speaking the blood must here be abstracted by leeches at the accession of the paroxysm ; antimonials must be used—cold must be applied to the shaved head—sinapisms and blisters must be applied ; but on the influence of calomel chief reliance must be placed. It must be given every three or four hours, with an occasional mild aperient in the intervals, until the dangerous symptoms shall have yielded; and this favourable state is often observed to be coincident with the mercurial influence, as evidenced in the odour of the breath, or on the gums. Dangerous symptoms such as are here described will sometimes arise suddenly, without any loss of time, or without any neglect in the treatment; and when such conditions are associated with yellowness of the skin, in persons broken in health, or of a feeble constitution, or of dissipated habits of life, or who may have undergone much mental distress, the chances of a fatal termination are imminent.

In the remittent, as in all forms of periodic fever, the stages of danger are those of the accession and of the decline of the paroxysm : in the first, the violence of arterial action may proceed at once, unless restrained by treatment, to destroy life by serous effusion; while in the second, so great a prostration of the vital powers may succeed to the previous tumult of vascular action, as to terminate in a feeble and irregular pulse, a damp coldness of the surface and of the extremities, despair, and death. I have seen one paroxysm of Bengal remittent fever, and of jungle fevers, cause death in each of these ways, within twelve hours; and the first instance, attended with very painful circumstances, occurred within a few months of my arrival in India. A young officer was seized with fever at 11 A.M.; but nevertheless he went into the China bazaar of Calcutta. He returned to his quarters in Fort William at 3 P.M., and placed himself under the care of a staff surgeon there. He was bled at 4, and he was dead at 7 P.M. The same operation, practised at noon, would probably have put an end to the fever.

When the spleen is affected with enlargement, either of the acute or chronic nature, mercury in all forms had better be avoided in the treatment of the fever ; for there is in the splenic complication a dissolved condition of the blood, with general cachexia, that should preclude the use of this powerful mineral. Bloodletting, general or local, when found necessary, should be cautiously used, and carefully regulated in these cases; and the oozing from leech-bites should be carefully and promptly arrested.

It is necessary to be on our guard against irregularities in the paroxysms of remittent fever, as they occasionally vary not only in their time of accession, but there may arise a double or anticipating night paroxysm, in addition to that of the forenoon. This will require a double attention, especially in respect of the time of visiting the patient and of using remedies.

A close observation is indeed necessary as to every event and circumstance which may arise in the course of these fevers; for upon the amount and accuracy of such knowledge will depend not only the selection and application of our means of cure, but the affixing of the proper time for using them—often a vital question.

The result of each paroxysm on the cerebral and abdominal organs should also be carefully noted; for by this knowledge we regulate both the force of our remedial means, and the frequency with which their application may be needed. Through such observations, also, we come to estimate aright the powers and capabilities of the patient; for the greater the number of paroxysms, the more the viscera are likely to be oppressed and congested, and the less power consequently do we find in the patient either to sustain him under further invasions of fever, or to bear him well through the operations of the necessary remedies. In such a case there will be a tendency to exhaustion, and, while we act with decision and calmness, we must be doubly watchful of effect. During life, even in persons of the sanguine temperament, we can neither measure the degrees of congestion or of inflammation existing in the organs of the abdominal or cerebral cavity, nor can we at all determine when or where congestion ends and inflammation begins. We must therefore relieve the congestion or the inflammation at the earliest possible moment, by active depletory or depurating means, using antiperiodics afterwards, without waiting for the settlement of theoretical or nice distinctions, whether of pathology or therapeutics. This doctrine applies with an especial force to the cerebral complications of plethoric Europeans recently arrived in tropical climates. In persons of an anæmic habit, again, whether young or middle-aged, whether of long residence or recently arrived in India, it is obvious that we ought not to deplete, and that we cannot actively depure. The tonic and antiperiodic treatment, therefore, with moderate nutriment, is that which is best calculated to guide the anæmic sufferer from remittent fever and its complications to a successful issue. The distinctions referring to the morbid states of the blood, and the varying treatments suited to them, require the most careful consideration on the part of all who practise in tropical climates.

I have preferred a simple narrative of the treatment of remittent fever, such as is here presented, to a detail of hospital or other cases; for I have seen that, in the treatment of fevers and other acute diseases, cases are too often seized upon and followed out to the letter, by young medical officers, to the disregard of the differences of circumstances, and to the exclusion of reason and reflection on the cases before them. Cases thus become a kind of pattern in routine, and the young naval and military surgeon is injured where it was intended to afford him help. He is thrown off his reasoning powers by an array of cases, and enticed into a groove of routine, from which it will require much exertion and firmness on his own part to extricate him. A case-book thus, while it purports to be a guide for the treatment of dangerous, varying, and violently acute diseases, carries with it, when used in the manner stated, sources of weakness, even to those whom it intends to benefit. It is otherwise in the ect of chronic lesions, the results of acute tropical diseases, in whic the constitution of the patient and the symptoms are at once more subdued, brought more into a common level, rendered thus less variable, and for the management of which ample time is given to the inexperienced for consideration of means, for reflection on their effects, and for consultation with the elders of the profession.

In chronic disease, again, no sudden changes occur, as the result of youth, constitution, influence of season, or of epidemic conditions —all which exercise powerful, immediate, and varying effects in acute disease.

We cannot put off to the morrow the treatment of a case of fever, dysentery, hepatitis, or cholera; duty requires that we should act on the instant; and to do so with justice to the patient requires at least a knowledge of general pathology and of the principles of medicine : we should not have to rely on a guide or casebook.

A detail of cases, describing the fevers and dysenteries of particular seasons and localities, will not represent faithfully or truly the fevers and dysenteries of other localities and seasons; neither can the treatment which may have been found applicable to the first-named, prove always justly so to the second. A careful detail of symptoms, and a treatment founded on general pathology and on general therapeutic principles, can alone represent remittent and intermittent fevers and dysenteries. Surgeons who purpose to deal with general principles, never write out prescriptions, and for good reasons : all treatment by means of medicines is but provisional; and the very reputation of many drugs is very variable and very much matter of fashion. Nothing, therefore, but well-founded principles can represent that just reason which, as our greatest historian assures us, is the same in all countries and in all ages.

Huxham, writing of the fevers of his time, says :—" I have given few or no FORMULÆ OR PRESCRIPTIONS; for, as Hippocrates says, he that knows the disease knows what is proper to its cure." This is, in fact, but giving expression in other words to the dictum of Rostan—that all medicine consists in diagnosis.

It is not by a routine detail of cases and of set formulæ that we may hope to advance those general principles of theory and practice which can alone give assurance and sanction to the name of Medical Philosophy—those principles of thought, observation, and conduct which, according to Sir Henry Holland, may most conduce to the progress of medicine, and to the honour and usefulness of those who profess it. Finally, fevers, endemic and epidemic, are frequently changing their types, but recorded cases always remain the same.

MANAGEMENT OF CONVALESCENCE.

I cannot conclude these observations without adverting to the importance of the management of convalescence from fevers, remittent and intermittent—not the least serious of the duties imposed on the naval and military surgeon. In all cases of recovery from fever, but especially in those wherein the complications have been severe, or where important organs have been affected in the course of the fever, or as a sequel to it, it is impossible to be too careful in the diet, and in attention to the activity of the secreting functions; and this vigilance must not be relaxed until perfect health shall be established. How often do we see patients who have been sufficiently well treated during the acute stages of diseases, but on whom a neglect of this important rule of practice has entailed enlargement of the liver and spleen, or other visceral diseases, requiring a protracted voyage at sea, or a return to Europe. I have, both in India and at home, seen much injury done by a too liberal and protracted use of quinine in convalescence accompanied by abdominal congestion. In such cases, and under such treatment, the liver often becomes swollen and painful, and the mucous digestive surface red and irritated. The proper treatment for such states is an emulgent and alterative course of treatment by alkalies with taraxacum, or by the nitro-muriatic acid bath, using a spare diet, and having recourse to change of air. In convalescence from fever and dysentery, quinine is very beneficial, if given in small doses and during a short period only, but when we exceed this measure we aggravate congestion, and sometimes we even produce it.

The just management of convalescence is a subject that should always be present to the minds of those who have the regulation and control of naval and military hospitals, wherein the perfect re-establishment of the sailor's and soldier's health, before their return to duty, should be a maxim never to be swerved from. It must not be supposed that with the medical management of acute diseases our duties towards those intrusted to our care have terminated.

It ought to be in the recollection, also, of medical officers, that, after every serious or protracted illness, the blood is necessarily impoverished—that all the organs and their respective functions are as necessarily enfeebled, sometimes nearly exhausted. To send a soldier in such a condition to the temptations, the diet, and the duties of the barrack, is an injury to the service, and a cruelty to the individual.

A small sick-list is pleasing to commanding officers, but the discharging of men from hospital in a partial state of convalescence, is a crime in the surgeon. The *medicina mentis*, and the benefits to be derived from change of air, ought to be as available to the soldier as to the officer; but they are matters that scarcely receive from us the attention they deserve from their great importance. In the latter stages of remittent fever, when the patient does not convalesce, owing to a slight feverishness towards evening, with warmth of the head, followed by restless nights and by increasing debility, then it is that the astonishing benefits derivable from change of air, and of gestation in the open air, are manifested. They save the patient's life ; and many are worn out and die for want of them, because the friends and relatives, and perhaps the medical attendants too, consider the patient "too weak to be moved." I never saw the fever patient that was too weak to be moved at the proper time ; and it should be remembered that movement does not here mean violence.

During the severe and fatal remittent fever of 1833 in Bengal, an eminent member of the Bench fell into the condition here referred to, so that I had little hope of his recovery ; and I directed his removal to sea. My friend, the late Mr. John Turner, the most able in the management of fever of any man I have ever known, said :—" You are mistaken in this instance ; he is so feeble that he will die before he reaches the boat, and all the people of Calcutta will declare that you have killed the Chief Justice." I persisted, nevertheless ; and the removal to the river, which was about 500 yards distant, was accomplished without accident. But, in the act of being hoisted from the boat into a 74-gun ship at Khidgeree, notwithstanding my warnings to the contrary, the head and shoulders were raised to near the sitting posture, when the patient fell back in a fainting condition, which for some minutes looked like death. But from this sunken state he recovered rapidly in the fresh breeze ; and in ten days he reached Madras, whence he was reported to be eating mutton chops. I have always been of opinion that but for the timely removal from malarious influences, this distinguished gentleman must have died.

Next to the benefits to be derived from early and effective treatment, come those which secure and maintain convalescence ; and this truth will be found to apply whether we refer to organized bodies of men, or to individuals. It is to the mismanagement of convalescence principally that we must refer the numerous and fatal relapses in the fevers and dysenteries of our seamen and soldiers, not to speak of ill health contracted through the sequelæ to those diseases, in the form of visceral affections. In India I have continually seen that almost all the relapses in fever, so often fatal to the soldier, were caused by mismanagement of the stage of convalescence, and by his too early discharge from hospital.

The mean age of a British regiment may be taken to be twenty-six years—a stage of life when the rallying powers of the constitution may be assumed to be at their acme, and when, therefore, the tendency of nature towards convalescence is at its height. But in the individual cases of older men, and with such of the

A A

young men as have been exhausted by the violence of disease and the activity of depletory measures of cure, wine, porter, and bitter tonics will be requisite, together with more time, and a longer exemption from duty, for the purpose of maturing health. This latter consideration is of great importance.

It is true that the authority of the naval and military surgeon does not extend beyond the hospital; but better days than those of Robert Jackson are coming, both for the soldier and the surgeon. Humanity is now at length pretty sure to have a powerful press on its side; and no governor or commander, by sea or land, can any longer venture to do or leave undone, the things which I have seen done and left undone.

When the disease is endemic, whether it be fever, dysentery, or hepatitis, the first means towards maturing convalescence, and obtaining the complete restoration of health is—a removal from the local and endemic influences.

This measure, coupled with great attention to diet, clothing, exercise, and bathing, will fill the ranks with healthy soldiers; while leaving them in crowded or otherwise unhealthy hospitals is too often but condemning them to wait for death. In all our intertropical possessions we should establish convalescent depôts, conveniently situated; and where practicable they should be in some near mountain range, or other elevated ground, or in well-selected positions on the sea, which latter are, I think, always preferable. I know that in the East Indies one or other of such positions may generally be found by the intelligent medical topographer; and, for the rest, everything will depend on the authorities, civil and military. Nor are the advantages of such positions to be confined to convalescence; for where the locality is pestilential, or where barracks, camps, or hospitals are badly situated, the sick should at once be removed to the elevated or other selected site. Such early removal will be found to modify the progress of disease, aiding thus the medical treatment, and saving the patient from those congestions which are so liable to occur in the progress of fevers, especially in malarious situations.

GESTATION IN THE OPEN AIR.

Gestation in the open air presents itself at once as one of the most refreshing restorative means for maturing convalescence, and it is seldom difficult of application under willing authorities. It should never be neglected in the late stages of fevers; for it gives tone and vigour to the flagging functions, and conduces to refreshing sleep where medicine has failed of securing rest. Of gestation in the open air, Robert Jackson observes that it is neither useful nor safe in the early stages of fevers, while plethora exists; but that in the late stages of concentrated endemic fevers, it constitutes the " last anchor of hope" to the sinking invalid. He complains justly that this powerful remedy has not been applied generally and systematically; for he had frequent opportunities of directing gestation in the open air, and of observing its beneficial results, in the first American war, in the West Indies, and in Holland. He says that "moving the body rapidly in an open cart or carriage through woods, or on the green turf; or in defect of woods, shaded, if in the daytime, with boughs of trees, exposed, if in the night-time, to all the freshness of the air, and all the dews of heaven, has appeared to do what no other means were capable of doing." Jackson considers that airings for an hour or two in carriages, where the subject is defended from the weather, or but partially touched by the salutary influence of the air, con- stitute but a feeble substitute for journeys of six or eight hours in open conveyances, even when the patients are exposed to wind and rain, to heat and cold, and other apparent disadvantages.

Where, as in the retreat through Holland, in 1795, this measure was adopted from necessity, he says that "it often succeeds; for the operation is continued till the effect is confirmed." Under all the disadvantages of this retreat, Jackson declares that the benefits to the sick were demonstrably felt. "Where due attention was bestowed in disposing the sick in waggons, the travelling was agreeable during its continuance even in cold and rainy weather; the good effect was strongly manifested at the end of the journey; even the most enfeebled acquired an evident accession of strength. Where the diseased action has actually ceased, but where the com- mencement of healthy movement is slow, and the healthy action imperfect, more benefit is visibly derived, and more strength visibly gained, by travelling for six hours in an open carriage, exposed to all the chances of weather, than by the best treatment that can be devised in a crowded hospital for a space of six days." The bene- ficial effects, he adds, are confirmed and rendered permanent by a continued application of the means.

This great authority expresses his regret that gestation in the open air—a means that has the smallest chance of any other medical appliance of doing harm—is not numbered among the regular means of physicians in the cure of fevers; and this regret must be shared by all who have seen and served in the sickly camp. The old 71st Regiment, or Fraser Highlanders, with which Jackson served during the first American war, was forced to retire before a large body of the enemy, carrying along with them a heavy sick list of men suffering from remittent fever. "The sick, during the march, had little opportunity of taking medicine; yet no one had died; some had got entirely well; and in others, indeed in all, where the disease had not yet ceased, the form was changed to that of distinct intermittent."

In the latter stages of fever, dysentery, and hepatitis, while morbid influences are in operation, medicine will do something, but will not cure; and it is here that change of air proves so supreme in effect, just where all other means prove unavailing.

"When, some years ago," says Boudin, "the French troops who had been in Spain were recalled, there were in hospital at Madrid about 160 wounded men labouring under *pourriture d'hôpital*, &c., who were deemed unfit to bear the hardships of a march, but who, at their own urgent request, were taken away. When after two days' journey the wounds were uncovered to be dressed, it was found, to the general surprise, that nearly all were healed, or rapidly healing, showing the effect of escape from the poisoned atmosphere of the hospital into the fresh air."

Those very few survivors who, like the writer of this work, marched with the miserable remnant of the European army orginally sent to Rangoon, during the first Burmese war, will never forget the drooping, attenuated form and haggard eye of the British soldier on the day we broke ground from the last-mentioned town, and the amended condition of the same man on entering Prome two months afterwards. Yet here the soldiers were moved under every conceivable disadvantage, excepting in the matter of diet; for, as we advanced into the interior of the country, we procured some fresh meat, and occasionally some fruits and vegetables.*

It may now prove both useful and interesting to take a glance at the prominent points of the treatment of tropical fevers by the following authors, all British but the first-named, in the order of their respective dates :—

1629. Bontius :—Bleeding, general and topical, and repeated as occasion required—purgatives—opiates—extract of saffron.

1751. Cleghorn :—Bleeding, repeated according to occasion—cathartics—bark.

1757. Dr. Bogue; Bengal :—Bleeding—emetics—purgatives—mercury—bark—camphor in the cold stage.

1757. Dr. Huxham :—Bleeding—purgatives—diluents.

1760. Dr. Huck :—Blood-letting, repeated according to occasion—ipecacuanha and tartar emetic, so as to vomit and purge—bark during the remission.

1762. Dr. James Lind—"Putrid and remitting marsh fever :"—cautious blood-letting—vomits of tepid water, occasionally of

---

* There perished, in the first year of the first Burmese war, at Rangoon alone, of the British portion of the force, 48¼ per cent., of whom 3½ per cent. were killed in action, or died of their wounds, being within one-half per cent. of the annual casualties from wounds in the Peninsular war, during forty-one months of the most active service. The total European loss within the Burmese territory, during the two years of the war, was 720 per thousand of the strength—being the greatest mortality of which as yet there is any record. I was very young when employed on that service; but it appeared to me as if I had lived many weary years in passing through the experiences, the personal sufferings and privations of those two dismal campaigns. My landing on the coast of Pegu was through an appalling shipwreck, and my departure, at the close of the war, was through a fever which nearly destroyed me : but all personal considerations vanished in the general scenes of which I had been an active witness.

emetic tartar and ipecacuanha—saline purgatives—cooling acidu-lated drinks—bark, speedily and freely administered.

1768. Pringle, Sir John :— Bleeding, repeated according to occasion—active purgatives—antimonials—bark, as an occasional means:

1784-1811. Balfour — "Putrid intestinal remitting fever of Bengal :"—Blood-letting, general and local, for the removal of "local affections"—calomel, 6 to 12 grains at bed-time, as a febri-fuge and cholagogue, followed in the morning by an active saline purge ; emetic tartar as a sudorific, every hour or two during the day; and this treatment to be persisted in so long as acute symp-toms remain—adding, " on the morning of the third day," bark and opium, so as "to throw in twelve drachms or two ounces before the expiration of the second day." Opium is added to the bark with the view to prevent vomiting or diarrhœa, while calomel and purgatives are used throughout the fever. Panada was given as diet, and great attention was given to purity of air and of dress.

1791-98, 1820. Robert Jackson :—Blood-letting, copious and repeated, according to the severity of the symptoms—the operation always performed in the recumbent posture, while the head and shoulders are dashed with cold water, and heat applied to the feet —purgatives followed by moderate doses of calomel, antimonial powder and cathartic extract, so as to keep up " effective evacua-tion "—bark—blisters, largely and freely applied when local con-gestions require them—gestation in the open air—change of air. In fevers with congestion of the cerebral and abdominal viscera, calomel as a remedy " of the first importance," one which " repairs mischiefs which no other means with which we are acquainted are capable of touching."

1795. Dr. Chisholm :—Calomel and opium to salivation.

1796. Dr. J. Hunter :—A strong saline purgative, followed by James's powder till remission took place—then bark freely admi-nistered throughout the disease, and during each remission—blisters—cordials—opiates—change of air.

1797. Dr. John Clark:—Mercurial purgatives—bark—anodynes.

1799. Blane, Sir Gilbert :—Bleeding—vomits and purges—su-dorifics—bark—anodynes.

1799. Dr. Lempriere :—Blood-letting—active purging by mer-curials and cathartics perseveringly used—diaphoretics—blisters —pediluvia—saline draughts along with the bark, to allay nervous symptoms—ether, camphor, and wine—in doubtful and dangerous cases, mercury to affect the system.

1804. M'Grigor, Sir James :—Emetics occasionally—blood-letting—cold affusion—calomel with purgatives—mercury to affect the system—blisters—nitric acid—opiates—bark.

1807. Mr. Curtis :—Evacuants and diluents, in the first stage—calomel, ipecacuanha, and purgatives in protracted cases.

1808. William Fergusson:—Early and copious blood-letting—calomel to affect the system—sudorifics—purgatives.

1811. Dr. Bancroft:—Bleeding—cold affusion—calomel—purgatives—bark.

1813. James Johnson:—Blood-letting, general and local—mercurial purgatives—diaphoretics—calomel, according to severity of symptoms, to affect the system—bark—change of air.

1816. Burnet, Sir William:—Bleeding both general and local—purgatives.

1818. Ballingall, Sir George:—Blood-letting, general and local—purgatives—cold affusion—moderate use of calomel—occasional emetics—bark.

1819. Dr. Dickinson:—Vomits—blood-letting—active purging—cold ablution—diluents.

1827. Dr. Geddes :—Blood-letting, mercurial and other purgatives—diaphoretics—diluents—opiates before the paroxysm—quinine.

1828. Annesley, Sir James:—Blood-letting, general and local—emetics—full doses of calomel—purgatives—diaphoretics—cold affusion and cold lotions to the head—bark during the remissions.

1832. Mr. Twining :—Blood-letting, local and general, repeated as occasion required—calomel, followed by purgatives—calomel so as to affect the system in severe cases—quinine in the remission.

1833. Dr. Joseph Brown—" Cyclopædia of Practical Medicine :"—Bleeding, general and local, aided by warm baths—mercurial purgatives—cold affusion—cold to the head—cold acidulated drinks—in the advanced stages opium—change of air.

1835. Copland—"Dictionary of Practical Medicine:"—An emetic—blood-letting, general and local—" full doses of calomel followed by purgatives"—evaporating lotions to the head—cooling diaphoretics—quinine during the remissions.

From the *coup-d'œil* here presented we learn that he who undertakes to determine this great practical question must be careful to separate real from spurious science; that to the cure of fever there is neither a short path nor a royal road, and that a disease so varying in its nature, so general and complicated in its influence on the system, is not to be justly treated by one remedy.   Bark and calomel, each a remedy of great power, will nevertheless not succeed in the cure of fever, if used exclusively ; and so it is with the most powerful of all means, blood-letting.   We must, therefore, give to each remedy its proper place in the treatment ; we shall thus be as nearly right as is possible.   No one can be found now-a-days to follow Dr. Clark or Dr. Chisholm in their exclusiveness.   Men of science cannot be induced to believe that because one practice is wrong, its very opposite must be right, thus meeting one extreme by another extreme.   The truth is, that exclusive doctrines and practices never take any general or permanent hold on the mind of the medical profession ; and even the names of Brown and Broussais have secured them but few followers in Europe. For the great mass of the profession extreme doctrines are "writ in water;" or, as Samuel Johnson says of Sterne's writings, "Nothing odd will do long." According to Dr. Forget, "Science, like representative government, is a system of balancing. Broussais dethroned Brown; and now behold Brown avenging himself on Broussais."

GENERAL REMARKS IN CONCLUSION.

If tropical fever and dysentery were always simple morbid actions, or mere inflammatory states of the system or of particular organs, no doubt bleeding and purging, as recommended by some writers, might often prove of themselves sufficient to the cure; but unfortunately, in both instances, we very seldom find this unmixed condition of disease in actual observation in Bengal, where, besides the morbid condition of the entire system, including a violent disturbance of the nervous and vascular systems in particular, we have in our fevers continually to combat dangerous abdominal complications, congestive and inflammatory; in the fevers of the hot season, too, the cerebro-spinal system becomes involved, and all these conditions demand a more or less complex and careful treatment, a speedy diminution of the force and frequency of the heart's contractions, and of the circulating current, followed by an unlocking of all the secretions and excretions of the body, which the most ample experience proves that bleeding and purging *alone* will not effect. Tropical fever, dysentery, and hepatitis are produced by the action of specific causes, and such diseases are nowhere cured by the exclusive use of blood-letting and purging, as in the instance of common or sthenic inflammations. Yet here, as in dysentery and hepatitis, bleeding is generally the standard remedy, subject to considerations of age, constitution, and length of residence in India. In acute hepatitis it is a necessity, if we would save the life of the sufferer. Bleeding, whether general or local, should in remittent fever be practised to the extent of reducing the force and frequency of the pulse, and of relieving the loaded and oppressed abdominal viscera. It precedes all other means of cure, both in order of time and in importance. The fevers of Bengal are not a mere inflammation, although they present the same types as both sthenic and asthenic inflammation; and also intermediate conditions between those types. Thus our fevers have for a length of time been treated according to indications grounded on explanation of the symptoms, on the physiology, and not on any exclusive plan. Accuracy of diagnosis and simplification of treatment, the true aims of the practical physician, have very generally been held in view; the symptoms being traced to their causes—in other words, the leading rules of practice being founded on general views of diseased function and structure, on general and special pathology, in fact. Pathological and therapeutical induction ought mutually to elucidate and sustain each other, so as to conduce to an assured hope of recovery.

Blood-letting has been had recourse to, to moderate the force and frequency of arterial action, and to relieve congestions; free purgation, by means of mercurials conjoined with cathartics, to remove accumulations or vitiated secretions, and to aid in correcting the latter; calomel with sudorifics to act on all the secretory and excretory functions: bark or quinine during the remissions, to arrest the coming paroxysm; cold affusion in the ardent continued fevers of the hot season—these have long been in use with us; and by their just application we may generally cure the fever, and obviate visceral disease—the token of bad practice—the measure of the insufficiency of the treatment.

Subject only to the limitations already stated, bleeding—early bleeding—whether general or local, *and always practised at the very onset of the stage of reaction*, is very generally necessary in the severer forms of Bengal remittent fever; then come full doses of calomel and sudorifics, short of producing salivation, with saline purgatives, antimonials, and refrigerants, and quinine in the intervals. If under such treatment the disease does not speedily yield, but, on the contrary, if the secretions become of a watery nature, or if they be suppressed, and the paroxysms recur at shorter intervals, or with increasing severity, leaving but imperfect remissions, then there is imminent danger, and inflammation or congestion, more or less acute, in some important abdominal or cerebral organ, may be more than suspected; indeed, the justice of the suspicion is continually verified in our examinations after death.

For the cure of this aggravated state, in addition to topical bleeding and cold applications to the head, when it proves the seat of disease, calomel in small and repeated doses, with antimonials, must be exhibited so as mildly to affect the system; its judicious use, and that of quinine, constitute the only known means of saving the patient by anticipating the destruction of some organ essential to life. I have seldom had occasion to urge mercury to the extent of salivation, during the whole period of my service in India; and where there is much irritability of the nervous system, or tendency to sinking of the vital powers, the union of camphor with the calomel, as recommended by the Indian surgeons of old, will be found useful. In such conditions it will be found more safe than opium, especially in the hands of the inexperienced; for it does not favour congestion or lock up the secretions as opium is too apt to do. But opium is necessary in some cases, and given with care and judgment, it will then save life. In treating seamen and soldiers suffering from tropical fevers and other acute diseases, we should very carefully inquire into the previous habits of the patient, for when these have been dissipated, including the free use of ardent spirits and tobacco, we must be on our guard against the complication of delirium tremens more or less masked by the fever. This is a delicate point to determine by the young surgeon; but, looking to the history of the man's life, and to the predomi-nance of nervous over vascular disturbance, he will soon perceive that tartar-emetic and opium, and not the lancet, are the remedy; the latter would indeed be fatal. Here the nervous system has been rendered feeble and irritable, while the blood has been de-praved, by habitual excess.

When, again, through the duration of the disease, congestion or inflammation has taken its seat in some important abdominal or cerebral organ, and the fever has established itself in the system, then measures less heroic, but more persistent and varied, must be employed, the fever having now become established and compli-cated. Here the physician must neither give way to a feeble timidity, nor to a reckless audacity—courses alike dangerous to the patient. We must remember, too, in laying down rules of treatment, as indeed in all medical reasoning, that we err not so much in the upholding of false views, as in upholding one truth to the exclusion of many other truths.

The tendency to sinking of the vital powers is another most important consideration, never to be overlooked in treating the remittent fever of Bengal. This impending event is the reason why all our active antiphlogistic measures of cure, as blood-letting, purgatives, and sudorifics, must be so cautiously regulated as to the time of using them; *for what was a saving means at the com-mencement of the paroxysm, is as surely destructive at the end of it.* In every fever, as in every battle, there is a decisive point, a de-cisive moment, which, once past, never returns. In remittent fever, that point and that moment present themselves only once, and that early in the first day—that is, if we would pretend to cut short the disease at once.

On the subject of blood-letting Robert Jackson's works abound in valuable injunctions, such as ought to be present to the recol-lection of all who undertake the onerous duty of treating tropical fevers. After the exposition of admirable rules as to the "just point of time" for the application of this most powerful means, he concludes by declaring that "the same remedy, after the delay of a few hours, not only ceases to be useful, but the application of it even sometimes becomes unsafe :" further on he adds, with equal truth, that "it requires much discernment in many cases to dis-cover the cause, a very correct judgment to measure the means, and even no small degree of knowledge to be able to ascertain that the end is attained."

That our fevers in Bengal alter their types under different seasons—nay, that instances both endemic and epidemic occur in which blood-letting is not only unnecessary but injurious, the pages of this work sufficiently attest, and death even from its ill-timed use has more than once come under the author's observa-tion ; yet the fact remains untouched that blood-letting, practised with the care and thoughtfulness which should mark every step we take in this disease—at the proper time, and apportioned to circumstances of constitution, age, sex, season, and length of residence in India—forms the principal means of cure in our severer endemic fevers, and of preventing those organic lesions which otherwise so frequently follow them.   We must, however, remember with care that the condition of the blood in the newly-arrived European and in the old Indian differs ; and that while the first-named bears and demands the free use of the lancet, the last does not always bear even moderate depletion ; and this, owing to anæmic tendencies, being frequently manifested.   Leeches are a ready and powerful means in the treatment of tropical fevers of every type ; but I would caution the inexperienced against this mode of abstracting blood as a general rule, or as a substitute for venesection ; and I would likewise place him on his guard against the ill effects of prolonged oozing from leech-bites, especially in the instances of persons at the two extremes of life—the very young and the aged.   I have seen the most serious results from carelessness in this respect.

The great and pervading tendency of malaria to deteriorate the blood has been commented on in various portions of this work. But, besides these acknowledged morbid operations, it has been alleged that in the cycles of years since the outbreak of cholera in the East, in 1817, not only has that very disease undergone changes there, implying a progressively greater depression of the nervous functions, but the endemic diseases of the country, as fevers and dysenteries, have been supposed also gradually and imperceptibly to have become less and less sthenic in their natures—the complications of these diseases having in like manner become less inflammatory and more congestive.   Analogous changes have been observed in England since the visitations of influenza and cholera in 1831-32.   Some generally depressing influence is supposed to have been in operation ever since, lowering the tone of the nervous system, and injuring the quality of the blood, here as in India, so as to cause a marked alteration in the types of fevers and inflammations—the former having become more adynamic, while the latter have assumed more of the erysipelatous and suppurative characters, general plethora being less frequent and anæmia more prevalent than formerly.   The great increase of population in our English cities—the great and rapid extension of the great town system—without any commensurate improvement in the sanitary condition of towns, these cases have doubtless contributed their shares to the general deterioration at home.   Altogether, the considerations here briefly referred to are of the highest interest and importance, as subjects to be attentively investigated ; for, if founded on truth, they must necessarily tend, in no small degree, to influence our estimate of the physiology, and modify to a like extent the principles of our treatment of all classes of diseases, at home and abroad.   Thus we perceive that, as years roll onwards, certain changes in our climatic ecliptic arise to view, suggesting changes in physiological and pathological doctrines, and in principles of cure, appropriate to their several epochs. But this great subject has need of minute and extended investigation, in order to its being verified. Dr. Watson states his conviction " that there are waves of time through which the sthenic and asthenic characters of disease prevail in succession, and that we are at present living amid one of its adynamic phases." The depressed condition of the public health is shown also in the altered nature of erysipelas, the acute phlegmonous form of the disease with inflammatory fever, familiar to our fathers, having disappeared. The unceasing competitions, the jar and bustle of an overcrowded manufacturing and trading nation, with their enormous wear and tear of the nervous system in "the battle of life," and the consequent excitements and depressions of the vital energies, must have their injurious effects.

In regard to the next most powerful remedy in paroxysmal fevers, namely, the Peruvian bark;—where the remissions are becoming sufficiently well marked, quinine should be given in full doses without waiting for a perfectly favourable condition of the system :—in bad fevers we should seize the very first dawn of remission to exhibit quinine in doses of five to eight grains every second or third hour, according to the urgency of the symptoms, and repeated up to the period of the next accession; but in any case not repeated more than four or six times. Some practitioners recommend that before this drug is used we obtain a clean tongue, natural secretions, and the absence of all heat of skin, and of local complication. I believe this to be a very dangerous practice : if we are to wait for everything favourable, we shall often have to wait too long, and till it has become too late. It is in diseases as in critical circumstances, political and commercial—everything is for him who can wait; but, unhappily, in the formidable remittents of the tropics we can wait for nothing, for there is not a moment to lose. I have always given quinine in the more favourable cases now under consideration, in disregard of certain abdominal complications (those of the cerebral cavity, in plethoric subjects, in whom inflammation or congestion is suspected, should exclude its use), believing that if I arrested the paroxysms, the progress towards curing the disease as a whole greatly outweighed any harm which the quinine could possibly do to the local affection, the treatment of which, by local depletion, by mercurials, or by counter-irritants, is not interfered with by the means in question. Again, all tenderness on pressure, or local pain, does not necessarily constitute inflammation : and even where such is actually present, its character is often so modified by age, length of residence in India, by malarious influences, and by anæmic states of the general habit, as to constitute a state very different from idiopathic and uncomplicated inflammations, such

with the care and thoghtfulness which should mark every step
take in this disease—if the proper time, and apportioned to
cumstances of constitution, age, sex, season, and length of resid
in India—forms the pincipal means of cure in our severer en
fevers, and of preventing those organic lesions which other
frequently follow then We must, however, remember wi
that the condition of te blood in the newly-arrived Euro
in the old Indian differs; and that while the first-named
demands the free use of the lancet, the last does not
even moderate depletion; and this, owing to anæmic
being frequently maniested. Leeches are a ready
means in the treatmat of tropical fevers of every t
would caution the inexperienced against this mode of
bloo'l as a general rul, or as a substitute for venesectio
would likewise place im on his guard against the ill effect
longed oozing from eech-bites, especially in the instan
persons at the two extmes of life—the very young and the ag
have seen the most seous results from carelessness in this res

The great and perving tendency of malaria to deteriorate
blood has been commnted on in various portions of this wo
But, besides these aclowledged morbid operations, it has bee
alleged that in the eyes of years since the outbreak of cholera m
the East, in 1817, not oly has that very disease undergone changes
there, implying a prcressively greater depression of the nervous
functions, but the endmic diseases of the country, as fevers and
dysenteries, have been supposed also gradually and imperceptibly
to have become less ad less sthenic in their natures—the complications of these diseas having in like manner become less inflammatory and more cagestive. Analogous changes have been
observed in England sice the visitations of influenza and cholera
in 1831-32. Some gnerally depressing influence is supposed to
have been in operatioiever since, lowering the tone of the nervous
system, and injuring te quality of the blood, here as in India, so
as to cause a marked teration in the types of fevers and inflammations—the former iaving become more adynamic, while the
latter have assumed iore of the erysipelatous and suppurative
characters, general plhora being less frequent and anæmia more
prevalent than former. The great increase of population in our
English cities—the gnat and rapid extension of the great town
system—without any ommensurate improvement in the sanitary
condition of towns, tese cases have doubtless contributed their
shares to the general cterioration at home. Altogether, the considerations here briefl referred to are of the highest interest and
importance, as subjes to be attentively investigated; for, if
founded on truth, the must necessarily tend, in no small degree,
to influence our estinte of the physiology, and modify to a like
extent the principles cour treatment of all classes of diseases, at
e perceive that as ears roll onwards,

certain changes in our climatic ecli
changes in physiological and patholog.
ciples of cure, appropriate to their severa.
subject has need of minute and extended i
its being verified.   Dr. Watson states his
are waves of time through which the sthenic n.
of disease prevail in succession, and that v a
amid one of its adynamic phases." The ep'
the public health is shown also in the alte d
the acute phlegmonous form of the dis se
fever, familiar to our fathers, having disa ;a.
competitions, the jar and bustle of an ove o
and trading nation, with their enormou we.
nervous system in " the battle of life," an the
ments and depressions of the vital ene ies,
injurious effects.

   In regard to the next most powerful med
fevers, namely, the Peruvian bark ;—wl e tl
becoming sufficiently well marked, quinine houl
doses without waiting for a perfectly favo able c
system :—in bad fevers we should seize th very fi
mission to exhibit quinine in doses of fiv to eigh
second or third hour, according to the urgen of the s)
repeated up to the period of the next acc sion; but
not repeated more than four or six times. Some prac
commend that before this drug is used w obtain a cle
natural secretions, and the absence of all h t of skin, a
complication.   I believe this to be a very dangerous pr.
we are to wait for everything favourable, e shall often
wait too long, and till it has become too la . It is in dis
in critical circumstances, political and con ercial—everyth
for him who can wait; but, unhappily, in tl formidable remit
of the tropics we can wait for nothing, for there is not a mom
to lose.   I have always given quinine in tl more favourable case,
now under consideration, in disregard of c rtain abdominal complications (those of the cerebral cavity, i plethoric subjects, in
whom inflammation or congestion is suspe ed, should exclude its
use), believing that if I arrested the p oxysms, the progress
towards curing the disease as a whole geatly outweighed any
harm which the quinine could possibly d to the local affection,
the treatment of which, by local depletio by mercurials, or by
counter-irritants, is not interfered with by he means in question.
Again, all tenderness on pressure, or loca pain, does not necessarily constitute inflammation: and even here such is actually
present, its character is often so modif d by age, length of
residence in India, by malarious influe es, and by anæmic
states of the general habit, as to const ute a state very different from idiopathic and uncomplicate inflammations, such

as may demand only the kind of treatment here immediately
referred to. On the other hand, the power of all antiperiodics is
quadrupled when exhibited *before* the advent of visceral complications; and hence the value of immediate recourse to antiphlogistic
means—to be followed again, immediately it has become proper, by the exhibition of bark, or other equally powerful means.
It is thus, if at all, that fever *may* be cut short; but the preparation must in such a case be a prompt, and not a protracted process. In respect to quinine, I have often combined it with calomel
and with sudorifics, and I think with advantage; where there
existed depression of the vital powers I have added small doses
of laudanum. It is also usual with us in Bengal to combine this
powerful antiperiodic with common purging mixture, a mode
whereby it applies itself to the entire and extensive surface of the
mucous digestive organs, so as materially to add to its influences.
When it is seen that, by such means, the periodical febrile movement has been checked, and that no recurrence takes place, then
quinine—no longer necessary in antiperiodic doses—becomes
nevertheless useful in smaller and less frequent doses, as a general
tonic, to promote convalescence, and to prevent relapse.

It is well known in the history of the treatment of the fevers of
India—a history so instructive that it ought to be known to all of
our profession who may serve there—that at different times bark,
calomel, blood-letting, purgatives, and sudorifics have, each in
its turn, been in almost exclusive favour with some individual
practitioners; but such partial plans of treating so formidable and
complicated a disease have never, for any length of time, held influence on the more thinking portion of the profession. Some
authors, again, have troubled themselves to prove that blood-
letting must in all times have been injurious;—an unprofitable
research—" a perverse idolatry." I would guard and caution the
younger medical officer alike against the adoption of exclusive
measures of cure, and against the over-treatment of fever, both
being equally mischievous. In truth, it is only by a rational and
well-adjusted plan, which shall call into operation all the aids
suggested by science and by experience, that such a disease as
fever can anywhere be justly treated.

At this time of day it cannot surely be necessary to write
chapters of heavy solemn dulness, to warn and convince well-
educated medical officers that generally or locally to bleed, or
otherwise reduce, old, worn-out, emaciated, or drunken men, or
infants—anæmic, scorbutic, or otherwise sickly persons—would be
neither good nor safe practice. If such persons were dying of
apoplexy, no well-informed surgeon would propose to bleed them
from the little toe—so carefully would he treasure up the watery
blood of such subjects. Huxham indicates the just principle of
action for all times and places, when he says that " each particular disease in every individual patient is to be considered by the

attending physician; not according to the *nomenclature*, but according to the nature, causes, and symptoms in that particular person." We must here, as in all other instances, be careful not to confound the abuse of a great principle with the principle itself.

Finally ; it cannot be too much or too often impressed on the Indian surgeon that it is on his careful attention to the phenomena and treatment of fever that nine-tenths of his usefulness depends. I have here presented the reader with a summary of the nature and treatment of the Bengal remittent fever : it will be found to correspond in most of its details with the history of endemic fevers generally, with the bilious remittents of the Indies, whether East or West:—they all have a pathological community, they are all fevers of locality, and do not by any means differ so much as medical writers of partial views and partial experiences would have us believe; their supposed differences, or nosological divisions, are more frequently the work of man than of nature :—they may and do differ in degree of intensity; but their essential phenomena, and the organs affected in their progress so as to endanger or ultimately to destroy life, are the same, and so likewise are the essential parts of their treatment.

The remittent fever of Bengal is a disease of much danger to health, and of no small danger to life also ; but, under a rational plan of treatment, I know of no disease in which the resources of medicine are more effectual. General principles in physiology, pathology, and therapeutics, so far as these may be understood in our time, ought to be the aim and purpose of us all ; and the difference between one physician and another must in all times and places consist in the relative power to balance and determine such principles. This is indeed all that the best of us can do.

I have now concluded this, the most important article in this work; and I trust that, provided I have treated the subject worthily, the reader will not consider that I have devoted too much space to the discussion of it ; for he who can successfully combat the formidable remittent fevers of tropical climates need not despair of acting with a like success in the treatment of the equally formidable dysenteries and hepatic diseases of those regions. The principles here inculcated will, if I mistake not, guide the medical officer to such favourable issues, under every variety of type and complication of remittent fever, as may reasonably be attainable in the present state of our knowledge. The means of cure recommended by me may appear to some persons to be of unmeasured power; but the more I consider the nature of the three diseases named, the more assured I feel that the measure of cure, to be effective, must at least come up to that of morbid action. A moderate and hesitating imbecility will never effect anything in medicine—and, least of all, in the treatment of tropical diseases. To treat effectively one of the most acute and dangerous of fevers, the

mind of the army surgeon must be prepared by much foreknowledge and reflection; for now the practical judgment must be
formed at once, there being no time for scientific deliberation. The
decision to be arrived at must be the result of such matured foreknowledge, in order that the patient may receive at once the
benefits of that compression of thought, instantaneousness of conception, and simultaneousness of grasp of the different bearings of
a practical question, which are so necessary to the army surgeon.

For the following table, exhibiting the comparative frequency
and the intensity, as shown by the relative mortality of remittent
fever, throughout the wide extent of climate occupied by British
soldiers, I am indebted to my friend Sir Alexander Tulloch :—

STATIONS.	Period of obser- vation.	Aggregate strength.	Remittent feVer.		
			Attacked.	Died.	Proportion of deaths to admissions.
Windward and Leeward Command.	20 years.	86,661	17,799	1,966	1 in 9
Jamaica....................	20 ,,	51,567	38,393	5,114	1 in 8
Gibraltar..................	19 ,,	60,269 { YF.* 314, 1,522		28, 423	1 in 11, 1 in 3⅗
Malta	20 ,,	40,826	384	16	1 in 24
Ionian Islands............	20 ,,	70,293	6,984	623	1 in 11
Bermudas	20 ,,	11,721 { YF.* 19, 277		6, 101	1 in 3, 1 in 2¾
Nova Scotia and New Brunswick	20 ,,	46,442	15	...	1 in 15
Canada.....................	20 ,,	64,280	294	18	1 in 16
Western Africa...........	18 ,,	1,843	1,601	739	1 in 2
Cape of Good Hope......	19 ,,	22,714	15	1	1 in 15
St. Helena.................	9 ,,	8,973	25	1	1 in 25
Mauritius..................	19 ,,	30,515	6	1	1 in 6
Ceylon	20 ,,	42,978	4,643	868	1 in 5½
Tenasserim Provinces ...	10 ,,	6,818	594	22	1 in 27
Madras.....................	5 ,,	31,627	1,139	54	1 in 21
Bengal	5 ,,	38,136	1,311	89	1 in 14¾
Bombay.....................	5 ,,	17,612	2,854	114	1 in 25

INTERMITTENT FEVER.

THE proportionate amount of sickness from intermittent fever, in
any given communities, will depend on the relative amount of
local sanitary improvement, or of the neglect of it, in the districts,
stations, and cantonments occupied by them throughout our intertropical possessions.   The geographical distribution of the class of

* The prevalence of epidemic yellow fever is here indicated.

fevers here treated of will be found to be very much the same with that of remittent fevers; where the one form of fever prevails, there we generally find the other likewise; and whether an European is to be affected by a remittent or by an intermittent fever will depend on length of residence in a tropical climate, on age, constitution, and previous habits of life, on season, and the intensity of the exciting causes.

Intermittents, which are most frequent throughout India in the rainy season, attack the European and the native soldier in nearly the same proportion, the mortality in both, according to Mr. Waring, approximating very closely. He adds that, in hot climates, the quotidian is by far the most frequent type, the proportion being greater in Bengal than in Madras: tertians rank next, and quartans are the least frequent. The proportion of deaths in quotidians exceeds that which is observed in tertians and quartans.

The usual history given by Europeans who have resided in malarious districts or stations is, that they had first been affected by remittent (jungle) fever, and that then followed the intermittent form.

Dr. Bryson, in his Statistical Reports on the health of the navy serving in the East Indies, says of the fevers of China:—" A large proportion of, or nearly all the cases of intermittent, were the sequelæ of fevers which had first appeared in the continued or remitting forms; still there were a few which seem to have been intermittent from the commencement, although it is probable they were connected with preceding attacks which were not observed, or had been forgotten."

In Calcutta, through the hitherto gradual improvements in its ill-chosen site, intermittent fever has become, for many years past, a mild and infrequent disease comparatively, especially among the better classes of society, and amongst Europeans of better habits of life. This simple fact strongly illustrates the beneficial influenees resulting from local sanitary improvements, while it constitutes a powerful inducement to the government and the public of the city in question, to proceed in the same course of amelioration which has already secured to its inhabitants so great an exemption from disease.

At home, and in our own capital, we find that the sweating sickness, scurvy, dysentery, malignant ague, and other formidable diseases, have yielded to the slow progress of sanitary improvement in modern London; so, in our Eastern capital, we have no longer "the obstinate putrid intermitting fevers" described by the older writers, with their cold stage of " *twelve hours*," and their long list of sequelæ in the form of tumid livers and spleens, diarrhœas, dropsies, &c. &c., a condition of public health which we now regard, even in the capital of British India, with horror.

Dr. Bogue, who practised in Calcutta in 1757, speaks of this form of fever " as the most fatal" of that time. It began with the rainy season, and continued with increasing violence during its continuance, and "for some time after," the paroxysm recurring daily, so that "the patients had not above four or five hours respite from it." Thus he says, " we had sick at the same time, in this place, one half of the men of the squadron under the command of Admirals Watson and Pocock."

The fevers here described would seem to have possessed the malignant character of the *febres intermittentes algidæ* of Torti, in which the power of generating heat was so impaired, that the patient died in the cold stage at the end of two or three accessions.

Immediately, our modern intermittents are in general not dangerous to life, but consecutively, the dangers arising from visceral diseases, in after years, are considerable. Of this latter fact I have had presented to me in England very numerous instances, and a very remarkable one will be found under the head of Chronic Diarrhœa. In certain districts of the East Indies, as in others of our colonies, the type of intermittent fever assumes a malignant form, and then the dangers of a rapid dissolution, or of visceral disease and a broken constitution, are very great.

I have said that ague is an "infrequent" disease in Calcutta, and strangers will read with surprise that I do not think I saw above a dozen cases in a year, on the average; and these occurred in persons who went into the neighbouring jungles on hog-hunting and other such excursions. But this disease is of frequent occurrence in the marshy and jungly portions of Bengal Proper, as well as of all such countries throughout India.

I remember attending a mercantile gentleman who contracted his ague in the Sunderbunds, about the middle of October. On his return to Calcutta, about the 26th of the month, he experienced a good deal of malaise, and took medicine from a chemist with partial relief. Towards the end of the month the native servants who accompanied him fell ill of ague one after the other, and on the 20th of November their master was seized with a violent paroxysm of the same disease. Here we perceive the superior power of resistance to the morbific influence exhibited by the European over the natives, as shown by the difference in the period of latency or of the abeyance of the fever in each, being more than thirty days in the former, as compared to ten and fifteen days in the latter. This gentleman was temperate in his habits, and inured to the climate; and both master and servants entered the Sunderbunds in good health, and neither had been previously affected with ague.

CAUSES.

That the emanations from marshes produce agues is the universal belief of mankind in all ages and countries; and the accordance of the medical profession in this opinion has always been quite as general.

Many authors believe with Cullen that, in the climate of England, this fever can alone be produced by exposure to marsh exhalations; and Sir John Forbes has shown, in a very able memoir on the medical topography of Land's End in Cornwall, "that neither impure air simply, nor wet, nor the alternations of cold and heat, nor all these combined, can give rise to fevers of this type." This I believe to be quite true in respect to a *first seizure*, but *after that*, and when the disposition to relapse is once established in the system, such a combination of influences will certainly, in tropical climates, prove an efficient cause; and even Cullen admits " the concurrence of other existing fevers," when the malaria is not " strong enough to produce disease." In support of this latter view I quote the following important passage from Sir James M'Grigor.

" After the effluvia from marshes or the exhalations raised by a powerful sun acting on a humid or luxuriant soil, we found that in those who were convalescent or lately recovered from agues, the causes next in power to reproduce the disease were exposure to a shower of rain or wetting the feet, exposure to the direct solar rays, or to cold, with intemperance and irregularity, or great fatigue. Many other causes would excite the disease in the predisposed, but these never failed to do it. In marching troops in a country where the disease is endemic, particularly if they have been lately discharged from hospitals, the above causes should by all means be avoided, since the whole of our experience in the Peninsula showed that relapsed cases seldom or never get completely well in the country in which they were contracted, under all the circumstances of a soldier's life. In making calculations of efficient force, this description of men could not be depended on for operations long continued in the field." Pringle, the father of British military medicine, writes to much the same effect :—" After the frosts of November the intermittents never appeared unless upon catching cold, and even then such only as had been ill of them in autumn were seized in that manner."

The important observation is continually repeated, also, by this great author, as to the excessive liability to attack of those who occupied the lower floors of houses and barracks, and this happened all over Flanders.

SYMPTOMS AND PROGRESS.

The symptoms of intermittent fevers are well known to consist, like those of remittent fevers, in paroxysms of three stages—a cold, a hot, and a sweating stage, the succession of such events following each other every day, when the fever is termed quotidian ; or every other day, when it is called tertian ; and when two days intervene, then it is termed a quartan ague ; the intervals being respectively twenty-four, forty-eight, and seventy-two hours.

The intermittent differs from the remittent fever in this, that in ague the stages are generally complete and well marked, while they are followed by a complete intermission of disease, or state of health, which allows of time and opportunity for the application of means of cure, having for their object the arrest of further progress of the fever. Unchecked by medicine, however, the paroxysms of intermittent fever recur at regular or irregular intervals, for weeks, months, or even years, so as eventually to prove more or less detrimental to health. The types of intermittent fevers change so that the quotidian becomes tertian, and this last again a quartan; and so likewise do the paroxysms occasionally change their hours of invasion—sometimes coming later in the day, when they are said to be postponed—while by coming earlier they are said to anticipate. In all fevers of the paroxysmal form the former is regarded as a favourable, while the latter is held to be an unfavourable event, in the progress of the disease.

All the types of intermittent fever are to be found in the East, but by far the most prevalent is the tertian; and we very generally find that the first seizure of this fever ensues upon an attack of the remittent form. It was so in my own person:—after a dangerous jungle fever, which I contracted on active service in the hill ranges of Gondwana, and from the violence of which I must have speedily sunk but for the profuse hæmorrhage from the nose, during the height of the two first paroxysms (the moment when I ought to have been bled, had there been any other medical officer present), I was left in a very emaciated and enfeebled condition.* In this state, while sitting to be dressed, near the door of my tent, a shower of rain came on, accompanied by a very slight reduction of temperature; and on the instant I was seized with violent shivering, which proved an intermittent fever. This disease in its tertian form harassed me greatly during eighteen months subsequently; and I only got rid of it by proceeding to the Isle of France, and by being absent from Bengal during eight months. But so severe were these fevers, that, in my after life, the susceptibility to malarious fever has remained so strong on me as never, up to this very day, to have left me.

The average duration of a paroxysm ranges from six to twelve hours, the severity of the disease, as well as its amenableness to treatment, depending very much on the duration of the cold stage; for where this last proves of two hours' duration, or more, and the disease is protracted, the patient incurs much risk of disease of the abdominal viscera.

PATHOLOGY.

All the organs and functions which are disturbed or oppressed during the paroxysm of remittent, are likewise more or less affected

---

* I was bled by Nature—an effort without which I must, like many others employed on this disastrous serVice, haVe sunk at ouce. An occurrence of this kind ought to suggest reflection, and imitation too. Nature bled me—at first not enough; but on the second day sufficiently to saVe my life.

in that of the intermittent fever. During the cold stage of the latter the brain is occasionally oppressed by congestion, while all the abdominal organs are similarly affected ; and in the succeeding hot stage the same organs and functions are more or less seriously disturbed in the tumult of vascular reaction. There is flushing of the face, headache, and sometimes delirium, the patient being at the same time distressed by general uneasiness, restlessness, and epigastric anguish. It is no wonder that morbid actions and alternations such as these, repeated during weeks, months, or even years, should result in organic diseases of a formidable character.

"The great influence of the malarious poison," says Dr. Golding Bird, "is in all probability essentially and primarily exerted upon the nervous system, especially on the organic or ganglionic struc- tures, which preside so importantly over the function of secretion. Thus all the secretions elaborated in the body become affected ; and, as is well known, a remarkable tendency to congestion is observed in the portal circulation, destined most particularly for the depuration of matters rich in carbon. There can be no doubt that the unhealthy secretions thus formed become active agents in keeping up in the body the impression of disease."

Agues which have become habitual by repetition will also im- part a character of periodicity to other ailments, such as neuralgic affections. A few years ago I became subject to facial neuralgia, which came on regularly at eleven A.M.—the very hour at which ague used to commence with me in India more than twenty years previously. Further, when the intermittent fever has been severe or long-continued, the disposition to recurrence of the same disease seems to last with many persons for life. After a residence of ten years in Europe I happened to pass three nights at the best hotel in Strasburg, at a time when ague prevailed in the garrison amongst the French soldiers who had served in Algeria ; and two days after quitting that town I was seized at the accustomed hour of eleven A.M. with ague, and I was the only person of the party who was so affected.

We have in the East not only every variety of type of inter- mittent fever, but every degree of intensity also—certain districts and provinces being noted for the malignity and fatality of their agues ; and even in Bengal Proper we have often to combat severe and obstinate visceral diseases, the sequelæ to these intermittents. Under neglect of early and effective treatment such cases termi- nate in permanently broken health, through disorganizations of the liver, spleen, or mesentery, or of all three. In the malignant intermittent fevers of Aracan and Gondwana, and of provinces of a like unhealthiness, we perceive such remote ravages of disease as to prove at once conclusive, both of the original intensity and danger of the disease, and of the ultimate serious consequences, even after the lapse of years. One such case I will adduce by way of illus- tration :—

Captain F——r contracted the intermittent fever of Aracan in 1837, which was speedily followed by great enlargement of both liver and spleen. At my recommendation he was sent from Calcutta to England for the recovery of health, whence he returned to India in 1839. His health continuing very indifferent under various changes of climate, he was constrained to resign the service in 1847. But even in England he was always an ailing person; and in October, 1852, I was consulted on the state of his health, which was then desperate. He died two months afterwards in a state of universal dropsy.

For the following post-mortem record I am indebted to Mr. Pollock of St. George's Hospital :—"The peritoneum was covered throughout its free surface with an opaque, white false membrane. This membrane was thin on the surface of the abdominal wall and small intestines, but was very thick elsewhere, as on the surface of the stomach, transverse colon and liver, from which viscera it could be peeled off. From the peculiar manner in which it was spread over and attached to these organs, when the abdomen was opened, the small intestines were the only viscera that could be observed. The large intestine, stomach, liver, and spleen were hid from view by the false membrane glueing them together; and the only indication of their situation was an irregular nodulated mass, covered with this membrane, and situated at the upper part of the abdominal cavity. The membrane on the right side was continuous from the abdominal wall over the ascending colon to the spine, and so bound down the ascending colon that, until the membrane was removed, the situation of the bowel was not ascertained. From the surface of the bowel the membrane passed to and attached itself to the mesentery of the small intestine over the vertebræ, in some parts thicker than others, so that it might almost be said to consist of bands, and, from their attachments, they must have much compressed the ascending colon. On removing the membrane from the irregular mass, the stomach, transverse colon, omentum, and spleen, with the liver, were brought into sight; but all these viscera had been compressed, as it were, into the mass by the false membrane spread over them—the membrane being strongest in this situation, and equal to three or four sheets of paper in thickness. The membrane here was readily removed. The liver was enlarged, but chiefly on its left side; and between the longitudinal fissure and the extremity of the left lobe and its anterior margin, there was a whitish yellow mass of hardened deposit, which dipped some two inches into the substance of the liver, and was some three inches broad. When cut into, it was firm and consistent, and appeared to consist of fibrous tissue, with portions of fatty matter, somewhat resembling the character of scirrhus, but less hard. The spleen was healthy, but larger than usual. The kidneys were healthy. The other viscera were not examined."

The reader will now be able to appreciate the original violence of the intermittent fever in this instance, and the necessity there was for the most active antiphlogistic means, including general blood-letting, to overcome inflammatory complications. Such means were not applied—or, if applied, they were of but insufficient power ;—and hence, assuredly, the unfortunate issue.

In all the severer intermittent fevers of India, such as that by which the European and Native force under General Morrison was destroyed in Aracan, during the first Burmese war, we find the sequelæ of diarrhœas and dysenteries to be very frequent also ;* and it is justly observed by writers on the diseases of Turkey, that where there is ague, dysentery is not far off. Congestive and inflammatory affections of the spleen and liver, diarrhœas and dysenteries, the results of intermittent fevers, are most frequent and most severe during the cold season in Bengal.

The influence, real or supposed, of splenic disease in keeping up the morbid train of actions of the original fever, and in producing relapses, is a subject well deserving the careful attention of the tropical practitioner.

M. Piorry, on his attentive examination of the state of the spleen in more than five hundred cases of ague, has come to the conclusion that that organ is invariably enlarged during the progress of the fever ; and he has ascertained with equal accuracy the fact that, by the use of quinine the spleen is diminished in size. M. Piorry states :—

---

* The devotion of the medical officers attached to this portion of our invading army was most notable. Mr. Grierson, of the Bengal Medical Department, says :—" Of the first five deaths that occurred among the European officers, four were in the medical branch of the service. This blank was severely felt ; but twice the above number were soon on the sick list ; and at length only eight medical officers remained for the whole duties of the division, the sick of which at that time amounted to near 5500 men, besides the sick of the various public establishments and the camp-followers." All who were not dead were in hospital. From this simple statement, the hopeless nature of the duties devolving on the few surviving surgeons of the army of Aracan may be inferred ; and it will be matter of no surprise that in a few months three-fourths of the entire force, European and Native, perished on the spot, while the suffering survivors were ruined in health.

Mr. Lewis Grant, of the Bengal Medical Department (brother to the gallant Sir Colquhoun Grant), was the principal medical officer. It is related of him that "he was attacked by the fever, and recovered. When told by the surgeon who attended him, that to save his life he ought to go, he replied, ' No, Sir, this is our post, and I will not set the example of leaving it.' He soon afterwards had a relapse, which proved fatal." The native officers of Gardiner's Horse tried to cause the authorities to interfere with their surgeon to take care of himself, and be less in hospital. "The death of a dozen of us does not matter," they said ; "but if he dies, the whole corps will perish."

Mr. T. C. Robertson, the humane and most able commissioner on the spot, says, in his " Political Incidents of the First Burmese War :"—" The devotion of all members of the medical staff to their duties was most exemplary. Not one of them, however ill, withdrew from the Province, where many of the number died. I have myself seen some of them, in the intervals of their own agues, wrapped up in cloaks and busied in visiting the sufferers under their charge." The commissioner, who subsequently rose to be Governor of Agra, might well designate the conduct of Mr. Grant as "a fine example."

1st. That the reduction in the size of the spleen bears some proportion to the quantity of the medicine taken.

2nd. That the effect produced by quinine upon intermittent
fevers is proportioned to the reduction of the spleen.

3rd. That the fever is cured simultaneously with the cure of the
splenic disease.

4th. That, on the other hand, the fever will be liable to recur
so long as the spleen exceeds its proper size.

M. Piorry believes that as the spleen attains its greatest size at
an early period in ague, the paroxysm does not produce the hypertrophy, but rather that the enlarged organ maintains the disease.
He and M. Bally are of opinion that no other remedy is so certain
or energetic in agues as quinine ; its powers being equally remarkable in the ascites that results from long-continued disease of the
spleen.

There are cases of intermittent fever, however, complicated with
hepatic and other engorgement, and which continue to recur
with deplorable perseverance and tenacity, despite of all means,
until a few doses of calomel, followed by purgatives, are administered : then the quinine, which before failed, will speedily cure
the disease.   It would thus appear that certain morbid conditions
of both liver and spleen will certainly produce and maintain the
tendency to recurrence of agues.   Ramazini relates the case of a
patient harassed by an obstinate ague, and who was cured by
mercurial frictions administered for syphilis.

" The cause which prevents the cure of ague," says Dr. Billing,
" is visceral disease, which may either have existed before the
intermittent, or have arisen during its continuance.   The ague
and the visceral disease, whether of bowels, liver, spleen, or lungs,
&c., act reciprocally as cause and effect—the ague aggravating the
visceral disease by causing congestion during each paroxysm ; the
visceral disease, by keeping up morbid sensibility during the intermission (or even a pyrexial state between the paroxysms, when
the disease is named remittent), which prevents the cure ; but if,
by mercury, or bleeding, &c., the visceral disease be removed, the
cinchona exercises its influence on the nervous system, and finally
arrests the disease."

Following out this principle, though by means of a different
class of remedies, Dr. Golding Bird shows how, in persons having
the sallow, dirty aspect of malaria, they may be made to exchange
it for the cleaner and brighter complexion of returning health, by
a course of alkaline treatment, including the *renal depurants*, and
how visceral engorgements may be overcome, and the sufferer
thereby prepared for the beneficial use of antiperiodics which had
been previously ineffective.   " *In ague*," he says, " nothing is more
easy, as every one is aware, than to check the paroxysm by means
of antiperiodics, especially quinine, and in many cases the patient
is cured by the remedy.   But any one who has had an opportunity

of seeing much of the effects of marsh miasmata, is perfectly aware that if a patient has been long exposed to their influence, although paroxysms of ague may for a time be checked with quinine or arsenic, the unhealthy state of the blood is not removed. The sallow aspect—the depressed health—the visceral engorgement—all indicate that the poison remains in the system and is continuing its work, although its influence has been blunted by our remedies. After a time, however, imperfect paroxysms, the 'dumb ague,' as they are often graphically called by the patient, appear again, requiring the antiperiodic to check their further development. This is a common history, and many persons are thus not really absolutely freed from miasmatic poison for months or years.

"I do not claim for the acetate of potass the virtue of an antiperiodic, but I do unhesitatingly declare that it will effect that which quinine and its allies cannot do. It will enter the blood, and as a *nascent* carbonate (possessing a far higher state of "chemical tendency" than ready-formed carbonate of potass) in the capillary network of the body, aids the metamorphosis and excretion of the unhealthy elements of the blood, and their consequent elimination by the kidneys.

"When to a person suffering from the effects of marsh malaria, this drug has been administered to the extent of two drachms in the course of twenty-four hours, largely diluted, and continued for two or three weeks, not only is no injury effected by the remedy, but the most marked benefits are observed to result. The patient's skin becomes less dusky, the expression more healthy, the dull aspect of the eyes changed for one of cheerfulness, the engorgements of the liver and spleen lessen, and the paroxysms of 'dumb ague' disappear, or merely require a few doses of arsenic for their complete cure, and thus to effect the complete restoration of the patient."

We now perceive that, whether we have to treat the acute malarious fevers of hot climates, or the dumb smouldering fevers, the sequelæ of the former, as they appear in temperate regions, we must, to obtain the full powers of tonic and antiperiodic remedies, first remove active or passive congestions of the abdominal viscera, and secondly, we must establish a free depuration, as necessary preliminaries. It is thus, and only thus, that we may justly combine the two objects we have in view, and lead to the safe and perfect cure of such diseases.

This rule of practice applies, indeed, to the use of all general tonics—their effective application requiring a certain amount of previous depuration. The principle is founded on the acquired experience of ages; yet it is not so well understood, nor carried out in practice, as it ought to be. Let us hope that a due consideration of its practical worth may never be lost sight of.

The course of treatment here recommended I have found to be

sound in principle and in practice during many years past, in the chronic agues of European climates, and in the cure of the sequelæ to the intermittents of the tropics.

We shall be led to the most effective treatment of intermittent fevers, by an early and close attention to their complications, such as the splenic and hepatic congestions, and the inflammatory affections of these and other organs, which occasionally arise during their progress, and towards their termination. The utmost attention should be paid, during and subsequently to each paroxysm, to the condition of the two important organs referred to, as well as to the state, whether congestive or inflammatory, of the cerebral and abdominal organs generally. It is easy in the average of cases to cure a simple uncomplicated ague; but it is not so when the type of the fever is malignant, or adynamic, or where the complications are severe. In every case of ague there will be more or less of simple turgescence of both liver and spleen during the cold stage, especially if this last prove of long duration; but this turgescence disappears in mild cases with the sweating stage of the fever. It is different, however, under concentrated endemic influences, and where the ague is consequently pernicious; for here the spleen and liver, if they do not become immediately affected, are sure to be so eventually. Repeated over a succession of months or years, even simple turgescence may terminate in organic disease, from want of early or of proper treatment. In truth, the difficulties encountered in the treatment of agues consist in the presence of the original malarious influence, and in the existence of the complications above mentioned. Wanting these two, or, in other words, under change to a purer air, and in the absence of cerebral or abdominal complication, agues are very easy of cure.

Emetics would seem to be indicated in the cold stage of this fever, with the view to restore the balance of circulation and relieve oppression resulting from congestion of the viscera; but here, as in the remittents of Bengal, emetics are not, and never have been in favour with practitioners in the East. Warm drinks, ammonia, ether, camphor, and other diffusible stimuli, and warmth externally applied, are preferred by the great majority.

When the hot stage has come on, a full dose of calomel with James's powder should be given at once, and in three hours this should be followed by a brisk cathartic—diluent drinks being freely used meanwhile, along with some cooling diuretic: the tartarized antimony with nitrate of potash answers the double purpose of determining the fluids to the skin and the kidneys. On the following morning, the intermission being complete, the sulphate of quinine is to be administered, at intervals of three hours during the day, the patient being kept in bed, and supplied with farinaceous food only. The treatment here briefly indicated will speedily cure a mild and uncomplicated ague. In the simple cases here contemplated it may not be necessary to administer mercurials more than once or twice; but active purgatives are always beneficial in relieving the full and congested state of the abdomen generally during the continuance of intermittent fever.

But where the disease is severe, and accompanied by præcordial oppression, pain, or fulness of the spleen or liver, or of both, or where there is severe headache, or headache with giddiness, or an oppressive fulness of the chest, a general or local blood-letting, or even both together, will be necessary as a means of present cure, and as a preventive of future ills. Measures of depletion are as necessary here as in remittent fever, and repeated applications of leeches, with several doses of calomel and strong purges are required, in these severe cases, to prepare the system for the anti-periodic power of bark, quinine, or arsenic.

" *Depletions,*" says Copland, " are almost indispensable preli-minaries to the quinine or bark, especially in the complicated and congestive forms ; for, without them, it will either not be retained on the stomach; or, if retained, will convert congestions, or slight forms of inflammatory irritation, into active inflammation, or into structural change." He adds that it is chiefly from a neglect of this practice that complications and unfavourable consequences so often follow the use of bark, quinine, or arsenic ; for these often interrupt secretion, and over-excite and inflame loaded, obstructed, or congested organs. As in the milder instances, mercurials with sudorifics, occasional diuretics followed by powerful cathartics, and quina, are here necessary ; and on their proper application the efficiency and the speed of the cure will depend. Blood should be drawn here, as in the remittent fevers, at the very onset of the hot stage, or that of reaction; and it should be regulated by the constitution, age, and habit of the patient, as already explained. By such timely depletion congestions and inflammatory conditions will be removed, and much future disease and suffering will be prevented.

Where, on the other hand, the intermittent fever assumes a low adynamic form, or where the subject is in a state of anæmia, with or without enlargement of the spleen, mercurials should be most carefully avoided in the treatment, and reliance placed on change of air, quina, chalybeates, and improved diet. Under the condi-tion of the general habit now referred to, mercury must not be administered for the cure even of hepatic enlargement :—the nitro-muriatic acid must be used instead, both internally and externally. Mercury would here be at once ineffective and injurious—indeed dangerous—while the mineral acids are most powerful to good.

"One of the great elements of successful treatment," says Dr. Golding Bird, "must of necessity be the depuration of the blood, and thus by freeing the system from the depressing influence of these vitiated matters, allow the vital powers to throw off the influence of the poison which for a time oppressed them. The influence of small doses of mercury in the treatment of ague is well known; by a gentle but persistent appeal of this kind to the liver, the patient is immensely relieved, and his ultimate cure expedited. Cotemporaneously with this, the aspect generally becomes less sallow, and sufficient indication of the liver becoming active in depurating the blood of carbon. Then, under the influence of that very curious class of remedies, the antiperiodic tonics, the paroxysms become less, or quite vanish, whilst ample evidence is afforded of the kidneys performing the important duty of filtering from the blood highly nitrogenized substances, in the rapidly increasing amount of solids existing in the urine."

Those who advocate the exclusive use of antiperiodic means appear to forget that in fever a poison has been imbibed, and that for its elimination—to subdue the resulting visceral complications, and to remove the poison from the system—we must, as often stated in this work, at first act upon, and through, the depurative functions; and that, without such preliminary process, we necessarily leave behind some form of organic lesion. To arrest the periodical movement of fever merely for a time, is not to cure the disease; and soldiers in this condition discharged the hospitals are harassed with relapses, and afflicted with abdominal congestions, too often to terminate in permanent injury to the structure of important viscera. When chronic disease of the liver eventually destroys life, the fatal result is principally brought about through the destruction of its depurative function.

In the low form of ague, in the anæmic habit, and where there is chronic enlargement of the spleen, with the splenic cachexia, blood-letting, general or local, should also be avoided; but even in weakly persons who are not anæmic, local blood-letting by means of leeches will be found extremely beneficial, under the cautions as to subsequent oozing already pointed out. In removing epigastric oppression or tenderness, or similar states of either or both hypochondria, fomentations followed by leeches will always, in a tolerably sound state of the constitution, be safe and proper, as will occasionally blisters. Warm-baths, used at bedtime, are likewise very beneficial.

The condition of the spleen should be carefully observed during the entire progress of intermittent fever. In persons of plethoric habit, leeches and purgatives in the stage of reaction, followed by quinine in the sweating stage, and in that of intermission, and given in a larger dose two hours before the attack, will conduct the patient through in safety; while, in anæmic patients, the quinine ought to be conjoined with iron, and animal food should take the place of depletory measures.

The sulphate of quinine is exhibited variously by various practitioners—some, as Maillot, giving very large doses, such as twenty and thirty grains four hours before the expected paroxysm—while others begin to administer the quinine on the subsiding of the paroxysm, and during the sweating stage.   But the most rational plan, so far as my experience extends, would appear to be that of ex-hibiting the quina every three or four hours during the apyrexy, and in such doses as the urgency of the symptoms may demand. In this manner a sufficient quantity of the antiperiodic will be best borne, while the risk of injury by overdosing will be avoided—seeing that during the intervals of exhibition we can watch and measure the effects.   I have always exhibited the sulphate of quinine in this manner, I believe with an average amount of success ; and it can hardly be necessary to observe here that I have seen, over a long range of years, and in various countries of the East, very severe types of intermittents.   To cure the patient by means of the quina is all that is wanted ; and to exhibit more of that medicine than is needful to this object, or to protract the use of it beyond the occa-sion, is to injure him.   I always administered the quinine in solution, with the addition of a small quantity of dilute sulphuric acid, and with the other occasional aids already mentioned.

In the instances of plethoric subjects, I conjoined the quinine with antimonials and diuretics ; and where the patient was feeble and irritable, with symptoms of exhaustion, I added small doses of tincture of opium to the antiperiodic.   In robust subjects, newly arrived from Europe, the calmative and depurative measures were thus advantageously followed by a cholagogue and brisk cathartic ; and then came the tonic and antiperiodic influence of quinine, in its proper time and place.   Several very able medical officers are in the habit of giving quinine in the intermittents of the East Indies, in doses of twenty-five to thirty grains "as soon as the patient begins to perspire freely after the hot stage." They declare that this plan has proved in their hands more effective, and more economical of the medicine.

Arsenic has for ages been known to, and largely exhibited by the Native doctors throughout India, in every form of fever, continued as well as paroxysmal ; and they are in the habit of exhibiting the mineral in very large doses, and for a long continuance—frequently with permanent injury to the health, as mentioned at page 341. When arsenic is preferred in the treatment of ague, it should be given in the College formula of solution, not in bitter infusions, as recommended by some writers, but in some aromatic water, with or without a few drops of laudanum to each dose of the arsenical solution, as may be deemed necessary.   From six to eight drops given in this manner, every three hours, during the apyrexy, and continued only for a few days, prove very effective in many cases.

Arsenic may also be given with safety during the paroxysm, as well as in the stage of intermission ; but the dose should always be taken after meals, as then the mineral is disseminated through the food and absorbed along with it, without the risk of causing irritation of the stomach. It will always be found to effect its greatest results where the spleen is not enlarged; and this is a fact of importance to note.

After the force of the fever has been broken by the use of quinine, or where relapses in lesser degrees of violence still harass the patient, the arsenical solution will be found a valuable aid and substitute; and this becomes an important consideration in the field of active service, where quinine may be scarce.

The Swietenia Febrifuga, and the kernel of the Cæsalpinia Bonducella, and the Chiretta, are much used by the native practitioners of Bengal, as antiperiodics and tonics.

Mr. E. F. Sankey, of Beckley, Sussex, has for some years treated the ague of his district with iodide of potassium, and he states, on his experience of a large number of cases, that he "has never yet failed in curing the disease very quickly." His formula is a drachm and a half of the iodide to twelve ounces of peppermint water; and of this mixture the patient took two tablespoonfuls every four hours. In chronic cases, where the patient was much reduced, two grains of quinine were added to each dose; but, in general, the iodide alone was relied upon.

Another treatment, and a successful one according to report, has been by chloroform. M. Delioux, professor in the French Naval Medical School, forms a syrup by adding five parts of chloroform to a hundred of syrup; of which he gives from one to three drachms in a mixture at the same intervals at which quinine would be given. The febrifuge powers of chloroform are stated to have received ample verification in the hands of this gentleman, in the cure of intermittent fever.

The question of the proper substitutes for quinine acquires great importance in the East Indies, owing to the great cost of the drug, to the difficulty of obtaining it in remote districts and stations, and to the extensive adulteration of it by the natives.

Where the intermittent fever has become chronic, or when as secondary results there is organic disease of the liver or spleen, or of both, change of climate becomes a measure of necessity; and it is one that should never be neglected in such cases. I trust I need not add to what has been written in the last article on this subject.

As, notwithstanding its scientific claims, fashion unhappily still holds some influence in medicine, and as bleeding in the cold stage of intermittent fever may again come under professional review, in the round of medical opinions and practices, I think it right to notice the subject. My own personal experience will not allow of my speaking in favourable terms of this practice; neither will a reference to authority prove more encouraging, as the following comparative quotations will show:—

DR. MACKINTOSH.

"The practice prevents debility in a direct manner by saving the vital fluid."

MR. TWINING.

"I may say that in all regular intermittents, with cold, hot, and sweating stages, and tolerable uniformity in the hours of accession, the practice of bleeding in the commencement of the cold stage, has proved always safe, and generally more successful than any other remedy."

DR. MACKINTOSH.

"I believe bleeding in the cold stage, conjoined with the occasional use of sulphate of quinine and laxatives, to be as certain a mode of treating intermittents as any other set of medicines can be said to be certain in the treatment of any other class of diseases."

DR. MACKINTOSH.

"The practice may be adopted in the first stage of all fevers."

MR. TWINING.

"The recent practice of bleeding in intermittents, as recommended by Dr. Mackintosh, not only accords with the acknowledged pathology of that class of fevers, but seems to bring our system of therapeutics, as applied to them, within the limits of those established principles adapted to the treatment of other fevers,

DR. ELLIOTSON.

"It is not at all right to take away blood, and thus impair the power of the patient;" when, as he adds, he "never saw a case which he could not cure by the sulphate of quinine."

DR. WATSON.

"I object to bleeding because it appears to me quite unnecessary; because it is not such as the nature of the symptoms would suggest; because it tends to produce subsequent debility, which we should not needlessly inflict; and because the experience of other sober-minded men, who have given the method a fair trial, does not bear out the statement made by Dr. Mackintosh in respect to its usefulness. If in this country bleeding be requisite at all, it is in the *hot* stage."

DR. STOKES

"Bled in the cold stage, and found it useless and injurious; and, after all, was compelled to give quinine sooner or later."

DR. ELLIOTSON.

"The quinine, which cures it best, interferes with no other measures."

THE CELEBRATED DR. GREGORY.

"Blood-letting, which at another period of the disease," namely, intermittent fever, "might have been proper, if employed in the *first stage* never fails to be attended with the most dangerous consequences; or it is, to use the words of Celsus, *hominem jugulare.*"

DR. COPLAND.

"In a case where I directed blood-letting before reaction supervened, the loss of three or four ounces caused profound and prolonged syncope, yet within four hours, when reaction had come on, fifty ounces were taken before any effect was produced upon the pulse; and before the sun of the same day had gone down, forty more were abstracted at one time, in all ninety-four ounces within twelve hours."

DR. DENMARK, PHYSICIAN TO THE FLEET.

"In these instances venesection was never had recourse to till the vascular system had fairly emerged from the depressed state incident to that stage of the fever, and reaction had clearly manifested itself by the returning glow of the skin, the filling of the previously shrunk

from which, formerly, intermittents were almost excluded."

and dejected features, and the firm though frequently oppressed beat of the pulse. Former experience not only taught me that an earlier abstraction of blood was never borne to an extent productive of ultimate benefit, but, on the contrary, seemed to be injurious by tending to protract the first stage of the paroxysm."

MR. TWINING.

" The safety and efficacy of this practice have been so far established by Dr. Mackintosh that I have not hesitated to adopt it." . . . . "The great advantage of V. S. in the cold stage of ague appears to me to depend on the prompt and decided relief it affords, guarding the patient against the ulterior results of repeated congestions of internal organs." . . . . " It appears to me that V. S. in the cold stage of intermittent fevers deserves to be classed among the best remedies which we possess for the effectual cure of many of the most obstinate cases of these diseases in Europeans."

DR. WATSON.

"Drs. Townsend and Law, of Dublin, found it fail in the majority of cases. In Dr. Stokes's hands the most usual effect of blood-letting was to check the shivering; and, next to this, to mitigate the severity without abridging its duration. In most instances no modification was produced of the hot and of the sweating stages. In Dr. Kelly's experience the general effect was to shorten the cold stage, and to render the hot one milder ; but in some cases it seemed to aggravate the symptoms. Mr. Gill found that although the blood-letting might cut short the cold stage, it appeared to lengthen the period of febrile disturbance."

DR. MACKINTOSH.

" Bark has been long in use, and although I never denied that it had virtues, yet when given in substance in the large doses which are admitted to be necessary, I have so frequently seen it do mischief that the question has often suggested itself to me, whether it was not more injurious than beneficial ? It seems to be injurious in many cases by overloading the stomach and bowels with indigestible ligneous fibre, and I have seen it cause serious intestinal irritation, as displayed by griping pains in the bowels, diarrhœa, and painful tenesmus. On examining the stools in these cases, they seem chiefly to consist of bark, with a considerable quantity of mucus occasionally tinged with a little blood.

" The preparation of bark, which is known by the name of the sulphate of quinine, is the greatest improvement in modern pharmacy, and the knowledge of its beneficial effects in simple intermittents affords sufficient proof of the virtues of the substance from which it is extracted ; yet this remedy, all-powerful as it is, is useless in the cold stage, and must also fail in cases complicated with organic disease. . . . . My youthful readers may rest assured that the same observations are generally applicable to the sulphate of quinine ; yet they will most probably meet with many practitioners who will assure them that they have never seen a case in which bark, exhibited in

DR. STOKES.

"Having now described the effects of the practice on the paroxysm and on the local symptoms, I must next mention some very untoward circumstances which appeared to follow the bleeding in the cold stage—these were *the occurrence of new local inflammatory symptoms, and the supervention of a low irritative fever.* From the examination of the cases, I apprehend that an impression will be received against the indiscriminate or even frequent use of bleeding in the cold stage of ague. It may be remarked that in the great majority quinine had to be administered before the disease was eradicated ; that many of them had an extremely slow and dangerous convalescence ; that in several instances the disease, so far from being relieved, appeared exasperated by the practice ; that local inflammatory affections occurred several times after the operation ; and lastly, that the bleeding appears to have a tendency to convert intermittent into continued fever. In one case, that of Caseley, death from pneumonia and softening of the brain occurred. In none of my cases did any bad effects from sinking of the powers of life follow the practice immediately ; but I am informed that in the practice of a highly respectable individual, there occurred two cases in which the patients did not recover from the collapse produced by bleeding in the cold stage. These facts should make

substance, or in any other form, has failed in their hands. When they hear such statements they may be satisfied that such practitioners never met with a severe case, or that there is some subterfuge. Some medical men, it is but charitable to suppose, are in the habit of deceiving themselves. In the instances which fell under my own observation, and to which I have already alluded, fever and violent cerebral symptoms succeeded, and, in *two or three instances, local inflammations.*"

us very cautious how we interfere with nature by means of the lancet in simple intermittent, where we have so certain, and as far as I have seen, so infallible a remedy as the sulphate of quinine. I do not deny that cases may often occur where venesection may be proper, such as intermittent complicated with severe internal inflammation ; but shall only remark, as these cases have not come under my own immediate observation, that to offer my opinion on a purely practical point connected with them would be wholly useless. I may mention that I have been informed by my friends, Drs. Townsend and Law, of this city, that they have given the practice a trial, and have found it to fail in the majority of cases."

MR. TWINING.

" In the early stages of intermittent fevers, or to speak with more precision, *within two* or *three weeks* of their commencement, in persons of robust habit, there is very often disorder of the functions and secretions of the digestive organs, and particularly of the stomach, co-existent with congestion of the brain, and attended in some cases with *tolerably distinct evidences of inflammatory condition either in the cerebral* membranes or in the brain itself."*

DR. JAMES JOHNSON.

"What kind of inflammation must that be which explodes, as it were, the moment the clock strikes a particular hour, and this for days and weeks together ? What kind of inflammation is that which, every second day, terminates in profuse *perspiration* from head to foot, and yet is renewed after an interval of forty-eight hours with the symptoms as before, and so on ? Do we see real and unequivocal *inflammations* pursue this course ? Never. Are the causes of these *intermittent phlegmasiæ* (if such an expression be not a solecism in medical language) of a periodical or intermittent nature ? No. They do not accommodate themselves to any particular theory."

DR. HUGHES BENNETT.

" I usually give five grains of quinine three times a day, and a scruple two hours before the occurrence of the attack, and have never seen a case which resisted this treatment."

Thus it appears, at least in Europe, that the treatment of intermittent fevers by blood-letting in the cold stage, whilst it has the show of being prompt and energetic, proves in effect haphazard, systemless, operose, and tedious ; and, from all that I have seen and heard in the East, the result there has not been more favourable. Modern science, indeed, is steadily though slowly achieving a signal victory, in the treatment of fevers especially—namely, that over exclusive systems. It is no longer with us as with the character in Molière—" A dead man is but a dead man, but rules

---

* The italics in the two last quotations are mine, and I have added them with a view to mark the vagueness and want of precision in both writers when they speak of inflammation, whether as affording an explanation of the physiology of this disease, as some writers would have it, or as applicable to mere occasional complication. It is to the former notion that Dr. James Johnson's observations apply.

are everything." Exclusive doctrines in medicine have become like exclusive privileges in common life—they cannot be maintained.

To conclude :—The rule of practice laid down by Pringle and Cleghorn has received little or no addition in more recent times. Where general blood-letting is had recourse to, in the treatment of intermittent fevers, whether simple or complicated, it should, as in the case of all other fevers, be performed at the very onset of the stage of reaction. Practised at this period of the febrile movement, it will diminish the force and frequency of arterial action, relieve venous congestion, usher in the sweating stage, and thereby pave the way for the administration of purgatives, sudorifics, diuretics, and quinine, on the just application of all which the prevention of recurrence must depend.

In the milder forms of ague, in feeble habits, or in the cases of persons who may have resided long in India, local depletion, by means of leeches, will answer every purpose.

THE CONGESTIVE CONTINUED FEVER OF THE COLD SEASON IN BENGAL.

This fever, like all the diseases of the cold season in Bengal, is dangerous from its insidiousness. It is a frequent form of disease ; and none are exempt from its seizure—not even the prudent of the better classes of Europeans. It attacks persons of all ages, and of both sexes ; but men are, from their habits of life, far more exposed to it, and that in its graver forms. Its approach, unlike the fevers of the hot season and rains, is very gradual, being generally but little noticed either by the patient or his friends ; or, if noticed, it passes for catarrh, or dyspepsia.

At this stage, the functions of circulation and secretion are but little affected ; yet, there is a harsh dryness of the skin, especially of that covering the abdomen, coupled with a sense of fulness and oppression at the epigastrium, which will not fail to attract the notice of the careful medical observer. In the course of a few days, provided these symptoms receive no professional attention and treatment, the circulation and respiration become hurried ; headache is present, together with lassitude and anxiety, loss of appetite and rest, the tongue indicating disorder of the digestive functions. The loss of more time brings with it serious complications in the form of abdominal and cerebral congestions, as indicated by increased fulness and oppression of the præcordia—tension of the whole abdomen—intense headache, with occasional delirium—and sometimes with yellowness of the whole surface of the body, jaundiced eye, and a surcharged state of the urine ; in short, there are present all those morbid conditions which we might, *a priori*, anticipate as likely to arise from neglect, under the influences described at pages 57 to 63, and which cannot be too deeply impressed on the recollection of all who have to encounter the cold season in Bengal; for the same neglect may, according to circumstances, induce the fever here described, dysentery, or the still more dangerous, deep-seated and insidious hepatic inflammation common to the cold season.

It is believed that in animals whose pulmonary system is comparatively less perfect, there is a greatly increased quantity of blood transmitted through the liver. In hot climates then, where respiration is less perfectly carried on than in such as are cold, owing to the greater rarefaction of the air in warm regions, according to Tiedemann and Gmelin, a vicarious decarbonization of the blood is established by an increased flow of bile; and hence it is that the liver, now weakened and rendered torpid, in proportion as its function has been unnaturally excited during the previous hot and rainy seasons, becomes disposed to congestion and inflammation of its parenchyma during the cold season, and thus are produced the dangerous states of disease noticed.

An irritable or inflamed state of the mucous digestive surface is a frequent complication; and these combined circumstances constitute the great dangers of our congestive fever of the cold season in Bengal, as well as those of the autumnal fevers of the more unhealthy countries of Europe.

The form of fever is generally continued; but, when protracted, it may and does frequently assume the remittent character, particularly where the patient has recently been exposed to malarious influences, as during the sporting excursions made during the cold season into the districts around Calcutta. In cases where we have to lament the neglect of early treatment, cerebral congestion with delirium prove occasionally long-continued and troublesome, especially when to these states are added retention of urine—all demanding much care and attention : but serious as these cerebral affections appear, I have generally seen that the patient recovered, provided they were not associated with abdominal complication of a grave nature. But when we have the attendants of yellow suffusion, parched and black tongue, jactitation, and a generally typhous condition, we must perceive that the condition of the sufferer is one of imminent peril.

The appearances on dissection are such as the nature of the disease and its complications might lead us to expect; various degrees of acute congestion, or of inflammation, with their results, being very generally found within the abdominal and cerebral cavities. In neglected cases we find hepatic abscess, and sometimes ulceration of the mucous digestive surface. This latter condition I found to be very prevalent amongst the labouring classes of natives, whom I had continually to treat at the Native Hospital

c c

of Calcutta on account of neglected fevers of from fifteen to twenty days' duration; and yet a large proportion of them recovered.

The treatment of the continued fever of the cold season in Bengal, amongst Europeans, is conducted on the same general principles which guide us in our management of those of the other seasons. We have to diminish arterial action, and relieve local congestions, by blood-letting, suited to the age, sex, and length of residence in India of the patient, and to the urgency of the symptoms. Having effected these primary objects, we proceed, without loss of time, to promote the secretions by a full dose of calomel with James's powder, followed in a few hours by active saline cathartics. Where no complications exist, one or two moderate bleedings, followed by brisk purgatives, and tartarized antimony with nitrate of potash, will suffice for the cure, when these have been accompanied and followed by total abstinence from food, and by cooling diluent drinks. But where the brain, or liver, or both, have become the seats of diseased action, then our remedial means must increase in vigour; the general and local blood-letting being larger in amount, and more frequently repeated—the calomel with antimony, and the purgatives, must be more largely and more frequently exhibited—until relief from the fever and from all local congestion shall be obtained, together with a restoration of natural secretion; for these are the only true signs of recovery.

It frequently happens in the course of this fever, that, with or without cerebral oppression, we have a sluggish condition of the bowels, with defective hepatic and intestinal secretions. In order to elicit these secretions, I was in the habit of combining plain scammony and the James's powder with the calomel, exhibiting them thus united overnight, and following them up in the morning by a brisk draught of infusion of senna with simple jalap powder; or, where viscid mucus impacted the bowels, by a terebinthinate draught. In the fevers of children especially, we often find that the most alarming cerebral symptoms, with a doughy, inelastic state of the abdomen and torpid bowels, are removed at once by the night exhibition of medicine here mentioned, followed in the morning by the rectified oil of turpentine.

When the patient is seen after having been many days ill, without previous medical aid, congestion having proceeded unrestrained within the cerebral or abdominal cavity, or within both, blood-letting, general and local, calomel, sudorifics with diuretics, and strong purgatives still constitute the means on which we must rely; and we shall frequently have to exhibit the calomel so as gently to affect the system. These means, powerful as they are, will not, under the circumstances of neglect here contemplated, prove so prompt in their results as when applied earlier; but, nevertheless, they must be used, powerfully and repeatedly in bad cases, otherwise the patient will be destroyed—all the functions being overpowered by the force of congestive disease.

Where, on the other hand, we have evidence of irritation of the mucous digestive surface, we must determine to the skin freely by mild diaphoretics in the form of antimony or ipecacuanha, together with warm baths, relieving the bowels when necessary by the most unirritating aperients.

Natives of Bengal were daily brought into the Native Hospital in the most advanced and neglected stages of this form of fever; with tumid abdomens, confirmed stupor, and tongues black and dry as charcoal; and it was surprising how many of these poor people recovered under the following plan of treatment, which, after a large amount of experience, became at length the settled management in such cases. On admission into hospital, the patient was put into a warm bath, while the entire surface of the body was purified by the free use of brush and soap—the head being shaved at the same time, and cold applied to it. A large sinapism was then applied to the abdomen; and where the state of the pulse admitted of it, a few leeches were applied to the epigastric region, or behind the ears, or to both regions, followed in a day or two by blisters to those parts. A very mild aperient draught was always administered on admission, aiding its operation by enemata.

A course of treatment was then commenced, of alkali, mild aperient and sudorific, all conjoined. The formula which I ordered was generally as follows:—

Sesquicarbonate of soda . . . . Əj
Powdered rhubarb. . . . . grs. v.
Powdered ipecacuanha . . . . grs. j to ij.

This medicine was exhibited three or four times in the twenty-four hours, according to the severity of congestion, while the diet consisted only of iced barley-water; and, as I have already stated, the result from these simple means was such as to surprise medical officers habituated only to the treatment of Europeans. The progressive recovery of sense, and gradual restoration to health, of persons who, a week or ten days before, had appeared in a hopeless state of disease, were very remarkable: but the natives of India will recover from wounds, and from advanced states of diseases resulting from fevers, which would destroy any European. The cases of fever here referred to were those of persons of the labouring class of natives, in whom fever had gone on unrestrained by any treatment for fifteen or twenty days, and in which, consequently, the period for more active measures of cure had long passed away. We were therefore content to work on gradually with nature—to see the patients improving; as any heroic endeavour to hasten the operation of cure would only have endangered their safety—so reduced were the powers of life.

To conclude :—it is scarcely necessary to urge that where this fever assumes the remittent character, whether in the instance of an European or native, quinine in proper doses, and administered during the remissions, will prove of signal advantage.

THE ARDENT CONTINUED FEVER OF THE HOT SEASON IN BENGAL.

I HAVE placed my notice of this fever last in order, because, though very dangerous to persons of irregular habits of life, it is yet by no means so frequent of occurrence as the forms of fever previously noticed. A consideration of what has been said on the general influence of a high range of temperature at pages 45 to 52, will have prepared the reader for an unusually severe and dangerous disturbance of the nervous and vascular functions, under the united influences of direct, and of long-continued solar exposure, especially where there has been intemperance of habit; and so we find it in the European soldier, in whom this ardent form of fever often merges in coup-de-soleil, or heat-apoplexy.

It cannot be necessary to enter into all the minute details of symptoms in the milder forms of this disease, seeing the graver type of remittent has already been described. It is always easy to bring the mind to the comprehension of simple and uncomplicated diseases, when once we have been rendered familiar with their concentrated and more complicated states.

The type of this fever is usually continued, but sometimes remittent: it seizes with suddenness and violence, the heat, thirst, throbbing and frequent pulse, restlessness and racking headache, coming in rapid succession. The complications are generally cerebral, with occasionally severe forms of gastric disturbance, as indicated by pain, oppression of the præcordia, and vomiting; sometimes the liver is involved. We have not here the tendency to collapse so characteristic of the true Bengal remittent fever, as it occurs in the rainy season, but the ardent rapid progress of the disease, together with the cerebro-spinal and gastric complications, render this fever of the hot season one of very considerable danger.

The appearances on dissection are such as might be anticipated from the symptoms during life; they consist of inflammatory and congestive states of the cerebro-spinal organs; and where the stomach, lesser bowel, and liver have been implicated, we perceive the morbid appearances common to our other fevers of the climate. Serous effusions are frequently found in the cerebral and abdominal cavities, more rarely within the thoracic cavity.

The treatment consists in active blood-letting, practised to the extent of allaying the vascular disturbance, relieving the pain of the head, and reducing the temperature of the body ; these are the tests and the proof that the operation has been successful.

Leeches applied behind the ears, cold affusions, continued cold to the shaved head, and calomel and antimony, followed by very active purging, will generally confirm the relief of the patient and complete his cure. In this fever, as in that of the cold season, the skin will generally be found harsh to the touch, compacted, hot and dry, so as to require a more free use of antimonials and refrige-rants, antimonial diaphoretics, united with cooling diuretics, than we find to be necessary in the fevers of the rainy season. When remissions take place, provided the head be relieved, quinine must be had recourse to for the purpose of preventing the recurrence of paroxysms ; and should symptoms of exhausted nervous power, or of delirium tremens, make their appearance, from half a grain to a grain of opium, united with calomel and antimony, will soothe and procure sleep. But here, as in all diseases which tend towards coma, we must be guarded in the use of opium : it masks the real state of the disease, deceiving both the friends of the patient and the surgeon. In this, as in the ordinary remittents of Bengal, where an anæmic irritable condition of the brain has become manifest, symptoms occur which prove very embarrassing to the young surgeon ; and the treatment of them by camphor, or by camphor and opium, becomes an important practical question. Let it be carefully noted, that the indication for the use of opium is, the existence of well-marked nervous symptoms.

"For the congested state of the nervous centres in fever," says Dr. Billing, "syrup of poppy, or a few drops of laudanum, will produce an effect equal to that of a larger dose of opiate medicine in other states of disease." The same authority observes that narcotics are frequently useful *during* fever, nay, necessary, as may be understood by referring to the essence of fever, and knowing that sleep is nature's restorer of deficient nervous influence. The obstinate wakefulness which takes place in some cases of fever must have a deleterious tendency to produce collapse, hence the benefit of gentle opiates.

Drs. Corrigan and Gordon, of Dublin, have for some time past exhibited chloroform internally to procure sleep in fever, to re-lieve pain in painter's colic, and to overcome nervous agitation and restlessness in delirium tremens.

"The affections of the cerebral functions," says Dr. Gordon, "frequently assume great importance in fever; their derangement is sometimes indicative of disease in the respiratory apparatus, or in the digestive canal ; more commonly, however, it is owing to the organic nervous influence produced by the fever on the brain and nervous tissue itself. One of the most prominent character-istics of this lesion is insomnolency, causing, or, at all events, followed by delirium, subsultus, &c." It is in such highly dangerous states of disease that chloroform internally administered produces the happiest effects.

Dr. Corrigan states truly that " the loss of sleep, if continued, is of itself sufficient to kill;" and he adds that, " if even the shortest sleep is procured, some advantage is gained." His formula, of which one ounce is the ordinary dose, is a follows :—

Chloroform	ℨv.
Pulv. glycyrrhizæ	ℨv.
Mist. camphoræ	℥ixss.

To afford sleep in fever, to relieve pain in painter's colic, the minimum dose exhibited is half a drachm of chloroform repeated every two or three hours. In delirium tremens the dose at first is a drachm, and is often increased to two drachms. It may with safety be given in larger doses, and, unlike opiates, it does not lock up the secretions.

Speaking of the use of wine in fever, Dr. Billing says, that the person who best understands the nature of delirium tremens will be the quickest to discern the propriety and necessity for the administration of wine and opiates in fever, erysipelas, &c. Even in inflammations occurring in debauched and debilitated constitutions, it is absolutely necessary to give more or less stimulants at a very early stage.

Where wakefulness threatens injury during the course of, or in the more advanced stages of tropical fevers, or where symptoms indicative of delirium tremens arise, opiates are not only safe but necessary; but the inexperienced medical officer must be on his guard against error in diagnosis. He should feel his way with small doses at first, given at intervals; for, as remarked by Dr. Latham, it is a fearful thing to strike a heavy blow in the dark, where the alternative is of such magnitude.

It is in this fever that cold affusion exerts its greatest power in abstracting heat and subduing nervous and vascular excitement. I remember the case of an officer who had been much exposed to the direct rays of the sun, and who was not subjected to treatment until the advanced stage of his fever. His sufferings and distress were beyond description, and he appeared to be rapidly sinking. His reduced state rendered blood-letting in any form inadmissible; but the skin being of a pungent dry heat, I had him soused with cold water, and the relief was, excepting in one other case already narrated, the most surprising of any that I have ever witnessed. This person, to all appearance lost, was, through cold affusion chiefly, speedily restored to health.

HEAT-APOPLEXY, COUP-DE-SOLEIL, OR SUN-FEVER.

HISTORICAL NOTICES.

ALLIED in some degree to the ardent fever of the hot season in Bengal, and frequently merging into it, is the disease above designated. Under the appellations of insolation, coup-de-soleil, mort subite, heat-apoplexy, heat-asphyxia, ictus solis, sun-fever, and erethismus tropicus, this fatal disease has been long ago noticed by various writers, British and French, as especially visiting Europeans of intemperate habits, with impacted skins and gorged viscera, during the hot and rainy seasons of tropical climates. It is one of the most deadly of the " thousand natural shocks that flesh is heir to." Two instances of this sudden seizure are related in the Bible :—" And Manasses was her husband, of her tribe and kindred, who died in the barley harvest. For as he stood overseeing them, and bound sheaves in the field, the heat came upon his head, and he fell in his bed, and died in the city of Bethulia." Again, we have the case of the son of the Shunammite :—" And when the child was grown, it fell on a day, that he went out to his father to the reapers. And he said unto his father, My head, my head. And he said to a lad, Carry him to his mother. And when he had taken him, and brought him to his mother, he sat on her knee till noon, and then died."

The exuberant nomenclature of this disease offers an indication of the somewhat various forms under which it makes its appearance; varieties in morbid association and complication rather than in essential differences, and resulting from the influences of locality and climate, of season, diet, clothing, and nature of the service on which the soldier may have been employed. The truth is, that the terms above cited have been applied loosely to designate physiological and pathological changes or alterations in the functional connexions of the organs principally involved—as the brain, lungs, and heart; and these vary in degree according to the sanitary circumstances under which the sufferers happened to be placed at the time. Not one of the terms can be said to be founded on a strict pathology; and this fact has been variously commented on, especially by the French authors. As justly observed by Mr. Marcus Hill, of the Bengal Army, " the nomenclature of the disease requires careful sifting." Dr. Dowler, of New Orleans, makes a distinction between " *solar asphyxia*" and " *solar syncope ;*"—adding that " solar asphyxia is always fatal;" but that " this might be curable if the patient were bled *instantaneously.*" A close and careful consideration, however, of the sanitary conditions, the history, and the pathology of the several recorded instances, will show that they have each and all been bound together by the one necessary condition of an unnatural sun-heat, more or less directly or more or less intensely applied.   The main errors, in fact, appear to have arisen from an inattention to the true medical topography and statistics of the disease; and these neglects, again, have led to an uncertain pathology, and a more uncertain treatment.   But we have still in medicine, as in less important branches of knowledge, observers by whom everything is assumed and classified before anything is known; and thus words take the place of things.   In defect of a more special and determinate pathology, it may be best, therefore, in respect of this disease, to leave its terminology to be settled by the results of future research; meanwhile, the terms are sufficiently copious for the purposes of selection, when the proper time for it shall arrive.

CAUSES.

When the strong S.W. monsoon ceases, and the sky becomes obscured by a film of dark, negatively electrified clouds, and the atmosphere hangs like a weight on the mind and body of the soldier, then it is, as remarked by good observers, that epileptic seizures have always been most prevalent in India.

In countries near the equator, where the heat throughout the year, though high, is uniform, sun-stroke is said to be of but rare occurrence :—a certain amount of variation in the temperature of the seasons would therefore seem to dispose to this disease.   For instance, in Sierra Leone, according to Dr. Winterbottom, sun-stroke is unknown, in the infant "not a month old," as in the parents, although in all three the head is exposed uncovered at all seasons ; while in the East Indies, children and grown-up persons are everywhere, but more especially in the more northern divisions, struck down by the sun, or, as they conceive, by the wind. "Even Europeans," says Dr. Winterbottom, "are not liable to sun-stroke in Africa;" and "when they are said to die from this cause," he concludes that it occurs more "from the abuse of those destructive liquors, ardent spirits," than from the sun.   This author states that in the year 1743, between the 14th and 25th of July, up-wards of eleven thousand persons perished in the streets of Pekin from heat-apoplexy. It is worthy of remark that sun-stroke is very rare in the pilot service of Bengal, whose members enter on duty very early in life, although exposed continually in the chains as leadsmen during the first five or six years, in a frightful glare, and under the direct rays of a sun, amounting in July and August sometimes to a heat of 140°.   Instances of sun-stroke, on the other hand, are frequent amongst the crews of ships from Europe, when being piloted up the river to Calcutta ; another confirmation of the fact that the newly-arrived and robust are most liable to attack. Officers of the Indian navy have assured me that, not-withstanding the terrible heats of the Persian Gulf, sun-stroke was rare amongst the European crews.

Direct solar exposure has been too generally and too exclusively assigned as the cause of this form of disease; but Campet speaks of it, under the term *mort subite*, as resulting in Europeans (given to excesses in eating heavy suppers, and in the use of wine and ardent spirits,) during sleep under a high temperature, especially if, by closed curtains, they rendered the imprisoned air polluted and suffocative, thus depraving the circulating fluid, and producing a mortal syncope. In the East as in the West Indies, direct solar exposure is not necessary to the induction of sun-stroke, men con-fined in-doors during the hot season being also liable, especially under intemperance in diet, and in a calm, sultry atmosphere. The able and experienced Mr. T. E. Dempster, of the Bengal army, speaking of the prevalence of heat-apoplexy in the Mooltàn divi-sion, under Sir William Whish, in the hot season of 1849, says: "During the first few marches, a number of men fell victims to that fearful disease, and it is here worthy of remark, that the fatal seizures usually occurred about three o'clock in the morning, and long before the sun was above the horizon."

Dr. Dick, of Bengal, in a letter to Dr. Duncan, published in his Commentaries so far back as 1785, describes this disease as having been prevalent in a detachment of European artillery then serving in the Carnatic. In April, May, June, and July, the land wind blew so exceedingly hot and dry, that life was hardly sup-portable at noon. The cholera morbus, dysentery, inflammations of the liver, and ardent, or what they call bilious fevers, became frequent in camp at this season. A species of apoplexy which seized the men when fatigued by marching in the heat of the sun proved, however, more fatal to the Europeans than any of the above. They complained first of great headache, in a few minutes a vertigo and bilious vomiting came on; they dropped down breathless, turned comatose, and unless immediate assistance was given, the face swelled, and turned almost black; the pulse, which was at first full and quick, sank; and after some hard struggles for breath, they expired. Such is the substance of one of the earliest descriptions of coup-de-soleil in the East Indies.

The increased feebleness of the heart's action, as the disease advances, has been noted by several of the American writers; and there can be no doubt that feebleness of the respiratory function advances in corresponding accord, so as speedily to overwhelm the sufferer. In a recent hot-weather campaign in India, it was prin-cipally amongst the newly-arrived corps, composed of young men, and who had been exposed to much fatigue, that the mortality was the greatest.

Regiments previously stationary, as in cantonments, or during the ease and inaction of a sea-voyage, when called into sudden

and active exertion, with loss of night-rest, especially under exposure to heat and malaria, and under deprivation of water, will
be sure to suffer on the march from sun-stroke.   These unfavourable conditions will receive much aggravation from heavy arming
and marching in close order of the soldier, and from unsuitable
clothing.   The dining and sleeping under the greatest diurnal
heats must also prove injurious to the digestive process, and favour
cerebral and other congestions, constipation of the bowels, &c.

TOPOGRAPHY AND STATISTICS.

While making an examination of the records in the office of the
Army Medical Department, to which, through the kindness of
Sir James M'Grigor, I had access, the clerk who assisted me said:
" Here, sir, are twenty-two admissions into hospital at Berhampore in one season from apoplexy, and twenty-one deaths."   They
were, apparently, examples of the most violent cerebral fever,
amounting in many cases to actual and deadly apoplexy.   The
history of these fatal cases, as given by Drs. Henderson and
Mouat, the able medical officers in charge, will afford a fair sample
of certain forms of this fatal disease.   " Where the line was to be
drawn," says Dr. Henderson, " between apoplexy and remittent
fever, is here hard to say."

The soldiers consisted of older men, of damaged constitutions,
who had recently returned from the first Burmese campaigns, and
of recruits but recently arrived from England.   The corps (H.M.
13th Light Infantry) was marched in two detachments from
Nuddea to Berhampore, a distance of sixty miles, during the hot
season—cruelly, because unnecessarily.   The recruits had been
drilled in the sun, in the approved cocked-hat system, three times
a day, before quitting Calcutta, so as greatly to injure their health;
in short, both classes composing the regiment were in but indifferent health on commencing this unfortunate march; and though
it was chiefly conducted *during the night*, with every care within
reach of the medical officers, the effects were fatal in a remarkable
degree; " *while none of the Natives were taken ill during the trip.*" *
Such of the Europeans as could not reach the ground of encampment by nine A.M. " were seen to drop down and instantly expire;
others, less severely attacked, were saved by a timely and copious
bleeding."   But presently Dr. Henderson became seriously ill, and
this day closed with a sick-list of sixty-three, and eighteen deaths,
out of the right wing alone; both the sickness and the deaths
occurring principally amongst the recruits.

Dr. Milligan, H.M. 63rd Regiment, describes a similar outbreak
of this disease, on the occasion of a military funeral at Madras—

* " 1 have never as yet met with sun-stroke affecting a negro, though told that
such cases are not uncommon in the South."—*Dr. Levick, of Philadelphia.*

as badly arranged an affair as the other. " The greater number of the men were in the prime of life; but there were amongst them some old soldiers who had served twenty years or upwards, some of it in the West Indies, and were much broken down by service and intemperate habits." The entire corps had just arrived from Australia, " where spirituous liquors were to be had on easy terms." The regiment landed in Madras in May; and from the date of the " untoward circumstance " of the funeral, " the hospital became filled with cases of fever." Two men dropped down dead on the very day of the funeral, and for several days afterwards the fever cases augmented considerably. " I have reason to believe that the effects of this exposure to the rays of the vertical sun did not rest here, but laid the foundation of future mischiefs in assisting to originate fever, hepatitis, and dysentery, from which the regiment afterwards suffered much." All these observations are highly important, as establishing the great value of sanitary precautions, and the fact of the functional connexions of the morbid condition induced by direct solar exposure.

Examinations after death were, unfortunately, impracticable in both the cruel instances cited, the sickness of many of the medical officers, and the harassing duties imposed upon all, leaving no time for these customary investigations.

During the fatigue and severe exposure of the Bengal detachments, it has been remarked that, while the Europeans suffered so fatally, " *none of the natives were taken ill ;*" and such will, I dare say, generally be the case. I recollect an instance, however, where morbid insolation proved the reverse of this in the Governor-General's body-guard of cavalry, with which I served during the two campaigns of the first Burmese war. We mounted at eleven A.M. of the 12th May, and, with one short halt only, we made a forced march of forty miles, under as powerful a sun as ever shone in Burmah. The heat oppressed us almost beyond endurance, and many powerful men, native officers and troopers, fell off their horses, vomiting, convulsed, cold, and covered with profuse clammy sweat. Where a tree could be found, I had the men placed under its shade, and they were dashed over with water, the detachment pushing on in pursuit of the enemy, leaving the men thus affected on the roadside ; *yet not one of us European officers, whether commissioned or non-commissioned, fell sick, either on the march or after it.* But we were all young, healthy, and temperate in our habits; in the high, hopeful spirits of an active pursuit ; we were also well seasoned to the climate ; and such men, it is well known, will bear with comparative impunity fatigue and exposure almost beyond belief. By seasoning no more is here meant than the gradual accommodation of the constitution, through the operation of physiological changes, to unnatural and extraordinary ranges of temperature, and which accommodation we everywhere observe to occur during the first few years of residence within the tropics, when sanitary considerations obtain a careful attention. This, and no more, is meant by the term acclimation; in short, as stated in the article on " Climate," it is the ill habits of life of the European soldiery, and the sanitary neglect to which they are exposed, that give such fearful activity of power to tropical heat. In the two wings of the 13th Regiment, for instance, we hear of no officers having fallen sick, excepting Dr. Henderson; and his fatigues of body and mind will sufficiently account for his illness. There was this difference in the probable and actual event, as observed by me in the body-guard: that had any of us Europeans fallen, our saddles would have remained unoccupied; whereas, of the natives, all were up (although feverish) and doing well, when next day we marched back upon Prome.

The dangerous character of the disease is sufficiently exemplified in all the medical narratives which speak of the sun-stroke, and is statistically shown, by Mr. Marcus Hill, in the fact that, out of 504 seizures, there occurred 259 deaths. Of the remaining number, this intelligent and promising officer (since killed by the mutineers) states that eight were doubtful; leaving the deaths to seizures at $51 \cdot 38$ per cent., while the recoveries were but $45 \cdot 03$ of those attacked. The statistics of Dr. Gordon, of the 10th Foot, are still more melancholy. Out of 28 cases treated by this able officer, but one recovered, and that imperfectly. He estimates the mortality amongst European soldiers at 80 per cent., and that of officers at $66 \cdot 66$ per cent. Dr. Lindsay, of Bengal, again, states that, "once seized, he has never saved a patient." His patients, and most of Dr. Gordon's, must have been beyond the reach of cure when cure was attempted. This would appear the only fair construction.

Let us but contrast these declarations with that of Dr. Castello, of the Bombay army, and we shall perceive at once how great the varieties, how vast the differences which occur, under different conditions of service. This officer says:—" Under the head of 'diseases of the brain,' a large number were sun-stroke. I have been fortunate in the treatment of these cases, not having had a single death."

During the mortal and ever-memorable struggle within the intrenchments of Cawnpore, under Sir Hugh Wheeler, where " death and mutilation, in all their horrors, were daily before the garrison," the sun did its worst by the British soldier. The heroic Captain Moore, writing " by order " of his commander, says : " Our loss has been chiefly from the sun and their heavy guns."

Colonel Liddell, of the Bombay army, told me, that in the action at Coonah, May, 1857, thirteen dogs perished in the field, convulsed, and with all the symptoms of sun-stroke.

Nowhere else, unless it be on the field of battle, do we behold so sudden and violent destruction of life as in the heat-apoplexy.

Here, indeed, "in the midst of life we are in death." As described by Mr. Straker, of the Bombay army, "life does not ebb, but rushes torrent-like away."

The suddenness and fatal character of the seizure, leading, as it so frequently does, to the speedy death of men previously in health and in the midst of active employment, necessarily implies a defective knowledge of the earlier and less remarkable symptoms and stages of the disease. First we have vertigo and headache, with sense of burning in the eyes, the conjunctivæ being injected ; a full and frequent pulse, vomiting, great heat, sometimes floridness, of skin, a devouring thirst, oppressed respiration, and swollen face. Then come lividness, sinking and running of the pulse, clammy sweat, exhausted nervous energy, faltering of the tongue, coma, convulsion, and speedy death ;— these constitute the course of events in the true heat-apoplexy : the tale is soon told.

The gorged, apoplectic condition of the lungs, as of the brain, is made apparent during life by the oppressed and difficult breathing, with the "curious catching at the chest"—a *besoin de respirer*— observed by various of our surgeons, and by the racking headache, lividness, coma, and convulsion, manifested in other cases. In such instances the pupils are contracted and insensible to light, and there is frothing at the mouth, while the abdomen is swollen and tympanitic. A medical officer, a survivor from two attacks of heat-apoplexy, has stated to me that his greatest distress arose from constriction and oppression of breathing. Overpowered by these feelings, he fell off his horse, but did not altogether lose consciousness. It would seem as if the sun-stroke in some persons produced pulmonary engorgement and apoplexy, and in others the cerebral form of that disease. Others, again, have mentioned pain along the spine as occurring with intense headache, and that the former pain proved the more enduring of the two, recurring on subsequent occasions of exposure to the sun, while the head remained free from pain or giddiness. There is great and peculiarly intense heat of the epigastrium, with much oppression of the respiratory and circulating functions, all indicating lesion of the great central ganglia, analogous to that of the most concentrated forms of remittent fever ; in fact, when the seizures are of the milder nature, the case proceeds into the stage of fever. The differences in the symptoms and progress of the ardent fever of the hot season in Bengal and of the heat-apoplexy, consist principally in the more defective aeration of the blood in the last-named ; in the consequent stagnation and spoiling of the blood in the lungs and brain ; in the greater rapidity of the processes which lead to destruction attaching to the disease. In the most aggravated forms of heat-apoplexy, the morbid changes run their course in a few minutes apparently, and in cases of less fatal tendency in a few hours; while in the most severe forms of ardent fever, those changes, whether favourable or otherwise, are much longer in arriving at their termination. In the worst forms of the former disease, death comes, in fact, with all the rapidity of strangulation or of suffocation.

PREMONITORY SYMPTOMS.

The persistent marching of European soldiers in the night, however necessary as against insolation, deprives them of refreshment by sleep, and thus disposes to the subsequent stupor of the disease. One entire night's rest, at stated intervals of time, should be afforded during the hot weather march, whenever the nature of the service may admit of it. The want of this natural refreshment, and the evils attending the withholding of it, are shown in the fact that lassitude, yawning, with urgent desire for, but inability to sleep, extreme dryness of skin, with frequent micturition, very small quantities of urine only being voided, drowsiness, with heavy sleep, leading to stupor, and extreme general languor, constitute the most ordinary of the premonitory symptoms. These disorders result from continuous marching in the night, but they are greatly increased when the march is protracted into the forenoon or mid-day.

THE AFTER SYMPTOMS.

These, often melancholy in their nature, are of extreme interest; and they, as well as the more chronic and subdued influences of insolation, throw much light on the pathology of the disease under consideration. From the actual sun-stroke I have seen the following results, after the return to England of the sufferers :—

1. Severe mental depression, with sense of weariness along the spine.

2. Impression of the sun being always shining on the person, with tinnitus aurium.

3. Distressing formication, sometimes accompanied by a peculiar and general eruption and desquamation of the skin.

4. Deafness, more or less severe, with impaired vision and inability to use the eyes in reading and writing.

5. Various paralytic affections, more or less general, as hemiplegia, and local palsies, as of the eyelids, cheeks, or upper extremities, with and without loss of sensation. Heaving and difficult breathing.

6. Distressing hysterical states of the nervous system, with absence of self-control in laughing and crying—the paroxysm being followed by great prostration of nervous power.

7. Interruption to natural sleep, with incapacity to any kind of business.

8. Impression of alarm on any sudden movements of the body, and upon the occurrence of sudden noises.

9. Sudden epileptiform seizures, without loss of consciousness, followed by great nervous prostration.

10. In India we are familiar with the acute sequelæ to sun-stroke, as ardent fever with acute delirium, remittent and intermittent fevers, complicated with dysenteries, hepatic inflammations and congestions—all more or less dangerous to life and to future health.

PATHOLOGY.

The post-mortem appearances in this disease vary remarkably; so much so, indeed, as to show that out of several casualties the causes of death are different, the inconstant nature of the morbid results depending on the constitution, condition of the blood, the duration and intensity of the solar exposure, the amount of fatigue, the habits of life, and the duration of the disease. In the French West Indian colonies, Campet declared justly that the cases in which false polypi were found in the heart and great venous trunks, constituted examples of the worst form of this terrible disorder. In other reports an absolute rise in the temperature of the blood and solid tissues has been stated; while others describe the blood as being fluid and frothy. Cases are again reported as " simple congestion, without any lesion of the brain;" while in others, " effusion of blood external to the membranes of the brain, extensive effusion of blood between the dura mater and arachnoid," also, " enormous venous congestion of the scalp, with blood extravasated between the membranes," are noticed.

The result of cerebral congestion must be to diminish and sometimes to overpower the functions of the brain, and thus to enfeeble the actions of both lungs and heart.

What is cerebral syncope, and what its effects on the nervous system, on the heart and lungs? It is curious to observe that the sardonic laugh is common to the extremes of cold as well as of heat. Examples of the former are frequently mentioned by the historians of the French retreat from Moscow. In India, alternate crying and laughing, of a hysterical character, is a subject of frequent observation, during the attack and in convalescence.

In all the recorded instances of heat-apoplexy, we have perceptibly presented a great, and, to the European, a most unnatural elevation of the external temperature, a proportional rarefaction of the air, and a consequently diminished supply of oxygen at each inspiration; a resulting deterioration or venalized condition of the blood; a depression of the nervous functions, with augmented animal heat, and an impacted skin. Malaria and other atmospheric impurities, with their consequences, are occasional accessories, with the superaddition, also, of fatigue and its results. These circumstances, often acting on a system previously injured by improper diet and other intemperance, by disordered or diseased viscera, defective excretion, and the deprivation of sleep in the night marches, will go far to account for all the phenomena of this suddenly fatal disease. The condition of the lungs, heart, and brain, immediately resulting from the extremely rarefied air and intense solar heat, appears to be one of extreme venalization of the blood, with acute congestion at first, proceeding rapidly to passive congestion and greater depression of the nervous and vascular energies, to consequent narcotism of the lungs, heart, and brain, and to exhaustion of nerve-power as the last event.

A great majority of the favourable cases which occur during a march under a May tropical sun, present a mixed condition, partaking of the sun-stroke, or cerebral syncope, at first proceeding rapidly to congestive apoplexy, and ending in feverish reaction, or sun-fever ; those who die outright being extinguished by the shock to the brain, heart, and lungs. In persons who are seized in the shade, or under cover, again, the symptoms generally advance with diminished rapidity comparatively, the patient complaining of feverish debility in the morning, and being found in a state of stupor in the afternoon. The more or less rapid course in each description of case will generally determine the *post-mortem* results : the first-mentioned cases, owing to the extraordinary force and quickness of the shock, and of the consequent cerebral syncope, presenting but slight traces of disease within the cerebral cavity, but exhibiting intense pulmonary engorgement, ending sometimes in pulmonary apoplexy ; while in the last-named cases we shall find the vessels of the dura mater gorged almost to bursting, and the lungs more or less congested. Sometimes we shall find a copious and extensive serous effusion on the surface and within the ventricles of the brain ; while in many of the cases tabulated by Mr. Marcus Hill, and mentioned by other authors, enormous congestion within and without the cranium was generally observed after death. I conceive that death may occur in one of two ways ; either by destruction of the functions of the brain by stagnant and venalized blood, or by stagnation of the circulating fluid in the heart and lungs, overpowering their actions by engorgement, or extreme distention.

In all the instances of recovery from this disease, and in all the milder seizures, the patients have passed through a more or less marked stage of feverish reaction, assuming the characters of the ardent fever of the hot season frequently, but occasionally, and along with it, the association of the paroxysmal or malarious sign. These are facts which appear on well-recorded evidence, and they are of high importance to the right apprehension of the subject. In Mr. Longmore's history of sixteen cases of heat-apoplexy in the 19th Regiment of Foot, which occurred at Barrackpore between the 23rd May and 14th June, 1858, he notices that, of " other prevalent diseases," fevers were by far the most common. During the period here specified there occurred ninety-four cases of fever, ninety of them having been admitted into hospital between the

23rd May and 11th June—the day on which a rain-storm with reduced temperature put an end to the progress of heat-apoplexy. Two circumstances are here worthy of notice:—that, out of the sixteen men seized with heat-apoplexy, six were at the time in hospital suffering from remittent fever, and that no case occurred amongst the officers. This last circumstance—the exemption of the commissioned officers—is so uniform of occurrence, that the thorough investigation of its causes ought to prove both interesting and important. The more temperate habits, the better ventilation of their quarters, and the more suitable dress of the officers, made much, if not all the difference. Thunderstorms have often been observed to arrest the progress and recurrence of heat-apoplexy in barracks and hospitals in which the disease had prevailed for days, and this even where the atmospheric temperature had not been reduced by the storms. I am not aware that any observations have been made in India respecting the amount of ozone.

The late Inspector-General Murray supposed an essential pathological difference to exist between morbid affections resulting from exposure of the *bare head* to the direct rays of the sun, and such as may result from over-exertion under great heat, or such as are induced by the same degree of temperature *in the shade*, the former producing strong excitement in the brain by the direct stimulus of the cause. The scalp being protected by hair, and peculiarly constructed, does not blister under the sun like other parts of the body, but its temperature becomes exalted, and the caloric traversing it and the skull, gives immediate rise to active hyperæmia. Heat in the shade, again, acting on the general system, the cerebral affection appeared to Dr. Murray to be induced in a different, but unexplained manner :—"At first there is nervous depression or collapse, and sanguineous congestion, upon which the reaction follows." This doctrine would ascribe to the brain the same susceptibility to palsy, and consequent congestion, that is now generally believed to constitute, in the great central ganglia, the essential cause of fever. It would appear probable, on the other hand, that the sun-shock to the cerebrum and central nerves may, on occasions of great mortality, have proved so sudden and violent as at once to paralyse the brain, heart, and lungs; and thus the numerous instances of quick death, which left no trace behind, may be accounted for. Such sudden extinctions of life have all the appearance of death by the shock of lightning.

My friend Dr. Julius Jeffreys believes, in common with many tropical practitioners, that the special heat by direct rays of the sun not only produces sun-stroke, but generates more remotely, fever, dysentery, and hepatitis ; while the long-continued application of general heat debilitates the cutaneous function, so as to predispose the system to the influences of malaria. "The skin's débility is malaria's opportunity." A venalized state of the blood, and general impairment of the functions of depuration, with suppression

D D

of the cuticular discharge, constitute the earliest appreciable features of the disease; some of the sufferers declaring that for days previously they had not perspired. Scorbutus, in which the blood is already spoiled, constitutes one of the most serious complications.

Dr. B. W. Richardson concludes that excessive heat destroys the magnetic power of oxygen and its power of combination—coup-de-soleil resulting from an asphyxia commencing in the blood.

Hitherto, the coup-de-soleil has been too exclusively regarded as a primary affection of the brain—as an inflammation or congestion of that organ, in fact; but the more recent and careful study of the *post-mortem* appearances would tend to show that the more general, prominent, and enduring affection consists in an extreme engorgement, leading to a true apoplexy of the lungs, the result of an imperfect aëration of the blood, the brain being similarly affected by congestion, although in a less degree. Mr. Hill states that in " a great many *post-mortem* inspections, where the lungs had been examined, there was found the most extensive congestion, often amounting to engorgement, and sometimes even to extravasation or pulmonary apoplexy;" and in a fatal case reported by this officer, the upper part of both lungs is stated to have been immensely congested, the bronchial tubes being filled with frothy, serous blood.

Dr. Russell, of her Majesty's 73rd Regiment, relates, that in three fatal cases of this disease he found the lungs " congested even to blackness, through their entire extent, and so densely loaded that complete obstruction must have taken place." Drs. Mortimer, Shanks, and Green, in various stations throughout India, record similar observations; and a pale, blanched, cholera-like condition of the mucous membrane of the small intestines has been noted in some cases by Mr. Hill.

False polypi, or fibrinous coagula, in the heart, are mentioned by Campet, thus constituting an association in pathology with the yellow fever of the West, and with the malignant remittents and intermittents of the East, as of Aracan in the first Burmese war.

The enormous transudation from the skin, with the subsequent collapse of its function, and dryness of the entire surface of the body, under great solar heat, cause a concentration and diminution of all the internal excretions, and a consequent diminution of the depurative functions. Referring to the action of the sun upon the skin, I have very recently seen a medical officer from Central India, in whom a strange erratic form of œdema appeared on different parts of the body, from head to foot. The œdema was somewhat solid, and of small, circumscribed extent.

An occasional burning heat of the epigastrium, complained of during life, and an unusual pungent heat of the surface of the body after death, have been noticed by various writers; and I had occasion to remark both, at the General Hospital of Calcutta, in the instances of European recruits landed from England in the month of May, and who had free access to the vile rum and arrack of the bazaars, and were seized with what was then termed the sun-fever. These reckless young soldiers exhibited in death the true *calor mordicans* of the older writers.

TREATMENT.

The treatment of this imminently dangerous disease, in a large proportion of cases, is in truth but, as in violent forms of cholera, an attendance upon death. Many soldiers die outright, or before the stock or neckcloth can be untied ; many more die within a few hours of being knocked down, and of falling insensible out of the ranks. All such cases are at once almost beyond the reach of our art to cure, yet we dispute about their treatment ; and the result being nearly the same, under every variety of management, we find fault with all alike. The American physician Dowler says, for instance, that there exists a distinction between *solar asphyxia and solar syncope ;*—adding, that " solar asphyxia is always fatal ;" but that this even " might be curable, if the patient were bled *instantaneously.*" Another observer will declare that if cold affusion had been but persevered in, the fatal result would have been averted ; and thus extremes meet. Campet, who practised in French Guiana a century ago, urges a careful attention to the habit and constitution of the patient, prescribing free and early general depletion in such persons as are of sanguine temperament ; adding a cautious regard to the practical maxim that blood-letting kills, if it do not cure, the disease, concluding with another maxim, that for great ills there must be great remedies. But here, as with Dr. Dowler, it is a question of time ; or, in other words, of rapidity of morbid progress. Campet bled, vomited, and purged freely, at the very accession of the disease ; and his measures in the latter stages were prudently measured to induce convalescence.

Dr. Dick, of Bengal, while serving on the Coromandel coast, "removed the patients under the shade of trees, bleeding them freely in time, and giving them water, which generally cured them ; but as the stomach and bowels were often overloaded with bilious and putrid matters, it was necessary to give them in the evening a small quantity of tartar-emetic dissolved in saline mixture, which answered better than any other evacuant." Dr. Dick concludes his practical observations by stating that, though the sufferers seldom required any other medicines, they were a long time thereafter unfit for duty. So much for the earlier notices of sun-stroke by Eastern and Western practitioners, who were more in accord as to the nature and treatment of the disease than we are at present.

That the treatment ought to be determined by the immediate pathological condition of each individual case, few will question ;

but to discern on the instant the actual morbid state is difficult, and rather than solve this difficulty, many of us seek refuge from it, and betake ourselves to any easy system of generalization in treatment.   Like other difficulties, this one must be fairly looked in the face.   We cannot blink it if we would ; and to blink a question is not at all to solve it.   Without believing with La Bruyère that "discernment is the rarest thing in the world after diamonds and pearls," I still think that to discriminate justly is not here so very difficult as many would have it.   With a full bounding pulse, a hot pungent skin, and a flushed or livid face, the patient ought to lose some blood generally or locally ; while, with a sunken countenance, a sunken arterial action, a passive venous congestion, and oppressed respiration, such abstraction would prove injurious.   Local depletion, as from the nape of the neck or temples, must act in direct relief of congestion, internal and external ; and such states are not difficult of being recognised. With a view to the treatment of persons under sun-stroke, we should first distinguish and separate the subjects which admit of depletion, and those which do not ; holding mainly in view the constitution, age, previous service, and previous health, habits of life, &c., of the soldier, and also the duration of the disease.   We can thus very speedily determine the *nature* of the treatment of each individual case, and the *extent* to which such treatment may be carried.   For want of such preliminary arrangement, much confusion has often arisen.

If the subject come under treatment before the advent of vascular oppression and nervous collapse, the application of leeches behind the ears, or arteriotomy, as preferred by some experienced surgeons, will relieve the cerebral and thoracic organs overpowered by congestion, give time and place for the influence of cold applications to the head, and for the derivative effects of heat, and of persistent friction with warm flannels applied to the extremities— all being aided by the exhibition of an active and stimulating purgative.   At the same time that local blood-letting is being practised, *diffusible stimuli*, with ten-minim doses of laudanum, should be administered, with a view at once to rouse and support the nervous and vascular energies.

The earliest evidences of successful treatment are, reduction of the temperature of the surface, followed by relaxation of the skin, restoration of the nervous and vascular powers, and of the functions of depuration.   When local blood-letting proves beneficial, it acts in relief of the head, heart, and lungs, oppressed as they were by the most overwhelming congestion ; but, to further and maintain this beneficial result, the diffusible stimulants, hot applications and frictions, already mentioned, must be perseveringly used.   But in too many instances the time for the application of active measures, along with the season for speedy reaction, has gone by ; and in such cases nothing remains in the way of remedial means but dashing the face, neck, and upper part of the chest with cold water, while stimulating enemata and stimulating frictions to the abdomen are used in aid of the internal means already indicated. On the tone which we may impart to the nervous and vascular systems, all must depend; and whatever is to be done ought to be done quickly.

A good way of applying the cold water is by a douche of moderate volume falling from the height of a few feet, while the patient is on a cot in the recumbent posture.

From the earliest notices by our Indian surgeons, as well as from the recent observations of M. Guyon, and other able surgeons of the French army in Algeria, it has been made sufficiently evident that active measures of cure, to have a favourable prospect of success, must be practised as soon as possible after the soldier has fallen out of the ranks; and the great balance of testimony speaks to the fact that, when thus used, the proportion of recoveries has been considerable, counting only such as were within reach of cure. But we must remember that minutes are here of vital importance, and that it is to the disregard of this circumstance, and to the use of blood-letting, general or local, after the time for its use has passed away, that we must refer the differences of medical opinion on this head.

The opening of the temporal artery, when practised at the proper time, is said to have proved very successful in the hands of the American practitioners, and I have seen this operation very efficacious in India in the febrile stage of reaction from sun-stroke, and when the brain was oppressed by congestion. Mr. Dempster's experience in Bengal accords entirely with that of the American physicians; and Mr. Scriven, of the same service, an able officer, and no friend to blood-letting in this disease, says—" Six leeches to the temples often give marked relief;" and in the case of a seaman, twelve leeches were applied by him on two separate occasions. Mr. Chapple, of the Royal Artillery, found that "in cases not treated by leeches to the head, the scalp, on being cut into, four or five hours after death, bled profusely; and in one instance more than twenty ounces of blood were thus poured out."

There can be no doubt that the Brounonian doctrines and practices, as lately revived in some of our schools at home, have had their influence, and an injurious one, on the younger, and upon the more timid of the older surgeons, in deterring them altogether from the use of depletory means in this and in other tropical diseases. But exclusive doctrines and practices, of whatever kind, have never maintained any permanent hold on the professional mind; and Brown must share the fate of Broussais in this respect.

But the course of the army surgeon on the field of actual service must not be one of mere theory, or of speculative suggestion. His difficulties are actual and great. At a moment of terror to the looker-on, he has with a deliberate and firm mind to determine on the instant what can be done and what cannot be done ; to be useful he must be considerate, prompt, and bold. He must at once balance all the circumstances of each individual case, and then he must use all the effective means which reason and experience suggest. In the treatment of sun-stroke he must not be content with too simple or too easy a generalizing course of sousing by cold water, applied without discrimination or distinction to all cases, to all constitutions and stages of disease—to all ages and conditions whatsoever, under the ever-varying conditions of climate, habit, and service. It is true that to use properly so powerful a means as blood-letting, requires all the mental qualities above-mentioned, especially if the abstraction be general; and so does its application to remittent fever, dysentery, and hepatitis. Indeed, all the unqualified, exclusive, and absolute arguments against depletion in any instance of sun-stroke (and they are very easy to adduce) are founded only on its ill-timed application—on its misuse in fact.

Even cold water, when applied in cases of exhaustion of the nervous system, is an agent for good or evil of much power, and therefore not one to be used without care, any more than blood-letting. That there are cases of sun-stroke which must be treated with cold affusion, and others which ought not to be bled, we all know ; but the two instances together do not by any means constitute the whole of the cases to be treated on any one field. I am here anxious to state that, far indeed from underrating the value of cold affusion, there may be danger of its recommending itself in the treatment of all cases, acute as well as passive, as a chief means of cure ; and this, with many persons, on the score of the ease with which it can be applied :—any one can do it, and it is quite as easy to rely upon it ; but such are not here the questions. That cold affusion has been misused and abused, in common with blood-letting, and continued too long so as injuriously to depress the nervous and vascular energies, and repress the action of the skin, is what I am assured of; and this is another serious error to be guarded against. There are cases in which the persevering appli-cation of heat and of stimulating frictions to the body and extre-mities has proved powerfully restorative under apparently hopeless aspects. Such cases, and they are not infrequent, would be de-stroyed by the protracted or over-use of cold. Oxidation being more or less completely arrested, and coma being one of the results of the deprivation of oxygen, were I again to treat a case of sun-stroke, I would use the nitro-muriatic acid internally and externally.

If the suitable abstraction of blood, cold applications to the head, neck, and chest, a full dose of calomel with antimony or Dover's powder, an active stimulating purgative, a free ventilation, cold drinks, darkness of the apartment, and rest, be employed early, and while the nervous and vascular systems retain sufficient tone, we shall, as in Dr. Henderson's practice, obtain a large amount of success.* But if the same means be put in practice later, and when the vessels of the lungs and brain have lost their tonicity, they fail of relieving the oppressive congestion ; and, so far from making a favourable impression, they tend powerfully to the contrary result. This is an all-important consideration to mark ; it is the case here, as in remittent fever, the measures which, if applied early, may save life, will, if misapplied, as surely destroy it.

When, on the other hand, the surgeon, on the most careful balance of all the circumstances of the case, sees that the constitution of the patient is unfavourable, or that the time for active measures has passed away, those means which, in the first or earlier stage of the disease, would have been but adjuvant, become the principal—indeed the sole means. Heat to the abdomen and extremities, sinapisms to the epigastric region, and cold affusion to the head and chest, must be perseveringly applied, while brisk aloetic and aromatic purgatives are being freely administered. The capillary circulation being stagnant, like that of the great internal viscera, frictions all over the body—such as shampooing— have proved of great efficacy ; indeed, the restoration of the functions of the skin is a cardinal point in the treatment. By such means, persistently used, cases wearing a hopeless aspect sometimes turn towards convalescence. For many years, both in the French and British armies, the course here described has been that generally pursued ; and we surely have not now to learn that, when a patient is anæmic, or when the circulation has ceased, the heart being filled with coagula, the functions of the brain having ceased, we are not to bleed the sufferers ; that we may not bleed dead men, in fact.

Finally, a reference to the recorded histories of this disease leads to the conclusion that the means of cure have long been, and are now, tolerably well known generally—as well known as the means of cure of most other diseases ; and it is on the relative value of each remedy, its time and place of use, that I apprehend any real difference of opinion to exist. One thing is absolutely essential to the due estimate of the results of treatment—viz., that we confine our statistical records to curable cases—to cases possible of cure ; for it is from the neglect of this necessary separation of the incurable from the curable instances, that a serious statistical error has arisen ; just as the neglect to determine the proper time for the application of active remedies has thrown difficulties in the way of a determinate cure.

* Such men as could not reach the shelter of the camp by 9 A.M. "were seen to drop down and instantly expire ; others less severely attacked, were saved by a timely and copious bleeding." Just so ; the first-named were death-struck, but the cases which were of a curable nature obtained relief and safety in the "timely" abstraction of blood. When, again, in the practice of Drs. Henderson and Mouatt, "sinking of the vital powers, or kind of collapse, occurred, a grain of opium was given to produce reaction, after the occurrence of which they were largely bled ; and with these precautions, although thirty were admitted into hospital after the first march, none died."

A notice of coup-de-soleil would be wanting in interest which should not refer to Sir Charles Napier's most able and characteristic account of his personal seizure and treatment when serving in Sindh:—" I had hardly written the above sentence ten days ago when I was tumbled over by the heat with apoplexy : forty-three others were struck, all Europeans, and all died within three hours except myself! I do not drink! That is the secret. The sun had no ally in the liquor amongst my brains. Unable to talk, I flung myself on a table, and luckily one of my staff came in. He called the doctors ; two or three were with me in a twinkling ; wet towels rolled round my head ; feet in hot water; bleeding, and two men rubbing me. I was so drowsy as to be angry that they would not allow me to sleep. Had they done so, it would have been hard to awake me."

PREVENTION.

Of all the means of prevention of heat-apoplexy, the avoidance of spirituous liquors and of excess in the use of animal diet must take the lead. In the language used by the great general, Sir Charles Napier, he gave expression to a physiological fact, the sug- gestion of his own acute perception. The sun and its various in- fluences, and the ill habits of the men and their consequences, con- stitute the causes and chief accessories. On the line of march, deficiency of water-supply stands next in order of evils to the sun itself. I believe that, with temperance in diet, avoidance of so much direct solar exposure as may be compatible with the nature of the service, attention to tent-covering and ventilation, and to head-dress and body-clothing, British soldiers may be made to march well under the hottest sun of India ; just as suitable pro- visions of a somewhat opposite nature might have saved the French army on the retreat from Moscow.

Sundry of the French surgeons in Algeria, and M. Scoutetten pre-eminent amongst them, urge the importance, and indeed the necessity, of wearing a neck-cover as a protection of peculiar effi- cacy against the sun's rays, declaring this article of dress to be as indispensable to the soldier who may have to serve in that country as the very head-covering ; and in this they follow the instinctive habit of the natives of hot climates.

On the subject of the quality and arrangement of the soldier's dress when serving under great heats, there can be no difference or question. The head-dress should be light, of slowly-conducting materials, and constructed so as to command ventilation. Dr. Jeffrey's helmet gives protection by slow radiation, slow conduc- tion, reflection, ventilation, and evaporation. The body-dress should be of cotton ; and from head to foot everything should fit loosely, to allow the most perfect freedom of respiration and to the movements of the body, so as nowhere, but especially about the neck, to press on or interrupt the circulation of the superficial vessels. Everywhere throughout the world, whether east, west, north, or south, the army surgeons urge the use of the flannel roller to protect the abdomen; and a complete dress (shirt and drawers) of flannel, to wear on coming in from the march and whilst the uniform is being dried in the sun, is no less requisite.

Parades, formalities, the majestic English march, "Regulations" and appearances, must here be utterly and at once discarded; for it is a question of life and death. The open, disorderly-looking order of march, however slovenly it may seem to the lieutenant-colonel, must here be used, the close order being nothing short of stifling and sickening the men "by Regulation." The genius of pipe-clay must here concede something. While on the march, the face and hands should be frequently bathed; and on such halts, which should be ordered every hour, the men should be urged to refrain from drinking the impure waters so general in the hot season. It is hardly necessary to say that the ordinary march should be conducted slowly, and always during the night, when the service will admit of it. In cantonment barracks and hospitals the most free ventilation should be secured. Mr. Longmore states that the greater portion of seizures and deaths of the men of the 19th Regiment at Barrackpore, in May and June, 1858, occurred in those who had occupied a low ill-ventilated building; while Dr. Butler, of the 3rd European cavalry, at Lahore, referring to May and June, 1859, notices that the barracks which were most crowded and worst ventilated, and least provided with punkahs, furnished the greatest portion of fatal cases.

In the French, as in the British army, the newly-arrived soldier from Europe, over-fed and over-drammed, has been observed to be the most subject to attacks; and this circumstance would indicate the necessity for an especial precautionary regard to the new-comer and the plethoric. Here, indeed, in the words of Marshal Ney, the attentions of all classes of officers to their men should be un-remitting. Temperance is the great point to be attended to. Tea for drink has been suggested by Dr. Edward Smith, since, by its powerful influence in increasing respiration and the action of the skin, without increasing pulsations, it is particularly fitted to counteract the influence of heat in its tendency to induce heat-apoplexy.

Dr. Edward Smith's researches on the influence of exercise and labour on respiration, possess an extreme interest in reference to our subject. He has shown that walking at one mile per hour will double the respiration; at two miles per hour it is increased two and three-quarter times; and at three miles per hour it is more than trebled; while at four miles per hour it is five times as great: in other words, one hour's walking at four miles per hour causes as much respiration as would have occurred in five hours of the quiet-lying posture.

As applicable to the march, the soldier carrying from forty to sixty rounds of ammunition, the law deduced by the author is as follows :—"For every pound borne at three miles per hour, there is an increase of seven cubic inches per minute in the quantity of air inspired ; but the pulsation is increased in a yet higher ratio. Thus, if a soldier carry thirty pounds, he will breathe 200 cubic inches in excess; or if sixty pounds, 400 cubic inches in excess per minute, the former being equal to one half, and the latter to the whole influence of the quiet recumbent posture.   But since in the carrying of weights the pulsation is increased disproportionally beyond any other exertion, it is fair to assume that respiration does not alone measure the whole effect ; and hence, although the wear of carrying sixty pounds at three miles per hour would be each hour equal to that of nearly four hours in the quiet-lying posture, as deduced from the respiration, it is probable that the true effect would be beyond that amount."

In a letter from a distinguished staff-surgeon serving in India in the hot-weather campaign of 1858, I am informed that in his force they lost in a month one hundred or more British soldiers by sun-stroke.   The men at length became absolutely terrified at the overwhelming power of the sun, though "not at all of the enemy, for whom they had a great contempt.   But all dreaded the sun, and the hospitals became crowded, as well with men really ill as with men ailing but little, and anxious only to escape solar ex-posure."   Here the moral and military effect of the protective helmet of Dr. Julius Jeffreys would be almost of as great value as its admirable chemical action : it would not only save the lives of some twenty men on the long day's march under an Indian July sun, but it would impart new courage to the drooping battalion. Its influence, small though it looks, would stand in fair comparison, in moral and military power, with that caused by the first sight of Larrey's ambulances on the grenadiers of the French revolutionary armies : " Behold," said they, as they ascended the breach, " we shall no longer be neglected in our wounds and our sickness." Dr. Jeffreys, speaking of his own admirable suggestions, says : " We know too well what the climate of India can do while im-perfectly opposed; we have yet to learn what may be the immu-nities conferred by the most perfect protection at our command."

The protective influence of temperance in diet, as against the dangers of insolation, was never so thoroughly demonstrated as during the recent siege of Delhi, and indeed throughout the hot-weather campaigns, everywhere, against the great Bengal mutiny. Officers before Delhi describe themselves as marching all day in the sun of June, July, and August, and serving in the burning trenches for weeks together ; and yet they preserved their health, under a temperature of 130° or more, through temperance, to a wonderful extent.

Dr. Barclay of the 43rd Regiment states, as the result of his observation, that men whose nervous system had been injured by previous intemperance " were much more disposed than any others to attacks."

When many men are struck down, and the healthy have become nervous and dispirited, change of locality should instantly be solicited ; and the benefits attending such change were exhibited in a remarkable manner in Baroda, in June, 1859,—a movement made at the instance of assistant-surgeon Chapple.

Here, as in every instance of endemic and epidemic disease, where mental depression results from the suddenness and frequency of death, the soldiers should be removed to the hut located within reach.

All experience, finally, points to the propriety of limiting the issue of the spirit-ration to the time of sunset—the proper hour, also, for the principal meal of the soldier in the hot months.

NOTE ON THE FEVERS OF THE NATIVES OF INDIA.

THE subject of the diseases of the Natives of India deserves a separate treatise, and I trust that the time is not distant when we may hope to possess one worthy of so important a question. But the scope, purport, and very title of this work do not admit of any further discussion on the subject than the most cursory. A knowledge of the diseases of Asiatics is intrinsically of great importance, while, contingently, it will present an interesting and extensive field of comparison with the diseases of Europeans, and their causes. The Natives of India generally are amiable and respectful in their intercourse with Europeans ; and towards no class of their rulers do they show more real kindness of feeling and gratitude than to such of our medical officers as may prove deserving.

British India, divided into four great portions—that of the Ganges to the east, of the Indus to the west, of the Dekhan to the south, and of that bounded by the great Himalayan range to the north—is inhabited by nations differing in religion, but supposed by some authorities to be descendants of the same great family ; they are distributed over the vast extent of what is termed the Peninsula of Hindustan—the widest extent of empire, with the smallest and most easily defensible line of frontier, of any existing on the globe. All the physical features of nature are in India truly colossal.

There is reason to conclude, from the notices by the Greek authors, that no change whatever has taken place in the institutions, character, or manners of the Hindus from the age of

Alexander to the time when they were discovered by the nations of modern Europe.

The extreme length of Hindustan from south to north is 1880, while its breadth from east to west is 1620 miles, or 27 degrees of latitude and 25 of longitude;—all its features being on the most magnificent scale. Washed by the Bay of Bengal on the south-east, and by the Indian Ocean on the south-west, it is bounded on the north and east by mountains of prodigious elevation, from whence the two great rivers of India have their sources, and flow to opposite points of the continent.

" India," says Professor Eastwick, " presents every imaginable variety of scenery, from the loftiest and most sublime mountain ranges to the gentle undulations and velvet swards of an English park. Its natural products are equal, if not superior, to those of any region in the world, and would furnish endless materials for the pen of the describer. It is rich in historical associations, and there is scarce a hill which is not crowned with picturesque ruins of some old fortress, little known, or altogether unvisited by Europeans, but bound up in the Native mind with many a strange tale and legend. India is a land of ruined cities, and in one of these the antiquities of a whole European province might be collected. The ruins of Bráhmanabad, the Pompeii of Sindh, extend for twenty miles, and wherever the mattock of the excavator falls, curious relics come to light. The deserted city of Bíjapúr presents from a distance the appearance of a populous capital, and it is not until the desolate streets are entered that the illusion is entirely dispelled.

" But Indian architecture can boast not only of what is curious and surprising, but also of what is eminently beautiful. The Táj excels all buildings in the world in symmetry and rich decoration. The temples of A'bu are not to be surpassed in ornamentation. The palace of Amber is a structure before which the Alhambra shrinks into insignificance.

" India lies between 8° 4' and 36° N. lat. and 66° 44' and 99° 30 E. long., and contains a million and a half of square miles, with about a hundred and eighty millions of inhabitants. This vast region, says our authority, is, more than any other, formed by nature to be the storehouse of the world. The magnificent chain of mountains that encircles it from N.W. to N.E., consisting of the Himalayas to the N. and N.E., with the Sulaiman and Hála ranges running down to the sea on the west, supplies abundant water to irrigate the whole of Upper India; as, in like manner, the Vindhayan range, joined eastwards by the Rájmahal hills and other lower ranges, and the East and West Gháts, furnish sufficient water for the requirements of the Dekhan or South India.

" Thus India exhibits a series of great water-sheds, in which, or on the adjoining hills, grain of all descriptions, rice, oil-seeds, coffee, sugar-cane, tea, indigo, cotton, opium, tobacco, pepper, cardamom, ginger, capsicum, coriander, turmeric, and all kinds of vegetables and fruits, are or may be produced in inexhaustible quantities. In its forests, India possesses resources superior to those of any country in the world. The teak-tree, the cocoa-nut tree, the sago-palm, and the sandal-tree are first of their kind in utility; and innumerable trees, only second in value, might be mentioned.

"Iron, the parent of all other metals, abounds; and coal exists in untold quantities. Precious stones of all descriptions are found in different localities; and in the number and variety of animals, no region of the earth is comparable with India. To man, the climate of India is less favourable than that of the temperate zone; yet, amid the variety of races which is found from the Himalayas to Cape Comorin, some are not inferior in beauty to any that exist, as *e.g.* the people of Kashmír, the Rajpúts, the Bilúchís, and Játs of Sindh, and some of the Bráhmans."—*Handbook for India.*

Our Eastern possessions are said to contain, independently of the descendants of conquering races and strange settlers—men conquerors in creed and banditti by profession—some fifteen or more indigenous nations, different in race, different in religion, and different in language. From the great elements from whence to recruit our armies, it might have been expected that during our hundred years of rule in Hindustan we should have associated, or fused by a rigorous discipline, or ranged in battalions according to religions and languages, an army, if not worthy our name and power, at least one deserving of some trust. It was indeed supposed that, although the formation of our Indian army had always been encumbered by a sort of foreign European chance-medley, so much of the better British element of skill, discipline, and unity of action had been imparted to it by its European officers, that its fidelity might be counted on; but recent events in India have shown such expectations to have been utterly fallacious. In India there is no nationality—no union, political or other—the nations and the individuals inhabiting Hindustan having about that kind of cohesiveness which belongs to marbles in a bag. The people have thus been the ever-ready slaves of despotism, civil, religious, and military.

Ethnologists have pronounced the races of the East and West to be one in origin; but how vast the differences and distinctions which have arisen in the progress of time ! What differences in religion, morals, government, diet, institutions ! How differently do the two races regard what is true l

Varying in physiology of constitution as they may be, divided by geographical distinctions of latitude, quality and elevation of soil, or by differences in diet, the natives are separated, Hindu from Hindu, and Hindu from Mahomedan, by impassable barriers of caste and of religion; yet, under British rule, this wonderful aggregation of subjects has attained to a degree and kind of union, such as no antecedent rulers, whether ancient indigenous Hindu, or more modern conquering Mahomedan, ever could conceive, far less accomplish.*

Out of the enormous mass of the population, every description of person enters eagerly into the various public employments presented by the British government, whether civil or military, and natives of every caste and class are thus brought into familiar and friendly communication with their European superiors. Not only is this the case, but natives, both Hindu and Mahomedan, undergo laborious and protracted courses of education, the better to qualify themselves for the various public duties offered to them; and here, to the honour of the medical profession, it has taken the lead, and accomplished a noble triumph of education. Always prominent in every endeavour to advance the moral and intellectual condition of the people, youths may now be seen by the hundred, trained and instructed by our medical officers at the three Presidencies, who but a few years back, had they touched a dead body, would have become outcasts. Now these youths are seen to go through years of the dissecting room, and to leave their colleges able physicians and expert surgeons.

The relative proportions of the followers of the two dominant religions of India, the Hindu and Mahomedan, may be taken as about eight of the former to one of the latter, for the whole of Hindustan; Pegu and the Island of Ceylon being inhabited by Budhists. It is estimated that, throughout India generally, there are 3400 Natives to one European; but insignificant as this proportion appears, the presence of the European offers to the Hindu and Mahomedan the only hope of ever attaining to truth in religion or in science.

The complexion, stature, bulk, and weight of the body vary in the several nations, as they may inhabit the south or the north of India, as they may occupy countries near to or far from the Equator; the advantages in all the above respects being generally much in favour of the northern nations. But of high or low stature, the trunk of the Asiatic, whether Hindu, Mahomedan, or Budhist, will be found slender as compared to that of the European. The Siah-Pòsh, an undoubted branch of Hindu race, and who inhabit the cold mountain region of Kohistan, have, according to Sir Alexander Burnes, arched eyebrows, a fair complexion, blue eyes, and Grecian features, while, on the contrary, the descendants of fair Persians and Affghans have, in the course even of a few centuries, become of darker and darker shades as we trace them into the farther south of India. Generally speaking, the Mahomedan, whether of Persian, Affghan, or Baluchi descent, will everywhere, but in the north especially, prove the

---

* The Mahomedan conquest of India was completed A.D. 1215.

fairer as compared to the Hindu; but this distinction will be found to have gradually disappeared under a foreign climate, and the fairer Mussulman will have become more and more dusky with advancing generations.

The various natives inhabiting Hindustan appear to differ from Europeans less in feature than in the more trifling circumstances of colour, size, and form.   They are nevertheless moulded by a great variety of climates, localities, habits of life, diet, occupation, &c., so as to constitute in reality a people varying exceedingly in moral and intellectual qualities, in physical powers and appearances.   The medical officer will therefore have peculiarities to investigate in almost every state and province throughout the whole extent of our Eastern possessions.   Placed under few of the rigorous necessities which, in northern latitudes, impart energy to the mind and body of the inhabitants, the people of the East are handed over by the richness of their soil, the power of their sun, and by climate and institutions of religion, to a state of indolence and inactivity as compared to western nations.

Of Caucasian origin, but exposed during countless generations to the same succession of external influences of high temperature and corresponding habits of life and diet, receiving the same reiterated impressions peculiar to climate and religion, an acquired temperament is formed which constitutes the Hindu and Mahomedan—men differing widely, morally and physically, from Europeans, while from each other they differ principally in religion and in diet.   These general causes, together with the premature development of the generative function, produce an excitability of the nervous system, diminished volume, enervation, and relaxation of the muscular system, as compared to Europeans, all which dispose the natives of India generally, and those of Bengal Proper in particular, to tetanic affections under wounds, surgical operations, and the impressions of cold and damp.

If we would understand India, we must study well its physical geography and its great influence on the habits and customs of its vast population.   In some countries everything tends to exalt the human race, while in India everything has tended to depress it.   The climate and the religion have together stimulated the imagination far beyond the cultivation of the intellect; thus allowing the imagination to run into licence, infusing into the people a spirit of reverence instead of a spirit of inquiry, and encouraging a disposition to neglect the investigation of natural causes and ascribe events to the operation of supernatural ones.   Improvement in Asia has been wilfully arrested by the self-imposition of an arbitrary standard, beyond which it is considered a dereliction or a supererogation to pass.   Hence the Asiatic too often limits the just growth of improvement by his habitual neglect of morality, honesty, and justice.* No Asiatic race has ever shown that it possessed the power of resistance or the power of progress.

Generally speaking, the agricultural and the mechanical arts are in but a rude state with the Hindus, both being supposed to have remained stationary for two thousand years or more. " India," says Dr. Royle, "vast in extent and diversified in surface, is remarkable as the cradle of one at least of the nations who earliest practised the arts and cultivated the sciences which characterize civilization, and from whence these travelled to the west, and perhaps also to the east. Its present inhabitants continue to venerate sciences which they know only by name, and to practise arts of which they know not the principles, and this with a skill not only remarkable for the early period at which it attained perfection, but also for the manner in which it has remained stationary for so many ages. This can be explained by the fact that the son was unable to add to the manual dexterity of the father, and could not improve an art which he knew only as a routine process. But when commerce was in its infancy, or dealt only in the most precious commodities, these arts could not have been practised unless India had contained within itself all the raw materials which art could convert into useful articles or elegant ornaments. Without cotton the so-called 'webs of woven hair' could have had no existence. Without numerous woods, barks, and flowers, dyeing could not have been practised, and calico-printing would probably not have been invented. If an *Indigofera* had not been indigenous, indigo would never have derived its name from India, nor have afforded us the proof, in the stripe of mummy-cloth, of the early commercial intercourse between its native country and Egypt. Neither would sugar have been arranged by the Greeks with honeys, nor the Indians described as those who ' *bibunt tenera dulces ab arundine succos*,' unless they had had the cane-like *Saccharum* as a plant of their country. Neither in Persia would the proverb of ' giving an Indian answer ' have been considered equivalent to a cut with an Indian sword, unless the Hindus had possessed the ore which enabled them to manufacture the far-famed wootz steel; and gunpowder is likely to have been invented at an early age only in a country where ' villanous saltpetre ' is abundant." Another ancient saying amongst the natives, repeated to this day with glee by the Sepoys of Bengal, exhibits alike the warlike character of the people, and their readiness at all times for mercenary service :—

"Jis ka Deg, oos ka Teg."

This popular and admired proverb is translated by Colonel Hodgson of the Bengal army, as follows—

"He who can keep the pot boiling,
Will neVer want for trenchant *blades*."

His salt is, in fact, the banner and the country of the native soldier.

* Buckle " On Civilization."

The mention of an Indian answer, wootz steel, trenchant blades, and gunpowder, brings us naturally to consider the native army of India, the proper subject in the present article.

The native soldier has been held to be brave, obedient, cheerful and patient under labour, fatigue, and privation, abstemious by religion and habit, honest and amiable in all his dealings, and possessing a very high sense of military honour; attached to his European officer, and grateful for kindness shown him, he never until now abandoned his colours; and when kindly and justly treated, and properly commanded, he has never disappointed the reasonable expectations of his commanders. He is cheerfully resigned in sickness, never exhibiting any unmanly qualities under suffering; he thus stands forth an object deserving the special and high consideration of his European medical officer. A fine example of the kindly feeling of the sepoy towards his surgeon was afforded after the battle of Mahidpore, when the Commander-in-Chief of the Madras army, Sir Thomas Hislop, on visiting the hospitals, was addressed by the wounded sepoys, who " made a personal request of his Excellency that he would now take care of the surgeons who had been so kind and attentive to them." Colonel Blacker, in his history of this war, referring to the " unanimous petition" of the sepoys, adds, that " unassuming merit could not have a more gratifying and appropriate reward, intrinsically more estimable than any formal commendations flowing from authority."* That the qualities here recorded of the men forming the native army of India are derived from the domestic circle and habit of civil life, shared by the sepoy with his brothers, is as certain as that all the qualities of a great military commander are civil qualities. A soldier is a citizen and something more; the addition being but the result of military discipline and military habit. To form a just estimate of the soldier, we must everywhere trace him back to the recruit.

How, after a century of faithful service, the Bengal sepoy came all of a sudden to rise in murderous ferocity against his master; treacherous, faithless, and fiendishly cruel; how the Bengal army, once so distinguished for good conduct, became a huge band of dexterous traitors and disciplined assassins, turning against us in all the wantonness of Indian ferocity, so as to disgrace even savage humanity, it is not the business of this work to relate. I can only say that we are painfully thrown back for our future guidance and practice upon the maxim of Bacon, containing a suggestion which must never again be absent from the minds of our statesmen and commanders:—" Neither is money the sinews of war, as it is trivially said, when the sinews of man's arms, in base and effemi-

* Colonel Blacker is quite philosophical and even kind on the subject of handing over the surgeons of his army for rewards to the bare contemplation of their own merits; but he does not say that, in his own person, he would prefer such mode of recompence to the companionship of the Military Order of the Bath.

nate people, is failing.   As for mercenary forces, which are the help
in this case, all examples show, that whatsoever estate or prince
does rest upon them, he may spread his feathers for awhile, but
he will mew them soon thereafter."

"If we look through history," says Lord John Russell, "we
shall find no parallel case, nor anything at all resembling the
native Indian army.   The Romans held Spain with a single Roman
legion.   With a like force they held Africa and Egypt.   It is
true that auxiliaries were attached to those legions, but the really
armed and effective body was the Roman legion itself, and the
Romans would never have dreamt of having a large native army to
rely upon in case of emergency."

The monstrous perils of the Indian army, as constituted on the
principle condemned by the Romans, and by all history, ended in
treason, havoc, and massacre ; nevertheless, "By the fame of our
conquered difficulties, by the discovery of the might that slumbered
in our arms unsuspected by ourselves, by the proof of the fiery
ordeal through which we have passed triumphantly, by all the
buffetings of a terrible experience, we are a greater nation to-day
than we were at the beginning of the struggle."

To have placed implicit confidence in Mahomedan mercenaries
was a most fatal mistake ; for no Mussulman who does not absolutely renounce his religion can ever be trusted by a Christian
government ; he must, as a Mahomedan and a native, hate our
race, our religion, and our rule.   The Hindus, on the other hand,
are tolerant on principle ; but the wall of caste separation between
the individual Brahmin and his British officer is impassable to any
consideration, human or divine, according to the natives' own
notion.   But, as regards the service of the state, high caste is,
in the language of Sir Charles Napier, actual mutiny.   When a
soldier alleges his caste as a reason for non-compliance with orders,
it is nothing more or less than mutiny ; and the word CASTE should
never again be so much as mentioned between the employer and
the employed.

In India we must not expect, for years to come, that "the
harmony and married calm of states" shall prevail ; and therefore
its armies must not only be in the main British, but they must at
all times be perfectly organized and equipped, and so placed as to
be ready for instant action.   Henceforth English hands must
guard what they have conquered.   "A population constituted of
two races, one of which was the victorious, and the other the vanquished race, each retaining its own religion, and habits which that
religion has imposed upon it—each to the peculiarities of religion
adding the peculiarities of blood, and both, moreover, impressed
with those distinct characteristics which a common origin has
transmitted to the whole Oriental family—this population, which
numbers 110 millions of human beings, which is scattered over an
area equal to three great European kingdoms, which for two

thousand years has been exhausting the experience of Eastern despotism, which has never known, nor till lately heard, of a standard of public morality or public opinion, which has grown up generation after generation in the abject awe of power and the abject adoration of its trappings, which has recognised revenge, and cruelty, and lust as the legitimate attributes of successful conquerors, or the legitimate retaliation of offended and triumphant tyrants—this population is to be governed by the deputy of a remote sovereign, whose crown rests upon the broad basis of law, freedom, and opinion, and whose European subjects apply to the government of her dependency the principles and maxims of Runnymede and St. Stephen's. To reconcile those extraordinary exactions—to govern India so that native subjection may not be jeopardized, or native respect destroyed, or native prejudice outraged on the one side, or English opinion offended, or even English fanaticism alarmed, on the other—so that we may still remain the lords of that varied and uncombining people, but without the reproach of the crimes which follow conquest—to make a gigantic empire not only not onerous and disreputable, but honourable and profitable—such is the task that the British nation devolves upon those on whom it confers the administration of India, and more especially upon the foremost man among them—the Governor-General."

Hitherto, and in our self-complacent notions of our "empire of opinion," and of the cordial "attachment" of the natives to the British rule, we forget Napoleon's wise estimate of Spanish attachment to French domination. "Remember," he said to King Joseph, "that what a nation most hates is another nation." The truth is that the empire of opinion never had any real existence in India. The native impression of our invincibility was the only public opinion which stood of avail to us, and which can avail to us for the future.

Having shown the chief cause of our recent dangers in a too well-organized native army, the best mode of obviating these dangers for the future by means of a well-appointed European force, and the difficulties at all times inherent to our dominion over India, I will now revert to more strictly professional considerations.

Medical officers in the East Indies, holding as they do military commissions, have been principally employed in the duties of the native armies; a certain small proportion being allotted, or "lent," to the civil department of the State, for conducting the medical duties of civil stations. But the great body of the medical corps, numbering for the three Presidencies of India about eight hundred officers, are under the direct and immediate orders of the Commander-in-Chief, and are thus placed much more in contact with the native soldiery than with the civil population at large.

Nor is the social position of the medical officer less befitting a man of science. Entering the Indian army with rank corresponding to that of lieutenant, his position is at once established as that of an officer and gentleman, and it depends on the conduct and character of the individual how he shall uphold such privileges. To secure the confidence and respect of his brother officers of the army, and to become distinguished in his profession, he must possess knowledge, indefatigable industry, judgment, energy, resolution, address, and an untiring patience; and to all these qualities he must add a courage not fed by excitement in the heat of conflict, nor buoyed by any hope—a courage that does not look to rewards, a courage of the highest order : in truth, " the two o'clock in the morning courage," which Napoleon prized so highly, is quite as necessary to the surgeon as to the captain.   To be useful, the surgeon must possess all the experiences of the camp.   Towards natives of all classes his conduct should be just, kind, and liberal ; while in his intercourse with superiors and equals of his own country, his conduct should be that of a modest unpretending man of science.   He must learn that familiarity in the mess-room or elsewhere is not friendship, and that such conduct is never supported by real friendship.   And let not these observations be considered irrelevant, for they have in truth much to do with moral as with professional efficiency.

Against a vain discontent with his position of army-surgeon, I would warn my brother officers, no state of mind being more useless or unprofitable.   To take counsel of the son of Sirach—to feel that " to labour diligently and be content is a sweet life"—is the most truly wise course, whether as servants of the State or as men of science.   It was the practical rule of life of Robert Jackson and Henry Marshall—medical officers to whom the British soldier owes more than to all the commanders who have been placed over him from Cromwell to Wellington, both included.

Excellent as are the native qualities of the sepoy, his usefulness to the British government depends mainly on good discipline, aided by a just and kind treatment on the part of his European officer.   Taken from the middle class—the pith and marrow of British society, whether for peace or for war—the officer of the Indian army is at once a gentleman and a soldier by profession ; but he is neither a titled amateur, a *dilettante*, nor a holiday soldier.   He is recruited generally not from the wealthier of the middle class ; and the less wealthy, the better soldier, provided he be still the gentleman ; but he is not of the class of fine gentlemen who dislike real soldiering.   He generally continues his studies after he has obtained his commission.   In the Indian army there is as yet, happily, no place for "the destitute aristocracy."   He does not enter the army to make it an amusement rather than a business ; he is not a moneyed idler ; and wherever he is placed in command, he is not found wanting.   Freed from the weaknesses of class or caste, which for a long time have damaged certain branches of the British army ; freed, also, from the democratic infusions of the armies of continental Europe, he stands in a middle position between the two extremes. He comes from the highly-educated, high-minded middle class of the United Kingdom; and if at any future time he is to exhibit well-intentioned weakness and incapacity, it will be from causes which are not now in operation in the armies of India. After fifty years' service in the British army, Robert Jackson declares that, "for any great purpose of peace or of war, the middle classes of the empire are the saviours of their country." From the earliest formation of the Indian army, its officers have remembered, in a proportion which does them honour, that in reading, and the command of that reading, which opens the mind to the abandonment of error and the adoption of improvement, consist the most important part of education, and that no officer can deserve the name without such mental discipline. They will therefore generally be found neither idle nor incompetent. On the staff, too, in which they serve through merit and with little support from interest, we seldom find the offensive peculiarities against which Shakspeare has warned us in your " dog in office." Nor are they of a class to depend on others for what is necessary; for they are continually under a necessity to make provision for the most minute details, and they never exhibit a childlike helplessness. They know that to be of ready resource and contrivance, that to make the best of difficulties, is the business of campaigning. In short, the staff and regimental officers of the Indian army rise in skill with the occasion—the true test of excellence everywhere and in all callings. This is very generally true in respect of Indian officers, especially in the junior grades, and well up even into middle life, notwithstanding the baneful influences of a system of seniority promotion.

Finally, the officers of the Indian army do not as yet know the contamination and degradation of official influences; and while for the display of their talents they enjoy a fair field and no favour, there is, at present, no power which can step between the wrong-doer and his punishment. In short, the officers of the Indian army, whether staff or regimental, do not regard military life as a mere dashing and casual pastime, but as " a serious and permanent profession." It follows from what has just been stated, that the medical officer who has the good fortune to serve in the Indian army will find the criticisms of its officers on his general and professional conduct, matters not to be disregarded.

But, with all these advantages, there remained until very recently a source of affliction and of debility to the medical officer of Bengal especially. The medical department was there ruled, as in the other Presidencies, by the three oldest men in the service. To attempt the defence of such an institution were to build its tomb; to endeavour to instruct members who counted forty years' service under tropical influences, or to make them understand the true purpose and object of their official calling, or even to comprehend their own true interests, were about as hopeful as to send forth missionaries to convert the Pope to Protestantism, or the Emperor of Russia to representative government.

The strength of the native armies varies with the exigencies of the State; that of Bengal, in 1825, mustered 152,843 men of the several arms, infantry, cavalry, and artillery; while, in 1832, the same army was reduced to 78,346 men.

The following is stated by Colonel Sykes to have been the distribution of castes in the Bengal army which revolted.

Christians.	Mahomedans.	Brahmins.	Rajpoots.	Inferior castes. Hindus.
1076	12,411	24,849	27,993	13,920.

Grand total . . . . . 80,249.

The average admissions into hospital of this army, during twenty years, was for each soldier one admission in two years; while the average mortality for the same period was 1·79 per cent., and the invaliding 1·5 per cent. per annum.

The strength of the Madras army varied from 71,488, in 1826, to 48,571 in 1837. The average mortality in this army, during twenty years, was 2·09, and in the invaliding, 1·96 per annum.

In the Presidency of Bombay, the strength of the native army varied from 49,873 in 1844, to 25,782 in 1833. Six-eighths of this army are natives of Hindustan, there being in the proportion of eleven Hindus to one Mahomedan; and low-caste men constitute about one-eighth. The mean per-centage of deaths during twenty years gives 1·29—a remarkable degree of health—while the invaliding during the same period was 3·31 per cent. per annum.

The mean mortality during twenty years, for the whole native army of India, as given by Colonel Sykes, is 1·80 per cent. per annum, and the invaliding as 1·93—exhibiting a remarkable condition of health even in troops serving in their native climate.

It is with native as with European troops in the East, fevers and bowel complaints constituting by far the greatest amount of sickness. The maximum of admissions into hospital of Bengal troops occurred in 1842, when 98,936 men were treated medically out of a strength of 113,020; the minimum occurring in 1827, when only 30,903 were treated medically out of a strength of 130,303 men.

In the three Presidencies of India we have the following mortality among the British and native soldiery per cent. :—

	Bengal.	Madras.	Bombay.
European troops	7·38	3·846	5·07
Native troops	1·79	2·095	1·29

Thus a European regiment is renewed in Bengal in ten years, in Bombay in twelve years, and in Madras in seventeen years.

To account for the circumstance that in the Madras Presidency the native mortality is greatest while the European mortality is the least, Colonel Sykes states that the constituents of the Madras native troops are the reverse of the other two Presidencies. In the Madras Cavalry there are from six to seven Mussulmans to one Hindu; and in the infantry there is one Mussulman to $1\frac{1}{2}$ or $1\frac{3}{4}$ Hindus; but amongst the latter there is a considerable number of low castes, without prejudices of caste; therefore the majority of the native troops of the Madras army can eat and drink like Europeans, and the mortality returns show us that they suffer from cholera as much as Europeans, and that the mean mortality from all causes is $2\cdot095$ per cent., or more than $\frac{3}{4}$ per cent. beyond that of the Bombay army for twenty years.

"I never followed," says Colonel Sykes, "a farinaceous or vegetable regimen myself in India, nor do I recommend it to others; but I ate moderately and drank little, and I have a strong conviction that much of European disease in India is attributable to over-stimulus, and that the mortality among the European troops will not be lessened until the European soldier is improved in his habits, until he is made to understand that temperance is for the benefit of his body, libraries for the benefit of his mind, exercise for the benefit of his health, and savings' banks for the benefit of his purse. The climate of India is less to blame than individuals; for in the case of foreigners, the people of a country being healthy, they should, to a certain extent, conform to the habits of the natives, to be healthy also."

The same authority adds :—" The natives of India are generally considered to be very temperate in their habits; but it is quite a mistake to suppose that they all live upon farinaceous or vegetable matters, and do not drink fermented liquors; it is equally a mistake to suppose that the general food of the people is rice, which is only very much the case in low lands subject to inundation, and along the coasts. In the interior rice is generally so much dearer than the bread grains, of which there are many (wheats, millets, the genera holcus, panicum, paspalum, &c. &c.), that rice is rarely consumed, at least in Hindustan and the Dekhan. The Hindustanee soldier lives almost exclusively upon unleavened cakes of wheaten flour, daily baked upon an iron dish, and washed down with water. On the other hand, all Mahomedans, and all low-caste Hindus are consumers of animal food, spirituous liquors, opium, ganja, or hemp-water; and many castes of the Sudras, the Mahrattas for instance, eat mutton and fish when they can afford to do so; but meat is not essentially necessary to health and strength. Liebig says, that only those substances can possibly be called nutritious which are capable of conversion into blood, and that farinaceous food has also this nutritious principle in high degree. The truth of this profound assertion of Liebig is established by the food of the great majority of the native soldiers of the Bombay and Bengal armies. I have shown that six-eighths of the Bombay army consists of Hindus, and considerably more than half of the whole army are Hindustanees. These men never taste meat, fish, or spirituous liquors, but live, I may from personal observation venture to say, almost exclusively upon unleavened cakes of wheat, or other cerealea, baked upon an iron dish, and eaten as soon as cooked."

In 1857, the year of the great mutiny, there were in the three Presidencies of India, 155 regiments of native infantry, the army of India being then composed as follows:—

Of Europeans	45,522
Of Natives	232,234

Henceforth the garrison of India will consist of:—

Europeans	about	70,000
Natives	„	140,000

being a reduction in the latter force, including military police, of 200,000 men.

The natives generally are very subject to the influences of the various climates contained within the British empire in the East, and none more so than the sepoys of the Bengal army, recruited as they are almost exclusively from the plains of Upper Hindustan; but wherever circumstances admit of the use of artificial means, both Hindus and Mahomedans, though born and bred on the soil, take greater precautions against both heat and cold than the stranger European. "To brave the climate" forms no part of native disposition or habit.

The climate of Bengal Proper is, for instance, most prejudicial to the health of the "up-country" sepoy; for although, according to Colonel Henderson, but one-fourth of the Bengal army is stationed there, the deaths of that fourth are more than a moiety of the whole mortality reported. Much of this mortality is doubtless due to the excessive humidity and to the malarious character of the climate; but much is also due to the great change of diet from wheaten bread to rice, which latter the sepoy will use, not because he prefers it, but because it costs so much less. The native dealers in grain, taking advantage of the sepoy's frugality, offer cheaper and worse qualities of rice, or mixture of rice and wheat flour; so that within two or three years' residence in the Lower Provinces, what with the injuries from climate and the inferior and imperfect nutriment, the robust sepoy wastes, and falls a sacrifice to the fevers, dysenteries, and diarrhœas of an unnatural climate; and thus it is in many of the low malarious countries throughout India.

As with the European soldier, so with the sepoy of Hindustan Proper transferred to the malarious low regions, both shared a common fate when, through the feebleness and incapacity o General Morrison of her Majesty's army, the united force under his command was planted by him in the marshes of Aracan, in the first Burmese war. Those native soldiers who did not perish on the spot sank soon afterwards from general cachexia and enormous enlargements of the spleen, followed by dropsical effusions, colliquative white flux, or lientery; in fact, all perished alike—the native and the European.

In Ava, again, in the same war of 1824-25, where I was witness of what happened, and where the climate generally was good, the sepoy, by a proper diet and clothing, was preserved in comparative health through two severe campaigns; but the British soldier, the instrument of the power and glory of the Government, was suffered, by its criminal negligence, to perish miserably through want.

Dr. Finch, of the Bengal army, in an able report on the effect of climate on the health of the native army of that Presidency, gives the following comparative view of the influence of the climate of Hindustan, and of Bengal Proper:—

	Years.	Average strength.	Average sick.	Average per cent. sick to strength.
Hindustan	{ 1835 1836 1837 }	. . 753	. . 354	. . . 46
Bengal Proper . . .	{ 1838 1839 1840 }	. . 899	. . 649	. . . 79

"During three years at Mynpuree," he says, "the corps lost by death but twenty-six men; while during its stay in Bengal Proper the casualties amounted to not less than 203 !"

The manner of locating native troops, with reference to the country of their birth, the period of service in climates which are unnatural to them, and the proper time for relieving corps and divisions, so as to preserve the soldier's health, are matters that as yet have not received from the authorities the attentive consideration due to them.

As with the European, so with the native soldier, the season of greatest amount of disease is from June to Jannary—cholera being most prevalent in April, May, and June. During the rainy season fevers, remittent and intermittent, prevail the most; and towards their decline, bowel complaints, which in low malarious situations prove very intractable, become frequently associated with splenic cachexia. Again, as with the European, so with the native soldier, fevers, remittent and intermittent, generally constitute the first inroad on his health; after which, successions of recurrences ensue, followed sooner or later by enlargement of the spleen and general cachexia—the disease which closes life being dysentery or diarrhœa.

Amongst the natives in civil life, the bazar preparations of arsenic and mercury, so freely administered by the bazar empirics, prove a source of much broken health, causing severe rheumatisms, diarrhœas, and dysenteries, especially during the cold season. Of all this I observèd much in the Native Hospital of Calcutta, of which institution I was surgeon during ten years.

The fevers of the natives, whether remittent or intermittent, present the same events in the same succession as in the European, differing only in degree; and in the Indian army the patient, like his western comrade, has the advantage of coming under the care of his surgeon on the instant he falls sick; and within the first twenty-four hours much may be done to place him in a position of security, and to prepare him for convalescence.

I generally began the treatment by an emeto-cathartic, composed of from one to two grains of emetic tartar, from three to four grains of calomel, added to two scruples or a drachm of compound jalap powder, according to the age and strength of the patient. This powder, placed dry on the tongue and washed down with water, produced a speedy and free action of both stomach and bowels, followed by copious perspiration, and a more or less complete remission of all the symptoms. Generally speaking, the patient was next day in a condition to use bark, quinine, or some of the native bitter tonics to complete the cure. Such of my servants as had served me long, and been with me when in the army, always asked for what they called "the fever powder" whenever seized with the disease, and the other servants soon learned to follow their example; and my European friends, whether civil or military, when going into camp, or on a long march, always carried with them a supply of the same medicine for the use of their native establishment. It continually happened that in the milder cases of fever no tonics of any kind were necessary, the triple action of the emeto-cathartic and sudorific proving sufficient for the cure; and this was especially the case in the sudden and acute febrile seizures of the hot season. I may here add that mercury in any form, beyond the first moderate dose, I seldom if ever administered. When heat at stomach, with urgent thirst, is complained of, the greatest relief will be obtained from the use of saline effervescing draughts.

Dr. Macpherson, of Bengal, in his excellent Essay on "Quinine and Antiperiodics," observes that he who does not know how to employ other medicines does not understand how to make the best of quinine. But he adds, that "in many instances a great deal more quinine is given than is at all required, and the slighter forms of fever can be satisfactorily treated without its aid."

The febrifuges of India, he observes, have been neglected :—" In truth, the great enemy of other febrifuges is quinine. It is so superior to others that it saves much trouble to use it in preference. But a numerous list of native tropical febrifuges, East and West, has now become familiar to us, of which the Rusut, or *Berberis Lycium*—' the most promising of our Indian febrifuges'— the *Swietenia febrifuga*, bebeerine, cinchonine, narcotine — an Eastern drug, for it is not known as the product of other opium— may be mentioned with confidence, in the treatment of intermittent fever; and we must agree with Dr. Macpherson in declaring that the power of all the native antiperiodics, notwithstanding their excellence, must be tested by their proved influence in arresting remittent fevers : this is the *experimentum crucis*.

The general practice by the natives throughout India of adulterating quinine to the extent of 30 and 40 per cent., will go far to account for the discrepancies observable in the reports on the use of quinine in the military hospitals, European and native. The patients had not the doses alleged to have been administered, by one-third or thereabouts. In Europe salicine is largely employed in adulteration, and the natives add magnesia.

Mr. Day, of the Madras army, treating of the intermittent fever of Mysore, as it prevailed in the 12th Native Infantry, concludes :—

1. That in the treatment by bark, or its preparations, those cases in which large doses of quinine are employed are the most easily cured; and that next in value come small doses — and lastly, bark.

2. That in the employment of quinine as a medicine, a saving in the expenditure is effected by using large doses.

3. That great saving of time and trouble to the subordinate hospital servants is gained by giving one dose of quinine only.

4. That by large doses must here be understood, five grains of quinine and upwards, given in combination with tincture of opium.

But in malarious countries adynamic forms of fevers, both remittent and intermittent, will occur, accompanied very generally by abdominal congestions with enlargement of the spleen. Here, in addition to bark and other tonics, warm aromatic aperients, chalybeates, improved diet, and change of air must be had recourse to. The sepoy of Upper India is bound by warm ties to his family, to which he never fails to remit his pecuniary savings. In sickness he eagerly looks to rejoining his relatives ; and, where the exigencies of the service admit of it, such indulgence should always be recommended by the medical officer, whatever the colonel may think.

In treating the fevers of the natives we must not expect to find in them the sustaining powers of constitution of the European ; acute disease subsides in the former much earlier than in the latter, requiring, therefore, antiphlogistic measures of much less energy in the case of the Asiatic, while a much earlier recourse may be had to quina and other tonics in conducting his cure. Whenever we feel satisfied also that acute disease has been overcome, an improved diet may be allowed at an early period—the native constitution not bearing a severe and protracted abstinence ; and condiments may be allowed, especially during the rainy season.

Finally, let the surgeon be careful that the sepoy is not discharged from the hospital too soon, out of a small, narrow, or mistaken notion of military efficiency, or of what an unreflecting adjutant or crack colonel may designate "keeping the effective list complete." The effectiveness of convalescents amounts only to deceptive numbers borne on the muster-roll; and such sham efficiency will bring disgrace on the medical officer, stamping him at once with want of knowledge, want of firmness, and want of humanity. The medical officer who would hold his place worthily in the army of India must possess other qualities as well as talents.

ACUTE DYSENTERY OF BENGAL.

THIS is at once a dangerous and a frequent disease throughout our intertropical possessions; so much so that no medical officer should be permitted to enter on the duties of the public services without a careful previous study of its nature and treatment. Dysentery has at all times proved one of the most severe scourges of our fleets on foreign stations, and of our armies in the field, even when campaigning in temperate regions. It is truly designated by William Fergusson an army disease. "The soldier," he says, "when in the field may escape fever, but never dysentery, if he lie on the ground." It is the disease of the famished garrisons of besieged towns, of barren encampments, and of fleets navigating tropical seas, where fruits and vegetables cannot be procured. Dysentery has occasionally been found to assume a malignant character in low damp situations, so as to prove very deadly; but on the sufferers being removed to elevated sites, and a better air, the disease has been rendered amenable to treatment.

In tropical climates dysentery, though most prevalent during the hot and rainy season, will be found to exist at all periods of the year; but in European countries it is almost exclusively a disease of summer and autumn: it stands thus associated with a high range of temperature, and atmospheric changes. The European soldier in India, as compared to the sepoy, is peculiarly liable to dysentery—eleven of the former to one of the latter being treated in the hospitals. The temperate man who holds a middle course appears here, as in fever, to be the least liable; but the chances of recovery are stated by Mr. Waring to be in favour of the man who observes total abstinence.

Sir Alexander Tulloch states, that out of an aggregate force of 25,433 men of his Majesty's army serving in periods of eight and ten years respectively, between 1823 and 1836, in the stations of Calcutta, Chinsurah, and Berhampore, all in Bengal Proper, there occurred 8499 cases of dysentery and diarrhœa; and though the years within this return were subsequent to the first Burmese war, still the proportion of dysenteric cases is excessive, making every proper allowance for such unfavourable influence. The climate of Lower Bengal has always been very unfavourable to European health, as compared to Upper India; but making allowance for all circumstances, including the ill habits of life of the soldiery, the amount of sickness from dysentery and diarrhœa here exhibited is enormous.

In the Presidency of Madras, again, out of an aggregate British force of 82,342 men, serving there from 1842 to 1848, there occurred 10,531 cases of dysentery, and 9189 cases of diarrhœa, making a total of 19,720 cases of bowel diseases, exclusive of cholera. It thus appears that, next to the malarious fevers of India, bowel complaints are the most prevalent diseases, while the danger to health and to life from these last is even greater than from fevers. There were admitted into the European General Hospital of Calcutta, according to Dr. Macpherson, in the years 1830 to 1850, 2044 cases of dysentery, of whom there died 457, or 22·3 per cent. The extremes of mortality were 14·8 in 1833, and 34 in 1845.

Robert Jackson regards dysentery as " one of the most important of the maladies that occur among troops, particularly in the West Indies, where, in some of the islands, it amounts to one-half, even to more than half of all the forms of acute disease which appear in the hospital return of sick." This great authority adds : " It is dangerous in itself; more fatal, in fact, among the military in the West Indies, either primarily or secondarily, than any other, the concentrated fever, as incident to strangers, excepted." The losses of the French army in Egypt were greater by dysentery than by the plague—the deaths by the latter disease being 1689, while by the former they amounted to 2468. During two years and a half only out of the time occupied in the war in Portugal and Spain, the British army, according to Sir James M'Grigor, lost 4717 men by dysentery. Of the diseases which destroyed the European portion of the expeditionary force in Ava, during the first Burmese war, dysentery—scorbutic dysentery—was by far the most prevalent and fatal disease.

" The per-centage of mortality," says Miss Nightingale, " in acute and chronic dysentery, was perhaps greater in the Crimea than ever has been known in any disease except the worst form of epidemic plague. It was no less than 7·8 per cent. of the cases. This, too, was of the scorbutic form principally, and was caused solely by bad food."

PREDISPOSING CAUSES.

Whatever causes predispose to fever will exercise a like influence in producing dysentery, but more especially the following :—The various duties of the fleet and of the camp, which necessarily expose seamen and soldiers to wet and cold, suppressing the secretions—to high ranges and to sudden and violent changes of temperature, causing checked perspiration especially ;—the use of crude, ill-prepared, indigestible, or otherwise unwholesome diet—excesses in the use of wine, spirituous liquors, or tobacco—the use of impure water—retained excretions—fatigue and privation—endemic, epidemic, and malarious influences—previous fevers, of the remittent and intermittent types especially—diseases of the liver or spleen ; all these circumstances will, severally or individually as may be, dispose the subject to the invasion of dysentery. The causes of scorbutic dysentery are :—Deprivation of fresh meat, vegetables and fruits—sameness in diet*—crowding—mental depression— hardship and fatigue—exposure to damp and foul air—the use of impure water. The salt-meat rations of old were a source of enormous aggravation of dysentery, if they did not actually produce the disease.

SYMPTOMS AND PROGRESS.

The immediate and urgent symptoms in tropical dysentery are— sense of constriction of the skin, followed by irregularly developed febrile movements, more or less marked according to the season of the year, the length of residence in India, the constitution and previous habits of the patient. The amount of attendant fever is very variable ;—in some cases it hardly excites attention, while in others it amounts to heat and dryness of skin, flushed face, furred tongue, and hard frequent pulse. Fever is most considerable in the hot season; while in that of the rains it is less declared, the tendency being here, as in remittent fever, to congestion and collapse. In some forms of malarious dysentery there is considerable fever, with but little hepatic complication comparatively; at least it proved so in China.   But here, as in all the diseases of the stomach and bowels, the power of the pulse rapidly fails as the disease advances.

Soon the patient experiences, during from twelve to twenty-four hours, the uncomfortable feelings attending upon frequent loose discharges from the bowels ; when at length irregular pains, at first of a griping nature only, along the course of the large intestine, becoming gradually more severe, shooting, or " cutting," as the soldiers designate them, with sense of heat ascending from the rectum, and pain extending sometimes to the hypogastrium, until the whole abdomen becomes involved in soreness and feeling of distress, accompanied by frequent purging, griping, and straining, all aggravated during the night and early morning, and leaving behind them the wearing sensation that there has always remained in the bowel something which has yet to be discharged.   At this time the discharges are generally scanty, and consist of mucus

* I have long been of opinion that sameness of mental occupation, prosecuted for a long continuance, proves as injurious to the functions of the brain as sameness of diet to the health of the blood. The unvarying character of the occupation, and the intensity of application required in arithmetical and mathematical pursuits, have, in many instances, appeared to prove most detrimental to the brain, damaging the entire nervous system in the most serious manner.

and blood, or bloody slime as the soldier calls it; and this is a matter of the utmost importance to investigate, as from the character of the discharge we derive important information as to the extent and nature of the disease.

Towards a right estimate of the condition of the tubular, as of the associated solid viscera, we may also receive much aid from a careful exploration of the cæcum and colon, including its sigmoid flexure; and a careful examination of these regions, as of those of the liver and spleen, should never be neglected; for pain, fulness, or thickening of the bowel may always be detected, unless the subject be inordinately stout. When pain and fulness are absent from the regions named, and there is, nevertheless, much local distress, such as urgent and constant tormina and tenesmus, with sense of fulness and heat along the bowel, and with strangury, the seat of inflammation and thickening will be found to be centered in greater degree along the rectum; but this circumstance does not render the case less severe, or less difficult of cure.

The matters voided in the dysentery of India consist at first of liquid fæces, generally of unnatural colours, streaked with blood or mixed with blood and mucus. If the disease advances in the absence of treatment, or in defect or insufficiency of it, then we shall find all the symptoms, constitutional and local, much aggravated, while the intestinal discharges contain more of blood and mucus, together with exudation flakes, shreds, or larger sloughs of mucous membrane, so as often to assume the appearance of putrid blood, or of the washings of raw meat. Scybala are rarely seen in the dysenteries of the East. When to symptoms such as these are superadded a pungent heat and dryness of the skin, with furred tongue, an urgent thirst, high-coloured and scanty urine, an increased frequency of the pulse, and an increased urgency and frequency of call to stool—all augmented towards night—they indicate considerable danger. When, again, patients suffering from the tropical dysentery present the further retrogression of a cold clammy surface, a cadaverous smell from the body and intestinal discharges, an anxious and oppressed countenance, and a sinking pulse with hiccup, and motions voided involuntarily, the case is generally hopeless.

Such are briefly the symptoms of acute dysentery, which will be found to vary in degree according to the severity of the inflammation; and of this last the medical officer will best judge by an attentive observation of the constitutional symptoms, together with a careful daily examination of the nature of the discharges from the bowels: this, indeed, cannot be done too often, or too minutely.

The duration of dysentery varies with the force of the predisposing and exciting causes, the age, constitution, length of residence in hot climates, the season, and other contingent circumstances. Some cases will go through their course even unto death

within three to five days; while others will be received into hospital after having suffered during periods of from five to twenty days,
with appearances the most unfavourable, and yet they recover.

The progress of the disease will, in fact, depend on the condition
and circumstances, past and present, of the individual case.   The
scorbutic form of dysentery may be recognised at once by the
dusky hue and dull melancholy expression of the countenance;
the livid complexion of the surface generally, but especially of the
extremities, which are cold and spotted over with petechiæ, which
the least scratch will convert into an ulcer.   The tongue is dark in
common with the gums, which latter are spongy, and bleed on the
slightest touch, or blood oozes spontaneously from them.   There is
a disrelish for the previously uniform diet, and especially for the
use of salted meats, while there is an urgent craving for vegetables
and subacid fruits of every description.   The pulse is feeble and
frequent; in short, all the symptoms, general and local, indicate
an extreme and aggravated cachexia—a dissolved, diseased condition of the blood.   The purging soon exhibits the true scorbutic
character, the discharges being composed principally of grumous
putrid bloody matter, and even the urine has a bloody hue.

The progress to recovery from dysentery implies a healing of
ulcerated surfaces.   Dr. Parkes accords with the German anatomist Sebastian, and others, as to the fact of the reproduction of
intestinal mucous membrane; while Dr. Bleeker regards cicatrization as the normal termination of dysentery; but the number
and extent of the cicatrices " may withal produce a condition of
the colon which renders it unfit properly to perform its function.
Cicatrices, be they ever so completely formed, cannot make good
the loss of the mucous membrane, with its absorbent and secreting
organs."

COMPLICATIONS.

Dysentery is found in all climates to complicate readily with the
prevailing fevers, and within the tropics it is frequently associated
with fevers, remittent and intermittent: it is also occasionally
complicated with scurvy.   The connexion between epidemic dysentery and various pestilences has been a subject of observation by
many writers in different ages and countries; and the severe and
fatal dysentery of London followed closely on the influenza of 1762.
In the East Indies we find that, either from the beginning, or
during the progress of the dysentery, diseases both functional and
structural are apt to arise in the liver.

Amongst the European patients in the General Hospital of
Calcutta, Dr. Macpherson found that, out of an hundred and sixty
acute cases, the liver was altered in eighty-four cases—containing
abscess in twenty-one cases—being enlarged in forty cases, &c.;
while in fifty-five cases of chronic dysentery the proportion of
hepatic diseases was nearly the same.   This able officer states

that, on a comparison of acute with chronic dysentery, the liver is more frequently altered in the latter, that abscess is about equally frequent in either form, that in acute dysentery the liver is frequently enlarged and soft, while in the chronic it is more generally small and indurated. He adds, that the stomach and small intestines suffer also more frequently in the chronic form, and the mesenteric glands are more frequently altered in it.

In the Madras Presidency, out of fifty-one cases of acute dysentery there were twenty-six hepatic abscesses; and in Bombay, out of thirty cases of acute dysentery, twelve cases of hepatic abscess occurred. "It is worthy of remark," says Dr. Macpherson, "that the liver has been found, in the General Hospital of Calcutta, to have been altered in 118 out of 215 cases; in the Medical College Hospital in thirteen out of thirty cases, while Sir James M'Grigor found it in India altered sixteen times in twenty-two cases, and in Egypt, as in India, he found it diseased." Dr. Arthur found the hepatic complication so prevalent amongst the soldiers of the Madras European Fusiliers serving in Burmah, that "on admission into hospital nearly as much attention was directed to the hepatic region as to the abdomen."

The hepatic complication can in some cases be perceived from the commencement of the dysentery, while in others it probably arises in the course of the principal disease. The daily exploration of the hepatic region, and of the course of the large intestine, will therefore be necessary in every case, to arrive at a just appreciation of all its attendant circumstances. It sometimes happens that enlargement of the liver is not manifested till after the disappearance of the dysentery; and we observe also that hepatic abscess is discoverable only after the cessation of the primary bowel disease.

The association of hepatic diseases with dysentery would seem to be most frequent in the climate of the East Indies, and in such as have a common influence. Dr. Morehead of Bombay found, that out of thirty fatal cases of dysentery, twelve were attended with hepatic abscess; and out of twenty-five dissections of dysenteric patients at Moulmein, in Burmah, Dr. Parkes found hepatic abscess in seven cases, while the same proportion of complication was observed in Ceylon by Henry Marshall.

"As functional disease," says Dr. Parkes, "implies a proportionate certain amount of change in the molecular structure of organs, either primary in the organ itself, or secondary to changes in the blood or vessels, the most delicate test of the condition of an organ will in time be the chemical constitution of its secretion, when this knowledge is obtainable. We already see this test beginning to apply itself in the case of the kidneys and urine. Judging from this test, the liver is found to be more or less diseased in every case of dysentery."

In the province of Oran, Algeria, the French surgeons state

F F

that hepatitis and consequent abscess were frequently coincident with dysentery. Of 157 deaths, in two-thirds of which diarrhœa and dysentery had prevailed during life, " there were in sixty-five cases notable marks of diseases of the liver, including twenty examples of abscess." The tendency to hepatic complication was found in Algeria to increase with age, and with the length of service in that country. The coincidence of disease in the cæcum and liver was noticed by me in the wards of the General Hospital of Calcutta; and, reporting on the diseases of Bengal in 1839, I find the following statement :—" I have seen many cases in which morbid action was co-existent in the liver and cæcum, and I would beg to call attention to the subject." This official record referred to cases which terminated in recovery ; and the " calling attention to the subject" had reference to the verification of the fact in dissection.*

Severe illness obliged me to quit Bengal before this opportunity had been afforded me; but the fact of the morbid coincidence in question has since been ascertained both at home and abroad. It is now established that disease is frequently " co-existent in the liver and cæcum"—that an intimate connexion exists in chronic cases between ulceration of the mucous membrane of this portion of the intestine and hepatic abscess, owing to suppurative phlebitis, to purulent absorption, and to contamination of the portal blood, in chronic cases. In diseases so complicated as dysentery and hepatitis it is often difficult, when the histories are uncertain, to determine with accuracy where morbid action begins; but the extension and coincidence of serious evil, in all the associated organs, is early discernible to the careful observer of symptoms in both diseases during life, and we can readily trace the results after death. Here, as in many other instances, we arrive at an ultimate fact, but can proceed no further with certainty :—we can see and examine the co-relation, and infer a common cause; but we do not, therefore, understand which is the cause, and which the effect. We know not, in too many instances, which of the diseases is the primary—that in the bowel, or in the liver. There are cases, and they are numerous, in which we can plainly discern hepatic disease and hepatic abscess as primary, concomitant, or secondary affections in the time of their occurrence ; but whether they are to be regarded as a cause, a concurrence, or a consequence of dysentery, it is not so easy to determine : practically, a prompt and accurate diagnosis is here of much importance ; for, by a speedy removal of hepatic disease, in the first and second instances cited, we may obviate suppuration of the liver while we cure the dysentery ; and by the early

* It is worthy of remark that in the only dysenteric case of a Hindu, in which " the cæcum, with its appendages, was totally destroyed by a sloughing ulcer perforating in some places all its coats—similar ulcers being formed in the colon and its ascending portion, and sigmoid flexure, as well as in the rectum," there were found, by Dr. Parkes, in the liver, " throughout its substance, numerous small abscesses filled with viscid pus."

healing of ulceration of the bowel, in the third instance cited, we may cure the dysentery and perhaps prevent the occurrence of hepatic abscess, or purulent deposit of any kind. I would direct the special attention of pathologists to the state of the lining membrane of the ducts and gall-bladder, as affording, perhaps, some clue to the pathology of hepatic abscess in association with dysentery.

Diarrhœa, easy of cure, occasionally results from vitiation or redundancy of bile; but not so dysentery, as suggested by Annesley. It is an every-day occurrence, on the other hand, to find that diseases of the liver, and consequent *suppression of the biliary function*, will cause both diarrhœa and dysentery.

The whole question, however, is still an open one. "The connexion between abscess of the liver," says Dr. Ballard, "and dysentery, as a clinical fact, is indisputable. Dr. Henoch, however, refuses his assent to the explanation of it by Budd, who views it as a result of phlebitis, the pus from which, carried by the portal blood, is arrested in the liver, and becomes the focus for the formation of an abscess. Apart from the debated question of the capability of the inner membrane of veins undergoing inflammation at all, Dr. Henoch considers, as opposed to this explanation, the fact that Dr. Parkes, on the most careful examination of such cases, never found the slightest trace of inflammation in the small veins of the intestine, while no direct proof has been advanced of the mediation of the portal blood in the process." Dr. Henoch concludes:—" I believe we must give the preference to that view which regards the two diseased processes, dysentery and abscess of the liver, as without mutual relation, but as running their course together, dependent upon one and the same cause; in favour of which view is the circumstance, that in hot climates abscess of the liver also very frequently occurs associated with remittent fevers, or consecutive to them, without dissection exhibiting any ulceration of the mucous membrane of the intestine."

When dysentery follows upon, or is associated with intermittent fever, the spleen will frequently become enlarged. We then perceive a general anæmia, or splenic cachexia, with a low asthenic type of dysentery. This complication augments the difficulties and embarrassments in treatment, and greatly increases the dangers of the original disease. A writer on the climate of the Danubian provinces observes justly, that where agues are present, dysentery is not far off. In temperate climates dysentery is found associated occasionally with continued and typhoid fevers, and then it becomes sometimes contagious.

The scorbutic complication may be expected to arise in seamen and soldiers, when, in tropical climates especially, they have been supplied for some length of time with unwholesome rations, or with such as consist in whole, or in chief part, of salted meat. Sir Gilbert Blane asserts that the disease " has been known to arise among prisoners of war living entirely on fresh diet, and solely imputable, therefore, to confinement in bad air, a dull uniformity of life, depression of spirits, and indolent habits naturally belonging to a state of captivity." The most terrible instance of suffering from this cause was that of the European portion of the force employed in Ava, during the first Burmese war, where they were fed on salt rations for six and a half months, and where forty-eight per cent. perished within ten months, principally by scorbutic dysentery.

The symptoms noted by all the medical officers were as follow : —swollen, loose, and livid gums, with ulcerated and sloughing edges, and fetid breath, pain and hardness in the calves of the legs, constriction of the hams, and purple discoloration of the skin of the lower extremities—œdematous swelling of the feet and legs— anasarca—ascites and hydrothorax. When to such a condition of the system, scorbutic dysentery was added, the speedy and fatal character of the disease may be inferred.

The bowel complaint was characterized by green, or greenish-yellow discharges, becoming by degrees sanious ; then dark, bloody, grumous, and putrid. A sudden and universal dropsy marked the latter days of the sufferers : I saw one of Her Majesty's regiments at Prome, in the second campaign, lose forty men in one night from this cause; and at Rangoon, in the first year, the Madras European regiment, containing many old, hard-drinking soldiers, was the first corps to be destroyed by this dropsy, which, from its suddenness and fatality, resembled the worst form of the Beribery of Ceylon.

From such a hopeless state of disease as has here been described, there are many grades, down to the very minor degrees ; and the medical officer who finds his men fed on bad, poor, and insufficient diet, under tropical influences, should be on the watch for scorbutic taints. They are all dangerous, and they mount rapidly from the least to the most aggravated grades.

PATHOLOGY.

As the symptoms of acute tropical dysentery, during the progress of the disease, will depend on the nature and power of the cause— on the condition of the general habit—on the amount of plethora, of congestion, or of actual inflammation in a portion, or in the whole of the abdominal viscera; so the results of these morbid actions will, after death, be found to vary with the form and degree of the disease. Acute tropical dysentery consists in inflammation, commencing generally in the mucous membrane of the large intestine —sometimes in the follicles—and proceeding rapidly to exudation, ulceration, and sloughing, if not promptly checked by art. The disease is always associated with disturbance of the functions of the skin and liver. " Dr. Parkes considers it to be a process of ulceration universally commencing in the solitary glands of the large intestine; others, with Mr. Raleigh, consider it to be a simple inflammation of the mucous coat of the large intestine; but if it were simple in its nature, it would be more amenable to treatment. Whatever of truth or error may be in these opinions, the appearance presented to us in uncomplicated Bengal dysentery, is that of an inflammation of the large intestine, which may be diffusive, ulcerative, purulent, hæmorrhagic, or gangrenous, according to circumstances!" . . " It should be borne in mind that the state of the solitary glands, as observed by Drs. Murray and Parkes, exactly corresponds with their usual appearance in cholera, and that all Murray's and most of Parkes' cases occurred in dysenteric patients suddenly carried off by that disease."—*Dr. Macpherson.*

The train of pathological events in acute tropical dysentery may be summed up as follows :—Congestion succeeded by inflammation of the follicles of the large intestine—lymphous exudation and infiltration beneath the mucous membrane—degeneration of the infiltrated fluids, and ulceration first of the follicles and then of the mucous membrane ;—all the morbid processes described, including diffused inflammation and softening, rapidly extending to the mucous membrane, so as to destroy by ulceration both its structure and its functions—those of the glands having first undergone the same injuries. In states of anæmia and scorbutus, or under epidemic conditions and typhoid associations, there will occur phagedænic and rapid destruction of all the textures, accompanied by an extreme amount of mortality. It is not at all a colonitis, as Ballingall termed it, but a disease of a specific pathological character, influenced by the epidemic conditions of the atmosphere, by malaria, by the previous habits, duties, and diet, and by the states of the blood resulting from such conditions and habits. Such is acute dysentery, specially and pathologically considered, without waiting here to describe various complications.

In the milder cases which yield to treatment within two or three days, we may fairly presume that diseased action has not proceeded beyond plethora, or the mildest form of vascular congestion or of inflammation of the mucous surface and glands.

In severe cases the inflammatory action, far from confining itself to the mucous membrane, extends to the serous covering, and even to the solid viscera, while ulceration, and even sloughing of the mucous surface and its glands, may be in extensive progress ; and all this, occasionally, without that amount of corresponding fever which might, *a priori*, be anticipated—a circumstance which gives a character of peculiar insidiousness to a disease already very dangerous in its nature. Abrasions, ulcerations, and sloughs are but varying degrees of the same morbid process, the sloughing sometimes involving all the structures alike. Again, ulceration is found to result from deposits of pus, lymph, and serum below the mucous membrane, as well as from inflammation of this tissue.

"Omental congestion or inflammation," says Robert Jackson, "accompanies dysenteric fever not unfrequently. The indications of its existence are obscure; and its foundations are not moved without difficulty—not without the most extreme measures in bleeding, blistering, &c."

When much tumidness with tenderness of the abdomen is associated with irritability of stomach and vomiting, inflammation of the peritoneal covering may be more than suspected, and *post-mortem* appearances will frequently confirm this view of the case. When again, from want of treatment, or through unskilful treatment, the disease has proceeded unchecked for a considerable time, the best that can generally happen will be the merging of acute into chronic dysentery—or imperfect healing of the ulcerated bowel.

Certain portions of the large intestine have always appeared to me to be more affected when the complication in dysentery has been of the hepatic nature—namely, the cæcum and the rectum. In the General Hospital of Calcutta, a government institution for the treatment of Europeans, I observed so frequently as to attract my special notice, that, when the cæcum was the principal seat of pain and swelling, the liver was generally enlarged; but whether as cause or effect I could not say. As with the natives of India, Hindu and Mahomedan, so with British-born subjects in their native climate, hepatic abscess is found to be but very rarely associated with dysentery; whereas with Europeans placed out of their native climate, and under great heats, as in the East Indies, hepatic diseases and abscess have been found to be very frequent complications in dysentery.

In the Millbank Prison, out of "many hundreds of cases," which occurred during seven years, "not one has been complicated with hepatic abscess," says Dr. Baly. These facts would lead to the conclusion that a foreign climate mainly, and its unnatural influences, and more particularly heat and malaria, produce the difference of result as respects British subjects; but it is most difficult here, as in other diseases, to determine what is cause and what coincidence.

The other seat of irritation and of aggravated disease, associated with, or derived from, the hepatic complication, I observed to be the rectum; and in this portion of the bowel two causes appeared to me to operate unfavourably: the first consisted in the arrest of circulation in the hæmorrhoidal veins consequent on congestion or enlargement of the liver, producing internal or external hæmorrhoids, or both: the other depended on the constant state of irritation in which the rectum is kept by the passage over it of acrid discharges. Through inflammation, thickening, and adhesion, the cæcum speedily loses its tone and contractile power, thus becoming the passive receptacle for the lodgment of vitiated and

decaying matters; while the angle of the bowel at its sigmoid
flexure becomes, through the incessant drainings of the same
matters over its surface, the special seat of soreness.   Much of the
suffering and distress of the patient may always be traced to the
irritated states of the sigmoid flexure and rectum, kept in constant tormina and tenesmus by the passage of such matters, often
with the addition of acrid scalding bile.   The same distresses I
have seen produced by the misapplication, or by the protracted use,
of calomel and drastic purgatives—by over-treatment, in short.

· Death being presumed to occur only in the severer forms of
dysentery, and in the worst cases only, we perceive, on removing
the abdominal parietes, a turgid and congested state of the vessels,
with adhesions of the serous coverings of the omentum, mesocolon,
and mesentery, with varied and more extended adhesions between
the different viscera ; enlargements and inflammations of the
glands of the mesocolon and mesentery, with occasional suppurations in them ; inflammation and its results, such as thickening of
the coats of the large intestines, softening, ulceration, or sloughing
of the mucous membrane of the ileum, or of a portion, or of the
whole of the larger bowel—the ulcers having the appearance of
variolous pustules, and being, in fact, glandular ulcerations, sometimes perforating the coats of the intestines into the general cavity ;
thickening of the coats, and contractions of the bore of the intestines, from effusion of fibrine and lymph, especially of the larger
bowel, and most frequently at its sigmoid flexure.   Adhesions of
the omentum to the cæcum, and abscess in the vicinity of the
cæcum, are occasionally observed.

In the hepatic complication the liver will be found congested,
inflamed, suppurated, or indurated, according to the degree and
duration of the disease.   In the dysentery of the Peninsular army,
under the Duke of Wellington, the spleen, liver, and mesentery
were generally found diseased ; and in the epidemic form of the
disease, as it prevailed in Ireland, the liver was diseased in half,
the spleen in a fourth, the small intestines in two-thirds, and the
colon and rectum in all the dissections ; but I do not recollect
any mention of hepatic abscess from phlebitis, purulent deposit, or
other cause, an event so frequent in the East.

In the scorbutic complication the post-obit appearances are
altogether of an asthenic character, indicative of a diseased condition of all the fluids.   The inner surface of the large intestine, and
of the ileum likewise, generally exhibiting extensive disorganization and decay, the bowel being in many cases filled with shreds
and sloughs of mucous membrane and grumous blood, while the
liver has a blue appearance externally, and when cut into, the
blood which flows is atrabilious and dissolved; but where hæmorrhage from the bowel has occurred, the liver will be found
softened and .anæmic.   The spleen crumbles under the slightest
pressure, like a mass of grumous blood.   Ecchymosed patches

are to be seen on the outer skin, on the external and internal surfaces of the bowels, while congestive patches of diseased blood and
softening of textures are found in the heart and lungs.   Appear-
anecs such as these indicate—either that the forces of diseased
action have been invincible in their nature, or that the treatment
intended for their removal has been inert or insufficient.

TREATMENT.

The first and greatest care of the medical officers of fleets and
armies should be directed to the *prevention* of this formidable
disease, by securing such attention from the authorities to matters
of diet, clothing, protection from weather, and the conduct of duty,
as may preserve the men in the vigour of health.   There is no
disease in which an early preventive and remedial attention is of
more importance than in dysentery—the very great mortality of
the disease in many of our tropical possessions being in considerable degree referable to the neglect of early measures of prevention
and cure.   Soldiers and seamen, when left to their own ways, will
go on with their duties under seriously advancing disease ; and it
is only when " bloody stools, with cutting pains," afflict them, that
they will " report sick."   It is here that the all-powerful influence
of commanding officers should be solicited by the watchful surgeon.   An inspection-muster, morning and evening, should be
ordered, with a view to the earliest detection of advancing
disease.   This simple measure will save vast suffering and many
lives.

But however watchful the sanitary precautions, a certain amount
of sickness from dysentery will always occur in naval and military
service within the tropics. It therefore behoves all who have to treat
this disease to bear in mind that the destruction of those placed in
their charge is at hand—indeed imminent—unless the disease is
promptly relieved by appropriate medical means.   Every consideration of humanity and of duty to the State should concur and
unite in directing our efforts to the speedy and effectual arrest of
the sufferings and dangers attendant on tropical dysentery.   For-
tunately we have, both in the army and navy, to treat men in
the vigour of life, with the further advantage that the patient
comes under our care immediately he falls sick. A speedy and
secure convalescence therefore results from a timely well-regulated
and decisive course of treatment, while chronic dysentery, with
lingering sufferings in hospital, or permanently broken health, will
follow on feeble and indecisive attempts at cure.   Let it be remembered also that cases, bearing the appearance of the mildest character of disease, are occasionally found to exhibit, in course of a
few hours, the real characters of destructive inflammation. Nothing
therefore but the most watchful care, guided by intelligence in
the selection and use of means, can lead to the patient's safety. In

the treatment of dysentery, as of fever, our first and most special regard must be given to the character of the type, whether sthenic or asthenic.

It will be found with acute inflammatory or congestive dysentery, as with fever, that a sufficient abstraction of blood by venesection, practised at the very onset of the disease, will simplify and render easy all the subsequent stages of the cure ; so much so that, in mild and uncomplicated dysentery, as in the violently acute and inflammatory type of the disease, blood-letting is the primary as well as the cardinal measure.   In acute uncomplicated dysentery, a moderate bleeding from the arm, followed by a full dose of calomel and James's powder, or ipecacuanha, say ten grains of the latter to ten of calomel, given at bed-time, a warm bath, or hot fomentations to the abdomen—a morning aperient, followed during the day by sudorifics conjoined with diuretics—the moderate use of demulcent drinks, allowing no other sustenance—will, in a very few days, bring about convalescence.

Where pain remains in any particular region of the abdomen, as that of the cæcum, sigmoid flexure of the colon, or the rectum, leeches should follow the general abstraction of blood, guarding carefully against subsequent oozing from the leech-bites, and using warm fomentations or poultices only when the bites have been thoroughly dried up.   While any irritation of the bowels remains, as indicated by frequent stools, containing mucus and blood, the nightly dose of ipecacuanha, diminished in amount as the symptoms mitigate, must be continued, followed during the day by cooling diaphoretics with diuretics, as recommended in the treatment of fever.   In the use or the withdrawal of calomel or blue-pill at night, along with the sudorifics, we should be guided by the presence or absence of fever with a furred tongue, and by the healthy or depraved condition of the intestinal discharges. Mercury ought not, in short, to be regarded, in every case, as a necessity in the treatment of dysentery.   It is not a remedy of necessity in all cases or in all climates : in the West Indies, for instance, the hepatic complication is by no means so frequent as in the East.

While the use of sudorifics, with some mild mercurial, is indicated by the continuance of dysenteric symptoms and hepatic disorder, with more or less vitiation of the secretions, a mild aperient in the form of castor-oil, or of compound powder of jalap, should be exhibited every second or third morning, while in this mild, as in every form of acute dysentery, the diet must be of the very lowest, presuming that the time required for the cure will not comprehend many days.

In the highly inflammatory type of dysentery, on the other hand, we shall find that, after free blood-lettings, the occasion for the use of calomel with the sudorific will depend on the amount of complication, and on the constitution of the patient ; and when he is youthful and robust, with fever, tumid abdomen, and furred tongue, the repetition of blood-letting, and that of calomel and sudorifics in full doses, will be called for ; the mercurial sudorific also must be repeated every night, reduced in dose as the disease yields, until the discharges from the bowels assume a natural appearance, when calomel may be discontinued, and blue-pill or mercury and chalk substituted, if any mercurial should still be necessary. The circumstance too that, in certain cases, much blood is voided by stool should not deter the surgeon from the use of the lancet; for, on the contrary, the early and free employment of depletion will greatly conduce to safety. Of blood-letting and mercury it must be observed also that, although they prove most beneficial when used early in the disease, they will still be found necessary, in their just proportions, where the disease has even existed for some time, or where treatment has been neglected. Blood-letting was repeated by Robert Jackson " until all that was expected from it had been attained." But all the circumstances of each individual must be so weighed, in reference to constitution, age, habits of life, and length of residence in India, as to guide the medical officer in the amount and measure of every means employed. It is impossible to fix an arbitrary rule or gauge for every case beforehand, and it is better that a young practitioner should reflect seriously on all that relates to his patient, and act on principle according to his judgment, than that he should betake himself to a pattern such as is occasionally afforded in narratives of published cases. He must learn that, in our management of an ever-varying disease, we are unable to lay down any catholic rules of treatment which shall be suitable to every case. When we feel assured that inflammation has been subdued, a full opiate may be added to the night dose of sudorific, or the two may be combined in the form of compound powder of ipecacuanha; and thus, provided we have been so fortunate as to see the patient immediately on his being taken with the disease, a few days of treatment, such as is here described, will prove effective of cure. Used in this manner, opiates conduce powerfully to the cure; and their free use, in the manner here recommended, should never be neglected. Robert Jackson frequently ordered the Dover's powder, in doses of eight grains thrice a day. In persons of a less robust constitution, again, and even in such as are of delicate habit, in whom dysenteric purging, griping pains, and pain on exploration of the abdomen are present, repeated abstractions of blood generally, and by means of leeches, will be requisite; the measure of blood-letting, as well as the occasion for its repetition, being estimated and determined by the amount and degree of the disease. In every case dysentery must be speedily overcome by treatment, if we would save our patient.

It was a maxim of Hippocrates that " in desperate diseases, desperate remedies, energetically pursued, are the most efficacious ;" and we everywhere find this principle ably supported by Robert

Jackson, who urges that " when the state is inflammation, and the termination congestion, suppuration, or gangrene, the physician must not hesitate in striking a balance between the chances of debility and the almost certainty of death. There is here no safety in half measures."

But while without blood-letting there is no safety for the sufferer so long as evidences of inflammation are in existence, no sensible person would, on the other hand, practise such an operation, or continue the use of powerful remedies, after the subsiding of symptoms has indicated the approach of convalescence ; and here we limit ourselves to the use of ipecacuanha as a sudorific, cooling diaphoretics with diuretics, mild aperients, cold water enemata, with or without lead and opium, anodynes by the stomach and rectum, warm baths, demulcent drinks, and farinaceous diet, all which means must follow upon depletion, and their exhibition must be persisted in until we shall have obtained to convalescence, but no further.

The most cursory view of the special pathology and of the associations of dysentery, ought to satisfy the medical officer that no one exclusive mode of treating a disease so complicated in its nature can be rational in itself, or successful in its results. Dysentery, as it may occur in the plethoric, hale, newly-arrived, or older European resident in India with damaged constitution, is often simple and inflammatory, and, after a few days, complicated by congestion or inflammatory states of one or more of the surrounding viscera ; it is to be seen associated with low adynamic malarious fevers, remittent, intermittent, and continued, with scorbutus, with phagedænic ulceration and hæmorrhage. Nay, in temperate climates, we find typhus and scorbutus engrafted on dysentery, as with the French troops in the Crimea, so as to present a mortal combination of all three diseases.

Under such varied aspects, it is obvious that our means of cure, to be appropriate, must be different, and grounded on the true pathology of each condition. In the acute inflammatory seizure of the young and plethoric European, whether simple or complicated, the abstraction of blood must be immediate, and so impressive as at once to arrest inflammation and congestion, after which come a few cholagogue doses of calomel, and a few aperients, sudorifics, opiates, demulcents. In the older European the same means will be necessary, but in abated vigour and force. In the adynamic associations of dysentery, other and opposite means must be employed, such as may constringe, support, give tone, and improve the condition of the blood.

When, after the removal of inflammation, soreness along any portion of the large intestine exists, with a suspicion of ulceration of the mucous membrane, the use of washed sulphur alone, or in combination with the bitartrate of potash, will prove the best aperient given every other morning. This combination seems to have a detergent and healing influence, and even the sulphur un-combined acts as a most gentle and soothing relaxant.   Enemata are here also most powerful to good, either in the emollient and anodyne form, given at bed-time, or as an astringent and refrige-rant in the form of cold water, having eight or ten grains of the acetate of lead, with two of opium, in solution.   This last form of injection, with diminished proportions of lead and opium, may also be exhibited three times a day where great tenderness and irritation exist in the rectum.   It is always desirable that the in-jections should be retained, and to this end they should not exceed three or four ounces, and the operation of injecting should be performed in the most gradual and gentle manner ; as to the temperature, whether cold or warm, we should be guided by the feelings and wishes of the patient, these being the true tests.

It is important to pay attention to such adjuvants, for tormina and tenesmus are very wearing and depressing to the nervous system, and they are aggravated during the night so as not only to prevent sleep, but by the frequency of the calls to stool the patient is exposed to the additional risks of checked perspiration and chills.   To guard against such evils it will always be proper, in the case here under consideration, to add the enemata to the night opiate, or Dover's powder.   Suppositories of lead ointment, with two grains of opium, will likewise be found calming of irri-tation in the rectum, and therefore very grateful to the patient.

On the subsidence of inflammatory action, when fulness, tender-ness, or thickening of the bowel exists at any portion of its course, blisters are always beneficially employed.   Robert Jackson states, where tenesmus is urgent, with pain and heat in the rectum, ac-companied by offensive discharges, he found the following powder very efficacious :—

Finely powdered charcoal	. . . . . .	Ðj
,,	,,	rhubarb	. . . . . .	gr. x.
,,	,,	ipecacuanha	. . . . .	gr. v.

A drachm of charcoal powder in rice-water he also states to be equally effective as an enema. " These," he says, " of all means known to me, have had the most instantaneous good effect in this form of disease.   When the subject has been prepared by previous evacuation, &c., two or three doses of the powder by the stomach generally effect a cure."   In severe cases he gave this preparation every five or six hours ; but he adds, with characteristic candour, that " where the action of the disease is chiefly upon the exterior membrane, or in the more remote organs within the abdomen, it was of no value."

The force of disease having been subdued by depletory means, Robert Jackson says, that " the application of very cold salt-water to the abdomen, particularly to the fundament by cloths or sponges ; or immersion of the lower part of the trunk in a tub of cold water

is singularly refreshing.   It allays the torments of tenesmus, and
gives a respite from local sufferings, which, if properly valued and
improved, lays the case open to the action of general remedies, so
as that the disease may be conducted to a safe and speedy issue
with something like calculable certainty."

In the instance of inflammatory dysentery, as already stated,
we cannot be too sparing in the use of food, or even in the use of
liquids.   Thirst is rarely urgent, as in fever, and there is no
craving for food.   We shall therefore do well to require the most
rigid abstinence on the part of the patient.   During the first ten
days of convalescence also, the most careful attention should be
paid both to the quality and quantity of the food, else relapse may
be apprehended.   The healing of ulceration and the absorption
of effused fluids are processes likely to be seriously retarded by
anything approaching to a full stomach.

When convalescence has been established, quinine, or some
other preparation of cinchona, should be exhibited as a tonic, conjoined with the dilute sulphuric acid, and with the tincture of
opium if necessary.   Exhibited in this manner, quina gives tone
to the digestive functions, and obviates adynamic tendencies.

A most dangerous form of hæmorrhagic dysentery appears occasionally under the influence of causes the most concentrated, remote, and exciting, and chiefly amongst seamen and soldiers of
reduced health, when exposed to the joint actions of the deleterious
compounds of intoxicating liquors sold in the bazaars of Calcutta,
and of severe exposure by night and day to the influences of the
climate.   This is the form of dysentery termed retrograde by
Robert Jackson.   So imminent is the danger, that death may take
place within a few hours of admission into hospital, or it may be
protracted to the third or fourth day; but, even in a disease so
frightful to behold, it is surprising how cases wearing the most
unfavourable aspect will sometimes recover.

The patient generally presents the appearance of collapse with
a sad, anxious, scorbutic-looking countenance, much restlessness,
a cold damp surface, a small quick and feeble pulse, and a cada-
verons odour exhaling from the body, the matters voided consisting of grumous blood, or of fluid largely tinged with blood, with
sloughs and patches of mucous membrane, and having an offensive
cadaverous smell.   Increase of collapse with hiccup, vomiting,
and the involuntary passage of copious bloody dejections, end in
speedy death.

The fatal hæmorrhagic dysentery in the Bengal European
Fusiliers and H.M.'s 80th Regiment in 1849-50, is said to have
been preceded by bad malarious fevers of various types; but the
fact of the dysentery being confined to the soldiery would imply
also the additional disadvantages of neglects in the food and drink
—neglects in the sanitary condition of the localities, resulting in

bad air, and other injuries. These circumstances resulted in a deadly dysentery, accompanied by sanguineous discharges from the gums, nose, fauces, and bowels.

On dissection, an excessive deposition of coagulable lymph is found between the coats of the large intestine, and most generally in the cæcum, sigmoid flexure, and rectum, while large irregular patches of sloughing ulceration pervade the mucous membrane, and sometimes give rise to large perforations of the bowels.

In treating this hæmorrhagic form of the disease we must have instant recourse to the most powerful astringents in the largest doses, aiding their effects by the free addition of opiates; and both must be frequently and freely administered by the mouth and anus. Lead may be used more liberally and more safely than is generally supposed. Dr. Christison of Edinburgh has given six grains of the acetate of lead daily for several months, without any ill effects, while Mr. Webber of Norwich states that, " in severe cases of bronchitis he administers from three to ten grains of the same medicine in pill, *with a mixture containing three drachm doses* of distilled vinegar every four hours till symptoms subside, which frequently takes place after the third or fourth dose."

In hæmorrhagic dysentery the lead should be given every two hours, so as speedily to establish its influence, while to each dose a grain or more of opium is added, using at the same time strong enemata of solution of acetate of lead with opium, thrown with sufficient force to enter the course of the colon; and this plan of treatment must be persisted in till the discharge of blood shall have totally ceased. Dr. Kenneth Mackinnon of Bengal has for many years advocated the use of large doses of opium in the sloughing and hæmorrhagic dysentery; and Mr. Taylor, surgeon to H.M.'s 80th Regiment, when treating of the hæmorrhagic and phagedænic types of this disease at Dinapore, Bengal, says: " The medicine of most constant avail in those cases is opium; and it is astonishing the great quantity of it required to produce any effect. Fifteen to thirty grains a day may be given without producing stupor or even headache. When the case is less severe, allowing of more time, quinine is resorted to by all who have treated this disease, showing the general suspicion of its febrile nature." This is a revival of the practice of Sydenham, followed more than fifty years ago by Sir James M'Grigor and others in the East Indies. In a form of the disease characterized by a rapid destruction of the organs immediately involved, and by general collapse of the nervous and vascular systems, such a diet must be allowed as may nourish while it supports the sinking powers of the patient; and with these views soups should be added to the farinaceous articles, while wine and even brandy with opium must be allowed, in order to guard against sinking. Convalescence will be greatly promoted by the exhibition of quinine with nitric or sulphuric acid, with the addition of a few minims of laudanum. The value of opium in sloughing phagedæna points it out *a priori* as an efficient remedy in this terrible disease, and so it proves in fact— opium and lead, with suitable diet, constituting the only means on which we can rely.

Dr. Wilmot, of Tunbridge Wells, in a severe epidemic dysentery of a scorbutic character, and attended by sloughing ulceration of the mucous membrane, while he exhibited by the stomach the decoction and compound tincture of bark with sulphuric acid, administered in the form of enema a drachm of creosote in twelve ounces of thin starch ; and to this latter means, exhibited every night at bedtime, Dr. Wilmot ascribes very decided results, as a stimulant, antiseptic, and styptic. Oil of turpentine, in small and repeated doses, has for many years been recommended as useful by Dr. Copland and others in hæmogastric and low typhoid fevers, in typhoid hæmorrhage from the bowels, in hæmorrhages from the mucous surfaces, dependent on an atonic state of the vessels, and in hæmorrhagic dysentery. The physiological actions of turpentine are, in fact, very analogous to those of creosote.

But whether we have to treat dysentery in its milder or most severe form, complications will meet us, either from the commencement of the disease or during its progress, and we must then be prepared to meet each contingency as it may arise ;—and first, of the hepatic complication. The liver will be found involved, in some instances, from the very commencement of the disease, while in others it palpably arises in the course of the dysentery. The daily exploration of the hepatic region, as well as of the course of the large intestine, will therefore in every case be necessary, to obtain a just appreciation of all the circumstances of each case. Here depletion, both general and local, must be carried to such extent as to remove congestion of the portal system, tumidness, and pain of the liver, while by the nightly use of calomel and ipecacuanha, followed by compound powder of jalap in the early morning, and diaphoretics with diuretics during the day, we relax the skin, emulge the liver, and restore the lost balance of circulation. The measures here indicated must be repeated so long only as the signs of general congestion and hepatic complication are present, discontinuing the use of calomel and blood-letting immediately on their disappearance. In this, as in every other instance where leeches are used, I would urge on the young surgeon the necessity of applying so many leeches as may be necessary, and no more, arresting the oozing from their bites without delay, while no poultices or fomentations should be applied until all oozing shall have completely ceased.

After the removal of acute symptoms, should fulness or tenderness of the liver still continue, the occasional application of blisters should be made over the region; and to advance convalescence, the nitro-muriatic acid, internally and externally exhibited, will prove eminently serviceable. It is necessary in the dysenteries of the East to have constant regard to the hepatic complication; for it may be that, by appropriate means, we can remove inflammation and consequent ulceration of the mucous membrane of the intestine; but if disordered function, congestion, or inflammation of the liver tending to abscess be going on, the cure will be postponed or prevented by any one of the circumstances named, or by the occurrence of dysenteric relapse—a condition to be vigilantly guarded against.

In the cure as in the prevention of scorbutus we have mainly to look to the avoidance of all exhausting and depressing causes—to the removal from damp, to care in the diet, cleanliness, ventilation, cheerful occupation, and change of air; while medically, and referring to the scorbutic complication in dysentery, our first indication of treatment is, by appropriate medicine and regulation of the diet, to restore the health of the blood.

The want of fresh meat, fresh vegetables, and milk has everywhere contributed to the induction of scorbutus.

In addition to the liberal use of pure lime-juice, vegetables and fruits should be abundantly supplied, and potatoes especially, as being eminently anti-scorbutic. During long voyages some reduction in the meat portion of the ration might be advantageously made, granting a proportionate increase of vegetables and fruits; for it is to the want of these last, even more than to the sameness of the diet and the salted meat, that the production of the scorbutic taint is referred. Scorbutus is not only a serious disease in itself, but its complication with fever and dysentery, and the greater liability of scorbutic persons to be affected with the various tropical diseases, malarious and other, render its prevention and cure a question of great importance.*

In scorbutic dysentery fresh lime-juice with opiates simply, or in the form of Dover's powder, will prove the best medicine, while a liberal allowance of fruits and vegetables should be granted, along with so much fresh animal food as the stomach will bear. When irritability of stomach exists, the chlorate of potash, the carbonates of soda and potash in effervescence, lime-juice being in excess, may be given with advantage; and when tormina and tenesmus occur, with bloody discharges from the bowels, anodynes and astringents combined, or lime-juice and opium in the form of enemata, should be employed, while the infusion of cinchona with the nitro-muriatic acid and opium are given by the stomach.

---

* Sir Gilbert Blane states that "the first ample supply of lemon-juice to ships of war was as long ago as 1757, to the squadron under Admiral Watson, in the East Indies, at the suggestion of his surgeon, Mr. Ives, a gentleman highly educated, of great merit and modesty; and we do not learn that he courted public notice, far less that he solicited a reward for doing what he deemed to be merely his duty."

When sloughs are discharged by stool along with grumous blood, the scorbutic taint being manifest, the danger to life is imminent. For the removal of the oozing which takes place in scorbutic dysentery from the gums and mucous membrane of the bowels, the astringent and tonic properties of the sulphate of iron, largely administered in solution by the stomach and rectum, and used as a gargle, will be found eminently serviceable; with the same view the muriated tincture of iron is recommended by Annesley and others, but it is not intended that either means should supersede the use of the direct antiscorbutics.

The combination of iron and alum will likewise be found of great service, as will the Sand Rock chalybeate water of the Isle of Wight.

In default of lime-juice, the medical officer must seek for substitutes in citric acid, and in all kinds of summer fruits. For more than a century fruits have been justly lauded by our army surgeons in the treatment of dysentery, and the physicians of Spain and Portugal, according to William Fergusson, have for ages employed the juice of lemons with good effect in the endemic and epidemic dysenteries of their respective countries. Dr. Cabbel, a talented young surgeon of the Peninsular army, used no other medicine in treating British soldiers; when severely attacked in person by the disease in Portugal, though attended by Dr. Fergusson, he refused all remedies other than lemons and oranges, and he speedily recovered. "In Trinidad, too, when a dysentery of uncommon malignity appeared there, Dr. Lynch O'Connor found that limejuice, administered by the mouth and in *lavement*, was the only remedy that could be depended upon."

Isambert, speaking of the antiseptic powers of the chlorate of potass, says that it has been found of use in scorbutus; and thus we find the materies returning by another route to one of the first affections the chlorate was recommended for, on the theory of deoxidizing the salt in the economy.

Pringle, more than a hundred years ago, used grapes freely in the treatment of dysentery, and there have been few since his time who may be regarded as better authorities. On the subject of the Bael fruit of Bengal, and on the use of fruits generally in the East Indies, I beg to refer the reader to what is stated respecting them in the article on chronic diarrhœa.

Dr. Kinloch Kirk, of the Bengal army, speaking of the sickly condition of the 78th Highlanders in Sindh, in 1843-44, states that the soldiers suffered from "large livers and spleens, and were weakened by continued colliquative purging." In this state, and suffering from a low fever, "the men found, from their own expericuce, more comfort and more advantage from the use of limes than from any other substance, and many gave back a portion of their rations to receive in lieu its value in limes." This intelligent officer, with an excellent power of observation and a rare practical tact, when serving in the same country with sepoys suffering in the same manner, made use of the *Phyllanthus emblica*, or Aoûla of the natives, and which is held by them in high repute. The fruit is used in various ways, preserved in its dried state, in syrup, or pickled, and is to be found in all considerable towns throughout India. "An infusion of two ounces of aoula in twenty of water was given to ten men three times a day, in conjunction with whatever else was necessary, as bark, quinine, opium, &c.; and I found this remedy as useful certainly as lime-juice, in cases where the spleen and liver were enlarged." Dr. Kirk found, on examination, that the fruit consisted of "citric acid, tannic acid, and pectin, or vegetable jelly." For years Dr. Kirk, unhappily killed in the mutinies, had been using lime-juice in the treatment of enlarged spleen, "with the most beneficial effect." This quotation is made from the "Pathologia Indica" of Professor Allan Webb, of the Calcutta Medical College, a work of the greatest value to all who are interested in the progress of tropical medicine.

In treating the complications of dysentery with fevers, remittent and intermittent, we must have regard to the type and prevailing character of the febrile movement, as well as to the paroxysms, in addition to the attention that may be demanded by the condition of the bowels. When the fever is of an ardent inflammatory, or of a severely congestive character, our antiphlogistic means must be applied with an energy proportioned to the violence of the disease; while in the low adynamic type we must have recourse to bark, quinine, opiates, chalybeates, the vegetable and mineral acids, improved diet, and change of air. In this latter form of the disease, the morbid actions are very liable to assume a low adynamic character—sometimes degenerating, in low damp situations and crowded camps, into the hæmorrhagic and sloughing type, followed by a terrible mortality. Here opium in large doses, conjoined with quinine, will be found to constitute the best treatment. Opium has been administered in the East Indies, in such states of disease, to the amount of from twenty to thirty grains in the twenty-four hours, without inducing narcotism. A rather generous diet, with wine or ale, will likewise be found necessary to the successful treatment of these cases; and by such course of treatment the nervous and vascular functions will be supported, pain and irritation will be relieved, while time will be afforded for the reparative processes of nature. When, on the other hand, malarious dysentery is complicated with congestive or inflammatory states of the liver, the combination of calomel with quinine and opium— preceded and followed by the means already indicated—will prove of excellent effect. In short, here, as in fever, to be successful, we must hold continually in view the prevailing type and character of the disease, and adapt our measures of cure accordingly.

Where, happily, convalescence has commenced, it may be both promoted and matured by the use of chlorinated solution and the nitro-muriatic acid.

In convalescence from dysenteries, acute and chronic, indeed and of every type, much active benefit will be derived from the external and internal use of the nitro-muriatic acid. When the spleen is found to be enlarged, whatever the stage of dysentery, and whatever the type of the fever, mercury must be carefully avoided, trusting rather to the means just named, and to all such as vivify and improve the blood. It is almost unnecessary to add likewise that the abstraction of blood, in the complication of these fevers with dysentery, should be practised only when the fever is of the acute or ardent type; the adynamic forms, as well as the splenic cachexia, not admitting of the use either of mercury or of blood-letting.

As regards the treatment of convalescence from dysentery, I would impress on the inexperienced a careful attention to all that has been urged upon that subject in the conclusion of the article on fever. There is not a word of caution there inculcated that does not apply with equal force to the management of the stage of recovery from tropical dysentery, as to that of convalescence from fever; and too much attention cannot be paid to either case, if we would protect the seaman or soldier from the dangers of relapse. It should be a rule with all medical officers to grant the seaman and soldier sufficient time to confirm convalescence and restore health, before returning him to duty. Time is necessary to the absorption of interstitial deposits, and for the cure of functional disorders, the results of acute disease; and it would indeed be a mistaken notion of efficiency which should cause a half-cured man to be sent to labour, whether in peace or war, not to speak of the inhumanity of such conduct.

So much having been offered on the treatment of dysentery, simple and complicated, I must once more urge upon the naval and military surgeon the value of time in dealing with such a disease. In treating fever as well as dysentery, it should again and again be remembered that time is either our most important ally, or else our most powerful enemy, just as we may use or neglect it. Time will often be turned into a dire enemy, both by the soldier and seaman, if permitted; and in civil life the same neglect will occur through the carelessness or the vices of individuals; so that the patient comes under treatment at all stages of the morbid progress. Excepting under the pressure of actual war, when dislocations and impediments will occur, it is happily in the power of officers in command to order parades of inspection conducted by the surgeons; and thus every man may be looked to on the instant of his falling sick—an incalculable advantage to the individual and to the state.

THE DIET.

As in fever, so in acute dysentery, the diet must be of the most spare during the first few days of active treatment; and what little is allowed should be of the most bland and unirritating nature, and consist of farinaceous fluid preparations. Under circumstances of returning health, milk with sago, arrowroot, or tapioca will be found an excellent addition; and, as convalescence becomes matured, soups and broths may be substituted, ending in gradual return to the accustomed and regular diet.

In the scorbutic, sloughing, and hæmorrhagic forms of dysentery, on the other hand, diet constitutes from the commencement of the disease a most important part of the treatment; and the same principle will apply when dysentery is associated with anæmic states of the system—in all these latter instances, a more or less nutrient diet, together with wine, will be found necessary to the cure. Medicines alone will not cure such diseases; and not to speak of the destitute condition of the troops in Burmah, I have seen, both in hospital and in private practice in India, cases of dysenteries such as are here referred to, which appeared to termi-nate fatally from want of the diet proper to them. Dr. Kenneth Mackinnon, speaking of the low adynamic jail-dysentery of the natives of India, says justly—"Give me the benefits of pure air and change of diet, and I would feel inclined to exchange for them all the drugs in the pharmacopœia."

If the patient is seen in the first stage, or simple inflammatory, or in the second stage, or that of exudation into the submucous tissue—Arrowroot with milk or with cream will prove the best diet.

I propose now, as in the instance of remittent fever, to present a catalogue-raisonné of the treatment of dysentery in different ages and countries. This, while it exhibits the limited views of some men, establishes with authority the comprehensive measures of cure of the majority of authors :—

1622. Bontius :—Bleeding, repeated according to occasion— vomit of ipecacuanha, and a purge—the extract of saffron, "the anchor of hope "— emollient enemata and fomentations — fruit diet.

1696. Sydenham :—Early blood-letting—opiate at night—active purge in the morning, repeated every other day, and followed by a powerful opiate—an anodyne with a diaphoretic every night, or every eight hours in severe cases—emollient injections, and injec-tions containing Venice turpentine.

1760. Dr. Huck :—Blood-letting repeated according to occa-sion—purgatives—ipecacuanha and tartar-emetic, in repeated and full doses.

1768. Pringle, Sir Joseph :—Blood-letting—vomiting—mercurial purges—ipecacuanha and opium—grapes.

1773. Dr. John Clark :—Full emetic of ipecacuanha and tartar-emetic, followed by mild purgatives—ipecacuanha and opium in small and repeated doses.

1782. Mr. Curtis :—Purgatives chiefly ; in the advanced stage, small doses of ipecacuanha powder—astringents and tonics.

1787-9. Dr. Moseley :—Blood-letting—antimonials freely administered—revulsion.

1791. Mr. Wade of Chunar :—Solution of tartar-emetic and purging salts—anodynes and sudorifics.

1791-1820. Robert Jackson : — Copious blood-letting during immersion in the warm-bath, "the sovereign remedy, without which nothing can be done with a fair prospect of benefit," followed by an emetic and mercurial purgative ;—the alternate use of evacuants and sudorifics, "Dover's and James's powders holding the first rank of the latter"—hot fomentations to the abdomen, with the local use of cold water, 'and "tonic applications in glyster" —warm clothing—change of air, especially a sea-voyage.

1796. Dr. Hunter :—Mercurial and saline purgatives, followed by opiates. In mild cases this constituted the sole treatment; in severe cases—draughts of infusion of bark with rhubarb—fomentations—blisters.

1799. Dr. Lempriere :—An emetic—warm baths and fomentations—emollient injections " as a necessary preparation to a purge" —active and persistent purging by common purging salts, by calomel and rhubarb, or by calomel and jalap—diluents—farinaceous diet.

1799. Blane, Sir Gilbert :—Blood-letting—vomit and purge at the beginning—ipecacuanha and opium—purgative salts—small doses of ipecacuanha powder.

1799. Dr. Whyte:—Profuse blood-letting—flannel roller over the abdomen—careful confinement to bed, the body being anointed with oil—no medicine.

1804. M'Grigor, Sir James :—Blood-letting—mercury with sudorifics—flannel roller round the abdomen—aperients—opiates —nitric acid internally, and in the form of bath—enemata of lead and zinc—demulcent drinks—antiphlogistic regimen—change of air.

1814. James Johnson :—Blood-letting, repeated according to occasion—calomel in full doses—sudorifics—occasional mild purgatives—anodynes—cooling antiphlogistic diet—warm clothing— change of air.

1817. William Fergusson :—Blood-letting—small doses of calomel with ipecacuanha--inunction, till the gums become affected— fomentations—warm clothing—the use of fruits—change of air.

1818. Ballingall, Sir George :—Topical bleeding—purgatives— infusion of ipecacuanha—opiates—warm baths and fomentations —enemata—blisters.

1818-22. The Dublin Physicians — Epidemic dysentery : — Blood-letting, general and local—calomel, antimony, and opium combined—emetics—enemata—counter-irritation—warm baths.

1819. Mr. Bampfield :—Blood-letting—cathartics—diaphoretics with mercury.

1822. Annesley, Sir James:—Emetic of ipecacuanha, followed by full doses of calomel, smart purge, and warm bath—then blood-letting, general and local, according to constitution and length of re-sidence in India—calomel and opium, alternating with purgatives and enemata—ipecacuanha, or antimony, with opium as a sudorific.

1823. Dr. Latham:—After the failure of all the remedies com-mon to European practice, including ipecacuanha—"calomel and opium became the settled practice."

1832. Mr. Twining:—General and local blood-letting, repeated according to occasion—simple powder of ipecacuanha with extract of gentian—purgatives.

1833. Dr. J. Smith, Edinburgh—Epidemic dysentery:—Scruple doses of calomel, given so as to fall short of salivation, "the more common measures having failed."

1833. Dr. Joseph Brown—Cyclopædia of Practical Medicine:—Blood-letting, general and local, repeated according to urgency, aided by hot baths and fomentations—gentle laxatives—mercury as a subsidiary to general and local bleeding, and combined with simple or compound ipecacuanha powder—sudorifics—opiates—enemata.

1835. Copland — Dictionary of Practical Medicine:—Blood-letting, general and local, repeated according to occasion—opiates "after depletion"—mild aperients—cooling diaphoretics—ipeca-cuanha and opium—blisters.

It is observed by Mason Good, that "the *principles* of Syden-ham's practice it is not easy to improve upon;" nor, indeed, have either his principles or his details of practice been much improved upon from his day to the present — blood-letting, sudorifics, opiates, and aperients remaining still at the head of our standard remedies.

There can be no doubt that the "putrid dysentery" of Clark, described by him as prevalent in Calcutta in 1773, was compli-cated, like the fevers of those days, with scurvy. The then pro-tracted voyages to India, the bad diet, the general sanitary neglect during the voyage, and, if possible, the greater sanitary neglects after landing in Bengal, left little hope to the British seaman or soldier when tropical disease was added to scorbutus.

It is stated on the authority of the records of the Calcutta European General Hospital, that even in more recent times the mortality by dysentery was as follows:—

	Treated.	Died.
1797. March, April, and May	37	21
„ June and July	58	35
„ August and September	22	16
„ November and December	21	15
1798. March, April, and May	17	7
„ June, July, and August	27	14
„ October, November, and December	25	8
1799. July, August, September, and October	31	11
Total	233	127

In those days the treatment of fever and dysentery was by calomel and opium, mercurial inunctions, bark, animal food, and wine.

Of the authors quoted in the above catalogue, those who speak most in favour of their success in treating tropical dysentery are—Boutins, Dr. John Clark, Dr. Moseley, and Mr. Wade:—a brief inquiry into the merits of their respective modes of treatment may therefore prove of some interest.

Boutius commenced with the abstraction of blood, and with vomits;—then came the extract of saffron, "than which, I dare to say, a more excellent remedy was never discovered by mankind; and I am fully persuaded that it is the most perfect antidote against this disease, even when of a malignant kind."

Dr. Clark merely wishes "to present facts; but he must add that he has given bark to one hundred and fifty fever patients in Bengal and other places in the East Indies; and of that number lost only one who took the medicine with perseverance." This gentleman was equally successful in the treatment of dysentery; for out of " a number of patients" he only " lost four."

Dr. Moseley abstracted blood likewise :—" Bleeding," he says, " being an operation of great consequence in the flux, the cure is generally begun with it, repeating it as symptoms authorize, observing only, *Non quæ ætas sit sed quæ vires sint*. After bleeding, a vomit of ipecacuanha is to be given, and then an opiate after its operation is necessary. This is to be followed by a careful and continued use of antimonial wine and laudanum combined, with a view to keep up a sweat proportioned to the violence of the disease, and not in the trifling way of giving them in small doses, whilst the patient is exposed, and their operation neglected." The Doctor goes on to relate that the eminent success of this plan was exhibited when the soldier had been suffering from " the worst condition of the disease, with blood running from him as in a hæmorrhage;" and he adds that this demonstration of his superior success had been made before " several of the officers of different regiments in the West Indies who were desirous to be spectators of a fact so interesting to the army." He concludes his triumphant narrative by exclaiming—" Such is the power of *revulsion.*"

The power of revulsion in the cure of dysentery is undoubtedly great, whether produced by agents internally or externally exhibited. I remember, when serving with the army in Ava, to have heard that a British merchant, while prisoner in the capital, was seized with dysentery. After days of unmitigated suffering, under circumstances of barbarous treatment, and when death appeared to him near and certain, an order arrived for the removal of the prisoners to a place of closer and still more severe confinement, where they were literally packed together. Here the sufferer was thrown into a violent perspiration, and from that time all his symptoms left him. Such, again, is the power of revulsion !

Mr. Wade of Chunar claims an amount of success unbroken, except by "two cases of unfortunate termination in the treatment of about four hundred cases of fever and dysentery." The treatment for both diseases was by a solution of purgative salts and tartar-emetic, followed by anodynes and sudorific night-draughts.

Mr. Wade observes, that "the medical world may draw their own comments on the cases which are submitted to their examination. The person who has treated and compiled them. shall defer his until the public may have formed some unbiassed opinion of them, he should only venture at present to vouch for their authenticity." This is just what has been done and said at all times by every writer of such cases, and by every pretender to extraordinary cures ; but it is a curious fact, well deserving consideration how it happens—and happen it always does—that those who in their day claim the greatest and most exclusive success in the practice of medicine should, in after times, be the least followed in their modes of treatment.

Some of the causes of error in reasoning and practice, as respects dysentery, are so well stated by Sir James M'Grigor, that I cannot do better than present them in his own words :—" My opportunities of seeing this disease have been no common ones. Rarely, I believe, has it fallen to the lot of an individual to see so very many cases of one disease in such a variety of climate and situation. In the 88th Regiment, during more than ten years, I saw the same man the subject of this disease on the continent of Europe, in America, in both extremities of Africa, and in India. Of late, it has afforded me not a little amusement to review my notes as well as my journals of practice in this disease, in all these quarters. . . I became convinced in Alexandria that, with change of country and climate, we had a different disease. This is one proof how improper and how unsafe it is for the practitioner of one climate to set down and describe the diseases of another. They only who have studied the same disease in various opposite climates can fully comprehend the extreme absurdity as well as the fallacy of this. From reasoning of any kind we are incompetent to decide on the identity of disease. Reasoning from analogy here always deceives. In many of the symptoms diseases may agree, but from thence to infer their identity is taking a very narrow view."

Dr. Macpherson of Calcutta, speaking of the comparative results of the treatment of dysentery by the free use of opium and other soothing means, observes with proper candour :—" Our obvious difficulty in arriving at safe conclusions is, that the disease itself varies so much in intensity in different years, as well as in different periods of the same year. Thus, her Majesty's 55th

Regiment lost at Secunderabad, in 1837, one in four and a half; in 1838, one in seven and a half; in 1839, one in ten; yet the treatment was the same, and conducted by the same medical officer throughout."

If dysentery and fever were diseases of an uniform character, having an uniform *cause* and *seat*, then perhaps they might be treated after an uniform plan; but a very slender experience of the two diseases, as they prevail within the tropics especially, and even within the British Isles, shows that this is not the case; for although, in the disease now under consideration, some portion of the larger bowel is universally implicated, yet, either from the accession, or during the progress of the disease, for we cannot often say which, the lesser bowel, the liver, the spleen, the pancreas, and mesentery frequently become the seats of plethora and of other morbid actions, so as greatly to complicate the disease and modify its treatment.

The pathology of our dysenteries, whether in southern or northern India, as described by our best authors, sufficiently establishes the fact that, in this formidable disease, morbid action is not confined here, any more than in Europe, to the course of the large intestine alone; but that all, or most of the associated organs are found after death to be more or less deeply involved, just in proportion to the extent and severity of the symptoms during life. The truth is, that the dangerous and fatal characters of tropical dysenteries are principally due to these complications. "I have been repeatedly astonished," says Dr. Macpherson, of the General Hospital, Calcutta, " to discover after death an immense extent of structural change in boys, whose illness could not be ascertained to have exceeded eight or ten days." It appears to me that to a want of just consideration of these inevitable pathological complications must we refer the system of exclusive treatment, so much reprehended by every author who has had varied and extended opportunities of observation in dysentery; these complications explain also the successive abandonment, by the surgeons of our fleets and armies, of every exclusive plan of treatment hitherto proposed, almost as soon as it has been tried. " In the treatment of no other disease, perhaps," says Dr. Copland, " has the baneful influence of exclusive medical doctrine been more fully exerted than in that of dysentery."

The adhesions of the peritoneum—the pink colour, thickening and softening of the omentum, the effused lymph, the adhesions between the different intestinal surfaces, the red and thickened state of the mesentery, with the enlargement of its glands—while they indicate the general amount and great extent of inflammatory action during life, leave the fact still demonstrated that, in causing death, the main force of the disease has been expended on the mucous surfaces.

He who would treat dysentery with success, while he shuns

exclusive means and the inertia of accepted conclusions, must assign to each remedy its proper value, and neither more nor less. Blood-letting, sudorifics, and purgatives constitute the most universal remedies; in simple uncomplicated dysenteries, of the inflammatory and congestive characters, and where applied early in proper subjects, they will prove all-sufficient. But when the abdomen is tumid, and there is pain in the liver, or in any other region, while the nature of the discharges indicates advancing inflammation, calomel conjoined with sudorifics, and repeated to meet the occasion, will powerfully aid the curative effect, through its influence on the depurative functions—on the circulation, in unloading, jointly with purgatives, the gorged vessels of the abdominal organs, on the blood and on secretions generally, and on the very sudorific function which we so much desire to excite. This, in so many words, I believe to be the real value of calomel in the treatment of dysentery; and the inexperienced have been led into much unnecessary doubt, and into no small amount of error, by some writers who regard calomel as a remedy of necessity, and by those who, on the other hand, would exclude its use altogether.

It is hardly necessary to repeat that while calomel is a most powerful agent in its place, as an aid to blood-letting, the pushing it to the extent of ptyalism is here by no means intended; nor should mercury in any shape be used in adynamic forms of the disease, in the splenic cachexia, nor in states of anæmia —for in all these conditions of the system its actions are most injurious.

Amongst the surgeons in Bengal blood-letting, general and local, takes the lead, and has done so for many years, in the treatment of dysentery. It is the standard remedy; and I believe that when the subject comes early and freely under this treatment, and the case is not complicated with hepatic or other congestion, or with inflammation, little else than a few doses of sudorifics and aperients, as aids to general blood-letting, will be needed for the cure. But, as in most cases of this formidable disease as it appears within the tropics, the morbid action going on in the large intestine is intimately associated with general abdominal plethora and individual complications, other and important means speedily follow upon the bleeding; and of these the first are those which act powerfully on all the secreting organs, internal and external—such as calomel with ipecacuanha, in full doses at first, and given at bedtime; followed by mild laxatives, sudorifics, enemata, warm baths and fomentations, blisters, and other minor adjuvantia. I believe this to have been for many years the course of practice in Bengal, and I have seldom seen calomel urged to the extent of producing salivation: neither do I think this degree of effect at all necessary to the cure. Several experienced medical officers have assured me that antimony in combination with the calomel proved, in their hands, quite as efficacious as ipecacuanha, but in my own practice I always preferred the latter.

When, after a few days, inflammatory action has been subdued by blood-letting, with the lowest diet, and intestinal irritation has been overcome by calomel, ipecacuanha, and aperients, then recourse should be had to milder measures, as a persistence in the stronger ones is no longer either necessary or proper to the cure; indeed, such persistence would prove eminently injurious.

The late Mr. Twining would appear to ignore the associated diseases of the liver, and in his clinical work he advocates the use of simple ipecacuanha powder combined with bitter extract, which plan of treating dysentery he states to have been very successful. As first assistant, and as officiating surgeon to the General Hospital of Calcutta, during Mr. Twining's service in that institution, I had ample opportunity of witnessing the results of his treatment, and I am not aware that his system was followed at the time, or since, by any of the other medical officers of that hospital; neither would his plan of treatment appear to be successfully imitated in the provinces throughout Bengal. Dr. Macnab, in an excellent practical report on the dysentery of the native soldiery of Hindustan, when serving in Bengal Proper, says, that "blue-pill with ipecacuanha and extract of gentian proved a complete failure, as has generally been the case in my trials of it. Indeed, I much suspect that Mr. Twining overrated the value of his favourite remedy, and that he may have also miscalculated the anti-emetic properties of the gentian."

On Mr. Twining's use of drastic purging Dr. Everard says:— "Twining has certainly overpraised repeated strong purging. The Deputy Inspector-General Murray informed me that in his tour of inspection he found some cases which *had been dysenteric, labouring under one-drachm doses of compound jalap powder given daily at noon, which got well immediately on removing the cause.*" Over-treatment is always a cruel infliction upon the sick, and so also is the cry to let well alone, which, in respect of disease, proves too often but the negligence which would leave ill alone. How much of close observation and of discernment do we require to apportion the means to the end! how much of both, conjoined with experience, must we exercise even in withdrawing and withholding our means of cure!

Ipecacuanha has been a favourite remedy in the south of India for nearly a century, although Mr. Twining, like many respectable practitioners, fell into the error of supposing that what he observed was new, while in truth it was very old. Speaking of his cotemporaries, Drs. Geddes, Mortimer, and Baikie of Madras, he concludes:—" In fact, ipecacuanha has been a favourite remedy with some of the medical men at the Madras Presidency;" and from the context it is evident that a very recent date is here meant. Dr. William Dick of Bengal says that in 1782-83 he used the ipecacuanha, in the form of infusion, with the most excellent effects. "Though it vomited the patient the first day, it seldom had that effect afterwards, and in general it occasioned more copious evacuations than many stronger purges. All medicines for this complaint ought to be given in a fluid state, if possible, as I find they irritate and gripe less than powders, however fine they may be; and I am convinced of no fact more than that oily medicines are hurtful, rendering the use of emetics more necessary than the irritable state of the stomach always admits of. I believe also, that a more sparing use of purgatives, and a freer use of glysters, would in general answer better." Dr. Whitelaw Ainslie, writing in 1813, after an experience of thirty years in Madras, and an extensive practice amongst all classes of Europeans, says of this drug that "it has no equal in simple dysentery, that is, dysentery not complicated with hepatic derangement; in such cases, given even so as to produce daily a little vomiting, it has the happiest effects." This is an observation of great truth, and practical importance consequently, and I believe that it impresses and fixes a just discrimination in the use of ipecacuanha. In speaking from a personal experience of two-and-twenty years in the East Indies, and from an extensive range of observation of this disease as it occurred in hospitals, European and native, and in extensive private practice in Calcutta—also as it occurred amongst troops serving in the unhealthy provinces of Orissa and Gondwana, and in the fatal campaigns of Rangoon and Upper Ava, in the first Burmese war—I should say with Dr. Ainslie, that it is alone in simple uncomplicated dysentery that ipecacuanha shows its best effects, administered as an aid to blood-letting and moderate purging.

In hepatic dysentery—a frequent complication in Bengal, especially during the cold season—calomel is absolutely necessary to the cure. I remember treating, for this form of the disease, an officer who had suffered severely from the fever of Batavia, contracted at the capture of Java; he was bled generally and by leeches, the depletion being followed by sudorifics and purgatives; but no amendment took place, and nothing was voided but mucus and blood; two full doses of calomel with antimonial powder were then given at bedtime, which produced copious biliary discharges, followed by immediate relief; a few doses of blue-pill and ipecacuanha, followed by mild aperients, concluding the treatment. There existed in this case no enlargement of the liver, nor uneasiness on pressure, but there was a total absence of biliary secretion, and until that was restored, the other treatment afforded no relief. In another case of very severe hepatic dysentery, requiring remedial measures of great activity, recovery was marred on convalescence by errors in diet; the liver became as enlarged and painful as ever, the dysentery recurring, and requiring a repetition of general and local blood-letting, mercury, &c., and this under circumstances of greatly reduced strength. This gentleman was sent to China, where, six months afterwards, and owing to continued errors in diet, hepatic abscess took place, from which he died.

Cases of hepatic complication, treated without mercury, frequently terminate in inflammation and abscess of that organ, even where blood-letting has been employed. It is not enough here to reduce the volume of the blood, nor yet, along with it, to diminish the force and frequency of the circulation; we must also emulge the gland involved in disease.

To such as prefer ipecacuanha in the treatment of dysentery it might prove desirable to ascertain the following circumstances :—

1st. Whether extract of gentian have any and what effect in preventing vomiting under the use of this drug. It is true that, after a few days' use, a comparative tolerance of medicine seems to be established, as in the case of the antimonial preparations; but altogether, as it appeared to me, unconnected with the use or disuse of bitter extract.

2nd. Whether the preparations of the Cannabis Indica may, from their sedative as well as from their powerfully anti-emetic qualities, prove serviceable in conjunction with ipecacuanha, or with antimonials. Unlike opium and its preparations, hemp does not lock up the secretions.

3rd. Whether four grains of ipecacuanha occasion as much sickness as ten grains, and if so, whether the larger dose should be preferred for the cure of dysentery. If the action of ipecacuanha be purely revulsive, or if, according to Dr. Paris, it be to abate both the velocity and the force of the heart's action, so as to affect " the whole series of blood-vessels from their origin to their most minute ramifications," we may do wrong by being sparing of our dose, in so formidable a disease as dysentery, if the stomach can be made to bear the larger quantity. This subject has not, I think, received the attention due to its importance, in reference to the subject here under consideration. " Ipecacuanha has long been usefully employed," says the *British and Foreign Medico-Chirurgical Review* for July, 1855, "in various morbid puerperal conditions. M. Legroux is said to resort to it with almost uniform success at the Hôtel Dieu, in sub-inflammatory and congested states of the uterus following delivery." I would recommend the powder of nux-vomica in conjunction with the ipecacuanha, as in every way a preferable adjunct to any of the bitter tonics, and as possessing powers of its own which are of great value in dysentery.

Referring to the above observations on ipecacuanha, originally published by me in Calcutta in 1837, and to the suggestion to use large doses of ipecacuanha, I have recently been gratified by the perusal of a report of cases of acute dysentery treated at the Mauritius by Mr. Docker, surgeon to the 7th Royal Fusiliers. He begins generally with an emetic, but invariably with a thorough clearing of the bowels by a purgative. He then commences the following course of treatment :—A sinapism to cover the abdomen, and immediately after this application, a drachm dose of laudanum is exhibited. " Half an hour after, when the irritability of the stomach has been diminished, the ipecacuanha is administered, generally in a draught, sometimes in pill or bolus, while a semi-recumbent posture is steadily maintained." The doses ranged " from ten to ninety grains ; rarely less than twenty grains. The larger quantity was given in urgent cases only, the ordinary dose being a scruple or half a drachm."

Mr. Docker states that in a considerable proportion of cases the medicine was not rejected, or it was retained long enough to do its work. If necessary, it was repeated until the stomach did retain a sufficiency for the cure. It was never used in the form of enema ; and where such large doses as sixty to ninety grains were given by the stomach, an interval of ten or twelve hours was allowed before repeating the dose ; and whenever dysentery ceased, so did the use of ipecacuanha. "The action of these large doses is certain, speedy, and complete ; and truly surprising are sometimes their effects. In no single instance has failure attended this medicine thus employed."

Out of more than fifty cases thus treated, Mr. Docker " lost but one." On the authority of this gentleman, as on all grounds of justice, this simple plan of treatment ought to have, and no doubt will have, the fairest trial. But here, as in every question referring to the treatment of disease, experience has to be waited for.

An extensive trial, and a successful one apparently, has been made in the Madras Presidency, under order of the Director-General there, and excellent reports have been recently published in the *Madras Quarterly Journal of Medical Science,* by Mr. Cornish and Dr. Blacklock.

It appears from tables furnished by Mr. Cornish, that those treated for dysentery, by thirty-four medical officers, throughout Madras, are as follows :—

Europeans	297
Natives	218
Total	515

The cases were not specially selected for experiment, but " Mr. Mee thinks that the type of the disease had become milder before the ipecacuanha treatment began."

Of the whole number of Europeans suffering from acute uncomplicated dysentery, four cases only proved fatal—giving a death-rate of 1·3 per cent. instead of 7·1 per cent., the average of seventeen years previously. In the newly-arrived 44th Regiment, forming the garrison of Fort St. George, there were admitted into hospital 104 cases of dysentery. Of this number 68 were treated " in the ordinary way, with a mortality of six, or of 8·8 per cent. ;" while of another party numbering fifty-nine, " treated with large doses of ipecacuanha," all recovered.

"Although the large majority of medical officers pronounce strongly in favour of this treatment only in the acute uncomplicated dysentery of Europeans, yet there can be no doubt, from the experience of others, that it has had a remarkable effect in some cases where disease had passed beyond the first stage, and where deposition in the submucous tissue, or ulceration, already existed. In such cases, however, the remedy requires judicious management, and its operation should be carefully watched. Further experience is required before we can determine how far it should be depended upon in cases which have advanced to the second stage before coming under treatment."

Dr. Blacklock says, that "ipecacuanha in full doses is undoubtedly a remedy of great value in the acute stage of sthenic dysentery, and in those sthenic intercurrent periods indicated by increased dryness and heat of skin, scanty evacuations of blood and glairy gelatinous mucus, with increased firmness and frequency of pulse, occurring from time to time in the progress of severe cases, after the first acute attack has been subdued; but its employment must be restricted to this state of the system. If this precaution be not observed, great disappointment will be sure to follow its exhibition on the first occurrence of an asthenic epidemic constitution, and it will quickly pass out of favour again, as it often has, since its first employment for the cure of dysentery in Paris in 1686." . . . "Like tartar-emetic, and all other evacuants, ipecacuanha induces, when continued too long, the very state of vessels we find in inflammation, sometimes in the bronchia, sometimes in the stomach and bowels, or in all these parts at the same time." . . "The great danger, therefore, from the large-dose treatment is, that the power of the heart may become so much impaired by its continuance, that the brain may soon be too sparingly supplied with blood, and general unmanageable prostration ensue, while at the same time the local congestion increases with the debility. We require, for the removal of the disease, that the heart's force should be reduced to that of health, and the capillaries be moderately constricted; but, if we permit the effects of the medicine to pass beyond these safe limits, or continue the medicine after the natural progress of the disease has materially modified the original type, we place the patient in an asthenic condition in which adynamic congestion of the diseased bowel will be as marked and as destructive as was the dynamic congestion we sought to recover, and far more difficult to treat successfully."

Although "the good and bad effects of ipecacuanha are best elucidated by carefully observing its influence on the symptoms daily recorded in cases," it is here admitted that "really acute dysentery seldom presents itself in a form to permit of its being successfully treated by any one remedy. But no single remedy, nor combination of remedies, has ever been of such signal service in the first stage of the disease as ipecacuanha, when administered in large doses. No other medicine so soon brings the system into a condition favourable to the restoration of healthy function in the diseased intestine, and by its employment we have the great advantage of being able to dispense with blood-letting, and other means which are, to say the least, very unsatisfactory in their consequences."

For the following interesting table, exhibiting the prevalence and the intensity of dysentery, as indicated by the mortality in various countries, I am indebted to Sir Alexander Tulloch:—

STATIONS.	Period of observation.	Aggregate strength.	Dysentery.		
			Attacked.	Died.	Proportion of deaths to admissions.
Windward and Leeward Command.	20 years.	86,661	17,843	1367	1 in 13
Jamaica	20 "	51,567	4,909	184	1 in 26⅔
Gibraltar	19 "	60,269	2,653	64	1 in 41½
Malta	20 "	40,826	1,401	94	1 in 15
Ionian Islands	20 "	70,293	3,768	184	1 in 20½
Bermudas	20 "	11,721	1,751	36	1 in 48⅔
Nova Scotia and New Brunswick	20 "	46,442	244	18	1 in 13⅗
Canada	20 "	64,280	735	36	1 in 20½
Western Africa	18 "	1,843	370	55	1 in 7
Cape of Good Hope	19 "	22,714	1,425	44	1 in 32½
St. Helena	9 "	8,973	751	69	1 in 11
Mauritius	19 "	30,515	5,420	285	1 in 19
Ceylon	20 "	42,978	9,069	993	1 in 9
Tenasserim Provinces	10 "	6,818	1,460	137	1 in 10⅔
Madras	5 "	31,627	6,639	559	1 in 12
Bengal	5 "	38,136	5,152	411	1 in 12½
Bombay	5 "	17,612	1,879	151	1 in 12½

CHRONIC DYSENTERY.

ONE has but to behold a soldier in hospital under chronic dysentery to grieve that a disease so destructive had not been cut short in its acute stage; for truly does William Fergusson declare that the sufferer exhibits "a spectacle of distress of as pitiable a kind as can be found in the history of human misery." Let the young naval and military surgeon ponder on the spectacle before him, and determine so to master the subject and manage the treatment of acute dysentery, as that he may have the least possible amount of the chronic to deal with. He will thus by one act cure the acute, and prevent the chronic disease.

Chronic dysentery, following upon.acute inflammatory dysentery, like visceral infarction consequent upon remittent and intermittent fevers, must be regarded, in a large proportion of instances, as the token of bad practice—the measure of the insufficiency of the means employed during the acute stage of the disease. It is different when the original dysentery has been of the adynamic, malignant, or scorbutic characters; for in such conditions there is much which the surgeon can neither anticipate nor control, his appliances often coming too late into use, and thus proving necessarily unavailing. The fault here is generally with governments, and with commanders.

It is not intended in this place to enter into the details of chronic dysentery, the reader being referred to an article on that subjcet in the second part of this work, and which describes the disease as it occurs in European invalids on their return from tropical climates. But chronic dysentery in · the East Indies differs from that disease as it appears in persons on their return to Europe in this—that in India a certain amount of congestive and inflammatory action still remains, both in the mucous membrane of the large intestine and in the associated organs, requiring moderate topical blood-lettings, mercurial alteratives and blisterings; whereas in the same disease, as it appears in England in the person of the tropical invalid, neither of the above conditions hold.

With the important exceptions stated, the treatment of chronic dysentery should be the same in both hemispheres; and in that of the East as of the West I would strongly urge the internal and external use of the nitro-muriatic acid, shielded by opium. It is a powerful remedy as a substitute for mercurials, powerful in maturing convalescence.

NOTE ON DYSENTERY IN THE NATIVES OF INDIA.

A LARGE proportion of the sickness and mortality of the native troops throughout India occurs from dysenteries and diarrhœas, originally contracted as such, or resulting from fevers remittent and intermittent; and this holds especially in respect of the troops recruited in the plains of Hindustan, when they are transferred thence to the low marshy countries along the course of the great rivers, or into countries abounding in jungle.

The late Mr. John Tytler, of the Bengal Medical Department, in an Essay on " a most melancholy disorder," which he terms Diarrhœa Hectica, states that "it is no exaggeration to say, that of the total deaths among the lower orders of Hindustan, three-fourths are the effect of this disease, either idiopathic or as a terminating symptom. It is the scourge of crowded jails, and of hospitals filled with harassed and fatigued sepoys; and it is the great avenue through which the swarms of naked and famished paupers and miserable infants that occupy the bazaars are continually vanishing."

Mr. Burnard,. speaking of the sufferings of the sepoys in Aracan, under General Morrison, says : " Dysentery and diarrhœa were the diseases which proved most fatal, not in their acute form, but ensuing as a consequence of fever; and their ravages, particularly amongst the native troops, were very great."

" The average mortality amongst natives in the Calcutta Medical College Hospital," says Dr. Macpherson, " has been 16·9, that among Europeans, 22·5. This accords with general experience, which has shown the disease in natives to be more amenable to treatment than in Europeans."

The symptoms of dysentery in the Asiatic races are precisely the same as in the European, differing only in degree of severity and in complications; and the same may be said as to the pathology of the disease.

The post-mortem appearances exhibit ulcerations in the large intestine, amongst the natives of India, as with Europeans; but the complications in the dysenteries of Asiatics are by no means so frequent nor so severe, if we except that of the spleen in malarious districts, in which dysentery and diarrhœa are commonly associated with the remittent and intermittent fevers of such localities. Here the ulcerations of the large intestine are always of an anæmic, atonic character.

Excepting in the instances of powerful and athletic sepoys, and those mostly of the better-fed Mahomedans, I seldom had recourse to general blood-letting in treating natives for this disease, leeching being in the far greater numbers quite sufficient. The same regard to measure holds good in the use of purgative and other remedial appliances, the mildest in moderate doses being effective to the cure; and mercury in any form is seldom required, unless it be to the more robust, especially the Mahomedan, to whom I had often to exhibit one moderate dose of calomel with ipecacuanha or antimonial powder, followed by a brisk purgative, with the view to remove jaundiced appearances of the conjunctivæ, indicative of hepatic congestion. If such indications were not present, I never had recourse to mercurials in any shape.

The great principle of treatment in the dysenteries and diarrhœas of the natives of India, in their acute stages, is what Mosely would term revulsive—sudorific; ipecacuanha, in sufficiently full doses, being the best means, aided by gentle aperients, farinaceous diet, fomentations to the abdomen, and warm clothing. When by such means we have overcome the more acute symptoms, the Dover's powder will very fitly complete the cure; and the assistance to be derived from proper diet and warm clothing should never be overlooked. Cold acts most banefully on the native constitution, and too much attention cannot, therefore, be paid to the subject of suitable covering by night and day, especially during the cold season.

For maturing convalescence from the ordinary dysenteries of India, the nitric, or nitro-muriatic acid in bitter infusions will be found very efficacious; but where convalescence is retarded by continuance of liquid discharges, the acetate of lead and opium will prove greatly effective, the lead being exhibited in full doses. I had recourse to the acetate of lead in treating the native soldiery, after the more acute symptoms had passed, very early in my service in India, and afterwards very extensively in treating the dysenteries of the natives of Calcutta, while surgeon to the Native Hospital of that city. My excellent assistant at this institution, Mr. O'Brien, has for more than ten years subsequently, as surgeon to the 4th Regiment of Native Infantry, Gwalior Contingent, carried out this plan of treatment with great success, from the very onset of the dysentery. The Native Hospital formula was acetate of lead, tincture of opium, and distilled vinegar. This treatment has continued to be very successful in the hands of Mr. O'Brien as well as in mine; and he says that " when the liver is complicated, appropriate treatment is directed to that viscus ; but acetate of lead is given at the same time without at all interfering with the other remedies. I do not mean to say that I employ lead *solely ;* for I employ leeches, aperients, and blisters, which are very generally indispensable." The sulphate of copper and opium are also an excellent combination in the chronic stage of the disease. At all stages, indeed, and under every degree of severity and of distress from this disease, we are limited, in the treatment of natives, to the use of medicines by the stomach alone, as enemata they will not consent to use—the very impression of death making no alteration in their fixed aversion to every such remedy.

ON THE DISEASES OF THE LIVER.

THE most cursory reference to the articles on fever and dysentery must satisfy the reader that, whether as original or secondary affections, inflammation, congestion, and chronic enlargements of the liver constitute in reality very frequent and very important diseases in the East Indies. Nor do the official returns, under the special heads of acute and chronic hepatitis, afford any approach to the actual frequency of hepatic diseases ; for when these last occur as complications with, or as sequelæ to fevers, dysen-

teries, diarrhœa, and cholera, the hepatic complication or sequel
remains unnoticed in the numerical returns—the cases being
classed and numbered under the primary disease, whether fever,
dysentery, diarrhœa, or cholera.   It thus happens that the numerical hospital returns do not yield anything like an approximation
to a true estimate of the existing amount of hepatic disease.   The
same observations will, I believe, apply with equal justice to the
returns of acute diseases of the West Indies, the West Coast of
Africa, the stations in the Mediterranean, and the French possessions in Algeria, although in a less degree.

· Referring to diseases of the liver in the Bombay European Fusiliers, Dr. Arnott says :—" The functional and organic diseases of
the liver amounted, during the years 1846-1854, to 572 cases,
which, compared with the cases of fever, will show one case of
hepatic disease to about thirteen cases of fever ; but the chance of
death is greater from one case of hepatitis than from thirteen of
fever."

INCREASED SECRETION OF BILE.

On the subject of the physiological influences of the climate of
India on the functions of the liver, I must refer the reader to the observations in the introductory chapter on Climate. It is there stated
as a generally received opinion, that an increased secretion of bile
is one of the ordinary results of the exposure of an European to an
unnaturally high range of temperature : and this opinion I believe
to be well-founded to the extent, first—that the exaltation of
function is not of long duration, and is very much confined to the
earlier years of residence, declining thence ;—secondly, that to a
certain degree, such increase of secretion is salutary ;—and thirdly,
that it is in part from the sudden suppression of secretion through
cold, that congestive and inflammatory states of the liver are
engendered, rather than through any serious injury from increase
of secretion—a process consisting more of acclimation than of
disease, and one which nature adjusts in the progress of residence
in India.   So much has been said by some writers on tropical
diseases as to morbid increase and vitiation of bile, that they have
altogether forgotten the more important but less notable deficiencies and suppressions of this secretion—conditions far more
serious in their results than mere excess of secretion.

Chemically, we have as yet ascertained nothing as to the
healthy or unhealthy qualities of bile ; and, practically, all we do
know is, that with certain symptoms there is a redundancy, and
with others there is a deficiency of this secretion.   We know
also, from the scalding sensations that accompany certain forms
of bilious diarrhœa, that the fluid in question is then of an acrid,
irritating quality ; and that is all.

Dr. Kemp, in his experiments on the functions of the mucous

membrane of the gall-bladder, observes with respect to the action of mucus :—

1st. That when left in the gall-bladder in contact with the cystic bile, it is capable of subverting the composition of the fluid.

2nd. That this change is much accelerated by even a moderately elevated temperature.

3rd. That when the contents of the gall-bladder are evaporated to a syrupy consistence, the bile, at first neutral, becomes alkaline, and broken up into several organic groups.

4th. That if the mucus of the gall-bladder be carefully removed by alcohol or acetic acid, and the perfectly fresh bile be then evaporated, these changes do not take place.

The following generalizations appear to Dr. Kemp to be legitimately deduced from his researches :—

" 1st. That the mucus of the gall-bladder is not merely a secretion destined to lubricate the interior of that organ, and protect it from the irritation of its other contents, but is an essential integral portion of the cystic bile.

" 2nd. That the gall-bladder is not merely a receptacle and reservoir for the bile, but an organ highly endowed with organic functions, and that the proper secretion of the liver is converted into cystic bile mainly through the agency of its mucous membrane."—*Proc. Roy. Soc.*

Dr. Helenus Scott believed that nitro-muriatic acid exercised a solvent action on viscid and impacted bile, and, referring to paragraphs three and four, such an opinion would seem to have some foundation.

TREATMENT.

If, along with an acrid and irritating bilious diarrhœa there be fulness and uneasiness in the region of the liver, so as to excite the suspicion of congestive action, a few leeches, followed by fomentations and warm baths, together with a mild mercurial and an aperient, will procure relief; but when heat and dryness of skin exist, with irritative febrile symptoms, effervescing draughts, containing antimonials and diuretics, will prove both grateful and curative.

In general, the disorder constituting increased biliary secretion, and those resulting from it, are sufficiently cured and prevented by avoiding the direct rays of the sun, by a strict attention to diet, exercise, clothing, bathing, and by the use of demulcent and subacid fruits, as the bael, pomegranate, orange, grape, &c., and by the occasional use of mild aperients.

With few exceptions, and these resulting from exposure to direct solar influences, or from ill habits of life, such simple means of treatment I have always held to be both suitable and effective; and I cannot but think much unnecessary confusion has arisen from wordy descriptions of what certain writers on tropical diseases, as Annesley, appear to regard as an affection demanding a complicated medical management.   They talk of " bile" as if it were a disease, and would cure it by " full doses of calomel at bed-time, generally for five or seven days, followed by Pil. Aloes and Myrrh alone, or with Pil. Hydrarg." Of such unmeasured, disproportionate, and unnecessary treatment of a mere functional disorder, it is to be hoped we have seen the last:—it is really worse than routine.   The real diseases connected with bile—and very serious they are, too—are those in which bile is altogether *absent*, and wanting to the cure !

CONGESTION OF THE LIVER.

Congestions more or less acute, according to constitution, previous condition of health, and season, are very common to all countries in the East.   Sudden changes of temperature, producing chills—the repeated cold stages of fevers, remittent and intermittent—an over-full and stimulating diet, together with the abuse of vinous and spirituous liquors—violent bodily exercises, especially those carried on in the sun, exposing the individual to the more ready influences of cold ;—those are the more ordinary causes.

The organ will be found enlarged, generally in its upper convex direction, but sometimes in all directions, as in malignant intermittents—the enlargement resulting from venous and biliary congestion, and the latter being produced by the pressure of the over-distended veins preventing the due diminution of the smaller ducts—a condition of the liver, I repeat, frequently associated with, and following upon, remittent and intermittent fevers.*

The bulging out of the liver—the evidence of severe vascular turgescence—is rarely accompanied by more than uneasiness on exploration, or of weight on getting into the erect posture :—the respiration on the affected side will be found more or less oppressed and impeded.   These symptoms will become well-marked when, as occasionally happens, the volume of the liver is much augmented; and when such is the case, we may fairly infer that stagnation and consequent viscidity of the bile will take place, both in the gall-bladder and ducts, so as to complicate and aggravate the disease.

The countenance and complexion will exhibit pallor, or else a dusky, livid, sallow hue, according to the temperament of the patient, or the duration of the disease—paleness, with sense of cold and shivering, being more characteristic of the immediate result of external cold or chill.   The tongue will generally be found coated—the bowels constipated—the intestinal and visceral excretions depraved—the appetite defective, with occasional

* Passive congestion of the liver, and torpor of that organ, as they appear in the returned Indian, are noticed in the second part of this work.

nausea or even vomiting, and more or less headache. The pulse is slow, oppressed, irregular, or quick and feeble, according to the age and constitution of the patient, and to the duration of the disease ; but the frequency of pulse will not be that of fever. Here, in short, the symptoms are obscure—not declared—and they must be taken in their collective characters, assemblage, and connexion, and not separately or individually.

When, through any or all the causes above enumerated, congestion of the liver has been of long duration, permanent injury to its structure and secreting function may result :—the disease in any form must, therefore, be regarded as one of importance. The signs in this, as in other diseases of the liver, are so obscure, that of such as we actually possess a knowledge, we cannot afford to overlook the least, if we would do justice to our patients, and to our own characters. On examination after death, the liver is found to be enlarged, principally upwards into the right thoracic cavity—dark from impeded circulation, and full of blood : and, when the disease has been of any duration, its texture will be found softened.

TREATMENT.

When from careful exploration, and a due consideration of all the attendant symptoms, we are satisfied that congestion of the liver does actually exist—for its existence must not be assumed—a moderate venesection, followed by leeches if necessary—a few doses of blue pill or calomel, with purgative extract and an antimonial, all three united—a few saline purgatives—hot fomentations to the region of the liver, and warm baths ;—these means, together with abstinence in diet, will speedily bring about a cure. Nor must we be deterred—all other circumstances being duly considered—by feebleness or oppression of the pulse, from the use of such antiphlogistic means in these cases ; for, under judicious treatment, the pulse will rise and expand under the use of these means, and general relief will follow.

Finally, convalescence will be matured, and an exemption from future attacks secured, by attention to diet, exercise, bathing, attention to clothing, and by avoidance of exposure to direct solar influences, as well as to chills by night.

HEPATITIS.

Amongst the better classes of Europeans, who are careful in their habits, this disease is not of so frequent occurrence as formerly, when the habits of life were different from what they are now; and this observation has special reference to the acute inflammatory or adhesive form of the disease. The cases seen in private practice are very much confined to those of fair complexion and lax fibre. European females of every class are far less subject to this disease, and to every form of hepatic affection, than their countrymen; and women of the better classes are rarely affected comparatively. Out of three hundred cases of hepatic abscess occurring in India, nine cases only were in females.

Amongst British soldiers, and Europeans who lead what is called a free life, and who incur exposure to the direct rays of the sun, and to the damps and chilling influences of the night, the disease, on the other hand, attacks men of all ages, and of every variety of con-stitution. It is a disease of great importance in a military sense, causing much immediate loss of life, invaliding, and ultimate in-efficiency in the European portion of the army. It would appear from various returns to which I have had access, that, of British soldiers attacked, upwards of half were lost to the service by death, by ruined health in India, and by invaliding to England. In the Madras European regiment, according to Dr. Geddes, 280 cases of hepatitis occurred in five years, out of an average strength of 570 men; and in the Bombay European Fusiliers, according to Dr. Arnott, there occurred, in eight years, out of an average strength of 957 men,

Hepatitis, acute and chronic 483
Jaundice 89
Total 572

In the Windward and Leeward Command, although hepatic diseases are by no means so frequent there as in the East Indies, they are nearly thrice as prevalent as among troops serving in the United Kingdom, and they occasion a mortality five times as high. Diseases of the liver vary considerably, both in prevalence and mortality, at the different stations of the West Indies; for instance, at Grenada they occasion three times the mortality that results in other islands, and that without any cause as yet ascertained. The mortality during twenty years, from acute and chronic hepatitis and jaundice, as given by Sir Alex. Tulloch, was as follows:—

	Admitted.	Died.	Proportion of deaths to admissions.
Acute hepatitis	903	79	1 in 11
Chronic ,, ...	902	76	1 in 12
Jaundice	141	6	1 in 23
Total	1946	161	1 in 12
Annual ratio per 1000 } of mean strength ..... }	22	1·8	...

In the Jamaica Command there occurred the following amount of hepatic disease and mortality during twenty years:—

	Admitted.	Died.	Proportion of deaths to admissions.
Acute hepatitis	336	27	1 in 12
Chronic ,, ...	109	20	1 in 5
Jaundice	94	4	1 in 23
Total.................	539	51	1 in 11
Annual ratio per 1000 } of mean strength ..... }	10	1·	...

The frequency of hepatitis amongst European soldiers in India, as compared to all the other colonies occupied by British troops, stamps the disease as essentially tropical. The proportion of admissions into hospital from hepatitis is stated by Mr. Waring to be much higher throughout India, and in Madras especially, than in all the other possessions put together; and the earlier years of residence in the East are those in which the disease is most frequent. The intemperate European appears to be twice as liable to hepatitis as the temperate and the absolutely abstemious.

The natives of India he regards as almost exempt from hepatic diseases, only five cases out of ten thousand convicts in the jails of Madras having been thus recorded.

SYMPTOMS AND PROGRESS.

The symptoms and progress of hepatitis vary much according as the inflammation is seated in the upper convex surface, on the exterior of the organ, or in its central parenchyma; but the nature and amount of the inflammation are assuredly the first and most important considerations to be determined, if we would successfully combat so dangerous a disease.

For practical purposes hepatitis may be considered, first—as consisting in a more or less superficial and adhesive inflammation of the organ; and secondly, in deep-seated suppurative inflammation of its parenchyma, of the nature termed congestive.

1. This well-marked form of the disease is ushered in by rigor, or sense of cold and constriction of the skin, followed by febrile reaction, the complexion being of a dusky, sallow hue, nausea and vomiting, urgent thirst, loaded tongue, occasional headache, loss of appetite, pain of the right hypochondrium, increased by pressure or a full inspiration, and more or less acute according as the peritoneal covering may be more or less involved; pain occasionally of the right shoulder, cough and oppressed breathing, difficulty in lying on the left side; such are the usual and more urgent symptoms. They will not all be present in any case; but so many of them will be manifested as to render diagnosis generally easy. There occurs frequently a loose state of the bowels, the matters

voided being pale or muddy, and watery; at other times the bowels are even constipated. The surcharged state of the urine in this disease is caused by the suppression of the excretion of carbon by the liver, and perhaps by the lungs also. The urine is always scanty, high, sometimes porter-coloured, with deep yellow tinge, and depositing a reddish-yellow sediment. When vomiting is urgent, with sense of heat and burning in the epigastrium, it indicates an acute state of the disease, involving the ducts, duodenum, and pylorus. But with a view further to confirm and establish the accuracy of diagnosis, the surgeon must be careful to explore the region of the liver by inspection, commotion, and general pressure, and by percussion in the sitting posture, pressure being likewise carefully made over the intercostal spaces corresponding with the liver.

As the disease advances, the pulse becomes frequent and hard, the skin is hot, dry, ånd constricted, the pain, cough, and oppression of breathing increase, there is occasional hiccup, with an anxious and desponding countenance, all indicative of advancing disease; and if this condition be not speedily arrested by remedial means, abscess of the liver, destroying life, or permanent enlargement of the liver, destroying the general health, will inevitably result.

In this formidable disease we should regard the severity of the hepatic and epigastric pains, and other distressing symptoms as really invaluable indications; for while they warn us of a pressing danger they explain everything, and thus relieve the mind from what otherwise would be a most painful state of doubt and anxiety. In the form of hepatitis which is attended with so much suffering as is here described, the fate of the patient is comparatively secure; for even the inexperienced will be induced to apply immediate and decisive remedies.

2. It is different in respect to the deep-seated, congestive, and suppurative inflammation of the parenchyma of the liver; for here the danger is even greater than in the former instance, with no salutary warnings from symptoms. It is one of the most dangerous of diseases, because of the total absence of urgent symptoms, and consequent insidiousness; the process which leads to destruction is here silent and rapid.

Of the various kinds of inflammation the suppurative is by much the most frequent, in Bengal at least. It attacks persons of both sexes, and those even of the most temperate habits; it not unfrequently terminates the career of the old Indian.

Whether occurring in the person of the older resident in Bengal, or in the new comer, this form of the disease occurs very generally in the cold season, and is caused by exposure to alternations of heat and cold, by such means, in short, as determine powerfully from the surface to the internal organs. I have seen cases where it resulted from the chilling thorough-draughts of the northern entrances to the Calcutta houses, on issuing from a ball-room, for instance; and other cases where it was occasioned by exposure to damp and cold before daylight for the purpose of hunting.

The disease is sometimes preceded by a perceptible falling off in the general health, indicated by emaciation, dry cough and embarrassed respiration, loss of appetite, or the complexion gradually assuming a muddy, sallow hue, but it more generally comes on in the midst of apparent health. We seldom indeed see the patient till inflammation has actually commenced; when he generally complains of a feeling of abdominal uneasiness, but more particularly of the epigastric region and that of the liver, with some degree of fever, preceded by slight rigor or ague; but all these may be so slight as too often to attract but little of the patient's attention. Perhaps he consults his physician on account of *diarrhœa* supposed to result from errors in diet; medicine affords some relief, and the patient proceeds in his ordinary occupations for days, or, when the action is less acute, for weeks, though under great depression of the mental and corporeal energies, till at length his altered appearance, hacking cough, permanently dry skin, invincibly rough furred tongue, and morbid taste, all expressive of a suppressed and depraved state of the secretions, attract some more serious notice on his own part, and that of his family. The real nature of the disease may still remain a secret to both patient and physician; and it may not be till actual tumour of the liver, a marked succession of rigors, or profuse and clammy sweats announce in unmistakeable terms the formation of abscess, that either party becomes awake to the impending danger; and then it is too late. A sense of uneasiness, hardly amounting to an obtuse dull pain, a sense of weight and oppression, may or may not exist in the region of the liver, according as the disease is centred more or less deeply in its substance or in its upper convex surface; when the former exists, the symptoms are more than usually obscure and insidious; in the latter case they are somewhat more of an acute nature. In this form of hepatitis it is seldom that we discover any pain in the shoulder.

I should say, then, that a rigor, or a diarrhœa, followed by feverishness, the peculiar harsh state of the skin, the tongue having the roughness of a coarse file with adherent coating, together with the local uneasiness already described, cough, scanty surcharged urine, often of a deep saffron colour, ought immediately to warn the physician of the suppurative inflammation which speedily leads to abscess. In every instance the diagnosis will receive material assistance from the external examination of the chest, especially when the upper convex surface of the liver is the seat of disease. Nor should the exploration of the abdomen be less carefully made: nothing should satisfy the medical attendant as to the condition of his patient short of the most painfully assiduous explorations often repeated; for we have here to deal with a disease deadly in its nature and rapid in its progress.

The causes of hepatitis will be found in the following circumstances :—residence in hot climates, exposure to high ranges of temperature followed by cold and damp, causing sudden arrests of the cuticular as well as of the internal secretions, the cold seasons of tropical climates, night exposure while imperfectly clothed, the exposure of the bivouac. These causes become very powerful when fatigue is added to them, and under irregularities of diet, and intemperance in the use of wine and ardent spirits especially. Dysenteries and fevers, remittent and intermittent, a too rich and stimulating diet, producing gastric and duodenal irritation, these are frequent and influential causes of hepatitis ; and more remotely may be numbered previous attacks, malaria, various forms of dyspepsia, neglect of the natural action of the bowels, the age of puberty.

When we take into account that " the absorption of nutritive matters is not solely the work of the lacteal vessels, but that a part of the food digested in the gastro-intestinal canal is taken into the blood through the portal veins," and that " the liver must be also regarded as the organ for the assimilation of substances which have been absorbed from the intestine" generally, we discover at once how the abuse of highly-seasoned food, wine and spirits, with the absence of due exercise, must tend to the production of disease in this the greatest and most powerful of the glandular organs.

Were the earliest morbid change in the liver ascertainable antecedently to actual inflammation, I have no doubt that that condition would in most cases consist in acute congestion; for, as in the well-known instance of hepatic congestion and consequent diarrhœa, both resulting from the sudden application of the cold damp of the Himalayahs, for example, so the pale, watery, premonitory diarrhœa is one of the most ordinary and immediate precursors of hepatitis ; it is generally the earliest and, indeed, the only symptom which attracts the notice of the patient ; and it should always receive the instant and close attention of his medical attendant. In two cases of hepatitis in recently-arrived Europeans, and which terminated fatally, Mr. Twining found " the internal membrane of the hepatic veins inflamed, and puriform matter in the right ventricle of the heart." Their complaints, he says, " began as common diarrhœa of a severe description." In the case of an European soldier in Burmah, treated by Dr. Murchison, and in which inflammation terminated in abscess, " an obstinate diarrhœa had been one of the most harassing symptoms in this case ; but no traces of ulceration were found either in the small or large intestine." These observations on the earlier pathological changes, refer to every form of hepatitis, but more especially to the deep-seated suppurative inflammation of the parenchyma of the liver ; and he who will best ascertain them at their commencement will least be taken by surprise in the progress and terminations of this disease. In the suppurative inflammation the earliest observable lesions I believe to be redness and softening, soon to be aggravated into the formation of abscess.

Mr. Twining declares that he has " never seen a case terminate in abscess without our being able, by a careful examination, to detect the disease that is in progress long before there was any reason to believe that suppuration existed." This may be generally true, *but then the examination must be most rigorous and often repeated, until we are quite satisfied as to the true nature of the case.* The patient's recovery or death will depend on the care and discrimination with which this examination is made ; a false diagnosis is here a death-warrant,—they are indeed but convertible terms. I remember that, in the cold season of 1837 alone, in Calcutta, I was consulted in four cases of suppurated liver, in which no such condition had been previously suspected.

The appearances on dissection of Europeans who have died of hepatitis will vary with the intensity and the duration of the disease. Various vascular discolorations of the peritoneal covering are observed, differing according to the degrees of inflammation, and the number of previous hepatic ailments—thickenings of the peritoneum, and effusions under it, being very generally discoverable. Adhesions of the liver to the colon, stomach, and diaphragm are also common.

Where inflammatory symptoms have run high, and death has ensued rapidly, there will be great enlargement of the liver, with much redness and vascularity of the organ, and depositions in the interlobular cellular tissue ; in other cases its colour will be dark, or even black—bleeding freely in both instances on section being made. In other cases the covering membrane is found of a pale hue, thickened and indurated—the structure underneath bleeding but little on being cut ; while induration, more or less extensive, with deposition of coagulable lymph, tubercles, and concretions are very general.

On the concave surface of the liver, the gall-bladder is often enlarged and filled with viscid bile ; in other instances it is diminished in volume, its coats thickened, and the body covered with false membranes.

The observations of Rose and Henry would seem to show that the quantity of urea excreted by the kidneys is lessened in suppurative hepatitis apparently in a degree proportioned to the extent to which the secretion of the liver was destroyed by the abscess. " If the statement be proved by future observation," says

Dr. Parkes, "it is, in my opinion, impossible to overrate its importance in a pathological as well as in a physiological point of view."

Since my return to England I have on several occasions tried to obtain from India information on this and on other important matters connected with the chemistry of the blood and of the secretions in tropical diseases ; but some officers said they were over-worked, others that they were situated too far from the Presidencies, and so on.   Thus I have failed in my object ; but I hope yet to succeed.

TREATMENT.

The maxims of De Retz that what is absolutely necessary is never dangerous, and that what looks the boldest course is generally the safest, are true in medicine as in politics ; nor is there here any real difficulty in perceiving either what is necessary to be done, or yet what is safe in the treatment of acute hepatitis ; it is likewise very easy to comprehend what it would be dangerous *to leave undone*—the greatest danger in reality being found in feebleness, irresolution, and in do-nothing plans.

However long the disease may have existed, and in whatever part of the liver the inflammation may be situated, *provided there be no symptoms indicative of suppuration,* general blood-letting, repeated as the symptoms may demand, and copious in relation to age, health, and length of residence in India, must be had recourse to ; and the sooner the better for the patient, the measure of depletion being, in all cases, a sense of local and general relief—*with softening of the skin.*   These are the only criterions of adequate loss of blood ; and it should be always held in recollection that inflammation, suppurative especially, and of the most deadly character, is present, and that, consequently, there is not an hour to be lost.

After the general blood-letting, a full dose of ten grains of calomel with five of James's powder is to be exhibited at bedtime, followed in the early morning by a strong saline purge, or a full dose of compound jalap powder ; and this course must be pursued —using leeches to the side, mercurials with antimonials, purgatives, and diaphoretics with diuretics daily, so long as they are called for by fulness or tenderness of the hepatic or epigastric region. The medical attendant must remember that the subsidence of local symptoms, together with a declared and satisfactory abatement of all the general symptoms, including that of the force and frequency of the circulation, and a permanent relaxation of the skin, with freedom in the secretions, can alone warrant the discontinuance of antiphlogistic means, including the most spare use of farinaceous food and drink.   If the bowels be irritable, and anything like diarrhœa threatens to distress the patient, the Dover's powder, or ure opium, must be added to the calomel, in lieu of the antimonial.

As regards the constitutional influence of mercury, the utmost that I found necessary, even in the worst cases, was the producing a gentle action on the gums, salivation being unnecessary, and in the instances of persons of a feeble or strumous habit, naturally injurious. The precautions already insisted on against oozing from leech-bites must here be carefully regarded ; while blisters will be found useful on the entire disappearance of inflammatory action.

Nor should the most strict abstinence in diet be deviated from, until, by the subsiding of all uneasiness, and tumidness of the region of the liver, and of the abdomen generally, by the cessation of all febrile movements, and by the restoration of healthy secretions, we feel assured, on these sufficient evidences, that convalescence is well established:—and even then, the return to accustomed habits should be made very slowly, so as to afford time, under great abstemiousness, for the absorption of interstitial deposits ; a reparative process which cannot take place under a full stomach.

Mild saline aperients in bitter infusion, the nitro-muriatic acid in bitter infusion—the bicarbonate of soda in large doses with bitter infusion, where there is much acidity—warm baths, and gentle exercise in the open air—all tend to the maturing of convalescence ; and, in the cold season, great attention must be paid to the clothing. Nor should the European soldier here, any more than under fever or dysentery, be permitted to return to the barrack life, or to duty, before his strength has been restored : it is to the neglect of this rule that many of the serious and often fatal relapses are due.

When convalescence proceeds unkindly, and there is reason to apprehend structural injury to the liver, a full course of the nitro-muriatic acid, as described in the second part of this work, will be found the surest and best remedy.

Mr. Twining relied too exclusively on blood-letting in hepatic inflammation, and too little, as appears to me, upon other remedial means. There are cases where inflammation will go on notwithstanding the most copious depletions, and others in which the same will occur with a debilitated constitution and a weak pulse. What, then, is to be done ? " What degree of depletion," says Dr. Billing, " will remove a node, or syphilitic iritis, without mercurial and other medicines ? What would venesection do for rheumatic pains without antimony, colchicum, opium, bark, mercury, and other medicines ? The question is not so much as to possibility, as expedition and safety to the constitution." Robert Jackson— no advocate of mercurial treatment in tropical diseases—admits that " mercury, after the condition has been prepared for its action, is the principal means of cure where biliary secretion is principally in fault."

Mr. Twining, who was in the habit of prescribing half-scruple doses of calomel at bedtime, in hepatitis, asks the following ques-

tion respecting the action of mercury in this disease :—" We have
been told that mercury is beneficial in hepatitis in the way that
the breast-pipe or pump relieves inflammation of the female breast,
when milk abscess is impending.   But a legitimate parallel cannot
be established in the action of the respective remedies ; the pipe
relieves the inflamed breast by drawing off the superfluous milk,
without exciting increased secretion.   Has the action of mercury an
analogous effect on the liver?"
. No : and if it had but the limited effect of the pump or pipe, it
would not be the valuable remedy which physicians and surgeons
have ever found it to be in so great a variety of inflammatory
affections, and in the deadly inflammation of the liver in particular.
It is for the very reason that calomel assists powerfully both in
" drawing off " accumulations, and in promoting " *increased secretion*," that it proves of such value in aid of blood-letting.   It is,
in fact, by this very double action, of purging and increasing
secretion at the same time, that calomel relieves the loaded and
inactive vessels of the diseased gland ; not to speak of the other
acknowledged physiological influences of this mineral, such as—its
increase of all the secretions and excretions of the body—its influence on the capillary circulation—its febrifuge effect—the
peculiar specific power ascribed to it by physicians and surgeons,
as an antagonist to inflammations, whether general or local—its
stimulant power over the absorbent functions—its power of unloading, at the same time that it gives a new impulse to, the
vascular system—its peculiar power in removing viscid and tenacious intestinal secretions—its antiphlogistic, solvent, and alterative
effects on the blood ;—these are the actions and uses ascribed to
mercury, when exhibited for the cure of acute disease, during a
few days only, by the ablest British practitioners and authors ;
and they are such as to place this remedy second only in order of
importance to blood-letting in all the more acute hepatic affections
of India.
That mercury enters into intimate union with the elements of
the blood is now an ascertained fact : it must therefore " modify
its plasticity, and influence all the organic functions to which it is
subservient."   Mr. Tyrrell, treating of acute iritis, says : " The
early stage of the disease may be arrested and subdued very readily
by mercury. . . As certain as mercurial action takes place, so certain
will be the arrest of the inflammation."   He adds that it " appears
not only to arrest the inflammation, but further to promote absorption of fibrin, which is the common product of the morbid action
in the iris, and which occasions changes destructive of vision."
That mercury has been, and is still, abused by ill-informed and
inconsiderate persons, is quite true, both at home and abroad ;
but to argue hence its disuse would not be either safe or wise.
In respect to remedial agents of acknowledged power, it is not
just to support either means alternately and neither effectually.

Neither is it just or true to prefer a certain evil to a remote or possible danger; for such an argument might be turned against anything, however necessary. What is there in medicine without some danger, either in what we do or in what we leave undone? How great, therefore, should be the knowledge and discernment of the physician.

It is of great practical importance that the real benefits derivable from the use of mercury be impartially set before the inexperienced tropical practitioner, and I have here endeavoured briefly to do so; I hope, with fairness to the subject, and to persons with whom I may happen to differ in opinion. Mr. Twining would appear to hold the language of congratulation as to the result, and of censure as to the means.

In the pride of pathological science we are sometimes induced to believe that, because we see and examine, we therefore under-stand, to the neglect of the science of pure observation so inestim-able to the physician; and thus, I think, it happens that matters are still in doubt with us which a more chastened and correct observation ought long ago to have fixed and settled; and that we are driven, or betake ourselves to solemn trifling, and to a huge German manufactory of big words, as an off-set to research; to the bondage of mere phrases—to hazy sounding transcendentalism. Our faith in our remedies must carry reason with it, otherwise we move in ignorance or in wilful error.

When inflammation has terminated in hepatic abscess, mercury given with the view to its general influence, is always highly in-jurions:—it aggravates the irritative fever and general distress, while its specific influence—so hopeful in the previous stage—now but aggravates the danger by increasing the suppurative process and the general debility, so as to retard or altogether to obviate the curative efforts of nature.

Shortly before I left Calcutta, a case came under my care, in the month of August, in which slight hepatic tenderness existed in complication with severe dysentery. From both diseases the patient speedily recovered; and to restore his strength, I advised a short voyage to sea, where, having exceeded in diet, the liver became tender and enlarged, there being no recurrence of dysentery. A second time he recovered, but being of a weakly habit, and now much reduced by disease and treatment, I sent him on a longer voyage to Pinang. Here again, despite the most careful written instructions, he took to excesses in eating and in the use of wine:—the result was that, in three months from his leaving Calcutta, an hepatic abscess formed, and discharged itself through the stomach by vomiting, soon after which he died. I mention this case as affording an illustration of the necessity for abstinence in diet, and to show that, even when the hepatic disease is but secon-dary, it may, and very often does, prove the ultimate cause of death by the formation of abscess.

I I

In 1837, a young staff officer consulted me on account of cough and emaciation, which he considered to indicate tubercular consumption, as some relatives of his had died of this disease in England. His respiration and pulse were very rapid, and he had profuse night-sweats; in short, I found that he was dying of suppurated liver. The history he gave me was to the effect that, six weeks previously, he drove in an open gig from a ball-room in Calcutta to Barrackpore, and that, on getting to his quarters, he was seized with shivering, followed by feverishness and diarrhœa; he continued to perform the duties of his office up to the day on which he consulted me, and the real nature of his disease had not till then been so much as suspected. He died in a fortnight, and the entire substance of the liver was found to be converted into a huge cyst filled with pus.

Well might Curtis, writing in 1781, speak of hanging up cases such as these " *in terrorem,* against the attacks of this insidious disease;" or rather, he might have added, as warnings against the crimes of heedlessness and inattention in cases of so pressing a duty.

I will now present a case the converse of the above:—In the cold season of 1836, a professional friend called on me to consult respecting the case of a patient of his; and just as he was taking leave, he said, as if by accident, that he had " *a pain in his back like lumbago.*" Being an able, experienced surgeon, I might well have said, " go home and take care of yourself;" but there was a something in his expression of countenance which excited a suspicion of disease, and so I made a careful examination. The result was the discovery of deep-seated inflammation of the liver, and that it had existed for three days, during which he had been living as usual, and using the cold bath every morning. All the patient had noticed was a slight shivering three nights previously, followed by feverishness and pain in the back; but he considered his symptoms of so little moment that he felt a doubt as to the accuracy of the diagnosis. I then referred him to our common friend, Mr. Nicolson of Calcutta, who concurred with me completely as to the nature of the disease. The patient was young and of robust habit, so that with the loss of about eighty ounces of blood in the first twenty-four hours, followed by calomel and antimony gently to affect the gums, strong purgatives, and total deprivation of food, he rapidly recovered; but I think he recovered with difficulty; a few more hours lost to the treatment, and it would have been too late.

The above case is interesting and important, as showing how very obscure and insidious are the symptoms, and how little they possess of urgency to cause a salutary alarm, even to the mind of a professional person. But it is always thus when the inflammation is centred in the parenchyma of the liver; and hence the absence of that acute pain and those urgent symptoms which characterize inflammatory states of the peritoneal covering of the gland, and which generally give ample warning.

HEPATIC ABSCESS.

From a table of 216 cases of fatal hepatic abscess, presented by Mr. Waring of Madras, it appears that the maximum both of admissions and deaths occurred in the cold months. The diseases which immediately preceded, or in the progress of which hepatic abscess supervened, were as follows : —

Hepatitis, acute and chronic	43 per cent.
Dysentery, acute and chronic	27 ,,
,, with hepatic complication . . .	4 ,,
Fever, continued form	4 ,,
,, remittent	1 ,,
,, intermittent	1 ,,
,, intermittent with diarrhœa	2 ,,

Other diseases are here omitted, as are fractions; but eight per cent. of the deaths from hepatic abscess resulted from fevers. Mr. Waring concludes that the proportion of cases of hepatic abscess occurring after or during the progress of hepatitis, dysentery, and fever, is not only larger than that of any other disease, but of all diseases put together. The formation of abscess in the liver, as already stated, is generally announced by irritative fever, increased towards night—rigors or shudderings, followed by profuse cold sweats—a tenaciously furred rough tongue—scanty and high-coloured urine, &c. &c.; when the abscess is large, by a perceptible tumour of the right hypochondrium—the mind being anxious and depressed. Jaundice is by no means a general occurrence in conjunction with hepatic abscess.

These symptoms vary in degree according to the extent of the abscess; and when that is extensive there is much oppression of the respiration, with restlessness. When, on the other hand, the abscess is small, the symptoms are displayed in a very obscure manner and degree;—so that it is from a careful consideration of all the circumstances already detailed that the judgment must be formed. It is probable that in some persons mere congestion with softening of the textures will terminate in a kind of chronic abscess.

I remember hearing of the case of a trooper of her Majesty's 11th dragoons, who fell from his horse on parade at Cawnpore, and was killed on the spot by fracture of the skull and laceration of the brain. On *post-mortem* examination, an abscess was found in the liver; and this, although the man had never expressed any feeling of indisposition, and had not for months been an hour absent from duty.

Soon after I went to India, I was requested by my friend Mr. Nicolson, and by Dr. William Russell, to assist at the examination of the body of a deceased magistrate of Calcutta. He had but a week previously returned from a hog-hunting party, feeling then slightly indisposed. There had been no fever, nor any symptom to indicate danger ;—so that his sudden death took his friends by surprise. The appearance of the body exteriorly was that of a powerful and healthy man ; but in the liver were found seven abscesses, distinct and separate, and varying from the size of a common nut to that of an orange. I was then very young, and this case left a deep impression on my mind as to the concealed dangers of such cases.

Mr. Twining fancied that " a greater degree of *tension of the right rectus abdominis muscle* than of the left," formed " one of the most undeviating symptoms of congestion with incipient deposit into the texture of the liver, which commonly goes to deep-seated abscess." The truth I believe to be, that the right rectus abdo-minis, like any other muscle in the body, will contract more or less, according as any organ beneath its fibres is in a state of suffering or of pain—no matter whether that pain be from inflam-mation, congestion, or other cause ;—but that the mere tension or partial contraction of a muscle could prove an "undeviating symptom" of congestion, of suppuration, or, indeed, of any one special or peculiar morbid change in a gland beneath it, cannot be admitted in any case ; neither have I ever seen it confined to inflammatory or congestive states only :—on the contrary, I have known many persons in whom it was a well-marked accompani-ment of hepatalgia, as well as of the painful affection of the bowels described by the late Dr. James Johnson, and in whom it con-tinned so for many years. The same symptom was noticed by Dr. Budd, in a case of jaundice from a closure of the common duct, and in a case where a cancerous ulcer of the stomach had eaten into the adherent liver; and by Dr. Graves, in an inflamed gall-bladder. Dr. Parkes, again, has seen this state of tension very prominent in a case of phthisical diarrhœa, in which there was extensive alteration in that part of the ileum situated imme-diately under the muscle ; while partial contractions of the abdo-minal muscles over a suffering part, are justly stated by Mr. Holmes Coote and by Dr. Kirkes to be frequent in jaundice and other affections of the abdominal organs.

We may therefore conclude with Dr. Watson, that this sym-pathetic affection is but one instance among many of that kind of protective instinct whereby a tender part is in some measure shielded against the infliction of pain by pressure.

TREATMENT.

It is little indeed that we can do for the unhappy sufferer from hepatic abscess. When the abscess is small, we may favour the efforts of nature at absorption by care in diet and clothing—gesta-

tion in the open air, and change of air—the use of the nitro-
muriatic acid with bitter tonics, &c. When the abscess has happily discharged its contents into the stomach or bowels, or externally, a more nutritious diet will be proper, with the view to
support the strength of the patient, and even a little wine may
now be allowed. But nothing should be done which may unduly
excite the nervous or vascular functions ; and mercury in every
form is to be carefully avoided, and even the mildest aperients
should only be exhibited under necessity. When hepatic abscess
has once formed, its treatment is to be conducted on the same
general principles as irritative fever induced by purulent formations in any other region of the body.

Of the instances of recovery within my personal knowledge,
the majority were amongst such as had discharged the pus by
the bowels ; and one married lady I remember to have recovered
health rapidly, after vomiting the contents of an enormous abscess.
I also saw several instances of recovery where the abscess had
opened into the bronchi—the direction which the most extended
observation in all countries points to as comparatively favourable.
Of those in whom the pus was discharged through the external
integument, the majority have within my knowledge died. But by
much the greater proportion of the instances of hepatic abscess
end fatally—either before the bursting of the abscess, or within a
few hours from its discharge into the peritoneal or thoracic cavity :
—and this brings me to the consideration of the propriety of
making an opening for the discharge of such abscesses through the
external integument. I have often seen this operation performed
in India, and I have myself performed it ; but in no instance that
I remember did the operation appear to me to result in eventual
good. I therefore agree with Dr. Budd, that " it is generally best,
when an abscess of the liver projects at the side, to allow it to
open itself. Nature performs the operation better than the surgeon. When the abscess opens of itself, it is usually by a very
small aperture, like those of worm-eaten wood, which never closes;
and the matter gradually oozes out as the sac contracts. No air
gets mixed with the matter of the abscess, and no violence is done
to its walls ; and, consequently, no fresh inflammation is set up.
The discharge is very gradual, and as small in quantity as it can
be. There is less shock to the system, and less drain from it than
when the abscess is opened by the knife. The prominent part
should be poulticed, and the matter allowed to escape in the
poultice, but should not be squeezed or pressed out."

These observations accord altogether with my own experience
in India, where, too often, young medical officers are urged, by the
pressing dangers of the case, and by the importunity of friends, to
" do something."

Dr. Budd is deserving of attention on another question connected with this subject. " In opening an abscess in the sub-

stance of the liver," he says, "there is another, and greater, and more unavoidable source of danger, which has not been noticed by the writers to whom I have referred. It is, that the solid hepatic tissue cannot readily collapse, so as to close the cavity when the abscess is opened. When, then, a free opening is made even into a recent abscess, air almost necessarily enters into the cavity, and from the sudden removal of pressure, or, it may be, from the manipulation employed to empty the cavity, violence is done to the walls of the abscess, and there is often some degree of hæmorrhage from them. Air and blood thus become mixed with the pus in the abscess, decomposition takes place, and the air, or the decomposed pus, sets up fresh inflammation of the inner surface of the sac. This causes, of course, a fresh accession of fever, and of other constitutional disturbance, and if the abscess be large, a profuse, and fœtid, and continuous discharge, which may soon exhaust the strength of the patient. The secondary inflammation thus excited by the presence of air, or by the decomposed pus, may even lead to gangrene, and speedily destroy life; and this happened in one of the cases that fell under my care at the Dreadnought. A similar case is noticed by Cruveilhier."

Of fifty-seven cases of hepatic abscess, real or supposed, recorded in the *Medical Journal* of Madras for 1844, the following were the terminations :—

Recovery took place	in 17 cases.
Of these the trocar entered the abscess . .	in 8 „
No pus obtained	in 3 „
Pus obtained on the 6th, 7th, and 11th days	in 3 „
No pus mentioned.	in 3 „
Death occurred	in 40 „

The proportion of recoveries to deaths in eighty-one cases of hepatic abscess, recorded by Mr. Waring, of the Madras army, and in which their contents were evacuated by operation, was as follows :—

Recoveries	15, or 18·519 per cent.
Deaths	66, or 81·481 „
	81 100·000 „

Referring to 300 fatal cases of hepatic abscess, of which the details are given by Mr. Waring, in the first part of his work, he considers that operation might have been applicable in the following proportions :—

Total number of cases	300
There was a plurality of abscesses in	108
	192
Of 177 cases in which abscess was solitary, there was more or less extensive ulceration of the large intestines in . .	76
	116

Thus it appears that "*the proportion of cases of hepatic abscess which hold out a reasonable hope of cure by the performance of an operation for evacuating the contents,* is much smaller than most persons are aware of." . . Out of the whole number above recorded, "only in 116, or little more than one in three, could the operation have been undertaken with any reasonable probability of success; and this number would, of course, be still further diminished by taking into account the cases in which abscess, though solitary, communicated with the lung, colon, or some other viscera, and those in which other organic disease existed."

The best surgery here is what Trousseau terms "armed medicine, neither more nor less"—the arms, however, being held in reservation for very special and appropriate cases only.

M. Rouis, Surgeon-Major of the First Class to the Military Hospital of Strasbourg, has published an excellent monograph, entitled " Recherches sur les Suppurations Endémiques du Foie (Paris, 1860)," giving the results of eleven years' experience in the climate of Algeria. The subject is considered under the various heads of pathological anatomy, symptoms and progress, modes of termination, duration, convalescence, complications, prognosis, diagnosis, causes, and treatment. An analysis is given of 203 cases of hepatic abscess which came under the author's own observation, and the history of 40 of the cases is recorded in detail. Of the 203 cases, 162 proved fatal, 2 made an imperfect recovery, and 39 recovered completely. From this it would appear that four out of every five cases died. In 179 cases, or about nine-tenths of the entire number, the abscess in the liver was preceded or accompanied by dysentery. Of the 203 cases, the pus escaped from the liver in various directions in 50 ; and of these 50 cases, the abscess burst into the bronchi in fifteen, into the peritoneum in fourteen, eleven times into the right pleura, five times into the stomach, three times into the transverse colon, once into the duodenum, once into the pericardium, once into the gall-bladder, and once into the bile-ducts. A circumstance which, however, has been noticed before, was, that of the cases where the abscess burst into the bronchi, almost as many recovered as died. Bursting of an hepatic abscess into a bronchus is, therefore, comparatively, a favourable occurrence. The pathology of hepatic abscess is discussed with great minuteness and ability. The pus contained in the abscess is described as being usually of a yellowish-white colour, like that from an ordinary phlegmon ; but in some cases it presented a claret or chocolate colour, owing to the admixture of blood-globules or the *débris* of the hepatic tissue. In the case of old abscesses, it often exhaled a peculiarly fœtid odour."

JAUNDICE.

This disease occurs in India, as elsewhere, as an acute affection, and as a distinct and separate disease—often unconnected with hepatitis, fever, or dysentery. But there is observed not unfrequently a congested state of the liver, which, with the morbid conditions of the duodenum and gall-bladder, demand a very careful examination. To prescribe for the yellow skin, as is too often done, is to dispense with the care and justice necessary to the occasion, and to bring discredit on the prescriber. In jaundice, as in every disease affecting the liver, the exploration of the region should be made carefully and repeatedly, until we become satisfied whether the organ be enlarged, inflamed, or congested; circumstances which may always be determined by a careful percussion— as may likewise enlargement and distension of the gall-bladder.

Jaundice is usually attended by mental depression and physical lassitude—dyspepsia with loss of appetite, nausea, a yellow furred tongue, and flatulence. In some persons there exist fulness and uneasiness on pressure of the epigastric region and that of the liver; while the amount of sallowness of the conjunctivæ, skin, and urine, together with the degrees of paleness and of absence of bile in the alvine discharges, will depend on the intensity of the cause of the jaundice. The characters of the disease will vary also with the age, constitution, habits, and length of residence in India—age and length of residence being circumstances that are certain to operate to the disadvantage of the patient, especially if visceral disease, or an anæmic state of the system, be present at the same time.

The existence of gall-stones obstructing the ducts may be inferred from the following symptoms :—A sudden seizure of violent fits of pain in the epigastric and right hypochondriac regions, accompanied by irregular transient shiverings, and severe fits of vomiting—the pain at times being excruciating. Feverishness of the irritative character now makes its appearance; and within twenty-four or more hours, sallowness over the forehead, extending rapidly to the trunk and extremities, becomes evident, while on the appearance of the jaundice pain usually subsides. It is well to note here, that the pain attending the passage of gall-stones far exceeds that even of peritoneal inflammation, and that the fever, when such is present, is of a subdued character, unlike the endemic fevers of India—diagnostic circumstances worthy the attention of the inexperienced.

In the East Indies, and as it generally appears amongst Europeans there, the progress of the disease, under appropriate treatment, is very generally of a favourable tendency—the cause being in most cases of a congestive or inflammatory nature, susceptible of easy removal : and we find that as convalescence proceeds, the urine gradually loses its icteric, saffron hue, while the skin also becomes fairer by slow degrees. More rarely, though the jaundice is plainly seen, so as to require no other diagnosis than is furnished by the complexion, the causes of this complaint are nevertheless very difficult to trace.

CAUSES.

Whatever causes may produce hepatitis, or more especially congestion of the liver, will give rise to jaundice :—so biliary gravel, followed by hepatic colic, is a frequent and familiar cause of jaundice. Certain affections of the brain have been known to excite this disease, as the extremes of despondency, and sudden bursts of passion; but by far the more ordinary causes are—cold applied to the surface of the body, or cold applied suddenly to the stomach in the form of iced drinks, when the body has been heated by exercise or other exertion. In an analysis of seventy-two cases of icterus typhoides, by Professor Lebert, one-third of all the cases occurred in November and December, or in two only out of the cold months. Previous attacks predispose powerfully to jaundice. Formerly, when extreme courses of mercury were used in the treatment of venereal diseases, what with the action of mercury on the hepatic function, and with the influence of external cold on the skin, jaundice was a frequent disease in our hospitals at home. In every case of jaundice that I have seen in England amongst the returned Indians, cold has been the immediate cause of the disease.

Jaundice, according to Dr. Budd, may be produced in two ways :—first, by some impediment to the flow of bile into the duodenum, and consequent absorption of the retained bile ; and, secondly, by defective secretion on the part of the liver, so that the principles of the bile are not separated from the blood. It is probable, he adds, that jaundice which follows closure of the common duct, does not result merely from absorption of retained bile, but also, in part, from the secretion of the liver being less active, so that the principles of bile are retained in the blood.

"But in many cases of jaundice, perhaps in the greater number, there is no impediment to the flow of bile through the ducts. In fatal cases, it happens not unfrequently that the gall-bladder and gall-ducts are found empty, and their mucous membrane is unusually pale, showing that no bile was secreted. The jaundice results solely from suppressed or deficient secretion."

I think it right to place before the reader the views of this able writer, as to the causes of jaundice; adding, however, that in India the more general causes are congestion and inflammatory affections, involving the gall-ducts more or less directly.

In jaundice the presence of bile in the serum of the blood is manifest, while the absence of the hepatic secretion from the alvine discharges is caused by the bile not finding its way into the duodenum.

Catarrhal inflammation, with temporary obstruction of the ducts, may be inferred as a frequent cause of jaundice, as may, also, an impaired condition of the secreting structure.

Jaundice in its more ordinary form results from obstruction to the excretion of bile; in other words, from the absorption into the blood of bile already secreted, but which is prevented by some mechanical impediment from escaping by the natural channels. The actual suppression of the secreting function of the liver is a rare cause of jaundice in any climate.

Frerichs states that we have become acquainted with three causes of jaundice:—

"1. Obstruction to the escape of bile.

"2. Diminished circulation of the blood in the liver, and consequent abnormal diffusion. Both these conditions give rise to an increased imbibition of bile into the blood, and in both cases the liver is more or less directly implicated.

"3. Obstructed metamorphosis, or a diminished consumption of bile in the blood. This cause is independent of the liver, and, so far as we yet know the matter, is chiefly influenced by the composition of the blood, and by everything which essentially limits or modifies the processes of metamorphosis within the vascular system."

PATHOLOGY.

As few persons die in India of uncomplicated jaundice, the opportunities for the examination of the liver and its appendages in such cases can only occur by accident, as when a sufferer from jaundice dies of another acute disease. Such occasions, however, have been sufficiently numerous to establish, on examination after death, the following appearances:—These consist in inflammatory states of the liver and of the gall-ducts; congestions of the liver; deposition of coagulable lymph within the capsule of Glisson, with enlargement, more or less considerable, of its absorbent glands; effusion of lymph into the areolar tissue about the gall-ducts; and the presence of gall-stones impacting the common duct. Morbid affections of the duodenum are also found to be associated with jaundice.

Dr. Henry Kennedy of Dublin, after narrating some cases of rapidly fatal greenish-yellow jaundice, in which the ducts were found quite pervious, and in which the discharges from the bowels, "though probably of a lighter colour than what is natural, were by no means free from bile," suggests that "a much deteriorated bile, the absorption of which would cause serious consequences," may have here caused death. Dr. Cathcart Lees, of the same city, has been led by the examination of the urine of jaundiced patients " to entertain the opinion that the absence of any symptoms referable to the nervous system in many cases of jaundice might be accounted for by the presence cholic acid in the urine, and its consequent absence from the blood." . . . "If the supposition be correct, I think the detection of cholic acid or its conjugates in the urine, may prove a very important element of prognosis in every case of jaundice, as assuring us against the supervention of cerebral symptoms in cases where it is present; while, if absent, it may put us on our guard, and possibly enable us to adopt a prophylactic treatment."

In a fatal case of jaundice reported by Dr. Lees, in March, 1856, the presence of the biliary acids in the blood which flowed from the cranial cavity was satisfactorily determined; while, in the liver, the hepatic cells were greatly diminished in size, and there was fatty degeneration. The case was one of acute yellow atrophy, in which terrible affection jaundice is caused by non-elimination of bile.

The patient died in a state of delirium and convulsion on the third day of his admission into the Meath Hospital. In the urine voided *after* the development of the first cerebral symptoms, *not a trace* of biliary acids could be found, but albumen was present, and the amount of urea was very greatly diminished, while urea was found in the blood and serum taken from the brain.

Dr. Budd suggests that in these fatal cases a kind of decomposition may go on in the liver, with absorption of the poisonous products thereof into the blood.

TREATMENT.

Before proceeding to treat this disease, we must weigh carefully the symptoms, and be well satisfied as to the probable nature of the morbid action producing the jaundice. Where we find tumidness and tenderness of the epigastric region, extending into that of the liver, with a harsh dry skin, feverishness, and a furred tongue, the constitution being sound, one general blood-letting, followed by leeches and fomentations, will generally relieve the more acute symptoms; after which a few doses of calomel, of active purgatives, saline diaphoretics, with diuretics and warm baths, will in a few days bring about a solution of the disease, the diet consisting of farinaceous articles, fruits, and diluents, soda-water being about the best drink. Convalescence will be matured in such cases by the continuous use of warm baths, a moderately low diet, and by the daily use of saline aperients in some bitter infusion. In treating the jaundice of the returned Indian at home, I have found no remedy in the early stage of the disease more serviceable than the warm bath used at bedtime.

In treating the calculous form of jaundice we must commence with the use of such means as allay pain and relieve the hepatic colic, as ethereal anodynes, chlorodyne, &c., followed by hot fomentations to the affected region, and both measures should be repeated until relief shall be obtained. By such means the violence of pain and spasm will generally be overcome, while a hot bath used to faintness, and followed by a dose of calomel and a strong saline purge, will conduce greatly to the relief of the patient, and prepare for the stage of convalescence.   Chloroform conjoined to the liquor potassæ, in doses of twenty minims each, has proved eminently efficacious in jaundice resulting from gall-stones—relaxing the spasm, relieving pain, and giving freedom to the discharge of calculi.   This combination may be repeated every hour until relief is obtained.   In a case of gall-stones accompanied by violent spasmodic and remitting pains—hepatic colic—Dr. Charles Kidd exhibited chloroform internally in ten-drop doses every half-hour. The pain subsided after the third dose, and a speedy restoration to health followed.

When hepatic gravel and colic are proved to be the cause of jaundice, alkaline drugs should be administered, and green vegetables and fruits, as solvents, and as calculated to obviate the formation of fatty substances, should be freely used ; while exercise, by which their combustion is promoted, should be regularly and systematically practised.

I have during many years, in India and at home, been in the habit of prescribing freely the extract of taraxacum with alkalies, in hepatic gravel, jaundice, and all the functional disorders of the liver; and these means persevered in, along with a spare diet, exercise, and warm baths, very generally conduce to a true recovery.   Such means are believed to saponify fat, render it soluble, and promote its combustion, while they eliminate the ducts and promote a healthy biliary secretion.   I have also found the greatest benefit from the alternate use of the alkalies and the nitro-hydrochloric acids, these last acting as tonics and eliminants.

Should congestive or inflammatory symptoms supervene, the appropriate antiphlogistic means already indicated will become necessary, including nauseating doses of emetic tartar.

When, on the other hand, the patient is anæmic, or long resident in India, with a flat abdomen and evidences of enfeebled health, neither blood-letting nor mercurials will avail to any good, but indeed the contrary.   We must here be content with saline purgatives, bitter tonics, diaphoretics, and the persistent use of the warm bath at bed-time.   Should drowsiness or tendency to coma appear, very active purgatives perseveringly used, sinapisms to the epigastric region, and blisters to the nape of the neck will prove effective, even in cases wearing an alarming aspect.   Death occurs not unfrequently from blood-poisoning or cholæmic intoxication, and from retention of the constituents of the urine.

When jaundice, whether simple or complicated, becomes chronic, I know of no means to be compared in effect to the persevering use of the nitro-muriatic acid bath applied to the whole body, under the influence of which I have seen cases of the most obdurate nature recover, both in India and at home ; cases which had the characters of disorganization of the secreting structures. As stated elsewhere, this powerful agent was first used in the treatment of hepatic diseases by the late Dr. Helenus Scott of the Bombay army, who, according to Mason Good, "plunged the Duke of Wellington in a bath up to the chin for a severe hepatic affection he was then labouring under, and thus restored him to health in a short time." It was through this means that General Wellesley was enabled to return to his command, and to fight what, in pro- portion to the numbers engaged, was the most bloody of his victories, the battle of Assaye, and thus to lay the foundation of his future greatness.

In all acute forms of jaundice of the congestive and inflammatory characters, severe irritation of the duodenum is an inevitable asso- ciation. Here refrigerants and saline aperients, with leeches and fomentations to the affected region, will be found to procure the most speedy relief from duodenal disturbance and portal dis- tension.

During the actual paroxysm of hepatic colic, so generally followed by jaundice, the means already indicated will usually prove sufficient; but it is proper to state that some practitioners rely ex- clusively on minute doses of morphia, as one-sixth of a grain every half-hour until relief is obtained. Dr. du Parcque, on the other hand, found remarkable benefit to follow the exhibition of the following preparation, given in tea-spoonfuls, well mixed, every half-hour :—

> Ætheris sulphurici . . . . 3j.
> Ol. Ricini,
> Syrupi Aurant., ana . . . . 5j.

CHRONIC ENLARGEMENT AND INDURATION OF THE LIVER.

Although the subject of this article is fully detailed in the second part of this work, I am desirous very briefly to notice this form of hepatic disease as it appears in Bengal. It is presented as the result of previous inflammation of the liver, more or less acute, of congestions of the organ, or as the sequel to fevers, remittent and intermittent, and to dysentery.

The liver is enlarged, rising above the fifth intercostal space, and descending below the margin of the false ribs, it is sometimes indu- rated in a perceptible manner, and its function is. greatly impaired, the biliary secretion being scanty and depraved ; that of the kidneys being similarly affected. There is frequently a hacking dry cough, dyspepsia in various forms, a despondent state of the mind, and much general ill health, a generally cachectic state, with a sallow pasty complexion and emaciation ; more rarely we find dropsical effusion into the great cavities. In this form of hepatic disease we occasionally find, also, an embarrassed state of the circulation in the form of excitement of the heart's action, or an intermittent pulse—these symptoms being prominent in proportion as the liver is more or less indurated. In both instances the disturbance would seem to arise principally from the impediment to a free circulation offered by an indurated liver. Whenever, therefore, I hear mention of an excited or intermittent state of the heart's action, I make a careful and searching examination of the hepatic region, the only kind of examination that is of any value. The perfunctory performance of this great duty is a real crime in the surgeon.*

· There is a morbid condition of the stomach and bowels described by the late Dr. James Johnson, which is very often mistaken, both in India and in England, for hepatic enlargement or other diseases; it is a mistake of consequence, inasmuch as the disorder is one of frequent occurrence, and the treatment usually employed, on the supposition of its hepatic origin, is very injurious to health.

· In both cases there is tenderness of the right side and epigastrium, increased by pressure, but here the resemblance ceases. There are, in the affection described by Dr. Johnson, none of the other symptoms characteristic of hepatic disease, and the tumidness, besides the difference in anatomical position and somatic relations to other organs, wants both the appearance and solid character of the real hepatic enlargement. Abdominal tumors, such as morbid growths of the omentum or peritoneum, and fæcal accumulations in the cæcum or ·colon, are occasional sources of mistake; but the situation and fleeting character of such tumours, together with the occasional and spasmodic nature of the attendant pain will, in general, point to the true nature of the case. In this state of the stomach and bowels there will generally be found a red, inflamed, or excoriated state of the tongue, gums, and fauces, indicating a highly irritable condition of the mucous digestive surface, the nervous system being much excited. There is occasionally, also, a continuous acceleration of the pulse, while at other times irregular attacks of feverishness occur, preceded by rigors, and followed by irritable dyspepsy.

Purgatives are borne with great distress, especially when of an acrid nature; and calomel, so often resorted to for the cure of the supposed liver disease, is but rasping the already inflamed or irritated mucous membrane of the stomach and bowels, so as frequently to produce discharges of blood and mucus, with great aggravation of all the symptoms.

Grievous, then, as are the errors of *omission* noticed in the article on hepatitis, where acute disease of the most dangerous nature is allowed to proceed undetected, and fruitful as they are in calamity, they are not surpassed in result by the errors of *commission* in chronic affections, where mercury, bleeding, and drastic

---

* Gentlemen who think that they may hurry through so important an examination, would do well to recal to memory the following very elementary facts :—

1. The superior limit of the liver should in health correspond with the line of the fifth rib (some say below the sixth), or about two inches below the right nipple.

2. The inferior border of the liver should correspond with the margin of the ribs.

purgatives are quite as injurious to health as they are necessary
to save life in the first-mentioned instance; in fact, there are no
mistakes more detrimental, nor any against which the inexperienced should be more on his guard, than the two here mentioned.
In my experience, however, such errors in diagnosis do not arise
so much from want of knowledge as from a careless and hasty
manner of examining the patient—an unpardonable negligence in
exploration.

The treatment of this disease is not well understood. Mercury
I believe to be improper: it injures the stomach and bowels,
already but too often over-drugged, without exciting any secretion
from the organ chiefly affected, and on which this mineral, from
repeated use, has lost its influence; indeed, in the great majority
of instances, the system is in a cachectic state, so as to render
mercury on any account inadmissible. Purgatives of an irritating
or drastic nature are especially injurious; in fact, it is often an
unmanageable disease, not readily amenable to treatment or
change of climate. It must be borne in mind that I am here
treating only of simple chronic enlargement of the liver unaccompanied by plethora, general or local, or by inflammation of the
gland. Where such tendencies exist, or where general or local abdominal congestion is present, antiphlogistic means must be used,
followed by the persevering application of the nitro-muriatic acid
bath.

This bath is the plan of cure that I have had recourse to for
many years past, both in India and at home. Like mercury, it
seems to act powerfully on both the excretory and absorbent
systems; and in the cases here under review, it acts with a power
and efficiency superior to any other remedy that I have used, or
that I have ever seen used.

If we admit absorption by the capillary veins and the absor-
bents, and their conveyance of substances rejected by the lacteals
directly into the vena portæ, to be transmitted to the liver, there
to "undergo a true and proper digestion, a hepatic digestion which
is as real as that effected in the stomach and duodenum," we shall
be at no loss to account for the powerful influence of medicinal
agents exhibited in the manner of the acid bath.

When from morbid dryness of skin the acid is not readily taken
up, I direct the occasional use of the vapour bath, or the warm-
water bath, with powerful friction to the whole surface, in order to
restore the exhaling and absorbing actions, always suspended or
suppressed in this disease, and, generally, with a view to stimulate
all the functions of the skin.

Out of many cases treated by me with success while in India, I
will select one of the earliest and worst. It was that of a gentleman of the Civil Service who had resided ten years in India, and
who had suffered three years previous to the illness now described
from a dangerous attack of remittent fever. The details are in the

words of the patient, a preferable mode when the sufferer is a
person of education; because we daily observe, with Gooch, that
"such is the nature of the human mind that cases *for* a precon-
ceived opinion are retained easier than those *against* it." Were
the example of Sir A. Cooper and others followed in this particular,
medical cases would stand better, and carry more weight with the
profession as authentic evidence.

"In November, 1829, I arrived in Calcutta, suffering from a
jungle fever contracted at Chittagong; my liver and spleen were
perceptibly enlarged, my limbs were much swollen, and so stiff
that I could with difficulty walk, and the least exertion occasioned
vomiting. Before my arrival at the Presidency, I had for many
months taken medicine. This plan was altered, and I was put
through a course of the nitric acid bath, taking a vapour bath every
other night for the first week. The nitric acid bath acted in a few
days very powerfully immediately on using it, and in about three
weeks both the liver and spleen could no longer be felt, nor did
pressure give me much uneasiness; the stiffness, too, disappeared,
and my skin became less tense and dry. I took an aperient
draught twice a week, and nothing else but the bath. I left Calcutta
in the end of December for Simla, and had little or no occasion
for medicine for two years afterwards, my general health being
completely restored."

This was a case of extreme and urgent danger :—there was
enormous enlargement of both liver and spleen; so much so that,
on using any drink, if the patient walked across the room the movement caused the fluid to pour from his mouth. There were ascites
and universal anasarca ; and, altogether, the case was regarded as
of a very hopeless nature.

In the cold season of 1838, this same gentleman again visited
Calcutta in a peculiar state of disease. There was an unnatural
dryness or suspended function of the surface of the body and of
the mucous intestinal membrane, with a doughy enlargement of
the abdomen, swelling of the hands and feet, and obstinate consti-
patiou, his excretions from the bowels being deficient in bile, pasty,
and peculiarly dry. He brought the following report from the
surgeon of his station :—

"Arrived at this station in January, 1836, in tolerable health.
During the cold season the digestive organs were much deranged,
with loss of appetite, obstinate constipation, distension, and hardness of the epigastrium, particularly after meals, acidity, and flatulence. The complexion was sallow and pale, and occasionally he
complained of a dull heavy pain in the right hypochondrium.
These symptoms continued till the cold season of 1837, when some
improvement took place; but on the return of the hot season all
the former symptoms recurred with increased violence, accompanied by excruciating headache, which for the time utterly incapacitated him from attending to the important duties of his office.

Towards the termination of the rains, the hands and feet began to assume a dropsical appearance; and for many months he was compelled to take drastic purgatives almost every day, without which no movement of the bowels could be effected."

Regarding the case now, as one of well-marked and extreme torpor of the liver, I directed the patient to go through a course of the nitro-muriatic acid bath, and vapour bath, as before, administering mild saline aperients. Presently the skin began to soften, the tumidness of the abdomen to subside; and with these symptoms, a more ready action of the bowels, so that, in about a month, a fourth part of his original dose acted as an aperient; and before he left Calcutta for the Cape of Good Hope, the bowels were for the first time during two years moved without purgatives, the discharges having become copious, dark, and pitchy;—in other words, the first outpourings of a long pent-up liver. This was a case of peculiar interest from its severity, "calomel, alternate courses of blue-pill, combined with purgatives and ipecacuanha, and strong irritating medicines," having, in the language of the surgeon's report, "utterly failed of doing any good."

In the chronic enlargement of the liver, change of air and of climate should never be omitted in the treatment. We have, in the protracted stages of tropical diseases, indeed, no adequate substitute for change of air. "In India," says Sir James M'Grigor, "when patients, whose condition of life permits them to take a voyage to Europe, are in this state of disease, they never fail to take it, and most commonly are recovered by it; but there is no hope for the poor soldier or sailor."

It is so likewise in the latter stages of fevers and dysenteries; and Dr. James Johnson, speaking of the sufferers from the latter disease, in our fleets and armies, says: "they waste away and die for want of the only remedy that possibly could arrest the hand of death—change of climate."

The distinction so feelingly pointed to by the eminent men just named, as between the seaman and soldier and his officer, has been partially removed in respect of the British soldier serving in the East Indies. The distinction, I repeat, is unjustifiable in principle, as it is cruel and barbarous in results; and I trust the day may not be distant which shall see both classes treated alike in their diseases. On any medical, moral, or just financial grounds, the distinction is, I think, unwarrantable. The natural affections —the desire to return home to see once more their families and friends—to recount to them their sufferings and escapes—to share in honours and rewards—these feelings are as strong with the peasant as the peer.

As in the articles on fever and dysentery, I conclude the present one with a table exhibiting the geography of hepatic diseases, furnished me by Sir Alexander Tulloch. It shows that though diseases of the liver are somewhat more frequent in the south of India,

they are more fatal in Bengal. It is remarkable in the geography
of this disease that, though there exists so great an apparent similarity between the climates of the eastern and western hemispheres,
there should yet be so great a dissimilarity of result in the comparative influence on the European constitution:—in the East
Indies generally, Annesley states that thirteen per cent. of the
effective strength of British regiments are attacked with hepatic
disease, while, according to Sir Alexander Tulloch's reports, but
2⅛ per cent. of the effective strength in the Windward and Leeward Command, and one per cent. only in Jamaica, are similarly
affected.

STATIONS.	Period of observation.	Aggregate strength.	Inflammation of the liver and jaundice.		
			Attacked.	Died.	Proportion of deaths to admissions.
Windward and Leeward Command...............	20 years......	86,661	1946	161	1 in 12
Jamaica	20 ,,	51,567	539	51	1 in 11
Gibraltar......................	19 ,,	60,269	759	22	1 in 34
Malta	20 ,,	40,826	857	47	1 in 18
Ionian Islands...............	20 ,,	70,293	1168	58	1 in 20
Bermudas......................	20 ,,	11,721	168	6	1 in 38
Nova Scotia and New Brunswick	20 ,,	46,442	384	10	1 in 38⅔
Canada.........................	20 ,,	64,280	488	12	1 in 40⅔
Western Africa	18 ,,	1,843	150	11	1 in 14
Cape of Good Hope	19 ,,	22,714	496	25	1 in 20
St. Helena	9 ,,	8,973	171	24	1 in 7
Mauritius......................	19 ,,	30,515	2508	122	1 in 20¼
Ceylon	20 ,,	42,978	4382	213	1 in 11
Tenasserim Provinces......	10 ,,	6,818	488	29	1 in 17
Madras.......................	5 ,,	31,627	3372	190	1 in 17¾
Bengal	5 ,,	38,136	2412	174	1 in 14
Bombay	5 ,,	17,612	1084	62	1 in 17½

There died in London, according to the reports of the Registrar-
General, during the fifteen years, 1840-1854, of the specified hepatic diseases as follow, and doubtless a goodly proportion of them
had their origin in the influences of tropical climates :—

Hepatitis.   Jaundice.   Disease of liver.
2270 . . . . 2091 7914   =   Total 12,275.

ON THE ENDEMIC CONGESTION OF THE SPLEEN.

CONSIDERING the frequency and fatality of splenic affections, amongst soldiers especially, both European and native, and amongst the European inhabitants of our intertropical possessions, it has always been matter of surprise that so little attention has been bestowed by the profession on the consideration of diseases of the spleen. But when we look to our imperfect knowledge of the anatomy and physiology of this organ, we shall cease to wonder that naval and military surgeons have refrained from disquisitions on what could only result, at the best, but in unprofitable speculation, and confined their attention more particularly to the cognate affections of the liver.

Mr. Gray, of St. George's Hospital, the most recent and most successful investigator of the structure and uses of the spleen, considers that the organ " serves to balance alike the *quantity* and the *quality* of the blood, and is especially adapted for this function by its connexion with that part of the vascular system which is concerned in the introduction of new material into the circulation."*

Mr. Gray, from numerous experiments, has come to the conclusion "that the weight of the spleen *increases considerably* during the time when the digestive process is near to its completion, at the time when the new material is about to be, or has become, converted into blood; and that it *decreases considerably* in weight at varying periods *after* that process has been finally completed." This conclusion, says Dr. Carpenter, is confirmed by the results of experiments upon highly-fed and upon insufficiently-fed animals of the same species; for the increase during digestion was carried in the former to an unusual degree, so as to give the organ more than twice its former weight, whilst in the latter no increase after feeding was observable.

The distinguished reviewer concludes :—" We are inclined to believe that the office of the *colourless* parenchyma of the spleen is not only to serve as a storehouse for the surplus albumen that finds its way into the circulation on the completion of the digestive process, but also to exert an *assimilating* action upon it, whereby it is rendered more fit for the nutrition of the tissues; and of this assimilating action we deem the generation of fibrine to be one of the results. And if it be true, as we have elsewhere suggested, that one special function of red corpuscles is to assimilate or prepare that peculiar combination of materials which is required for the nutrition of the nervo-muscular apparatus, the disintegration of these corpuscles in the splenic parenchyma may answer the two-

* Review by Dr. Carpenter, "Brit. and For. Med.-Chir. Rev." for January, 1855.

fold purpose of regulating their total proportion in the mass of the blood, and of diffusing through the liquor-sanguinis the materials which the nervous and muscular tissues are to draw from it for their own development." If such be the functions of the spleen, we can readily perceive how diseases of that organ may, and actually do, spoil the blood, and produce a state of general cachexia.

The tumid or turgid spleen—the congestive enlargement—as it appears in Europeans who have resided in low marshy districts in Bengal, or as it comes under observation in hospital among the children of indigent Europeans, and as seen in British soldiers who have campaigned in unhealthy countries, appears to consist in passive congestion, or hyperæmia of that organ, and is found in its most severe forms during the cold season. It may, and does, occur as a primary disease, the result of mere residence in malarious localities, but far more generally congestion of the spleen is found, in India at least, as a complication of, and à sequel to fevers, remittent and intermittent, and especially in their adynamic types, as on the West Coast of Africa, Walcheren, parts of Italy, Aracan, and other malarious countries in the East. When complicated with endemic fevers, it may be regarded as in its more acute stage; but with the subsidence of the primary disease, this condition gives place to that of passive congestion, or simple hypertrophy. Why the worse term "engorgement" was preferred by Mr. Twining to the more truly expressive and old one, congestion, does not appear; but certain it is that the altered form of expression has in no way added to, or improved, our knowledge of the obscure pathology of congestion, whether of the spleen or of any other organ. In the medical, as in other sciences, terms ought not to be changed, unless they express relations established as certain which have not been determined before; whereas here we have but a distinction in words without any difference in fact. A German phraseology, now too much in use at home, threatens to become a fashion with us, overlaying our terse and manly language, while it is but ill calculated to fill up the voids in our knowledge. The Germans have reduced the art of talking about disease to a system.

In the fevers of the West Indies, Robert Jackson found that the spleen was " generally distended, sometimes even to rupture."

Hyperæmia and a softening of the spleen are found also to be very general complications in the congestive typhoid fevers of our own country, and of those of the continent of Europe—the fact being demonstrated in the most extensive *post-mortem* examinations.

SYMPTOMS.

In the more acute form of the disease we have present some febrile action—a sense of dull pain in the left hypochondrium, extending to the shoulder of that side, accompanied by fulness and increased uneasiness on pressure—all indicative of something more than mere vascular engorgement—the disturbance of the abdominal functions being referrible to congestive fever, and to its splenic complication.   The symptoms of splenic diseases, whether acute or subacute, are always more or less negative in character. Whether this form of splenic enlargement be the result of fever, or the more gradual influence of malaria, it is a very important affection, owing to the unfavourable state of the constitution which invariably accompanies it.   As a complication with fever, too, it is unfavourable in itself, and as putting an instant bar to the use of mercury, however desirable the exhibition of that mineral might prove, as a means of equalizing the circulation—of eliciting increased secretions—or of relieving local congestions in other organs.

To the practised eye, the very countenance of the sufferer bespeaks his condition.   The expression is dull, the mind apathetic ; the complexion is of a dirty lemon-colour, the integument being puffed up and bloated, the eye pale, and of a peculiar clearness, the lips, tongue, and fauces blanched and bloodless ; in short, we have here a concentration of cachexia of systematic writers—the very type and essence of anæmia.   A wound or trifling abrasion, which at another time would escape notice, now becomes a foul and sloughing-ulcer, owing to the depraved state of the blood, and the generally diseased state of the system :—hæmorrhages arise from slight causes—sometimes spontaneously ; and so altered is the character of the blood—from want of red globules apparently— that when performing surgical operations of immediate necessity, at the Native Hospital of Calcutta, I always became aware of the presence of splenic disease on making my first incision—the hue of the blood being demonstrative of the fact.

In addition to the depravation of the fluids, we have excessive muscular debility, bodily inertness, and mental despondency— the whole morbid assemblage tending to impair the functions of respiration, assimilation, and secretion.   It can be matter of no surprise, therefore, that when fatal terminations occur, they should be preceded by dropsies, hæmorrhages, or gangrenous ulcers of the cheeks and gums—conditions to which persons suffering from splenic disease are peculiarly liable.

CAUSES.

Of all the known causes of splenic disease, the most influential is malaria.   The long-continued application of the ordinary endemic influences, without causing acute disease of any kind, will, as already observed, produce anæmia, enlargement of the liver, of the spleen, and of the mesenteric glands.   But the most ordinary cause of splenic congestion, whether active or passive, will always be found in the malarious fevers of the East—remittent and intermittent—which, for longer or shorter periods, and by the recurrenees of their cold or congestive stages, for months or years together—disturb, or eventually destroy, the balance of the abdominal circulation, and with it the integrity of the abdominal functions.

When to these morbid conditions we add destitution—the absence of comfort in food and clothing—the residence in low, cold, and damp localities—mental depression—those causes, in short, which contaminate the blood, and determine its flow into the abdominal organs ; all these causes will powerfully tend to the production of splenic disease. Previous inflammation and acute congestion are often found in India to terminate in chronic enlargement of the spleen.

PATHOLOGY.

" Dr. Henoch of Berlin recognises two forms of chronic enlargement of the spleen. The most common form is a true *hypertrophy*, a mere increase of the natural elements of the organ. In a large number of cases, however, he considers the enlargement is due to excessive interstitial exudation of plasma, probably of a character unfit for healthy nutrition, and he consequently regards this kind of tumour as the result of chronic splenitis."*

The appearances on dissection vary from the firm and friable condition—congestion with fibrous hypertrophy—to the indurated and banded texture approaching to scirrhus—the degree of enlargement varying according to the intensity of the malarious and other external influences, and to the duration of the disease. The substance of the spleen is often found of a dark purple on being cut into, and composed chiefly of granular matter. Dr. Sieveking found crystals interposed among the granular matter, which were soluble in acetic acid ; also yellow spots with tuberculous-like deposits.

In the softened spleen we find its substance reduced to the condition of a grumous mass, indicating a diseased state of the constituents of the blood. Thickening of the investment and adhesions of it to that of the surrounding parts, are more generally found in the native than in the European subject.

There is reason to conclude that endocarditis is a frequent and serious concomitant of the more active diseases of the spleen, inflammation of the interior lining membrane of the heart, together with vegetations on the aorta and valves, coagula, and other appearances demonstrative alike of endocarditis and of a diseased condition of the blood, being often observable after death. I have no doubt that the numerous sudden deaths of both Europeans and natives of the army of Aracan, in the first Burmese war, during apparent convalescence, arose from the causes just noticed ; the fever which destroyed the army having been a malignant adynamic intermittent. Sudden deaths from the same causes are found to occur in yellow fever.

* Dr. Ballard, "Brit. and For. Rev." for July, 1855.

· Infarctions of the spleen occur much more frequently as the results of intermittent than of remittent fevers, and in the latter than in typhus.   According to Dr. Tebault of Virginia, the presence of enlarged spleen gives to typhoid fever a paroxysmal character.

TREATMENT.

In splenic congestion of recent occurrence, *where the system is sound*, and exhibits an inflammatory action, or an acute state of congestion, whether of the abdominal vessels generally, or of those of the spleen, a moderate blood-letting, general or local, repeated according to occasion, and followed by brisk cathartics and sudorifics, will conduce powerfully towards convalescence.   On the cure of the fever, indeed, we shall generally find that the splenic complication will subside; but if tumidness of that organ still remain, by the continued exhibition of quinine and brisk purgatives, followed by chalybeates and change of air, congestions, both general and local, will be removed.   But, on the other hand, if the type of the fever be adynamic, and the state of the general health anæmic, opposite and tonic remedies must be used ; every indication of cure resting on the two radical conditions—the local or endemic influence existing at the time, and the sanitary condition of the individual.

Within a few years of my arrival in India, I suffered severely from the dangerous remittent fever of Gondwana, followed by malignant, adynamic intermittent.   For the recovery of my health, I was sent to Calcutta, where, notwithstanding the best advice and care, ague recurred twice or thrice every month during a year and a half, when I was ordered to sea.   There was then enlargement of the spleen with œdema of the lower extremities.   I made a voyage to sea, and was absent but eight months from Bengal ; and although I used not one grain of medicine, all my ailments disappeared.   The truth is, that there are fevers, dysenteries, and chronic forms of hepatic and splenic disease, of malarious origin, which no amount of medicine *can* cure, but which change of air *will* cure with some degree of certainty.

When the more acute local symptoms have subsided, and the disease has become a simple chronic enlargement, we still find that no corresponding improvement takes place in the health ; and in general, according to the duration of the disease and the size of the spleen, so do we find a complicated parabysma and the consequent cachectic state to prevail; softening and relaxation being prevalent in the nervous, vascular, and glandular structures. Again, we occasionally see cases where enormous spleens, occupying two-thirds of the abdominal cavity, cause but surprisingly little disturbance of the health apparently—the patient complaining only of sense of weight in the left hypochondrium ; but this state of passive toleration does not last long, the general health being sure to suffer in the end; while in other cases, and with varying degrees, we have all the unfavourable disorders of the system already described as concomitants of the more acute stages of splenic disease. When the disease seizes upon the children of indigent Europeans, who are unable to command change of air or removal to Europe, we find every function in life—the development of the mental faculties—the building up of the corporeal frame—every constituent part stunted and retarded in growth; and without any precocity in youth, there is an actual precocity of old age.

In the chronic enlargement of the spleen, measures of depletion can but very seldom be required; and even those of a local nature should be used but sparingly. The general practice in Bengal is a steady use of the tonic aperient of Mr. Shulbred, formerly surgeon to the Native Hospital of Calcutta, aiding its operation by quinine, chalybeates, stimulant and rubefacient liniments to the affected region, and change of air. The formula of Mr. Shulbred, and the watery imitation of it by Mr. Twining, are as given below:—

MR. SHULBRED.	MR. TWINING.
Pulveris Jalapæ,	Pulveris Jalapæ,
,, Rhei,	,, Rhei,
,, Calumbæ,	,, Calumbæ,
,, Scammoniæ,	,, Zingiberis,
Potassæ Bitartrat. aa ʒj.	Potassæ Bitartrat. aa ʒj.
Ferri Sulphatis, ʒss.	Ferri Sulphatis, Əj.
	Tinct. Sennæ, ʒiv.
	Aq. Menth. Sativæ, ʒx.

Of Mr. Shulbred's powder a sufficiency is given to move the bowels twice or thrice daily. It has for half a century been a favourite remedy in Bengal; and Mr. Twining's formula is given to those who prefer the fluid manner of exhibition. He recommends a chalybeate with purgative extract overnight, followed in the morning by powder of myrobalan and the black salt of the bazaar;—this as a change of treatment. The kala-nimuk, or black salt of the bazaars throughout India, is composed of the following ingredients in one ounce:—

Muriate of soda	444 grains.
Sulphur	14 ,,
Muriate of lime	12 ,,
Black oxide of iron	6 ,,

The natives have long been aware of the beneficial effects of acids as well as of chalybeates and bitters in the treatment of the common tumid spleen, for which the bazaar doctors prescribe the undiluted sulphuric acid in doses of one drop at a time placed on a bit of plantain, or more generally five drops in cold water night and morning. Another native plan of treatment is by a mixture of aloes, vinegar, and garlic with a small portion of the bazaar sulphate of iron, " kuzees :"—this latter formula is said to be very successful. The decoction of the seed of the *Carum nigrum*, with the addition of acetic acid or lime-juice, is also used by the natives, and it is said with a marked benefit.

I found, in treating both Europeans and natives, that severe irritation of the mucous digestive surface was often present, attended by a low irritative form of fever.   Here the spleen medicines in ordinary use were altogether inadmissible, as causing increase of irritation or dangerous diarrhœa.   In such cases, and they were of frequent occurrence, after subduing intestinal irritation, I had recourse to pure chalybeates, as the saccharated carbonate of iron, the muriated tincture of iron with tincture of iodine, frictions with croton oil, warm baths, &c.   In this manner cases having a very unpromising appearance recovered; and the largest spleen I ever saw was cured by the iodide of lead internally administered.   It was that of an European boy in poor circumstances.   His health had been much reduced by an eruptive fever, when he was seized with ague, for neither of which diseases had he any treatment : the consequence was enormous enlargement of the spleen, and for which the iodide of lead alone was used, internally and externally.   The treatment was continued mildly for four months, when the spleen was no longer to be felt; and during the whole process of cure he never took so much as one aperient.   The enlargement in this case had come on very suddenly, but when I first saw the patient it had existed during several months.

In the case of a gentleman from Demerara, treated by me in consultation with Mr. Henry James Johnson of London, and in whose management we had to contend with extreme cachexia and sloughing ulceration of the penis, the iodide of lead was persisted in for two months, to the extent, indeed, of producing lead colic, when the spleen, previously of enormous bulk, was reduced to the natural size.   Iodide of potassium, warm baths, gestation in the open air, stimulating frictions to the affected region, are all beneficial ; but in the chronic enlargement of the spleen, with cachectic states of the system, blisters are apt to slough; and as to leeches and mercurials in such instances, they are most destructive—generally certain death.

In Europeans the liver is very often involved in disease along with the spleen, and then there is no remedy which, in my experience, can at all be compared in power and efficacy to the persevering use of the nitro-muriatic acid bath, using the combined acids internally at the same time with bitter infusions, and keeping the bowels freely open.   Here, owing to the hepatic complication, quinine and chalybeates prove ineffective to the cure of the splenic, while they injure the hepatic disease.   At pages 495–6 will be seen a remarkable instance of rapid cure, by the acid bath, of enormous disease in both liver and spleen associated with universal dropsy.   It was . one of the earliest cases treated by me after this manner, and I regard it as one of much interest and importance.

A practical fact of some importance, and which I found to take place in India as in this country, is this—that the acid bath acts more speedily and with far greater power in the hotter than in the colder months. Following out the suggestion afforded by this fact, I always directed the use of a warm-water or vapour bath twice or thrice a week at the commencement of the treatment in the winter months, with the view to open and purify the pores of the skin, and to increase its absorbent and exhaling functions.

It is almost unnecessary to urge the necessity of attention to the diet in every stage of this disease. So long as heat of skin or any febrile movement exists, the diet must be of the lightest and easiest of digestion, being limited to articles of a farinaceous nature; and even in the chronic stage animal food should be used but once in the twenty-four hours.

Some eminent French physicians have used large doses of quinine for the cure of enlarged spleen, exhibiting the salt to the extent of from forty to eighty grains in the twenty-four hours, the quantity of the drug used being in direct ratio to the extent of the disease. When the stomach did not retain the large doses exhibited, the Continental doctors administered the quinine in the form of enemata carefully retained in the bowel. Dr. Elliotson, in his lectures, recommends a similar plan of treatment; but I am not aware that this mode of cure has been anywhere established on the foundations of success. From all I have personally observed and studied I am disposed to look mainly to the emulgent plan by nitro-muriatic acid, internally and externally applied, for the cure of splenic diseases, aided and followed by purgatives, quinine, and chalybeates. This important subject is recommended to the careful attention of our intertropical practitioners; recollecting that "some of the greatest improvements in medicine have resulted from researches made in hot climates, and that there is not a single fact observed or a single disease investigated on the banks of the Ganges or the Mississippi that does not bring its quota of utility to the practice of medicine in our own country."

The following table but ill represents the prevalence of splenic diseases in any of the military commands specified, such affections being too often "lumped under the head of other diseases." I have been unable to procure any returns for the three Presidencies of India; and in the naval force in the East Indies, forming an aggregate strength, from 1830-43, of 40,512 men, only thirty-nine cases are returned under the head of splenitis.

We may nowhere hope to find any record of the splenic complications of fever and dysentery, although these last form together by far the most prevalent forms of the disease.

STATIONS.	Period of observation (inclusively.)	Aggregate strength.	Number admitted into hospital.	Number died.	Proportion of deaths to admissions.
Windward and Leeward Command	1817—36	86,661	104	3	1 in 34
Jamaica	1817—36	51,567	59	...	0 in 59
Bahamas	1817—36	535	5	...	0 in 5
Honduras	1822—36	320			
United Kingdom (Dragoon Gds. & Dragoons	1830—36	44,611	5	...	0 in 5
Gibraltar	1818—36	60,269	21	...	0 in 21
Malta	1817—38	40,826	21	...	1 in 10¼
Ionian Islands	1817—36	70,293	133	4	1 in 33¼
Bermudas	1817—36	11,721	2	...	0 in 2
Nova Scotia and New Brunswick	1817—36	46,442	19	...	0 in 19
Canadas	1817—36	64,280	25	...	0 in 25
Western Africa	1819—36	1,843	166	7	1 in 23¾
St. Helena	1818—21 / 1836—37 (6 yrs.)	5,908	1	...	0 in 1
Cape of Good Hope (Cape District)	1818—36	22,714	49	...	0 in 49
Cape of Good Hope (Eastern Frontier)	1822—34	6,630	5	...	0 in 5
Mauritius	1818—36	30,515	17	...	0 in 17
Ceylon	1817—36	42,978	50	...	0 in 50

In the very able report of a committee assembled by order of the Governor-General of India, to ascertain whether the Great Ganges Canal, which now unites. the Ganges and the Jumna, would tend to increase disease, and thus prove not a blessing but a curse to the inhabitants, we find a test proposed by my friend, Mr. T. E. Dempster, which seems to yield positive and satisfactory conclusions, and the value of which appears to have been fully established. Mr. Dempster examined the spleen in a certain number of individuals, and by the presence or absence of an enlargement, he determined whether or not the resident in a certain locality had previously suffered from endemic fever. The following table contains a summary of the whole inquiry.* It will be observed that in each subdivision of the table, the smallest number of spleens and the corresponding small number of previous fever cases, occur in the inverse ratio of the proximity to the river or the canal.

* "Brit. and For. Med.-Chir. Rev." for October, 1855, pp. 353-54.

			Per-centage of enlarged spleens. Adults and children of all classes.	Per-centage of adults suffering from fever.			Average depth of water from surface of ground, in feet.	
				1844.	1845.	1846.		
Irrigated from the Western Jumna canals.	Delhi branch	Within half a mile of the canal	58	51	45	41	11	
		Distant more than half a mile	49	51	49	40	18	
	Rohtuk banch	Within half a mile of the canal	44	47	38	27	28	
		Distant more than half a mile	29	34	34	27	48	
	Bootana branch	Distant more than half a mile	16	41	36	22	102	
	Hansi branch	Within half a mile of the canal	39	50	41	22	92	
		Distant more than half a mile	18	40	31	16	118	
	Northern division	Within half a mile of the canal	20	27	39	27	8	
		Distant more than half a mile	22	37	47	30	13	
Irrigated from the Eastern Jumna canals.	Central division	Within half a mile of the canal	59	63	54	31	8	
		Distant more than half a mile	47	60	53	33	14	
	Southern division	Within half a mile of the canal	35	48	40	17	24	
		Distant more than half a mile	18	47	30	14	34	
	Irrigated from wells in the high land of the Dooab		8	37	31	20	24	
	Sikh states	Connected with the canal	44	47	52	26	0	
		Unconnected with the canal	29	43	61	30	0	
	Delhi territory	Unconnected with the canal	11	32	28	11	88	
Uninrrigated.	Northern Dooab	High or bungor land*	3	32	30	13	46	
		Ganges khadir†	21	41	42	28	25	
		Near head of Eastern Jumna canal	6	35	43	27	0	
	Naturally malarious localities	Nujufgurh jheels‡	44	42	59	57	15	
		Valleys of Jumna and Hindun	34	46	42	31	14	

* Bungor : The high and firm bank of the river bounding the khadir.
† Khadir is the belt of moist, low, and often fertile land found alternately on one or other side of large rivers in these provinces. During the rainy season much of this land is submerged, and in it the river frequently alters its channel.
‡ Jheels ; Shallow pools of water, often very extensive during the rainy season.

EPIDEMIC CHOLERA.

FROM the contemporaneous writings of Hippocrates and the Chinese physicians, as well as from those of the later Hindu and Roman medical authors, it is evident that epidemic cholera was well known and accurately described in their respective times.

The first notice of this disease we have by an European writer is that of Bontius, physician to the Dutch East India Company, and who wrote in 1629, in Batavia. " The cholera morbus," he says, " is extremely frequent: in the cholera, hot. bilious matter, irritating the stomach and intestines, is incessantly and copiously discharged by the mouth and anus. It is a disorder of the most acute kind, and therefore requires immediate application." In its severer form " the animal spirits" are described as speedily " *ex- hausted, and the heart, the fountain of heat and life, is overwhelmed with putrid effluvia ; those who are seized with this disorder generally die, and that so quickly, as in the space of four-and-twenty hours at most. This disease is attended with a weak pulse, difficult respiration, and coldness of the extreme parts: to which are joined great internal heat, insatiable thirst, perpetual watching, and restless and incessant tossing of the body. If, together with these symptoms, a cold and fetid sweat should break forth, it is certain that death is at hand.*" Bontius treats of the " cholera morbus" and " spasm" as separate diseases ; yet it is presumed that both were frequently united, and that, in reality the spasm was a common complication with cholera, as indeed he describes it in the case of Cornelius Van Royen, who " was suddenly seized with the cholera, about six in the even- ing, and expired in terrible agony and convulsions before twelve o'clock at night."

I shall now lay before the reader, in as condensed a form as possible, the results of inquiry instituted by order of the Govern- ments and medical authorities of Bengal, Madras, and Bombay, with a view to obtain the best possible information as to the his- tory, nature, and cure of epidemic cholera. It was thus that they endeavoured to discover what noxious agencies were to be avoided, and how nature could be assisted.

How ably the medical services of the three Presidencies re- sponded to this call, need not now be pointed out ; neither is it necessary to dwell on the original merits of the author of the " Essay on the Influence of Tropical Climates on European Con- stitutions," further than by stating, on the authority of Dr. Cop- land, that " the nature and treatment of the disease were very imperfectly known, until Dr. James Johnson described its symptoms, and pointed out a more successful method of cure than had previously been employed."

In the reports of the medical boards of Bengal, Madras, and Bombay we find the following notices :—

BENGAL REPORT.

1781. In March of this year a disease, in all respects resembling the recent epidemic cholera, seized on the Bengal force under Colonel Pearse of the Artillery, while marching through the Northern Circars to join Sir Eyre Coote's army. Seven hundred men died within the first few days, and three hundred convalescents were left behind ; this out of an original force of five thousand men.

"Men in perfect health dropt down by dozens : and those even less severely affected were generally dead, or past recovery, within less than an hour. Spasms of the extremities and trunk were dreadful ; and distressing vomiting and purging were present in all."

1783. Cholera is said to have broken out at the sacred bathing spot of Hurdwar on the Ganges, in April of this year. It happened to be one of the twelfth years deemed peculiarly propitious by the Hindus, and the assemblage of pilgrims was consequently far beyond the common annual average, amounting, it is said, this year, to nearly two millions.

"The disease broke out on the springing up of an easterly land-wind during the night, and carried off innumerable persons." In less than eight days, twenty thousand victims are said to have fallen ; yet so confined was its influence, that it did not extend beyond the place of bathing, and ceased on the dispersion of the multitude.

1790. In the middle of April of this year, a fatal cholera of the spasmodic form attacked the detachment under Colonel Cockerell, marching from Bengal to Seringapatam, in the same country in which it had previously proved so fatal to the

MADRAS REPORT.

1774. The "true cholera morbus" is described by Dr. Paisley of Madras as being "often epidemic" amongst the natives, whom it destroyed quickly. In the first campaigns, it proved very fatal to both the European and native troops. He describes it as "operating on the system as a poison, and brings on a sudden prostration of strength, and spasm over the whole surface of the body." The pulse he found to "sink suddenly, and bring on immediate danger."

Sonnerat speaks of "an epidemic disorder which reigns" on the Coromandel coast, and his observations embrace the period from 1774 to 1781.

After describing the symptoms, and that the poorer and more negligent classes are most obnoxious to its seizure, he states that "above sixty thousand people from Cherigan to Pondicherry perished." "The Indian physicians," he says, "could not save a single person."

One epidemic is described as peculiarly severe. "Those who were attacked had thirty evacuations in five or six hours, which reduced them to such a state of weakness that they could neither speak nor move.

"*They were often without pulse; the hands and ears were cold ; the face lengthened ; the sinking of the cavity of the socket of the eye was the sign of death ; they felt neither pain in the stomach, colics, nor gripings. The greatest pain was a burning thirst.*"

1787. A disease is reported as prevalent this year at Arcot, "similar to an epidemic that raged amongst the natives about Palicola, and in the army of observation in January of 1783, in the Bengal detachment at Ganjam in 1781, and several other places at different times.

The characteristic marks were spasms of the praecordia and sudden prostration of strength.

The treatment consisted of stimulants and hot baths, supporting the vis-vitæ.

1782-90. During this period, cholera under various names, but always with the same symptoms and results, would seem to have prevailed in various parts of India.

"The mort de chien, or cramp," pre-

force under Colonel Pearse—the Northern Circars.

̄ The above three notices, two of which refer to seizures beyond the bounds of the Bengal Presidency, are all of which any record could be obtained by the talented author of the Calcutta Report. Rumour, indeed, had spoken of severe cholera in Bundlekund some forty years previously to the date of Mr. Jameson's report, or about the year 1780, and of another some time near the end of the last century; but as no authentic history exists respecting their nature, no attempt is made to trace them.

The Bombay Report enters into no history of epidemic cholera, beyond a casual reference to a letter from Dr. Taylor, who gives an account of a disease, taken from a Sanscrit work, "which leaves very little doubt that it has not only been long known to the natives, but proves its identity."

vailed in Sir Ed. Hughes's fleet in 1782. The sufferers were "*soon brought to great weakness, coldness of the extremities, and a remarkable paleness, sinking and lividity of the whole countenance.*" There was "*great thirst, or rather a strong desire for cold drinks, but there was no headache, or affection of the sensorium commune throughout.*"

From July to September, 1782, Mr. Curtis describes the same disease in the Madras Hospital, and in the fleet.

1782. Mr. Girdlestone describes a disease exactly similar, as destructive to the newly arrived troops from England, more than fifty of whom were carried off by it "within the first three days after they were landed."

1787. Dr. Duffins gives details of the symptoms and treatment of "cholera morbus," which then prevailed at Vellore with great violence—a disease "so rapid in its progress, that many of the men are carried off in twelve hours' illness."

The same epidemic prevailed fatally at Arcot, to which station Mr. Davis, member of the Hospital board, was deputed to investigate its nature. *He understood, from the regimental surgeons, that the last disease had proved fatal to all who had been attacked by it.*"

Mr. Thompson gives a similar account to that of Mr. Davis, both having remarked on the singular contraction and emptiness of the bladder on dissection, it being found no larger than "a walnut."

1814. Two notices of cholera are found in this year—one by Mr. Wyllie of the 24th Regiment, and the other by Mr. Cruickshanks of the 9th Regiment, in which it appeared with great severity.

"The disease in the 9th Regiment, in 1814, resembled in every particular, with exception of the heat at the præcordia, the cholera at present" (1819) "so common, although it could not be called epidemic." It appears to have broken out in a brigade of Native Infantry, while on the march from Jauinah, about the 10th of June. The patients "*exhibited all the symptoms, now so well known, of persons labouring under the ad-*

vanced and fatal stage of the epidemic cholera, the skin cold and covered with a cold perspiration, the extremities shrivelled, cold, and damp, the eyes sunk, fixed, and glassy, and the pulse not to be felt. These persons all died, and I find, on referring to such notes as I have preserved, that, influenced by consideration of the vascular collapse, and total absence of arterial pulsation, I had denominated the disease asphyxia."

The report of Mr. Cruickshanks is peculiarly valuable on many grounds, as well as for an early notice of one of those singular and unaccountable features which it has frequently manifested since, namely, that of the two corps composing the brigade, apparently under similar circumstances, one only was attacked, while the other escaped altogether.

Two distinct and separate notices of the epidemic cholera, one twenty-five years, and the other thirty-four, previously to 1817, are given by Mr. Staff-Surgeon Hay. These visitations were in the Travancore country.

Dr. Burke, also, in a report from the Mauritius in 1819, where he was chief of the medical staff, states that a disease in all respects similar to the recent epidemic is reported to have occurred in that island in the year 1775. "*The symptoms, fatal and sudden effects, and duration of the disease would seem to be the same.*"

It thus appears clearly that epidemic cholera prevailed at various remote periods, and at many of the principal stations throughout British India, sometimes coming as a wide-spread pestilence, and at others desolating only particular localities. That the disease, in its epidemic form, was not altogether unknown to our forefathers in Europe, is rendered more than probable also by the writings of various of the older physicians; and many of the cases described by Sydenham, in 1669, would seem to have been of the true spasmodic nature; but as none of the visitations described by former writers approached in duration, extent, or severity that which took its rise in Bengal in 1817, no detailed record of them is preserved. From the date of its first outbreak on the shores of the Ganges, till in its course it embraced those of the Indus, Euphrates, Nile, Danube, Volga, St. Lawrence, and Mississippi, this great epidemic has visited every nation of the earth, independently of all climates and vicissitudes— bound to no soil—circumscribed or limited by no prevailing wind; and whether it fastened on the delicate frame of the Hindu, or that of the robust European, the disease has been essentially of the same nature, nor have the results of medical treatment differed much. Everywhere throughout Asia, Africa, Europe, and

America it has been thus, no difference of race, climate, or temperature exercising any very marked influence on its nature and
progress.

Condition of life, as in all other epidemics, has everywhere
manifested its vast influence for good or evil; amongst the poorer
classes, in their greater liability to this deadly disease, and
amongst the wealthier classes, in their comparative exemption
from disease and death.

In each and all the countries traversed by this scourge, certain
low, damp situations, filth, destitution, and misery, have exercised
their usually fatal power; while the more comfortable conditions
of life *acted as powerful preventives*.

It was amongst the poor, ill-fed, ill-clothed, and crowded inhabitants of Jessore that epidemic cholera made its first appearance; and it is under similar circumstances, and in similar localities, that the disease has ever since, and in every country, proved
most rife, most virulent, and remained the longest.

The cholera epidemics which have ravaged various parts of
Hindustan since 1817, have always originated *in*, and issued
forth *from* India. They have never, in any instance within my
knowledge, been even supposed to have been imported *into* any of
the ports of India, by ships from infected countries, or through
any other manner of human intercourse. It may therefore be inferred, that the cause of the disease, however latent or submerged
for a time, is never actually absent from the soil of India, or from
some of its localities.

Without disputing the possibility of contagion in cholera, even
in the midst of and notwithstanding the thorough ventilations prevalent throughout India, I am bound to say that, although I may be
said to have lived in the midst of the disease during many years, I
have never seen anything which, in my opinion, warranted the belief; nor have I ever communicated with any Indian medical officer
who believed in the contagiousness of epidemic cholera in India.

In the European General Hospital of Calcutta, in which I
served as assistant-surgeon and surgeon, it was well known that, of
the five native keepers and washers of clothes who had during
twenty-five years kept and washed the hospital clothing, not one
had cholera; nor had those who assisted them. The same immunity attended the native dressers, averaging from twenty to thirty
men, who, during the same number of years, were in constant and
close attendance on the cholera sick all day and all night; nor
were the sweepers who washed and dressed the patients, and
who removed the matters vomited and ejected by stool, ever
affected with cholera.

I served in the General Hospital in March, 1827, the time
referred to by Mr. Twining, when the house was filled with cholera
patients, and when all of us, European as well as Native, including
Native medical students employed for the occasion, were ex-

hansted with the labours of attendance on the sick; but none of us suffered from the disease.

Out of some 250 to 300 medical officers, most of whom saw the disease largely, Mr. Jameson states that only three were attacked, throughout the Presidency of Bengal, and one only of these cases proved fatal. The same circumstance held in the Bengal Fusiliers in 1848, where, according to Dr. Bruce, not one medical attendant, European or Native, " ever showed the least symptom of cholera;" nor was there " even a case of bowel complaint among them," although numbering a hundred persons in constant attendance on the cholera-sick, "from May till September."

To exhibit the epidemic influence, it may be observed, again, that women in their secluded and guarded residences, men secluded in the desert, and others in ships and boats, have been attacked with the disease; while, on the other hand, in all countries, certain villages, and other localities, in unrestrained communication with notoriously infected places, have altogether escaped. The truth would appear to be that cholera, like certain fevers, is ordinarily propagated by other agency than reproduction in the human system, and yet at other times can be so reproduced, and be thus occasionally communicable from person to person; but the latter circumstance is very rare in its history, and, even where the disease is presumptively contagious, it cannot be localized by quarantines.

To these facts many others of the like nature might be added; but, in respect of contagiousness, who shall dispute the possibility of occasional exceptions, under peculiar susceptibilities, and under different circumstances of climate and other contingencies. Contagiousness is a condition difficult to disprove of any disease which spreads epidemically.

GEOGRAPHICAL PROGRESS.*

The epidemic cholera, which originated in the delta of the Ganges, in July, 1817, true to its birthplace, the town of Jessore, with its low, marshy, jungly, crowded, and ill-ventilated conditions, spread rapidly from villages, towns, and cities in no better sanitary state than their prototype; and from that day to the present, epidemic cholera has proved greatly more fatal in Asia than in Europe. In most countries it is said to have shown a marked preference for tertiary and alluvial soils, while it rapidly deserted the ancient formations.

It commenced its march from Bengal in August, 1817,
Reached Bombay . . . 10th August, 1818.
And Astrakan, where it died away, 18th September, 1823.

---

* It will be seen that, in the body of the following article, I have made free use of, and quoted largely from the admirable works of Dr. Farr, of the Registrar-General's office, and from those of Drs. Baly and Gull, framed by desire of the College of Physicians.

In Persia several local epidemics appeared at intervals in the seven years, 1823-30. The great epidemic that traversed Europe is said to have sprung up in June, 1830, on the low western shores of the Caspian Sea. The velocity of the two epidemics only differed in Asia; it was the same in Europe. The epidemics of 1830-31, and of 1848-49, travelled at the same rates westward, as appears from the following table:—

Astrakan . . . . July 20, 1830	June 1847
Moscow. . . . . September, 1830	September 18th . 1847
Petersburg . . . . . June 16th, 1831	June 1848
Berlin . . . . August 31st, 1831	June 1848
Hamburgh. . . . . October, 1831	September . . . 1848
Sunderland . . . . October 24th, 1831	October 4th . . . 1848
Edinburgh. . . . . January 22nd, 1832	October 1st . . . 1848

The progress of the disease did not stop here; it ravaged the nations again and again, its cause, like that of the epizootics, blights, and mildews, being altogether unknown. Infection has not been proved to have had any share in its general progress and propagation; on the contrary, it has marched onwards through an inscrutable atmospheric and terrestrial agency, uncontrolled by all opposing physical obstacles, and by all the efforts of man. Nor does there exist any means of modifying its force, other than such as are well known to lessen the power and duration of all epidemics, viz., the removal of all those conditions, whether natural or artificial, that produce and maintain impurity and stagnation in the atmosphere we breathe and in the water we drink, conditions that everywhere, and in all times, have opened the human frame to the admission of disease, endemic and epidemic.

NATURAL HISTORY, ORIGIN, AND LOCAL CAUSES.*

We have never before had the opportunity of securing for the benefit of succeeding generations an authentic record of the commencement, mode of progress, and propagation of a great and universal pestilence. The ravages of the " Black Death" and of the " Sweating Sickness" occurred in a comparatively unenlightened age, and first made their appearance among rude and semi-barbarous nations. The history of epidemic cholera is, on the other hand, the most complete of which we have any record— its very origin in Bengal having been observed and recorded by men still living. That such observation and record have not thrown more light on the obscure subject of epidemic diseases generally, or on this one in particular, is only another instance out of many of the inherent difficulties of the subject of epidemics.

* In the summary here being presented of what is known of the natural history of epidemic cholera, I have quoted fully and freely from the various articles on the subject in several numbers of the " Brit. and For. Med.-Chir. Rev.," and more particularly from the numbers for April, 1856, and January, 1857.

In the present state of science we must, in our endeavours to explain the causes and mode of propagation of cholera, be satisfied with compromises between the two extreme opinions as to the contagiousness and non-contagious nature of the disease, and with an enumeration of the several theories as to its remote causes.

1. The present opinion of the medical profession is, that epidemic cholera is induced by a special poison of Eastern or foreign origin, certain local conditions, and predisposition in the inhabitants of a given place being necessary to the propagation of the epidemic poison.

2. Diarrhœa, dysentery, and other fluxes, all of them congeners of cholera, have preceded the advent of the true epidemic, and thus the disease has found the population in a state of congeniality for its reception.

3. After the subsidence of epidemic cholera, the mortality from various alvine fluxes never entirely receded within its former limits; and similar antecedents and consequents were observed to prevail in London for some years prior and subsequent to the Great Plague of 1665.

4. It is supposed that during the second quarter of the present century the population of the United Kingdom has been undergoing a morbid change, as regards the tendency to diseases of the flux character; but whether this change be produced by the extension of the great-town system, or other cause, is not determined.

5. According to Dr. William Farr, whilst the materials were smouldering in England, the flame which threw the mass into combustion has been of Asiatic origin; in other words, the local causes of insalubrity which grew up amidst and around us require the combined influence of a certain atmospheric condition to produce the pestilence.

6. Dr. Barton of New Orleans designates the two causes of epidemic pestilence, whether yellow fever or cholera—the terrene and the atmospheric—as "the shears of Fate." When the agencies are apart they prove inert, but when they meet, the excitement of true cholera, or of yellow fever, is presumed to result. Whilst an epidemic state of the atmosphere exists over the whole country, the disease will only be developed where there exists also, in more or less intensity, the localizing conditions of filth, moisture, stagnation of the air, &c.

7. Mr. Glaisher enumerates the following as the meteorological phenomena of the three visitations of epidemic cholera in England. 1832 : In the summer, when the disease was raging for the first time, the barometer was high, the temperature below the average, the quantity of rain small, the direction of the wind N.E. and S.W., the air not in much motion, the sky particularly overcast,

and there was a seeming deficiency of electricity. 1849 : The pressure of the atmosphere was great, the temperature high, the sky overcast, the direction of the wind N.E. and S.W., the atmosphere misty and thick, the velocity of the air less than one-half the average. When the epidemic was at its height, a calm prevailed, with a thick mist at all places, which was sensibly more dense and torpid in low places ; the weather was dull, thick, and oppressive; no rain ; temperature of the Thames above 60° ; weak positive electricity ; no electrical disturbances. 1854 : The pressure of the atmosphere was great ; the temperature generally high; sky overcast ; direction of the wind N.E. and S.W., and the velocity of the air was less by one-half than its average for some time before ; and at the time of the greatest mortality from cholera, the barometer reading was remarkably high, and the temperature above its average ; a thick atmosphere, though at times clear, everywhere prevailed ; weak positive electricity; no rain. In low places, a dense mist and stagnant air, with a temperature in excess ; temperature of the Thames water high ; a high night temperature in London; a small daily range; an absence of ozone, and no electricity. Such an assemblage of circumstances, along with a still, heavy atmosphere, must have impeded the diffusion of the products of decomposition into space, and detained them in the vicinage of their origin, so as to strike with aggravated violence.

8. On a return to a healthy state of atmosphere, especially in respect of reduced temperature, and a free circulation of air, the epidemic declined.

9. The chief results deducible from Mr. Glaisher's observations are, that in cholera years the meteorological conditions are such as have a marked tendency to favour the chemical decomposition of organic substances, and to render the season defective in those atmospheric changes which, by decomposing or disposing into space the products of decomposition, renew the purity of the air. This distinguished authority has stated that "the crisis of the disease occurred at the droughtiest periods," the rainfall having, on occasion of the three great epidemics, been either wanting or very deficient.

10. These evils are in London greatly aggravated by the foul vaporous exhalations continually arising from the river surface, detained to a considerable extent by the still atmosphere, and the hills which bound the metropolis on two sides, and which hang like a veil over the city, obscuring the sun's rays by day and retarding the radiation of heat by night.

11. This is especially applicable to times when the temperature of the river, being higher than that of the circumjacent air, the former, which can be regarded only as the main common sewer of London, is converted into a seething, simmering caldron of foul

impurities, the emanations from which consist not simply of watery vapour, but contain also the products of this unwholesome decomposition. This is just the reverse of what would occur if the river were freed from its vile contaminations, for the water would then absorb and carry off some of the atmospheric impurities necessarily incident to the existence on its margin of a densely-peopled city.

12. No evidence of so precise and accurate a character on the meteorology of cholera as that furnished by Mr. Glaisher and Dr. Barton is procurable from any other source or from any other country; but abundant corroboration of the same general facts is met with in the Reports on Cholera from the East and West Indies, where languor, oppression, and stifling feeling were often experienced, the atmosphere feeling as if too thick for respiration.

13. It therefore would appear that a certain distemperature of season favours, if it is not necessary for the production of pestilence, the precise character of which will depend on the existence of some local or social condition, without the co-operation of which an epidemic pestilence cannot arise. Meteorological observations thus assume a peculiar importance, especially when we consider how much electricity, magnetism, light, and heat have to do with the tone of the nervous system, and with the vitality of the blood.

14. As regards England, certain aggregate meteorological phenomena would appear to constitute, in the language of the older physicians, the pestilential constitution of the year, and to have very generally accompanied the outbreaks of cholera. Allowing for the differences of contrasted climates, and the influences of varied localities, it has been proved that the atmospheric conditions under which cholera prevailed abroad have been almost identical.

15. The conditions referred to were, a variable but elevated temperature, a still and peculiarly oppressive state of the air, being more oppressive than the mere elevation of the thermometer could account for, and a certain amount of moisture. Such conditions of the atmosphere are rarely, if ever, confined to narrow geographical limits; yet it must be remembered that the condition of the locality greatly aggravates them, lowness of level and structural defects of arrangement in the streets and houses adding also to their morbific force.

16. But certain places, on the other hand, which partake apparently of the same meteorological and seasonal influences, are observed to escape the epidemic visitation, at the very time when other localities in the immediate neighbourhood are suffering severely from the pestilence; and it has often been noted, that whilst the occupants of certain streets and masses of houses are

being decimated, other streets and houses closely adjoining escape altogether. The causes of these differences have nowhere, as yet, been satisfactorily determined.

17. It was found by Mr. Simon that the mortality from cholera in 1849 was 19 in 10,000 inhabitants in the north-west district of the City of London Union, and 47 in 10,000 in Cripplegate district; and so on throughout various quarters of the city. But such differences must be referred, not to differences in the epidemic constitution in the atmosphere, but to some unascertained circumstances in the conditions of the localities themselves, or in the sanitary condition of their inhabitants.

18. In all countries, temperate and tropical, seasons presenting all the characters which conjointly form what we term the pestilential, have frequently occurred, without any pestilences. Dr. Barton states, as the result of his observation in New Orleans, that the atmospherical causes of pestilence are more or less present there every year, yet neither yellow fever nor cholera recurs annually in that city.

19. The localizing causes of cholera are further evidenced by the fact that, in the strictly analysed histories of cholera epidemics, we find them to be made up of a succession of partial and local outbreaks, and this not only as regards different districts, but even the same place. On the other hand, it has often occurred that the pestilence has lingered in some few favourite haunts through the entire course of the epidemic; and now and then, after attacking a place at the commencement of the visitation, it has returned to it again, after an interval of complete immunity, before its close.

20. The tendency of epidemic cholera to return at a subsequent visitation to the same towns, parts of towns, and even houses, which had formerly been affected by it, affords strong additional proof that local circumstances have great influence in determining its seat. In Chelsea, in 1848, the earliest case of cholera occurred in White-Hart court, and there the disease continued until the end of the epidemic in 1849. Again, in 1854, the first case of the disease was seen in the same place, if not in the same house. Similar facts were observed in Augusta-court, in which the three earliest fatal cases in Chelsea occurred in February, 1832.

21. In Dr. Acland's most valuable memoir on cholera in Oxford, in 1854, it is stated that every yard and street in St. Thomas's parish, with one exception, which had been attacked with cholera in 1832 and 1849, were visited by the disease in 1854. Thus, whatever other conditions may be necessary to the development of cholera, it is evident that some local circumstance plays a very important part in its evolution.

22. The existence of local causes of insalubrity is universally considered necessary to the evolution of a cholera epidemic,

although great diversity of opinion exists as to the part they bear in the production of the pestilence. By most persons, the unwholesome conditions to which the dwellings in unhealthy districts are habitually exposed, are believed to produce a low state of the general health, and proclivity to disease, which disable the inhabitants from resisting the exciting cause of the epidemic.

23. Dr. Carpenter surmises that these influences, and also other causes of a more personal nature, produce a condition of the blood itself which predisposes it for zymotic action, the precise character of which depends upon the nature of the exciting cause with which it is brought into relation ; the special poison of smallpox, scarlatina, typhus, and cholera, for example, being each capable of exciting its peculiar fermentation in the blood already charged with organic compounds in a state of retrogressive change.

24. It may fairly be doubted, however, whether the action of the exciting cause of cholera be not rather simply toxical ; and if fermentation has anything to do with its production, whether this does not occur externally to the organism, and produce rather the exciting cause than form the cause itself. That persons arriving from a pure atmosphere and in sound health, have so frequently shown themselves peculiarly prone to suffer from a brief exposure to the epidemic influence is, moreover, altogether at variance with the opinion that the supposed condition of the blood is a necessary predisposition for cholera.

25. Dr. Barton considers epidemic pestilences, as yellow fever and cholera, to be the direct consequences of the co-operation of certain meteorological conditions with the local cause. The local cause he believes to be "filth, moisture, and stagnant air," and especially the emanations arising from extensive upturnings and exposure of soil impregnated with the results of organic decomposition, of which latter influence he furnishes several illustrative examples. He believes cholera to be caused by a poisonous miasm, while this miasm he regards as altogether of indigenous origin.

26. Pettenkofer, on the other hand, believes that the introduction of a ferment from without is necessary for the production of cholera, but thinks that this ferment can only act where it meets with suitable local conditions. Arguing from this and other presumed facts, he confidently asserts that we must abandon all idea of the air and water as the nidus of cholera, and seek for it in the soil alone.

27. Whilst Dr. Carpenter believes that the foulness of localities taints the blood of persons exposed to inhale their emanations, and thus produces in them a personal predisposition for zymotic disease, Pettenkofer is of opinion that the special "leaven" sets up a zymosis, or series of decompositions in the impure soil itself, and that the special poison of cholera is a miasm generated by this earthy fermentation.

28. He considers the presence of a special ferment as essential to the production of a cholera epidemic, and he insists, also, on the existence of certain local peculiarities. These consist of a damp subsoil sufficiently porous to be penetrable by the decomposition products of human and animal excrement. It is only in such soil, thoroughly impregnated with this peculiar organic matter, that the special cholera-poison is generated.

29. The ferment supposed by Pettenkofer to be necessary to set up the peculiar decomposition of which the cholera-poison forms one of the products, is the matter of the dejections of cholera patients. His notion is that the cholera germ-bearing excrement, which spreads itself in the damp porous soil already impregnated with fæcal matters, produces, by means of the fine division which it there undergoes, such a modification in the process of putre-faction and decomposition, that, in addition to the gases already formed, a cholera miasm is produced, which becomes diffused through the atmosphere of dwellings in common with other exha-lations.

30. Thus, although the cholera miasm is formed in the ground, the air is the vehicle for its transmission to the patient; and Pet-tenkofer adduces several instances in which he supposes cholera to have been imported by means of the dejections of persons suffering either from diarrhœa, cholerine, or cholera; for he views these diseases as mere varieties, and infers that if the dejections of cholera patients be capable of originating the pestilence, those persons suf-fering from either of the milder complaints most probably produce the like results.

31. The physician just quoted says that the most intimate com-munication between places may occur without leading to the intro-duction of cholera; while, on the contrary, this disease has often broken out in places whose communication with the cholera sick could not be demonstrated. The former fact he explains on the supposition that the requisite soil relations were wanting. Facts such as these, and others previously referred to, which occurred in this country, point rather to the spontaneous production than to the extrinsic origin of cholera.

32. The several opinions above cited, however much they differ in other respects, agree in considering some local condition or other as necessary for the production or development of cholera, save only that Dr. Carpenter believes the predisposition to zymotic disease—and he considers cholera a zymotic disease—may be in-duced by personal as well as by local causes.

33. Pettenkofer's view of the nature of the local cause of cholera is sufficiently definite and simple, and to it there must be no further reference; but, with the exception just mentioned, nothing can well be more vague and unsatisfactory than the opinions that have usually been expressed as to the nature of the localizing causes of

cholera. Unmindful of the proposition that every effect must spring from some definite cause, it has been common with sanitary inquirers at once to refer the same effect to several causes, and several effects to the same cause, instead of endeavouring to trace each result to its proper origin.

34. It has frequently been said that cholera and fever arise and are localized by the same causes—that they run the same track, and haunt the same localities; the truth being that it would be easy to point to localities which have been alternately the seats of both fever and cholera—fever being rife and cholera passing over; cholera being prevalent and fever rare; but such facts point to no necessary connexion in the etiology of the two diseases.

35. Setting aside, then, most of the presumed local causes, as appearing in no ascertained degree necessary to the development of cholera, let us concentrate our attention upon impure water, lowness of site, and the emanations arising from the decomposition of animal refuse.

36. That impure water has a powerful influence over the intensity of cholera outbreaks is unquestionable, as shown by Dr. William Farr, Dr. Acland of Oxford, and by Drs. Sutherland and Snow; but large as is the influence of this contamination over cholera epidemics, impure water will not alone constitute a necessary factor of cholera. It is either an accidental and occasional vehicle for conveying the poison into the system, or, when impregnated with organic impurities, acts like unwholesome food, or the injudicious use of purgatives, as a determining or aggravating cause of cholera during the epidemic visitation.

37. Impure water probably acts chiefly, if not exclusively, by aggravating individual cases of the pestilence, causing such as might otherwise have been cases of simple diarrhœa to pass rapidly into the state of collapse. A careful consideration of the history of the sudden and severe outbreak in the district of St. James's, Westminster, in 1854, which was apparently connected with the dietetic use of water from the Broad-street pump—found at a later period to have been vitiated by the leakage from a cesspool—appears to support this supposition; but it must be remembered that when this visitation, and similar outbreaks at Rotherhithe and other smaller districts, took place, the pestilence was at its height.

38. As regards elevation of the soil, it has been shown at home and abroad that from the rise of a few hundred up to nine thousand feet, the influence ou the disease, so far as elevation is concerned, has relation more to the local conditions, and that where the population is dense, the supply of water bad in quality and deficient in quantity, or the drainage and sewerage imperfect, elevation, however advantageous along with other high sanitary conditions, will not suffice to protect of itself.

39. The influence on the alimentary canal of atmospheres contaminated by effluvia arising from decaying organic matter, was observed by Cullen, who regarded such vitiation as the efficient cause of diarrhœa—a remark confirmed by modern observation. It is probable that both the nature of the decomposing matter and that of the transformative process it is undergoing, are important elements in regard to the effect on the human constitution. Mere putrid odours, for instance, will not of themselves produce either diarrhœa or cholera ; but it is sufficiently proved that persons have suffered from the latter epidemic in proportion to the contamination by "privy odour" of the air they breathed, and that immunity from this particular foulness of the air appeared to secure immunity from cholera.

40. Of the two influences—impure water and impure air—the weight of testimony is on the side of the greater morbific power of the latter, both at home and abroad; and when to such local conditions we add the meteorological circumstances necessary, then cholera in its epidemic form will be developed. That local outbreaks of a sporadic nature, both of diarrhœa and cholera, have resulted from such contaminations of the air, would appear to be more than probable.

SYMPTOMS AND PROGRESS.

There are two circumstances which render the assault of true cholera both insidious and dangerous in the extreme :—it is preceded by a *painless diarrhœa* of more or less duration, according as the epidemic may be at its height or decline ; and its seizure is generally by night or in the early morning. It thus happens that, too often, the real nature of the case is mistaken by the patient for some slight disorder of the bowels.

When once the true cholera has fastened on the patient it proves the most unmistakeable of diseases—one case being the counterpart of all others—so that an error in diagnosis is here scarcely possible. The disease in its most malignant form is the same in all countries. It is ushered in by muscular debility, tremors, and vertigo, occasional nausea and spasmodic griping pains in the bowels, and marked depression of the functions of respiration and circulation, and sense of faintness. These signs are speedily followed by copious purging of serous fluid, and this again by vomiting, with sense of burning heat at stomach, coldness and sweating, dampness of the whole surface of the body, coldness and lividness of the lips and tongue, cold breath, a craving thirst, a feeble rapid pulse, oppressed and difficult respiration, suppressed urinary excretion, extreme restlessness, blueness of the entire surface of the body, a sunken and appalling countenance, a sunken and peculiarly suppressed voice, a peculiar and indescribable odour from the body, partial heats of the præcordia and forehead;—such are the signs of a fatal collapse.

Such is the ordinary course of this fatal disease in its most virulent form, or at the onset of its epidemic invasion. But in less concentrated visitations, or towards their decline, there will be found a precursory diarrhœa, varying in duration from three to twelve hours, or more, to be followed by true cholera. During the stage of diarrhœa the quantity of serous fluid voided is sometimes immense, and in one case noted by Dr. Parkes, in which the patient had but seven stools, eighty-eight ounces of fluid were discharged from the bowel.

But the relation between purging, vomiting, and cramps, and the final algide collapse, is exceedingly variable. In some cases the patient will have been purging for twenty-four, forty-eight, or more hours, before vomiting, muscular cramps, and collapse occur; while in other instances the whole duration of the disease will have been gone through unto death in seven or eight hours, with marked collapse almost from the commencement of the seizure.

A Hindu, attended by Dr. Parkes, lived 108 hours from the time of the first stool, and ninety-one hours after the positive development of algide symptoms, the patient having voided altogether twenty-one stools. Another Hindu, in contrast with the above, and who had only four stools, died in ten hours from the first discharge. All observation in India goes to show that the more concentrated, and malignant the disease the less purging and vomiting; and so also in the worst and most rapidly fatal cases, muscular cramps are very rarely observed as prominent symptoms.

After an indefinite duration, and varying infinitely in the degrees of severity of the several symptoms, we find, in favourable cases, that the oppressed functions of respiration and circulation begin to show signs of more freedom of action;—feverish reaction commences, to be developed into actual and sometimes severe fever, accompanied by headache and gastric symptoms—the results of previous congestions and arrested functions of secretion.

PREDISPOSING CAUSES.

Although it be quite true that the cholera poison requires no definite predisposing conditions in the system to enable it to produce its effects, and that it proves fatal at all ages, and nearly equally so to both sexes, and that neither the weakness of infancy, the vigour of manhood, nor the decrepitude of old age, is a safeguard against its inroads;—still, in common with fever and dysentery, it may be truly said that whatever depresses the constitutional powers will predispose to the invasion of cholera; as the use of crude, indigestible, or ill-prepared food—fatigue, want, filth, and misery,—but, above all, intemperance in the use of spirituous liquors, so common to the lower orders of English in all parts of the world. It was found by Dr. Farr that on Saturday, Monday, Tuesday, and Wednesday the deaths from cholera in London and other cities were above, and on Thursday, Friday, and Sunday, below the average. The week's wages are generally paid on Saturdays; and the Mondays are days on which a certain proportion of the population indulge in intoxicating drinks, the Fridays being days of comparative abstinence.

It thus appears that the depression of the nervous system and the derangement of the digestive organs following immediately upon occasional intoxication, had a marked predisposing influence. But it is difficult to estimate separately the various noxious influences which in large cities are naturally associated with intemperance. This vice soon entails all those conditions which not only impair the vigour of the body, but favour the dissemination, and probably the generation of the cholera poison. There is, indeed, sufficient evidence that not only habitual drunkenness in itself, but also the immediate effects of an occasional carouse, will induce a predisposition to an attack.

The influence of long marches in predisposing to cholera in India, would appear to indicate something more powerful than mere physical depression resulting from the labour of marching; for in the laborious trades and occupations of civil life the mortality from cholera in England has not been proved to have been necessarily high, or to have been in any manner associated with excessive labour.

It has been proved in India, and recorded by Mr. Orton, Drs. Balfour and Lorimer, that troops, both European and native, suffer more from cholera on the march, or soon after it, than they do at the military stations. Dr. Balfour has proved, that of the native soldiers of the Madras army 32 died of cholera in cantonment, and 86 when marching, to an average of 10,000 of strength. The attacks were respectively 85 and 200 in 10,000. Dr. Lorimer's reports show that the troops were more frequently attacked on long than on short marches:—thus the troops in 219 marches of 20-40 days were attacked 39 times; while in 14 marches of 100-120 days they were attacked seven times. If we take a hundred marches as the basis, they were attacked 18 times in about 30 days, in the one case; while in the other case they were attacked 50 times in about 110 days—that is, at the rate of 14 times in 30 days. This is no proof, says Dr. Farr, that *fatigue* increases the liability to attack;—it only proves that, on the long marches, the men are exposed a longer time to the causes of disease. We would assuredly expect more men to be wounded in a battle of three days', than in a battle of one day's duration. When a march is conducted with undue haste, in heavy order, or under direct solar exposure, in hot climates, it will produce fatigue and other injurious results:—but in general a well-ordered march is conducive to health; and there are well-known instances in which the health of an army has even improved materially on the line of march.

Soldiers are exposed to many injurious influences during long marches which frequently lie by rivers, on low marshes and jungly grounds; and when to these circumstances we add sleeping on the ground, we perceive many causes other than fatigue in operation. As elsewhere observed, camp beds, which should raise the men off the ground, would prove a great advantage; and so would a light order of march, and short marches.

. But referring to the special subject of this section, I believe that we are seldom so much in error as when we would ascribe sickness and mortality to *one cause only;* while in reality disease and death are always, and under all circumstances, justly to be referred to the assemblage of many causes. In truth, the medical topographer, when investigating the difficult and obscure causes of disease, must ever hold in recollection the requirement of Cabanis—to inquire into all the circumstances, natural and physical, in the midst of which we live in a given place.

THE SIX THEORIES AS TO THE CAUSE AND PROPAGATION OF EPIDEMIC CHOLERA.

The varieties of opinion as to the remote cause of Asiatic cholera, according to Dr. Baly, and the causes of its spreading are very numerous; but all that need be referred to may be reduced to six principal theories, which must be briefly stated, since it is only by reference to them that the value and import of the facts to be examined can be estimated.

" 1. The first theory is, that the disease spreads by an ' atmospheric influence or epidemic constitution,' its progress consisting of a succession of local outbreaks, and that the particular localities affected are determined by certain ' localizing conditions,' which are, first, all those well-known circumstances which render places insalubrious; and, second, a susceptibility of the disease in the inhabitants of such places, produced by the habitual respiration of an impure atmosphere.

" 2. The second theory, following the analogy known to be due to morbid poisons, regards the cause of cholera as a morbific matter which undergoes increase only within the human body, and is propagated by means of emanations from the bodies of the sick, in other words, by contagion.

" 3. The third theory—that propounded by Dr. Snow—gives a more specific form to the doctrine of contagion. It supposes that the poison of cholera is swallowed, and acts directly on the mucous membrane of the intestines, is at the same time reproduced in the intestinal canal, and passes out, much increased, with the discharges; and that these discharges afterwards, in various ways, but chiefly by becoming mixed with the drinking water in rivers and wells, reach the alimentary canals of other persons, and produce the like disease in them.

" 4. The fourth theory assumes that the cause of cholera is a morbific matter or poison, but supposes that it is reproduced only in the air, not within the bodies of those whom it affects, and that its diffusion is due to the agency of the atmosphere.

" 5. The fifth theory is a modification of the fourth. It admits that the cholera matter is increased by a species of fermentation, or other mode of reproduction in impure, damp, and stagnant air, but maintains that it, nevertheless, is distributed and diffused by means of human intercourse; it being carried in ships and other vehicles, and even in the clothes of men, especially the foul clothes of vagrants and the accumulated baggage of armies.

" 6. The sixth theory combines the second and fourth, assuming that the material causes of the disease may be increased and propagated in and by impure air, as well as in and by the human body."

Of the six theories above-mentioned, that alone is supported by a large amount of evidence which regards the cause of cholera as a matter increasing by some process, whether chemical or organic, in impure and damp air, and assumes that, although, of course, diffused with the air, it is also distributed and diffused by means of human intercourse.

This theory explains much that would otherwise seem capricious in the course of cholera; and it elucidates the relation subsisting between cholera and other epidemic diseases. Several epidemics of cholera have sometimes been immediately preceded in some countries or cities by the prevalence of fevers or of diarrhœa and dysentery; and this has been made an argument in support of the vague notion of an " epidemic constitution." For it has been supposed that this epidemic influence, in the course of its development, gives rise at one time to fever or diarrhœa, and at another time to cholera. It has been imagined, therefore, that the prevalent diarrhœa preceding cholera resulted from a slighter amount of the peculiar atmospheric influence which subsequently produced the more formidable epidemic. But it is not by any means a general rule that an increasing prevalence of diarrhœa, or of any other epidemic disease, precedes the appearance of cholera; and the occasional association of cholera with such diseases is capable of being otherwise explained. The fact in question, and the similarity of the local conditions favouring cholera and epidemic diseases generally, together with other facts examined, seem to agree best with the view that these several diseases are caused by different

poisons, all of which find their means of increase in similar states
of the atmosphere, though there probably are modifications of the
atmospheric conditions more essential or more favourable to some
of these diseases than to others.

In the statement that the theory above indicated is the only one
supported by a large amount of evidence, it is not implied that this
theory is adopted to the exclusion of all others.　For the possibility
that cholera is occasionally communicated by a virus produced in,
and emanating from the sick, has already been admitted; and
other questions relative to the means by which the cause of the
disease is disseminated, and its introduction into the human body
effected, have been left open for further inquiry.

PREVENTIVE MEASURES.

The ultimate object of an inquiry into the subjects treated of
are stated by Dr. Baly to be—the discovery of the means by which
the onward progress of cholera may be stayed—its increased diffusion moderated, and individuals protected from its attacks.　The
partial attainment of this object is all that at present can be hoped
for; but the principles by which endeavours to attain it thus
partially should be guided, are, for the most part, free from
doubt.

" From among the great features of a cholera epidemic three
stand forth as of paramount importance :—one, the undoubted influence of locality and of the sanitary condition of towns and
dwellings on the degree of severity with which the epidemic visits
them ; a second, the equally certain influence of season and temperature, together with some unknown condition of the atmosphere
on the general prevalence and rate of extension of the epidemic ;
and a third, the share taken by human intercourse in determining
not only the progress of the epidemic, and the direction of its advance across a continent, but also its extension from continent to
continent, and most probably its communication from one town to
another in the same country, and from one locality to another in
the same town.　This third feature of the disease is less generally
admitted than the other two ; but the question here is not whether
the evidence is so complete as to compel belief, but simply whether
it amounts to so great a degree of probability that it cannot merely
be neglected in the consideration of the measures to be taken for
the prevention, arrest, or mitigation of a destructive pestilence.

" 1. With regard to the *first* of the features of the epidemic, there
cannot be a doubt with regard to the course of action which it
calls for, as the duty and interest of every portion of the community.
The more fortunate classes are, it is true, exposed to proportionably
little danger, since they are often able to leave the neighbourhood
of spots in which the disease is raging, and usually dwell in more

elevated, open, and airy parts of towns, and in more spacious and cleanly and less-crowded houses.

" But it is also true that the power of the disease through a town is increased in proportion to the degree in which the conditions of insalubrity referred to are present in various parts of it; and not merely the poor, who live in the spots where moisture and foul air feed the cause of the disease, but all the inhabitants, are exposed, by the existence of these evils, to a greater risk of becoming its victims. And further, it is certain that the more intensely the epidemic prevails in a large town, the more does the whole district for miles around suffer, and the more danger is there of its being propagated to other districts.

" By improving the drainage in low parts of the town, opening close courts, thinning the buildings in the more crowded parts, putting a stop to the burial of the dead in large cities, keeping even the smallest streets constantly free from filth, covering drains and sewers, and abolishing cesspools and other sources of foulness in the air and soil; by improving the dwellings of the poor in respect of ventilation, giving them the means of maintaining a due warmth in their rooms without excluding the external air, promoting the general substitution of good water-closets for open privies, inculcating cleanly habits among the poor, and affording them that most important requisite, an abundant and constant supply of good water, by means of which they may attain cleanliness; by adopting these measures, it cannot be doubted that the ravages of the disease would not only be lessened among the people dwelling in the localities thus improved, but they would also greatly weaken the force of the epidemic over a far wider space. All these things should be done by the public authorities before the pestilence comes, and in the time of its presence, it would further be wise to enforce cleanliness and ventilation even in the interior of houses by a *house-to-house inspection*.

" These principles seem now to be more generally understood, and happily are being more widely acted upon than at any former period. But as public functionaries are apt to direct their efforts too exclusively to the removing evidences of dirt, and to think all must be well where the eye finds cleanliness, it may not be superfluous to call special attention to the fact, that mere overcrowding and want of ventilation have in several instances enabled cholera to exert its worst effects. This want of ventilation is especially common in workhouses and other pauper establishments, and in public lodging-houses, in which the number of inmates ought to be strictly limited, and in a time of pestilence reduced.

" 2. The consideration of the *second* great feature of the epidemic teaches that the efforts to restrain and overcome it, though less obviously needed, might be more successful in the cold than in the hot season. In the winter the diffusion of the disease takes place slowly and with difficulty, human intercourse being probably, in

certain states of the atmosphere, the sole means by which its propagation from place to place is effected. Hence the disease at
this time gradually becomes limited to a few isolated spots; its
cause exists for the most part only in the interior of inhabited
buildings, and in these it ought to be attacked. Wherever cases
of cholera occur during the winter, those measures of purification
which at all times would be proper, should be put in force with
the more energy, from the consideration that during this season
they are likely to be attended with greater success.

"Free ventilation is, perhaps, the most efficient means of destroying the cholera poison, especially in winter, for there is reason to
believe that in fresh cold air the poisonous matter soon becomes
inert. The removal of all obvious dirt, and the thorough cleansing
of every surface of wall, floor, or ceiling, with the unsparing application of lime and of disinfecting fluids, the washing of furniture,
and the exposure of it to the open air, the destruction of foul
clothes, even of those worn by inmates of the house who are yet
healthy, as well as those which belong to the sick; all these measures might reasonably be enforced during the winter, since at
that season so great a result as the entire eradication of the pestilence might possibly be attained. This result, however, can be
hoped for only from the systematic adoption of such measures in
all infected parts of the country simultaneously. For, if the disease be allowed to maintain itself in a single district throughout
the winter, and the early months of spring, it will most probably
increase there, and soon spread widely, in spite of all efforts to
restrain it in the ensuing summer season; the renewed warmth
and other qualities of the air more frequently attendant on a high
than on a low temperature, enabling the poison then to maintain
its morbific power, or even to increase, in its passage through the
atmosphere.

" May not other means of preventing the extension of the epidemic, whether in the winter or the summer season, be suggested
by the facts relative to the share borne by human intercourse in
its diffusion ?

" If the march of the epidemic is dependent mainly on human intercourse, and if foul ships and barges, bodies of troops, dirty
vagrants, and foul clothes, are the means by which the infection is
most frequently carried from one country to another, surely some
measures might be devised which would be at the same time
effectual in checking the propagation and extension of the disease,
and consistent with the other great interests of society.

" Quarantine can no longer be adopted as the means of preventing the entrance of cholera into England, for it is incompatible
with the present state of commercial intercourse, and with the
well-being of a commercial country. Moreover, quarantine has undoubtedly often failed of its object, partly from its being evaded by
the crews of infected ships, partly, perhaps, from the ships being

placed so near to habitations on shore that the infected air of the ship would be carried to them by atmospheric currents; and in some cases, probably, because clothes still containing infectious matter were conveyed on shore during, or subsequent to, the period of quarantine.

" For similar reasons sanitary cordons around towns are now impracticable, and have at former times often, though apparently not always, failed to prevent the diffusion of cholera. But if the ordinary regulations of quarantine and sanitary cordons are relinquished, it is the more desirable to adopt other measures which shall oppose some obstacle to the importation of cholera, and to its propagation from one town to another in this country.

" It cannot be doubted that ships are more or less fitted to convey the disease or its cause from port to port, in proportion to their want of cleanliness, defective ventilation, and over-crowded state, and that if these evils, of which the two former are so flagrant in the smaller trading vessels, and the two latter in ships carrying passengers, could be removed, the danger of importing cholera would be greatly lessened. While, therefore, it is much to be desired, on general grounds, that measures should be adopted for inculcating and enforcing attention to cleanliness and free ventilation in the whole mercantile marine, the especial application of measures of this kind to ships coming from ports where cholera prevails, as far as may be practicable, is imperatively called for. A close inspection of all such vessels should be made on arrival in port; and it would not be unreasonable to require that, in con·sideration of the restrictions of quarantine being abrogated, there should be brought with each ship coming from an infected port, an official certificate of its having been inspected, and found cleanly and not over-crowded, and the crew healthy at the time of its sailing.

" On the arrival of ships having persons ill of cholera on board, or having had deaths from that disease during the voyage, more active measures must be adopted; and the best that have been recommended seem to be—1, the removal of the sick to a hospital ship, moored at a distance from the other shipping in the harbour, or to a special hospital in an isolated and airy situation on shore; 2, permission to the rest of the crew to land after exchanging their dress for fresh clothes provided from the shore; 3, the thorough exposure of all articles of dress and baggage to the air and disinfecting agents before they are removed from the ship; and 4, the thorough cleansing of the ship itself, with the free use of disinfecting agents in every part of it, but especially in the parts occupied by the crew and passengers, or their baggage.

" If, notwithstanding such precautions as these, cholera finds its way into the country, then the low lodging houses frequented by vagrants, and the vagrant-wards of workhouses, should be narrowly watched. For these especially are the places in which the dis-

ease is fostered, and whence it seems to be distributed widely to
other localities.   In these establishments, then, the most scrupulous cleanliness and free ventilation should be maintained, and
even the personal cleanliness of the inmates as far as possible enforced.

" When cholera appears in the places referred to, or within
dwellings of the poor, intercourse with the surrounding population
cannot of course be interdicted.   But still it is possible to adopt
measures which would not only check the extension of the disease
among the inhabitants of the infected houses, but greatly diminish
the risk of its propagation to other localities.   Of these the most
important is the provision of spacious and well-ventilated build
ings in airy dry sites for the reception of the inhabitants of the
infected spot, while their dwellings are cleansed and disinfected.
These " Houses of Refuge," it cannot be doubted, have saved
many lives from destruction by cholera, both in this country and
on the continent.   No considerable town should be without one ;
and several should be prepared in the environs of the larger cities.
The " Houses of Refuge" would receive the healthy, but for those
already labouring under cholera other asylums must be found.

" There has been much difference of opinion respecting the desirableness of establishing Cholera Hospitals.   But it surely cannot be disputed that those struck with cholera amongst the poor
ought to be carried to some hospital, if they are at all in a fit
state to be removed.   They cannot be properly treated at their
homes, and mere change to a purer air offers them a better chance
of recovery.   Moreover, in the rooms in which the poor are struck
with cholera, those who nurse them, and in a less degree those
who visit them, are exposed to danger, probably not from contagion, but in most cases from the pestiferous atmosphere of the
locality ; while, if the sick are placed in the spacious and well-
ventilated ward of a hospital, nearly all danger from approaching
them is at an end.   Wherever, therefore, general hospitals do not
exist, or cannot afford sufficient space, cholera hospitals should be
established.

" The buildings selected for the purpose should, if possible, be
situated in the least crowded parts of the towns or districts in which
they are needed. They should have spacious rooms, with provision
for permitting the free circulation of air through them ; and during
their occupation the most strict attention should be paid to their
ventilation and cleanliness ; otherwise they may prove an injury
rather than a benefit.

" In the general hospitals, too, the same conditions of ample space,
free ventilation, and scrupulous cleanliness are the essential requisites.   If they are provided, it is probably a matter of little moment whether the cholera patients are placed together in special
wards, or dispersed among the ordinary patients in the general wards
of these establishments.

" Whether the sick be removed to cholera hospitals, or to wards of general hospitals, it should equally be an object of care to prevent the accidental introduction of infection together with the patients, and with this object it is desirable that the clothes brought with the patients should be removed from them in a special receiving-room, or at once be either destroyed or subjected to a disinfecting process. And even in the case of the healthy removed from infected dwellings to houses of refuge, care should be taken that the foul clothes be not carried with them, and that the clothes they wear should as soon as possible undergo an efficient cleansing.

" The propriety of adopting measures founded on the belief that human intercourse aids in the dissemination of cholera, has been urged upon those who may still doubt the propagation of the disease in that way. And, on the same principle, other precautions, suggested by the view that the discharges from the stomach and intestines contain the cholera poison, must here be recommended, although the theory based on that view has been found generally untenable, and, at most, susceptible of very partial application. The precautions referred to are, the immersion of the soiled linen of the patients, and subsequently of their bedding, in water to which some disinfecting liquid has been added ; care that neither the food nor the drinking water can in any way be contaminated by the discharges of the patients, and especially that care on the part of nurses and others about the sick be taken to wash their hands before taking food ; to which may be added, as a measure more feasible in hospitals than in the dwellings of the poor, the placing a small quantity of chemical decomposing liquid in all the vessels into which the discharges of the patients are received.

" One other method of combating the pestilence has been proposed and partially carried into effect; namely, the house-to-house visitation of infected districts, with the view of discovering and treating all cases of diarrhœa, some of which may be presumed to be cases of cholera in an early stage. This measure, however, is based on principles which do not properly belong to the subject of this report. It would, therefore, be out of place here to inquire into the amount of success with which it had been attended."

Dr. Bryson states that in the navy epidemic cholera has never been known to go on extending for more than one or two, or at most three days in any ship of war at sea, provided the decks were properly ventilated and the sick kept as much as possible from the healthy.

Throughout the capital and in the provincial towns of Denmark, the removal of the healthy inhabitants from their houses into tents pitched in chosen localities, thus separating them from the sick and from local influences, was followed by the most gratifying results ; while the house-to-house visitation, although it had been carried out with more energy and system than in any other country, was far from being so favourable in result.

PREVENTIVE MEASURES IN THE ARMY.

The following "Instructions," framed by desire of Sir James M'Grigor, the venerated Director-General of the Medical Department of her Majesty's Army, were issued under authority of the Secretary-at-War, and dated War Office, August 31st, 1848. "These Regulations are to be considered as General Orders, and are to be observed as such by all persons to whom they may apply:—none of them are to be modified or disregarded, unless special reasons shall exist for so doing, and even not then without the consent of the Director-General, unless the delay which would be necessary to obtain that sanction was likely to be the occasion of injury, either to individuals or the public. In the event of there being reason to anticipate the latter, the alterations considered necessary may be effected, but their nature and extent must be immediately reported by the medical officer who adopts or advises them."

When Cholera shall have been officially reported to be prevailing in the Country, but distant from Military Stations, the following IN-STRUCTIONS *are to have effect:—*

1. Medical officers will exercise more than common vigilance in the discharge of their professional duties; they will devote more than ordinary attention to the interior economy of their corps, the constitution of the men, and to every circumstance, however remotely affecting their health. They will be expected to be cognizant of every military arrangement involving the health of the troops, and to put themselves in communication with their commanding officers on any alteration of arrangements in the ordinary duties, which they may consider beneficial or likely to afford greater security.

2. Every possible precaution must be taken to guard against intemperance, crowding in small, ill-ventilated rooms, use of unwholesome food, deficiency of clothing, bedding, fuel, &c.; and, if found to exist, measures must be taken to correct or remove them.

3. Medical officers are to attend the ordinary parades, and observe the health of the men, without exciting suspicion.

4. Great attention to personal cleanliness is to be enjoined, and the men cautioned carefully to avoid unnecessary night exposure and damp, and to change their clothes when wet.

5. Especial care is to be observed in the cooking of vegetables; and lamb, pork, and stale fish interdicted.

6. Roasted or baked meat is to be provided twice a week, instead of boiled meat.

7. Drains, dustholes, privies, and the removal of accumulated filth, are to be specially attended to.

8. The barrack-bedding is to be aired daily, but not in the open air in winter; and great caution observed as to the perfect dryness of fresh supplies.

9. As attacks of the disease seem to be frequently determined by exposure to wet, damp, unusual intemperance, and other irregularities, every means should be taken to prevent those.

10. At this period all ailments, particularly diarrhœa, require the strictest attention; and the commanding officer should explain to the men the importance of immediately reporting themselves when they feel in any way unwell.

11. Where there is any suspicion of the approach of cholera, immediate steps are to be taken to establish a separate ward in hospital, to which every case not strongly marked is to be sent on admission.

12. An abundant supply of hospital bedding, dresses, and medicine is to be kept in readiness.

When the Disease has appeared among the Military of a Station, or the Inhabitants in its immediate Vicinity.

13. The avoidance of all unnecessary alarm cannot be too strongly enjoined; and it is hoped that medical officers, by their own example, will endeavour to allay apprehension in those suffering from, or in any way connected with the disease.

14. On the appearance of cholera in a corps, health-inspections are to be made at morning and evening parades, and a daily inspection of every individual attached to the regiment.

15. Each soldier is to be provided with two cholera-belts, as part of his necessaries. Flannel-waistcoats, if thought necessary for individuals, are to be provided at their own expense.

16. Married men (if out of mess) should each be provided with a ration the same as the single men; and it is also desirable, in barracks in which the disease exists, that the women and children should have sufficient and regular meals.

17. Soldiers should be cautioned against intemperance; and drunkards, and all men of weakly or susceptible habits, should be limited to a certain quantity of liquor at the discretion of the medical officer.

18. As a precautionary measure, but particularly in infected localities, drills, parades, and duties generally, should, as much as consistent with discipline, be reduced, and favourable hours and weather chosen for them; but, above all, the number of sentries, especially at night, should be diminished, so that in no case shall the men have less than three nights in bed.

19. Good fires are to be provided in the barrack-rooms, to increase ventilation, and to diffuse a cheerfulness,—which last should be promoted in every way.

20. Coffee or warm drinks are to be provided to the men before morning and night duties. A hot evening meal enforced, and breakfast, if possible, supplied at the usual hour to every man before leaving his barrack-room.

21. In the event of the appearance of cholera among the civil population in the neighbourhood, the troops should be confined to barracks, and all intercourse prevented. When the disease prevails in a corps, it may be found beneficial to encamp it—a proper site being selected for the purpose.

22. During confinement to barracks, the minds of the men should, as much as possible, be amused and occupied; and, under proper regulation, occasional marches into the country, and trap-ball or other games, in an adjoining field, permitted.

23. Officers' servants are to be under the same restrictions as others, and no person from the town to be admitted into barracks.

24. If practicable, a considerable reduction of the numbers in barrack should take place, as well to insure a purer atmosphere and more thorough ventilation, as to make room for the accommodation of women and children, and, if necessary, for a temporary hospital, or observation ward. Over-crowding, under any circumstances, is to be avoided—great attention paid to cleanliness and ventilation, and the floors and passages dry rubbed, not washed.

25. Personal washing, and that of clothes, is to be done in sheds or storehouses appropriated for the purpose, and not in the barrack-rooms.

26. The quality of the beer to be used by soldiers is to be ascertained by a competent person, and the acid in porter or ale corrected by chalk or carbonate of soda.

27. Where cholera is present in the neighbourhood, the women and children are to be accommodated in barracks, or aired houses in the vicinity, and to be put under similar restrictions as to intercourse. Where this cannot be done, soldiers with their families who are permitted to live out of barracks are to be excluded therefrom, or placed in a temporary barrack until it is considered safe to admit them—their quarters during this separation being frequently inspected.

28. Where a house is hired for the women, they may be required to pay their usual rent, and coals supplied by Government at prime cost.

29. Diarrhœa, either as precursory, co-existent, or prevailing by itself, should, as a measure of safety, be regarded as closely allied to cholera; and where bowel complaints prevail in a corps stationed in an infected district, a spare room should, if possible, be set apart for the accommodation of the healthy of any room that may become unusually subject to that complaint; and the room thus vacated must be whitewashed, cleansed, and fumigated, so as to be ready for any similar occurrence. This applies still more

strongly where cholera actually exists in a corps. Cases of common cholera are to be removed to the Observation Ward.

30. The regimental hospital is to be appropriated to the treatment of cholera, and the ordinary cases of sickness accommodated in barracks; or, where this cannot be done, in a hired house, the authority of the Director-General for the latter arrangement being previously obtained.

31. The appearance of cholera in places where troops are stationed is immediately to be reported to the Director-General, without waiting for its being officially announced by the local Board of Health.

32. From the moment that a case of common or spasmodic cholera occurs, a daily report is to be forwarded to the Director-General until further orders.

33. A full report of each case among the troops, with detail of previous habits, intercourse, diet, exposure to cold, wet, &c., and other particulars, is to be forwarded to the Director-General.

34. Daily reports of the progress of cholera among the civil population where troops may be stationed, will be required from medical officers.

35. Cases among women and children in barracks are to be admitted into hospital; those in quarters to civil hospital, under such regulations as may be adopted in parishes; for the former, a separate ward, or barrack-room, is to held in readiness.

36. Cases among the troops of the East India Company are to be admitted into hospital, as also those specified as entitled to medical attendance in the hospital regulations.

37. Medical officers are to visit their hospitals frequently, and to state the hours of visit in the monthly sick report. They will be required to be always available for any sudden call of the service; and when cholera prevails in the corps, are not to leave the barracks, except on imperative duty.

38. Smoking, to those habituated to the indulgence, may be permitted.

39. Corpses are to be removed to the dead-house without delay, buried as soon as possible, and conveyed in a covered cart—not on men's shoulders.

40. *Post-mortem* examinations are not to be discontinued, but performed under such modifications as the occasion will readily suggest.

41. Bodies of patients dying of cholera are to be sprinkled with chloride of lime, to be wrapped in a coarse sheet steeped in a strong solution of the same, and some of the powder should be put into the coffin.

42. Medical officers are not to visit civilian patients in town, and are to conform to the same regulations and instructions as other officers.

43. In infected places, Divine Service should preferably be performed in barrack, instead of marching the troops to church.

44. The old clothes of recruits are to be washed and fumigated ; or, if necessary, destroyed, and new clothes issued.

45. The clothes and bedding of cholera patients are to be immersed in cold water for forty-eight hours, then washed and steamed in boiling water, and dried in the open air.

46. The place whence a patient is taken is to be thoroughly washed, the bedding and bedstead removed, and fumigation made by chlorine gas, if possible, if not, by nitric acid gas, or fumes of vinegar.

47. The barrack bedding is to be removed with cholera or suspicious cases to the hospital, or Observation Ward.

48. Provisions brought from town should be delivered at the barrack gate.

49. Deserters, recruits, and men from escort or furlough, on rejoining, should be separated from the other soldiers for a period varying from seven to twenty-one days, according to circumstances.

50. Attention is called to Her Majesty's orders, in the Book of Instructions for Regimental Hospitals, on contagious diseases, extraordinary sickness, inspection of barracks and quarters, ventilation, and fumigation.

51. For the purification of drains, privies, clothes of recruits, &c., chloride of lime will be issued by the Ordnance Department, on the requisition of the commanding officer.

52. Bearers are to be applied for to the Ordnance Department, and a horse and covered cart hired for the conveyance of the sick, should the distance from the hospital require it.

MORBID APPEARANCES AFTER DEATH IN COLLAPSE.*

In the former, as well as in the latter epidemic, it was noted by several observers, that the icy coldness of the body, in the stage of collapse, passed away after death.

Rise of temperature, &c. No precise thermometrical details were given; but the surface of the body was observed to have become actually warm. Latterly, it was proved by Dr. Barlow, of Westminster Hospital, and others, by careful measurements, that a rise of temperature on the surface of the body did occur after death. In one case, in which the coldness of the surface during life was very marked, the thermometer indicated $102 \cdot 12°$, two hours after death ; in another case, ten minutes before death, the temperature in the axilla was $103 \cdot 1°$, and five minutes after death, it rose to $104°$; in a third case, the temperature of the uncovered body, twenty-five minutes after death, was $89°$; forty-five minutes after death it was $90°$; and fifty minutes after death, it rose to $91°$

* I purpose here to present such extracts as are deemed necessary, from the report of Dr. Gull, on the Morbid Anatomy, Pathology, and Treatment of Epidemic Cholera. "The design" of his portion of the work "has been to set down the principal ascertained facts, and to draw such conclusions as were possible from them."

Among the phenomena presented by the body Muscular con-
after death from cholera, are the well-known contrac- tractions.
tions of the muscles, which often occur to so great an extent, and
last for so long a period, as to excite horror in the ignorant, and
add in such minds a further mystery to this disease. The muscles
affected were principally those of the extremities, but contractions
were occasionally observed in the other voluntary muscles ; the duration of the contractions varying from a few minutes to two hours.

This phenomenon was observed more commonly in those who
died rapidly of the disease, in the middle period of life, when the
muscular system was vigorous and well developed, which will,
perhaps, account for their greater frequency in males than in
females.

Cadaveric rigidity often supervenes very quickly ; Rigor mortis.
in one case it began at the end of an hour, and in another after forty minutes. Its occurrence was not retarded by the
high temperature which the body retained.

Cruveilhier says that putrefactive changes were Putrefactive
slow, as in all cases where much blood has been lost, changes.
and adds—" In the alimentary canal, on the contrary, decomposition was rapid, as commonly occurs where the
digestive organs are the seat of considerable sanguineous congestion." Most observers confirm the former part of this statement ;
but with respect to the intestinal canal, the conditions were variable, and often the contrary of that noted by this great authority.

The stomach was pale, and generally more or less Stomach.
distended. It contained turbid mucoid fluid, grey
or colourless, or tinged of a chocolate or reddish-brown hue, by
admixture with blood. The surface of the mucous membrane was
covered with tenacious mucus, having in some cases a puriform
character, from the large amount of exfoliated epithelium. In
some instances it was pale ; in others, hyperæmia, in different
degrees, existed.

The membrane was generally rather thickened and opaque, the
texture firm, and the surface mammillated.

The state of the œsophagus and pharynx was not Pharynx and
generally reported. In one case, fatal after twelve œsophagus.
hours of acute symptoms, it was observed that the
lower part of the œsophagus was deprived of its epithelium.

The small intestines had generally a pink or rose Peritoneum.
external tint from hyperæmia of the portal venous
system. In some instances they had a remarkably dark colour, the
venous trunks being large, and full of pitchy blood. The different
tints soon changed upon exposure to the air.

The coats of the small intestines were thickened Small intes-
and pulpy, from œdema of the mucous membrane tines.
and sub-mucous tissue. The duodenum and ileum
were more commonly affected, and to a greater extent than the

jejunum.　In some instances the mucous membrane was pale throughout; in others, the lower part of the ileum only, or the duodenum only was hyperæmic.

The vascularity of the mucous membrane presented itself under two conditions, as uniform arborescent venous injection, affecting large tracts of the intestine, particularly the lower part of the ileum; or as patches of variable extent, in which the redness was punctate, and of a bright colour, frequently with spots of ecchymosis, and an exudation of tenacious mucus.

The villi were also small and prominent from œdema, especially throughout the jejunum.　Their appearance, and the condition of the epithelium covering them, were minutely described by Böhm, during the last epidemic of 1832-33.　Quoting Dr. Gairdner, the report says :—" The most frequent of all the abnormal conditions of the mucous membranes was the prominence of the intestinal glands, both of the aggregated and solitary, but especially of the latter.　This condition, the ' psorenteric' of some French writers, was found in about two-thirds of the cases."

The patches of Peyer.　The changes in the patches of Peyer were similar to those occurring in the villous surface of the mucous membrane generally, and in the solitary glands. They were often thickened and prominent, from infiltration of serous fluid, and the included glands, when visible, presented the conditions found in the solitary glands of the mucous membrane elsewhere.　There is no evidence that they were the seat of morbid changes peculiar to them in kind or in degree.

Large intestine.　The large intestine was more rarely affected with hyperæmia and ecchymosis than the small intestine. In many instances it presented nothing abnormal beyond a greater distinctness of the solitary glands.

The solitary glands.　In only four, out of thirty-four cases, were the solitary glands prominent throughout the whole extent of the large intestine; in eleven others they were slightly enlarged about the cæcum and ascending colon.　They were often translucent, from distension of their cavities with serous fluid; sometimes their distension had been followed by rupture, producing an appearance of a small rounded ulceration.

The spleen.　The state of the spleen is noted in twenty-three cases fatal in the algide state :—of those, in three it was of a natural size, and in eighteen it was small, or very small. It weighed but two ounces, two and a half, and three ounces, in seven cases recorded.　In most cases there was no obvious change in the tissue, beyond that arising from a want of blood, giving its capsule rather a wrinkled appearance, and enabling it to resist laceration, the texture being often described as pale, firm, and dry.

The liver.　After death in the algide stage, the liver was generally diminished in bulk, the tissue flaccid, and the capsule finely wrinkled.　The larger veins, both the hepatic and the portal, but especially the latter, were often full of dark viscid blood. The lobular appearance of the secreting structure was indistinct, and the whole tissue of rather a lighter red than usual; but to this rule there were exceptions.

The secreting structure, on a microscopical examination, presented nothing abnormal.

The gall-bladder was usually distended with dark bile, generally viscid, but sometimes more watery than natural. Gall-bladder. In most cases, the gall-ducts were not obviously affected. The mucous membrane of the gall-bladder and ducts was healthy, except in some rare cases, where it was the seat of morbid changes, similar to those occurring in the intestinal mucous membrane. In some cases, again, the gall-bladder was found very much distended with semi-transparent, slimy, pale, orange-coloured fluid, rendered turbid by boiling, and by nitric acid.

The kidneys were of the natural size, their surface was mottled by arborescent venous injection, and, on dissection, the same venous hyperæmia gave a dark colour to The kidneys. the cones. The secreting structure rarely presented any obvious morbid change.

The contents of the pelvis were mostly turbid, with exfoliated epithelium and free nuclei. The mucous membrane was generally pale, but in some instances it presented patches of venous injection.

The urinary bladder was empty, or contained but a small quantity of turbid fluid, like that in the pelvis of the kidneys, coagulable by heat. The mucous membrane was occasionally hyperæmic.

In the majority of cases fatal in the algide stage, no other morbid change existed than engorgement of the lower and posterior parts of the lungs with dark The lungs. blood. In some instances this was so complete as to cause portions of the pulmonary tissue to sink in water. The anterior and superior parts were drier than natural. In only one case reported was there any degree of œdema. In certain cases the pulmonary tissue throughout was full of dark blood.

The pleura was healthy, or sometimes covered with a trace of slimy albuminous secretion, as in the peritoneum.

The bronchial tubes were normal in appearance, or their mucous membrane was congested. They contained a small amount of frothy serum, sometimes tinged with blood.

In the cases reported, the pericardium generally contained a small quantity of serum, varying from a drachm to half an ounce, or an ounce. The colour of the fluid Pericardium, heart, &c. was mostly a pale straw or citron, but in some instances it was decidedly sanguinolent. On the adherent pericardium, about the base of the heart, small ecchymoses were not infrequent.

The physical condition of the blood in the cavities of the heart
The blood. and large vessels varied with respect to the degree
and mode of coagulation, but most observers admit
that it was more commonly dark and fluid, or less coagulable than
in other diseases. In nearly half the cases of fatal collapse
tabulated, the blood was fluid, either entirely so, or with but a few
masses of fibrin; in less than one-fourth of the cases did the
coagulation approach the normal condition. This accords with
the observations made by Dr. Parkes upon cases in India.

With respect to the chemical constitution of the blood, the committee was unable to institute any new series of observations; but,
according to Schmidt, the effects of the abnormal transudation
of fluid from the capillaries of the intestine in cholera upon the
remainder of the circulating fluid may be thus summed up:—

1. The density of the blood, and of its morphological elements
(blood cells and intercellular fluid), is increased in proportion to
the duration of the process of exudation from the intestinal capillaries. It reaches its maximum in 36 hours, and then falls again
as water is re-absorbed.

2. The solids of the blood and of its morphological elements,
left after evaporation at 248° Fahr., are relatively increased in a
marked degree, according to the time from the commencement of
the exudation of the saline fluid from the intestinal capillaries.
They reach, after 36 hours, nearly one-half more than the normal
proportion, and afterwards sink as fluid is again absorbed.

3. This increase relates only to the organic constituents (albu-
minates) of the blood and its morphological elements, and not to
the inorganic salts, the absolute quantity of which, although indeed
increased directly after the onset of severe symptoms, appears to
be subsequently diminished.

The degree of concentration of the organic constituents, resulting from the exudation of the saline fluid from the intestinal
capillaries, regularly rises according to the interval from the beginning of the attack, and reaches the highest point 36 hours from
the onset, after which, even in fatal cases, a re-absorption of fluid
occurs. This increase of inorganic salts at the beginning of the
disease, owing to the large amount of fluid poured out, reaches its
maximum after four hours; they afterwards, within a few hours,
fall to the normal quantity; after 18 hours, sink much below it;
and after 36 or 40 hours, are still further diminished, according to
the time which has elapsed.

The sinuses and veins of the meninges were more or less loaded
Encephalon. with dark blood. In most cases, this was the only
morbid appearance. In some cases the vessels of the
pia mater were loaded with blood, while in others, effusion into the
lateral ventricles, sub-arachnoid effusion, a soft watery condition
of the brain, and œdema of the pia mater, were observed.

After the exposition, of which the above is an abstract, Dr. Gull proceeds to describe the morbid appearances where death occurred after reaction; but as, in general, these last do not appear to have had much of important distinctness and of difference from the morbid appearances already described, I must here refrain from quoting them. In the instances of persons dying during the febrile reaction consequent on the cholera collapse, we should naturally expect to find congestions of the gastro-intestinal mucous membrane, with hyperæmia and serous effusions in the brain.

PATHOLOGY.

" The first unequivocal symptoms of cholera indicate that the gastro-intestinal mucous membrane, with its ganglionic nervous centres, are the focus of the morbid action.

" The morbid appearances characteristic of cholera are most marked in the small intestine, duodenum, and stomach, and the general symptoms indicate an early and severe depression of the ganglionic nervous centres of these parts.

Pathology of the cholera process in the intestines.

" The principal phenomena which arrest attention are the œdematous state of the mucous membrane, and the more or less extensive patches of capillary and venous hyperæmia, and ecchymosis. These, together with the character and amount of the fluid effused, demonstrate an important lesion of the circulation through the affected parts. How this is produced can at present be no further elucidated than by the hypothesis of a specific poison, acting upon the ganglionic nervous centres, or upon the mucous membrane itself. The former appears to us the more probable supposition, from being more in accordance with some other phenomena of the disease, as the profuse sweating and the sudden and severe collapse, which, as will be seen hereafter, are not in a necessary and constant relation to the discharges from the mucous membrane. Either would, however, suffice to explain the altered condition of the circulation, since it is well known that if one of the agencies in operation in the capillary circulation be abnormal, there will be a corresponding change in the ease and rapidity with which it is sent through the tissue. In this respect nearly the same result is produced, whether the blood be unfitted to stimulate and nourish, or the nutrition in the part itself be perverted or defective, or the vessels be deficient in nervous supply. We no longer look for mere mechanical causes of vascular retardation; and whatever light may hereafter be thrown upon this stage of cholera, it will no doubt come from a more intimate knowledge of the pathology of the capillary circulation.

" These morbid changes in the first stage of cholera are of the simplest kind;—the tissue is infiltrated, and the glandular follicles are distended with the same watery fluid as escapes into the cavity of the intestine:—the epithelium, by this maceration, readily separates after death, and to a certain extènt during life, but not so largely as Böhm supposed. Exfoliation of the epithelium appeared to this excellent observer to constitute an essential part of the primary morbid action, but further investigations show that during life it occurred to only a very limited extent, and was in itself an unimportant change. The coats of the capillaries and smaller veins are often ruptured, giving rise to ecchymosis:—this, with the punctate and stellate character of the hyperæmia, denotes a want of tonicity in the vessels.

" As death occurs only when the phenomena reach their greatest intensity, and when the circulation in the nervous system generally is much retarded, the ramifications of the intestinal veins in particular are often distended with dark blood.

"An examination of the fluids effused from the mucous membrane gives no evidence of active plasmatic changes taking place in them. On the contrary, the large amount of fluid thrown out, its low specific gravity, and its other physical characters, indicate an almost passive exosmosis, as through a dead membrane. Some observers have referred the morbid changes to a *catarrhal condition*, others have regarded the disease as a form of *serous hæmorrhage*, and the Berlin pathologists, whose attention was particularly arrested by the occurrence of amorphous granular fibrin in and upon the affected surface of the mucous membrane, designate it a *destructive diphtheritic inflammation*. We believe that, for the present, such generalizations, however plausible, are of little value, and that we arrest inquiry by their adoption. The depression of the capillary power—the extreme exhaustion of the great ganglionic nervous centres in the abdomen—the passive character of the lesions of the mucous membrane—its normal action being reversed to a fatal exosmosis—are peculiar to cholera, and give it an individuality which forbids our merging it for the present in any general category.

" Although the intestinal tract is the principal seat of the morbid actions, they are not limited to it. The kidneys, at an early stage, are sometimes affected; the urine having been found albuminous prior to its suppression, and the secreting tissue and the lining membrane of the pelvis present occasionally, after death, lesions of the same character as those observed in the intestine.

" In the female the uterine organs are similarly affected; the lining membrane of the uterus and vagina being frequently much congested and ecchymosed, with commencing diphtheritic exudation upon it.

" The liver is free from disease, except in some rare cases, where the lining membrane of the ducts and gall-bladder is the seat of the cholera process, their contents being then of the rice-water character. The distension of the gall-bladder with bile is nearly constant, but cannot be referred to as a pathological indication of any moment, as such a condition is common when the digestive function is long interrupted, and indicates a passive rather than an active state.

"There is a hypothesis regarding the nature of cholera, based upon the supposition of a suppression of the hepatic secretion and consequent congestion of the liver; this is altogether unsupported by anatomical facts. The absence of bile from the evacuations is not a necessary phenomenon of the early stage of cholera. In a large proportion of cases the diarrhœa ceases to be bilious only when the more intense symptoms set in, and even then the rice-water fluid often gives, with re-agents, distinct evidence of the presence of bile; but when it is no longer passed in the evacuations, the secretion is not altogether suppressed, as shown in the contents of the gall-bladder and ducts after death. The hepatic function does not appear to be subject to any further derangement than that which naturally *follows upon* the retardation of the circulation during the stage of collapse.

"It would have been unnecessary to advert to this hypothesis had it not widely influenced the treatment of the disease. Dr. Ayre, the great advocate of the administration of calomel, gives the following rationale of the cholera process. He says :—' Now, there is one condition which is uniformly and conspicuously present in malignant cholera, and is, indeed, characteristic of it— namely, a suppressed or suspended secretion of bile, as shown by the diminution, and at length the total disappearance of it from those watery discharges which are poured so profusely from the stomach and bowels. As a consequence of this cessation of the hepatic function, an accumulation,' he adds, ' will take place in the liver, of venous blood, and an impeded circulation result from it, producing` a congested state of that organ, and subsequently, by a retention of the blood in its course through them, of those abdominal organs whose circulation is associated with it. Now the congestion thus produced in the portal venous system of the liver and its associated organs, constitutes the stage of collapse, and under various modifications and grades of intensity, whose real nature and amount are unknown, forms the essence of it in all.'

"Such a train of reasoning is unsupported by any evidence. The serous rice-water character of the cholera stools is obviously due to special pathological changes in the mucous membrane, and not to any merely mechanical congestion of a secondary kind, as here stated. What these pathological changes are, we have endeavoured to show, and have referred them to a specific action of the cholera poison operating through the blood; a more minute account we are unable to give.

"The appearances, after death, in the chest and cranium, show that the viscera in these cavities were not primarily affected. The occasional emphysema of the lungs, their emptiness of blood, except at the posterior and inferior parts, and the inelastic compressed character of their tissue observed in some cases, are explicable by the state of the respiration and circulation at the last stage of life. The congestion of the veins, and the effusions under the membranes and into the ventricles of the brain, are referrible to the same cause."

Cholera has been classed among zymotic diseases, but its clinical history and morbid anatomy are opposed to the theory of its being due to a zymosis, in a strict sense of the term. In a zymotic disease certain plastic changes are induced, from which results its augmentation. In cholera we have no evidence of such changes; the alterations in the blood, so far as they are known, being referrible to the loss of its fluid parts, in accordance with the physical laws of exosmosis. The local morbid action appears to be of a negative rather than of a positive kind. The marked depression of the organic functions, and the morphological characters of the effused fluids, as well as their general physical properties, indicate a passiveness almost peculiar to cholera. In cholera, the onset of an attack is frequently sudden, and the effects apparently direct, such as would follow the immediate action of an extraneous poison upon the body. The zymotic process is more gradual, and the symptoms follow a more constant rule with respect to them.

Is cholera a zymotic or contagious disease?

Cholera appears to consist of but one single series of actions, which may vary in intensity through every gradation, but, throughout, maintain the same character of passiveness. There is no febrile stage to which zymotic changes, as ordinarily observed, and the production of a *materies morbi* may be referred.

Certain prodromata of a general kind have been enumerated as occurring prior to the symptoms which arise from the local morbid action in the intestinal mucous membrane, such as vertigo—headache—general malaise— muscular fatigue — faintings—wandering pains in the limbs— cramps—gripings in the abdomen—sense of weight at the præcordia—and nausea. A cursory inspection of such a category suffices to show that, even if generally present, these indications would be unsatisfactory. Many of them arise from mental emotion, so prevalent during an epidemic, and others are not so much premonitory of an attack as the first symptoms of its onset, and the result of the morbid action already begun in the abdomen.

General prodromata.

In most cases, a painless diarrhœa, lasting for a variable time, precedes the more characteristic symptoms. Although all observers admit the frequency of this precursory stage, there has been some difference of opinion, and much unfruitful discussion about its pathology, whether it be a part of the disease, and due to the action of the poison, or merely a common diarrhœa, upon which the specific effects may at any moment be engrafted. There are no characteristics which enable us to draw these distinctions with any certainty.

Precursory diarrhœa.

Experience has sufficiently shown that during the epidemic the stages from a mild and apparently simple diarrhœa to the rice-water purging and collapse are not definable, and that the former, if unchecked, does, in numerous instances, gradually pass into the latter, with its attendant collapse and fatal results. The diarrhœa which prevails when cholera is epidemic is due to the same cause as cholera itself.

Numerous replies were received, all serving to establish the frequency of a stage of diarrhœa, lasting from a few hours to several days. A table fixing the period definitely of the duration of premonitory diarrhœa, exhibits a range of from one hour to ten days. *Frequency of precursory diarrhœa.*

The evacuations were generally more profuse and liquid than usual, but otherwise of a natural appearance, often unaccompanied by pain, and passed without effort, the painlessness and passiveness giving a false security to the patient. It was not until the nervous *Is the precursory diarrhœa characteristic?* system began to be depressed, and the feculent character of the stools was lessened or lost, and they became alkaline, watery, and flocculent, that they were distinctive. On this point the experience of the profession appears to be uniform, and hence we may draw the following conclusion—that during the prevalence of the epidemic every case of diarrhœa arising without obvious cause, may be regarded as a probable result of the specific poison.

The cholera poison is not known to produce its fatal effects without the characteristic affection of the intestines. Cholera sicca, in a strict sense, does not occur, for although the disease may be fatal without any evacuation, the intestines, *How far collapse depends upon loss of fluids.* after death in such cases, have been found to contain the rice-water fluid. In some cases which came under our observation, on a *post-mortem* examination, the larger intestines contained healthy fæces, whilst in the upper two-thirds of the small intestine the mucous membrane presented the ordinary changes induced by the cholera process, and the rice-water effusion was abundant.

As many of the symptoms of the stage of collapse depend upon the loss of fluid, it has been too absolutely inferred that the general phenomena of the disease are always in a necessary relation to the amount of these effusions.

THE TREATMENT.

It is well ascertained that in the largest proportion of cases, at least in European countries, the poison of cholera produces its first effects on the system *gradually*, as indicated by diarrhœa, varying in duration from a few hours to several days before the intense symptoms supervene. This period may be called the period of invasion.

The numerous communications received by the College establish

Treatment of the period of invasion.   the importance of recognising this stage at its commencement, and render it highly probable that the morbid effects may then be often successfully combated.

The popular theory that the discharges are an effort of nature to throw off a *materies morbi,* is not only unsupported by any known facts of the disease, but, when applied to practice, is found to increase the violence of the symptoms.

At present no antidote or specific medicine is known to neutralize the cause of cholera, or with certainty to arrest its early effects; but the communications received show that the diarrhœa was, in a large number of cases, arrested by various combinations of such remedies as generally suppress discharges from the intestines, and prevent the exhaustion of nervous energy.

Opium was an almost constant ingredient, and was given in conjunction with astringents, aromatics, and diffusible stimuli.

A recumbent position is proved by experience, and also from the nature of the case, to be a most important measure. It prevents exhaustion, favours the circulation, and lessens the frequency of the evacuations. It is highly probable that cases, which otherwise resisted the action of medicines, would have readily yielded, had the horizontal position in a warm bed been strictly enforced. Enemata were not, as might have been anticipated, of much service, since the small intestine and duodenum are the principal source of the effusion.

The indications of treatment in this stage are formed entirely from the mucous membrane itself, independently of any hypothetical derangement of the liver. This organ does not appear to be in any way the cause of the symptoms; the diminution of the bile in the evacuations, as they become more and more fluid, being an ·effect, rather than a cause of the disease. The character of the fluid thrown out—the attendant symptoms—the absence of pain— the passiveness of the evacuations, and their occasional retention to a large amount in the intestine, indicate a depression of all the energies of the affected surface.

The amount of success attained by early treatment is not yet determined; there is a general opinion that it was very great, but this must be received with some limitation, as the facts upon which it is founded are not unequivocal. By far the greater number of cases of diarrhœa would probably never have passed beyond this stage if no medicines had been administered; and, on the contrary, in many instances the symptoms were uninfluenced by any treatment, and fatal collapse came on in spite of every effort to prevent it.

Notwithstanding this uncertainty, the general results of preventive measures were apparently very favourable, as shown by the small proportion of cases which passed into the severer forms of the disease subsequently to early treatment.

The following are the results of the house-to-house visitation in the metropolis from September 1 to October 27, 1849 :—

Cases of diarrhœa discovered.	Cases approaching cholera discovered.	Cases which passed into cholera discovered.
43,737	978	52

In various cities, as Dumfries and Glasgow, the same favourable results attended the system of house-to-house visitation; and it is no longer matter of doubt that the earlier the disease is encountered, the greater, in an infinitely high ratio, are the advantages under which medicines are employed to counteract it.

On this division of our subject we can do little more than point out, according to the evidence before us, what forms of treatment seem to have been of some service, or useless, or injurious; and by thus clearing the ground, prepare the way for better directed efforts. *Treatment of impending and complete collapse.*

An enumeration of all the means proposed for the treatment of this stage would be useless; it is, therefore, only upon the principal of them that we shall make any report.

Calomel stands foremost, from having in this country been more fully used than any other remedy. The theory of the disease which has chiefly led to its employment, is not supported by anatomical facts. The absence of bile from *Use of calomel.* the evacuations appears to be merely a subordinate result. Calomel can be administered only on empirical grounds, and its value must be determined by the results so obtained; for there appears to be no argument in favour of its exhibition either from analogy or pathology.

The results in 365 cases treated by this remedy in small and frequent doses were 187 deaths, and 178 recoveries.

The numbers given by Dr. Ayre to the College of Physicians, do not sustain his favourable opinion of the treatment of cholera by small doses of calomel. The deaths were 365 out of 725 unequivocal cases.

Under various and opposite plans, the recoveries, even in severe cases, averaged from 45 to 55 per cent., according to the period of the epidemic; they should therefore exceed the highest of these numbers before they can be adduced in proof of the value of any particular method of treatment.

In general, no appreciable effects followed the administration of calomel, even after a large amount in small and frequently repeated doses had been administered. For the most part it was quickly evacuated by vomiting and purging, or, when retained for a longer period, was afterwards passed from the bowels unchanged. Salivation but very rarely occurred, and then only in the milder cases.

We conclude that calomel was inert when administered in collapse ; that the cases of recovery following its employment at this period were due to the natural course of the disease, as they did not surpass the ordinary average obtained when the treatment consisted in the use of cold water only.

This is termed the "rational method" of treatment, and was intended to combine those remedies which seemed best fitted to fulfil the supposed indications of this stage. The calomel was given to restore the functions of the liver, and as an alterative of the morbid action in the gastro-intestinal mucous membrane ; the opium to allay irritation and arrest the discharges ; and the stimuli to counteract the depression of the nervous system. Experience did not confirm the theory : the results were unfavourable, and not altogether so indifferent as when calomel was exhibited by itself.

Treatment by calomel, opium, and stimulants.

Although opium and diffusible stimuli, brandy, camphor, and ammonia were useful at an early stage of the disease, as collapse set in, they not only failed to produce any favourable result, but often aggravated the symptoms.

It seems well ascertained that opium in large doses was at this period injurious, by increasing the cerebral oppression, and embarrassing the system during reaction. It was probably less and less applicable as the disease advanced to its characteristic development.

Stimuli, especially the various preparations of alcohol, did not act as restoratives in collapse, but even increased the irritability of the stomach, and added to the sense of oppression at the præcordia.

The expectations excited by the early success apparently obtained by the use of chloroform, were not realized in its subsequent employment. It not unfrequently allayed the vomiting and cramps, but did not in any degree arrest the course of the disease.

The perchloride of carbon in five or ten grain doses, and a solution of camphor in chloroform, acted as powerful stimuli, but the results did not indicate that they possessed any specific therapeutic value. Although they produced symptoms of reaction, this apparent improvement was generally, in severe cases, but transient, and their continued use seemed to exhaust the little remaining power rather than to restore the patient.

The obvious requirements of the system, and the urgent thirst, were sufficient indications for the use of diluents, and the experience of the profession appears to be uniformly in favour of permitting patients to gratify their appetite for them. Cold water was generally preferred, and good results were often observed when it was taken freely in repeated and copious draughts, although it excited vomiting. In smaller quantities, and iced, it was refreshing to the system, and allayed the irritability of the stomach.

The use of cold water and ice.

Ice was generally grateful to many patients in impending or approaching collapse, and probably acted favourably upon the mucous membrane, and served to arrest the discharges. The use of ice and cold water appears, in most cases, to relieve the burning thirst, while it favours reaction. Dr. Arnott administered a mixture of ice and salt in large quantities, and in the cases of two patients so treated, both recovered; but there is no further experience respecting this mode of treatment.

Salines of low specific gravity were sometimes given instead of common water, the intention being to restore to the blood a fluid similar to that lost in the early stages of the disease. We have no evidence that they possessed any influence over the local morbid action in the mucous membrane. It was not until this surface had in part recovered its function of absorption, that any good resulted from their employment. When given at an early period, and in a more concentrated form, they appeared to favour the discharges.

The treatment by salines.

Emetics were sometimes given at the onset of the disease, with the intention of cutting short the morbid action, by distributing the blood to the surface, and relieving the congestion of the intestinal mucous membrane. It is probable that, when administered early, they were occasionally of service; but the results appear to have been too uncertain to admit of their forming any part of a routine system of treatment. In collapse they were inadmissible, being often followed by increased exhaustion; and even when they appeared to produce symptoms of reaction, this effect was but of short duration.

Emetics.

Bleeding was employed in the premonitory stage of cholera, for the purpose of arresting the discharges by relieving the congestion of the intestinal mucous membrane. This was not much resorted to in the last epidemic; and the communications to the College contain but little mention of it. The only reports in its favour, by Annesley and other writers on the disease as it occurs in India, have not been confirmed by further observation; and hence, except in rare and exceptional cases, it is not usually had recourse to in the premonitory stage, or at the onset of the more severe symptoms. Its general inadmissibility is to be inferred from its almost entire disuse in the last epidemic.

Blood-letting.

Even in the consecutive fever blood-letting in any form requires much caution. Leeching the epigastrium and temples, or cupping the back of the neck, were sometimes of service in obviating the cerebral congestion of this period; but if carried to any great extent, were injurious by exhausting the patient.

The general inference, from all we have observed of the disease and collected from the experience of others, is, that large losses of blood, in the consecutive fever, are injurious; but that occasionally good results follow its local abstraction, according to the indications of the symptoms.

Quinine, strychnia, arsenic, sesquichloride of iron, nitrate of silver, nitrous acid, chlorine water sulphur, sulphuric acid, bichloride of mercury, char-coal, &c. &c. The failure of these methods of treatment, which, from being based upon some supposed indications of the disease, may be called rational, led naturally to the employment of almost every active medicine in the materia medica.

It is notorious, that the results have been discouraging, notwithstanding the bold assertions to the contrary. The communications made to the College contain no data for determining the inquiry, nor is anything deserving the name of evidence in favour of the value of these means, to be gathered from the numerous journals and published treatises in this country, and on the Continent. This part of our report must, therefore, be defective, although an unlimited amount of time and labour has been bestowed upon a perusal and comparison of the statements brought before us.

The report goes on to say, that the therapeutic history of cholera leads the authors to guard against the submission of remedies to what is termed a " *systematic trial* in a *series* of *cases*," by expressing their conviction that for empirical inquiry to be pursued to a good end, the most favourable opportunities are required for noting the state of the patient at the commencement, and at different stages of the treatment, by which alone discrepancies in the results can be reconciled.

Again, the employment, without definite scope, of one remedy after another, with the vague hope of at last finding a specific, is to be deprecated, not only because it can lead to no good result, but because it deprives the patient of that assistance which established experience affords.

The state of the patient in the collapse of cholera is so unfavourable to the absorption of medicines, that even if we knew the remedy in itself most appropriate, we could not anticipate great results from its administration by the mouth at this period. Every consideration of this formidable malady urges upon us the paramount importance of obviating the causes which give rise to it, and of arresting symptoms at the onset.

The application of heat to the surface has been largely tried. The hot bath alone, or with mustard or salt, &c., the vapour bath and the hot-air bath, have been principally employed. It appears to be the uniform experience of the profession, that in collapse these means are but of little value.

In the earlier stage of the disease, or when it is less severe, and the pulse indicates some degree of power, the hot and vapour bath may allay cramps, and prove grateful to the patient; but when the nervous and vascular functions are greatly depressed, and the surface cold and clammy, although heat may be imparted to the body, it rarely excites reaction in the system itself; on the contrary, it is oppressive to the patient, and increases the exhaustion.

It is not found by experience that the degree of reaction, which may be sometimes excited by such means, and by internal stimuli, is of any permanent advantage, nor was this to be anticipated from a consideration of the conditions of the system in the collapse of cholera. The state of the blood, and the extreme depression of the nervous power, necessarily render abortive such attempts at restoring the circulation. The whole tendency of the evidence yet acquired from the treatment of this stage, is towards a more restricted use of powerful excitants of the kind alluded to.

On the Continent, in the former, and in the last epidemic, cold affusion was highly spoken of as a means of producing reaction. The patient was placed in a warm hip-bath, and cold water poured or thrown over the head, back, and chest. This was done quickly, and the patient then placed between two warm blankets. If the first application was followed by any improvement, the operation was repeated every three or four hours. The results appear to have been, on the whole, more satisfactory than from the hot bath. *Cold affusion.*

The "wet sheet envelope" was more commonly used in this country. The effect varied according to the state of the patient; and in the milder cases it favoured reaction, but when the disease was severe, it was useless or injurious. The sweating caused by it added to the exhaustion, and had no influence in arresting the intestinal discharges. *The wet sheet.*

In the milder cases, stimulating epithems of mustard and turpentine were of some use in relieving local symptoms, and for obviating nervous depression. Frictions, chloroform liniments, and warm fomentations allayed the cramps. In severer cases these means were quite ineffective. *Stimulating epithems.*

Two cases are reported in which oxygen was inhaled in the stage of collapse with asphyxia, at the same time galvanism was employed to stimulate the respiratory function. The effects upon the circulation and respiration were such as might have been anticipated. The heart's action was, for the time, increased, and there were slight symptoms of general reaction, but no permanently-favourable influence was exercised, by these means, upon the course of the disease in the majority of cases. *Oxygen and galvanism.*

This method of treatment was not much investigated during the last epidemic. The results were, as in 1832-33, generally unfavourable. Its nature, however, cannot be determined by statistics collected from various sources. The operation in all its details is a delicate *Saline injections into the Veins.*

one, and requires not only a careful discrimination of the cases to which it is applicable, but also an exact attention to the physical characters and composition of the fluid to be injected, and other collateral circumstances. Until these points receive greater elucidation, the results obtained can form no sound basis for an opinion respecting its merits.

Medicated venous injections.
The arrest of the function of absorption in the stage of collapse, and the consequent inertness of all medicines administered by the stomach at this period, naturally led to the suggestion of injecting them into the veins. The trials which have been made in this way are too few to admit of any deduction from them. In the former epidemic, laudanum, camphor, quinine, &c., were used unsuccessfully.

From the discovery of the circulation to the present time various experiments of this kind have been instituted by different observers, which prove that medicinal substances can thus with safety be employed.

Treatment of imperfect reaction.
Of those who resist the fatal influence of the cholera poison in the stage of collapse, a large number yet fall victims to its protracted effects. Probably half the cases fatal after the first forty-eight hours of severe symptoms belong to this category.

We may, therefore, infer that much care is required during the early period of reaction, since circumstances, in themselves apparently trifling, may at this time determine the issue. A strict observance of the horizontal posture, moderate external warmth, stimulating applications to the extremities, region of the heart, or epigastrium, and the administration internally of diffusible stimuli in small quantities, with the free use of ice, cold water, and other diluents, appear to constitute the principal part of the treatment as far as it is yet determined.

The cerebral oppression and delirium of this period are probably due to exhaustion and the asphyctic condition of the capillary circulation, the blood being imperfectly aërated and deficient in water. The state of the brain which gives rise to these symptoms is to be distinguished from that which occurs at a later stage from retention of the urinary excretions. It is not benefited by local or general depletion, but is slowly removed as the circulation is re-established.

Treatment of " consecutive fever" or uræmia.
The fruitless search after specifics which occupies the mind in the preceding stages of the disease is now tacitly given up, and we are content to be guided by the pathological indications, as in other diseases. But whilst our attention is directed to the local and more tangible complications, it must not be forgotten that they are the effects of an agent which has remarkably depressed the whole of the vital powers, and, consequently, rendered neces-

sary modifications in the activity of the measures otherwise adapted to their removal.

The next important indication for treatment is the depuration of the blood from the urinary excretions. The conditions following collapse are favourable to their retention, viz., the blood is of high specific gravity, the circulation is embarrassed, and lesions of the kidneys are frequent.

The treatment must include such means as allay irritability of the stomach and promote absorption, restore circulation, and remove the lesions of the kidneys. Of these may be enumerated the use of ice and cold water, effervescing draughts, or weak solutions of the alkaline salts, the warm bath, emollient enemata, dry-cupping to the loins, and counter-irritation over the stomach.

Stimuli are sometimes necessary for the purpose of counteracting the nervous depression; but their employment, whilst the system is poisoned with urea, obviously requires careful regulation. Stimulating diuretics, as squills, cantharides, &c., are not adapted to the great majority of the cases. The spontaneous occurrence of profuse diuresis, when the intestinal mucous membrane recovers its functions, shows that the matters to be excreted are, in themselves, sufficient to stimulate the kidneys, if the conditions favourable to their action be present.

Occasional doses of mercurials, followed by laxatives, were found to be useful, probably by quickening the circulation through the liver and promoting absorption, as well as depurating the blood, but their use was necessarily limited, whilst the excretive function of the kidneys was defective.

During the consecutive fever, the intestinal tract is frequently, in different parts, the seat of persistent   Muco-enterite.
congestion with diphtheritic inflammation and ulceration. The termination of the ileum is most commonly thus affected, and is the frequent source of the bloody stools observed during reaction. In some rare instances, limited sloughs of the mucous membrane result from effusion of blood into the submucous tissue. Such have been observed in the large intestine and in the stomach. The character of the local action indicates a want of reparative power.

The treatment of these lesions is probably that generally employed with success in other forms of gastro-enterite, such as gentle support, ammonia, serpentaria, and a moderate allowance of wine.

Such is an abstract, as copious as I could render it, of Dr. Gull's ably-conducted portion of the Report to the College of Physicians.

EPIDEMIC CHOLERA IN CALCUTTA.

There is no branch of medical inquiry more interesting, nor any more important, than the history of epidemics, nor one, the accurate observation of which would prove more useful to physicians,

in every climate. How true it is in our day, as in that of Sydenham, that no one has treated this great question in proportion to
the dignity of the subject.

An accurate history of epidemics in Bengal would prove of
great value, as enabling us to trace their connexion with changes
of climate and condition of the surrounding localities, or with the
social condition of the people, European and native. Had such a
history existed, it would have helped to an earlier establishment
of general principles, and to a more rational plan of treating the
local fevers especially; for, though all the epidemic fevers within
my personal recollection differed from the ordinary endemics of
the country, still, there was in most of them so much of the savour
of the soil (if I may be allowed the expression), as to render a
knowledge of their history and treatment a matter of interest and
importance.

It is these sweeping epidemics, aggravated by endemial and
social influences, that swell the bills of mortality in our Eastern
metropolis, and that did so in former times more especially, to so
fearful an extent: in truth, endemics are very often the parent-
stock upon which epidemics are engrafted.

Under a system of local sanitary improvement, such as has for
years past, at the original instance of the author of this work, been
established in Calcutta, the endemic sources of disease will be
gradually diminished, and along with them the force of epidemics
may also be reduced, so as greatly to improve the health and enhance the value of European and native life, within that rising
emporium. Let want, filth, crowding, and misery be removed,
and epidemics will have lost their chief power. It is these and
other well-known sanitary defects that everywhere, but especially
under tropical influences, give such destructive power to endemic
and epidemic agencies, and that gave rise to the observation of
Cabanis—that the effects of climate are not the same with the rich
as with the poor.

CHOLERA-FEVER OF 1834.

As bearing on the subject of this article, I would briefly mention
a form of epidemic fever which visited Calcutta in 1834, and which
we termed the cholera-fever.

It arose in May—the worst of the cholera months—and continued through that and the following month, disappearing only on
the full establishment of the rainy season.

Its symptoms were, heat and dryness of skin, frequent soft
pulse, clammy white tongue, and generally a slight diarrhœa.

So mild a fever I seldom recollect to have seen; yet it was most
dangerous to treat—the irritable condition of the bowels, which
formed so prominent a symptom of the epidemic, being readily
aggravated into fatal cholera whenever purgatives of a saline or
drastic nature were exhibited.

At first the peculiar character of the fever was not known ; and I remember hearing at the time that several deaths occurred where strong purgatives had been exhibited *over night;* indeed, one such case came accidentally under my observation. It was that of a gentleman, the patient of a professional friend, into whose house I was called in haste on passing at 6 A.M. His countenance and voice at once testified to the collapse of cholera, and to his approaching end. He had been feverish during the previous day, and had taken a drachm of compound jalap powder at nine o'clock of the previous night.

Others fell victims, in like manner, to the hasty exhibition of purgatives ; but within a few days, and when the nature of the epidemic became generally known, it proved a manageable form of disease, and after that few deaths occurred.

A stout mercantile gentleman, whom I treated with a moderate dose of castor oil, had fifteen stools between 8 and 11 A.M.—the former having been the hour of exhibition. Had the above dose, small as it was, been administered at bedtime, the result to the patient would have been fatal.

Not only was the peculiar fever here noticed prone to merge into true cholera, but I had to remark, on three several occasions in Calcutta, that when the cholera poison was present in a concentrated form, we were for the time precluded from treating the cases of ordinary remittent fever of Europeans in our usual manner. Moderate blood-lettings were now liable to be followed by extraordinary collapse, and purgatives could not be administered over night, lest the fever should be changed by morning into a deadly cholera. The state of the system here indicated, showed that the fevers, and also the diarrhœas of the country, did, under epidemic or other peculiar influences, merge into the true cholera, the cholera poison being at the moment the more powerful influence. In times like these we found it difficult to persuade ourselves that the endemic and the epidemic diseases were absolutely " caused by different poisons."

No fever of the nature of the epidemic just noticed, affording as it did an example of choleraic remittent, had been known in Calcutta previously ; nor has it recurred since the year specified. The treatment I adopted was by mild doses of calomel and James's powder, with a grain of opium, exhibited at bedtime, and an occasional mild aperient in the forenoon.

All the epidemics of which I could trace any record occurred in the hot months of March, April, or May ; and thus they correspond, as to time of occurrence, with almost all the known European epidemics. Andral states, that of fifty epidemics known in Europe, thirty-six occurred in summer, twelve in autumn, one in winter, and one in spring.

INFLUENCE OF HIGH TEMPERATURE.

Independently of the proved influence of heat in promoting the existence and continuance of epidemic cholera, it is remarkable that this disease should have so frequently commenced in Bengal at the season during which ventilation is most free and effective. In Europe we are told that a free ventilation is the most efficient means of destroying the cholera poison; yet, in Bengal, the epidemic has been seen very generally to commence about the middle of March, when the south-west monsoon comes sweeping with power and purity over the plains, fresh off the Bay of Bengal. The freedom of ventilation at all seasons in India will account, I think, for the circumstance that so little suspicion of contagion has at any time arisen in that country—from the first origin of the epidemic to the present day. It is a fact that, " of between 250 and 300 medical officers in Bengal, most of whom saw the disease largely, only three were attacked, and only one attack was fatal." In Calcutta, as in London, the highest range of temperature was that of greatest prevalence of cholera. " The reader of the meteorological tables," says Dr. Farr, " will not fail to observe that in the thirty-sixth week of 1854, when the cholera raged, and the deaths from all causes rose to their maximum (3413), the average daily range of temperature was 30°·9, consequently the greatest in 'the fifty-two weeks ; the *highest* temperature of the week was 81°·2, the *lowest* was 43°·1, therefore the entire range was 38°·1." It is worthy of remark, says the same authority, that in the hot season of 1846, when the cholera epidemic acquired great force about the Indus, summer cholera and diarrhœa prevailed with great violence in England.

THE INFLUENCE OF SEASON.

The following tables are interesting, as exhibiting the influence of season on sickness and mortality from epidemic cholera amongst the inhabitants of Calcutta, native and European.

Mortality by Epidemic Cholera of Hindus and Mahomedans for each Month during Seven Years, from 1832 *to* 1838 *inclusive.*

MONTHS.	Hindus.	Maho-medans.	Total.	Remarks.
In 7 Januarys	572	125	696	Mean temperature, 66°·2. Dry.
7 Februarys ...	620	196	816	,, ,, 69°·8. Rain.
7 Marches	1,873	439	2,312	,, ,, 80°·0. Dry.
7 Aprils	2,707	482	3,189	,, ,, 85°·4. Dry.
7 Mays	2,170	464	2,634	,, ,, 85°·$\frac{7}{15}$ Rain.
7 Junes	615	217	832	,, ,, 83°·7. Rain.
7 Julys	914	133	1,047	,, ,, 81°·8. Rain.
7 Augusts	806	146	952	,, ,, 82°·0. Rain.
7 Septembers ...	785	121	906	,, ,, 82°·8. Rain.
7 Octobers	1,030	198	1,228	,, ,, 79°·$\frac{2}{15}$ Dry.
7 Novembers ...	1,687	230	1,917	,, ,, 74°·2. Dry.
7 Decembers ...	1,425	161	1,586	,, ,, 66°·6. Dry.
Total	15,204	2911	18,115	

In the jails of Bengal, according to Dr. Kenneth Mackinnon, there died of cholera, during ten years, in the months of March, April, May, June, and July, 2434 prisoners; while in the remaining seven months of the same years the casualties amongst the prisoners amounted to but 1046.

It thus appears that while the proportion between the Hindu and Mahomedan inhabitants of Calcutta is but 2½ to 1, the ratio of mortality amongst the former is to that of the latter, as 5½ to 1. This great difference in favour of the Mahomedans can only be ascribed to their better habits of life—to their better diet, clothing, habitations—comparatively.

The influence of the highest temperature of the year on epidemic cholera is exhibited in a still more striking manner on the sickness and mortality of Europeans; for, by the following table, it appears that for the twelve quarters ending 30th June, there were admitted into the General Hospital of Calcutta, 492 cases of this disease, of whom 220 died; while, for the remaining 36 quarters, there were but 311 admissions and 152 deaths. This is a remarkable fact.

Table of Admissions and Deaths of Europeans from Cholera into the General Hospital of Calcutta, for each Month during Twelve Years :—

Range of observation.	Total admissions.	Total deaths.
In 12 Januarys	28	11
12 Februarys	8	5
12 Marches	56	34
12 Aprils	86	57
12 Mays	268	125
12 Junes	138	38
12 Julys	32	6
12 Augusts	37	18
12 Septembers	10	5
12 Octobers	49	27
12 Novembers	59	32
12 Decembers	32	14
Grand total	803	372

It should be observed that the patients admitted into the European General Hospital of Calcutta are—soldiers belonging to detachments, invalid soldiers from the Upper Provinces, soldiers forming the garrison of Fort William, European townsmen, and men belonging to the shipping in the river. With exception of soldiers on duty in garrison, all the Europeans sent into the General Hospital are exempted from that salutary regulation and discipline which prescribes that every man shall come under medical control the instant he falls sick; and hence, doubtless, a great increase of deaths from cholera, as well as from all other acute diseases within this institution.

The results of an extensive series of observations, ranging over twenty years, show that, in the Presidency of Bengal, the annual mortality of European soldiers from epidemic cholera is about 1·15 per cent., while of the Bengal sepoy army it is but 0·22. This remarkable difference, so opposite to the popular belief, is worthy our careful investigation. Here we perceive that the boasted strength of the European does not serve him. On the contrary, in his power to resist this terrible scourge he stands vastly below his comparatively feeble native comrade. Why is this? We can only refer it to the habits of life of the British soldier, to his habitual indulgence in an over-full animal diet, and to his abuse of ardent spirits, thus keeping the digestive, nervous, and vascular systems in a constant state of over-excitement. He is thus rendered more prone to collapse of the vital powers; for, whatever lowers these last, reduces the general nervous energy, deteriorates the blood, or interferes with the processes of digestion and nutrition, will dispose to attacks of cholera.

PREDISPOSING CAUSES.

Some of the predisposing causes, as already stated, have been ascertained with some degree of accuracy, but not yet the existing cause. Here, despite our science, all is mystery, alike in the fleet on the ocean, or in the army on the march—all is inscrutable. Why does the epidemic come in one year and at one season, and not for years or seasons thereafter? These and such questions no one can answer.

The number of instances which I observed in Calcutta of Epsom or Seidlitz salts leading to profuse serous diarrhœa, and subsequent fatal cholera, is a circumstance worthy of notice. The dose was always taken in the early morning, and the patient had gone through his ordinary avocations throughout the day, mistaking for the operation of a saline aperient what was in reality the induction of choleraic diarrhœa, true cholera, and deadly collapse.

In the end of March, 1833, I was requested to visit the head partner of a large house of business—a healthy and powerful man. The note, which was not expressed with any urgency, was delivered to me at 5 P.M., near to the house of the patient, so that I was with him within a few minutes of its being written. I found the gentleman at his desk, at work. His countenance and voice at once expressed fatal collapse, and he died at eight o'clock that evening. He stated that at five o'clock that morning he had taken a dose of Seidlitz, his health previously having been quite good.

PRECURSORY DIARRHŒA.

I have never attended a case of cholera in which precursory diarrhœa, of longer or shorter duration, had not been plainly manifest; but I have seen people—villagers and camp followers—struck down with sudden death on the line of march during April and May, in the deadly jungles of Gondwana, and there the relatives and attendants declared emphatically that there had been no antecedent purging or vomiting whatever. All I observed personally was, that the persons lay dead by the road-side, and that there were no evidences about them of there having been any diarrhœa or vomiting. The cholera was raging at the time in our moving camp, of which I had charge.

A gentleman of the civil service, describing to me the fatal outbreak of cholera which visited Calcutta in 1842, says:—" It some time in March took quite a new character,—those attacked had not the usual purging and vomiting, but it came on with a sort of faint sinking—the strength was, without outward effort or apparent cause, totally prostrated, and the patient died without suffering, as if labouring under the effect of poison." In the terrible epidemic which seized on Her Majesty's 86th Regiment, at Kurrachee, in June, 1846, and which destroyed within sixteen days 238 men out of 399 who were attacked, it was noted that " the peculiarity in many cases was, that there was neither vomiting nor purging, and in the latter cases, by no means profuse. Also, among some of the first cases, before the natural hue had been replaced by the livid look so characteristic of the disease, the pulse at the wrist was almost imperceptible, the eyes turned up, and the voice hollow and feeble. In an hour after, such cases were dead." Others are described as attacked of a sudden, " and the collapse preceding the vomiting and purging of serous fluid." Dr. Lindsay, of Perth, declares that " cases of cholera undoubtedly occur without any rice-water evacuations: nay, it does not appear essential to cholera that there should be intestinal evacuations of any kind."

In the onset of many epidemics we learn that sudden deaths occur, apparently from the concentration of the poison: men are thus struck down at the outbreak of yellow fever and plague, as well as in cholera. During the onset of epidemic plague, almost all who are attacked with it perish—death occurring in from twenty-four to forty-eight hours; while, after a little time, death is deferred to the fourth, sixth, fourteenth, and even to the twentieth day—many cases recovering health: at length the pestilence loses its malignity altogether.

It has been held that in a practical sense diarrhœa cannot be held to be premonitory unless it have been of such duration as to allow time for the action of remedies; for where vomiting, purging, and collapse have followed each other in rapid succession, neither the vomiting nor the purging can be justly said to have been " premonitory." There is here no premonition; for persons have died of collapse without any marked symptoms, in whom the intestines were found filled with serous fluid. There is in recent discussions on premonitory diarrhœa in cholera, much of what our forefathers termed word-catching.

In the onset of the cholera epidemic which afflicted our army in Bulgaria many men were, according to Dr. Hume, " death-struck ;" and Dr. Williams observed that in those worst cases " there was no premonitory diarrhœa." The truth is, that we must regard the painless and colourless diarrhœa as the most characteristic and important symptom of commencing cholera ; as the first stage of the disease, in fact, and as that which is easy of cure in the average of cases.

PATHOLOGY.

The first circumstance that will strike the observer in cholera is the astonishing and fatuous prostration of the mental sensibilities, on all questions relating to the disease, and to the condition of individual danger belonging to it. The person who, before the seizure, was all anxiety, alacrity, and alertness on the subject of cholera, both as affecting himself and others, is now fatally apathetic; the feelings of hope, sympathy, and fear having vanished, and that of self-preservation even being deadened by the morbid impression of the poison on the nervous system. With all this, the faculties of the mind are in perfect integrity for the arrangement of business and the disposal of property—the patient making his will with a cold indifferent justice—the mind being as benumbed and prostrated as the body.

The first impression of the morbific cause would appear to be made on the system of the organic nerves and their functions ; for almost immediately we have the vital actions of circulation, respiration, the generation of heat, secretion and absorption, conspicuously depressed; and that probably, amongst other causes, through some unknown changes in the proportion of oxygen, or in the electric condition of the atmosphere. We have here, to use the language of John Hunter, the death of the blood. This condition of the circulating fluid produces torpor of the brain : the voice is veiled, as when great hæmorrhages occur, and very soon cyanosis becomes complete, the complexion assuming a lavender hue. To the prostration of the nervous system, and to the death and viscidity of the blood, we may refer the rapid destruction of life in cholera.

Fevers, both symptomatic and idiopathic, are referred by Dr. Billing to the loss of the functions of the nervous centres—the citadel of life, as they have been termed—and subsequently to that of the organs depending on them.

In all the severer visitations of this epidemic, we have symptoms at the very onset of the disease which, as it appears to me, can be referred to no other circumstance than this primary influence of the poison of cholera on the great nervous centres—giving the death-blow to the organic functions. All the secretions are suppressed, and in their place we have a general and exhausting transudation from the bowels and skin. In short, all the great functions of life are first altered and perverted, and then com-pletely and fatally arrested. The very stomach and bowels seem dead-drained of their *serum sanguinis;*—all now tends, in fact, to death. It is a common saying with the European soldiers in India, when they have felt the sun's power, " it has taken me in the pit of the stomach ;" and there, in seasons of the epidemic, the symp-toms of cholera make their immediate appearance.

The shock to the nervous system, paralysing its functions, causes the blood to be detained also in the great trunks, and thus the functions of secretion and excretion become additionally suppressed —the power of generating heat to be lost—and eventually the death of the blood, as John Hunter termed it. The livid hue on the surface of the body is due to the non-arterialization of the blood in the process of respiration.

TREATMENT.

In respect of plague, yellow fever, and cholera, we shall do well to study their natural history, with a view to the discovery of the most efficient means for their prevention; for as to their cure, we may not, in our time at least, hope for a knowledge such as can lead directly to so desirable a result. The instances are without number, in the East Indies and other countries, in which the prompt use of alterative mercurials with opium and spices have arrested precursory diarrhœa, and thus prevented cholera ; but in the stage of maturity, and in that of collapse, who amongst us can conscien-tiously count his cures ?

It is indeed impossible to say anything satisfactory on the treat-ment of a disease which would seem every year to become a subject of greater difficulty to medicine. Like the pestilence of the fifth century before the Christian era, described by Arnold, this epidemic has in a manner travelled up and down over the habitable world, unaffected by human endeavours, returning often to the same place after a certain interval ; pausing sometimes in its fury, and appear-ing to stop, but again breaking out on some point or other within its range, till, at the end of its appointed period, it disappears—we dare not say—altogether.

Dr. Elliotson declares that " if, as respects this country, all the patients had been left alone, the mortality would have been much the same as it has been. We are not in the least more advanced as to the proper remedies than we were when the first case of cholera occurred."

Certainly, every year makes us more and more familiar with the phenomena of the disease; but this circumstance has in no way improved our acquaintance with the means of checking its progress in the human frame, or of effecting its cure. It is indeed in the *prevention,* rather than in the cure of cholera, as of plague and common typhus, that medical science will at all times prove most conspicuously beneficial in this disease. If measures of cure be in a large proportion of instances beyond the reach of the sufferers, or of but little avail when applied, we should devote our energies with redoubled force to the prevention of cholera; for here it is ascertained that our power of beneficial action is great.

In the stage of collapse, the disease has too often proved to physicians what traumatic tetanus is to surgeons—a disease, according to Hennen, which, once fully formed, tended more to show him what he could not trust to, than what he could place the smallest reliance on.

But we have every day presented to us, in every form and variety, what are termed new views of the causes, pathology, and treatment of cholera; yet of each and all of them how small a portion, if any, is really true. It is better to argue from cause to effect, than from effects to infer causes; and if we are to arrive at any just pathology, or successful treatment of this disease, it will probably be through such course of investigation. Certainly, the search after specifics does not appear to be a promising course.

Reasoning, for instance, would lead us to expect some aid against the desperate stage of collapse from the conjoined use of the oxygenated gases and galvanism; but it does not appear that any persevering trials have been made of them.

In 1827, at the General Hospital of Calcutta, I ordered the inhalation of pure oxygen gas in the case of a robust European soldier who was dying in the stage of collapse. The effect for a time appeared very promising, the skin becoming warm and the pulse being restored at the wrist; but, from defective means, I was unable to pursue the experiment.*

To decarbonize the surcharged blood globules, and rouse the capillary circulation, Dr. A. C. Macrae of Calcutta had recourse to the nitro-muriatic acid bath; and the results were so interesting, when used by him in the Howrah Seaman's Hospital in 1851, that further trial of this powerful agent is anxiously looked to.

"The patient when in the worst stage of collapse, with cold, blue, shrivelled skin, pulseless and voiceless, moribund, was stripped and wrapped up in a sheet taken from a vessel containing the bath prepared according to your formula, occasionally made a little stronger. Over this was placed a blanket, and the attendant was instructed to wet the sheet every few minutes by means of a sponge, taking care to replace it carefully when thrown off by the restlessness of the patient. He was instructed to continue this treatment until reaction decidedly set in, the period of which varied from one to six or eight hours: the signs of it were first seen in the conjunctiva, which, changing from the dull leaden hue so characteristic of cholera collapse, became of a brilliant red, simu-

* Oxygen gas may easily be produced by intimately mixing chlorate of potash with one-sixth of its weight of black oxide of manganese, and throwing the mixture on an iron shovel heated to dull redness.

lating acute ophthalmia. The same change, though in a less marked degree, took place in the skin, the blue colour giving place to a general erythematic blush. With these signs of improvement, others speedily were manifested, as cessation of cramp, of incessant thirst and general restlessness, until reaction fairly set in, and so far the patient was saved."

This able officer treated twenty of the worst cases after the manner here described ; " and the result was most encouraging, the proportion of recoveries being greatly in excess of that from any other mode of treatment."

When first I entered on military practice in Bengal, the disease had some marked points of difference in character, and in the means used to combat them, from those of more recent visitations of the epidemic. Formerly simple mucous congestion of the most aggravated nature appeared to form the more essential feature of the disease ; and the consequent spasm, which was of a clonic character, could be referred to the oppression of the nervous energy following on concentrated cerebral and spinal congestion. It is on the supposition that this condition formed the leading feature of the disease in its earlier visitations, and of the organic nervous function being there less involved, that I would account for the efficacy of blood-letting during the first six years of our acquaintance with cholera ; for, latterly, there seems to prevail a depression of the vital actions which has greatly embarrassed our treatment, and deprived us almost altogether of our former great resource, general blood-letting.

The first European whom I treated was a stout young soldier of Her Majesty's 59th regiment stationed in Fort William. There was incessant vomiting and purging of a watery fluid, with spasms so violent that four men were required to hold the patient in his cot. I bled him largely, and in a few hours he recovered health. What a simple matter did the treatment of cholera then appear to my sanguine and youthful inexperience, and in how few years had I to think and act differently !

The efficacy of blood-letting, even on the approach of the stage of collapse, we constantly observed ; and we practised it as if under direction of the great physician of congestive disease—Robert Jackson. In 1822, when serving in the Governor-General's body-guard, I found the European farrier-major of the corps apparently dying of cholera. During the night he had voided enormous quantities of fluid by vomit and stool, and when I saw him in the early morning his appearance was surprisingly altered. He was cold and livid, his countenance shrunk and shrivelled, his voice veiled, the circulation flagging in the extremities. I opened a vein in each arm, but it was long ere, through the aid of diffusible stimuli, frictions, &c., I could obtain but a trickling of dark treacly matter ; at length the blood flowed, and by degrees its darkness was exchanged for the more florid hue of nature. The farrier was not of robust habit, and had resided long in India ; but nevertheless, I bled him copiously, when he, whom but a moment before I regarded as a dying man, stood up and exclaimed, " *Sir, you have made a new man of me.*"

The changes in the course of disease here spoken of are another example of that depressing influence operating on the nervous system, which has been observed in many countries where, through epidemic constitutions of the air, or other causes, epidemics have engrafted themselves on the endemics, as on the parent stock of the soil. Here, for instance, we have, to appearance, the same symptoms in the same order, but these signs are fallacious ; and the treatment which proved most successful on the first appearance of cholera no man will now venture to put in practice. It would appear that in the more recent visitations of the epidemic in Bengal, we have, from the very onset of the attack, a greater depression of the organic nervous function, and a more rapid loss of vitality in the blood, than was observable in its earlier history. It is in the manner here indicated that dysenteries, fevers, and other endemic diseases come, in the progress of years, to alter these characters.

After what has just been stated, it may appear almost beneath the dignity of medicine to speak of cures in such a disease ; yet I believe the thing is to be done, with some degree of success, too, if only undertaken in time. Cholera being the most acute of all acute diseases, medicine, to have any chance of success, must be applied at the earliest moment of its invasion.

If the first impression of the morbid cause be to depress the innervation of the ganglionic nerves, and thus to paralyse all the great functions of life, the indication of treatment should be to excite and restore the healthy powers of the nervous centres. In my own experience, this indication has best been fulfilled by the exhibition, at the very onset of the disease, of large doses of calomel and opium ; and where, nevertheless, the disease still proceeded, the repeated use of smaller doses of calomel with highly diffusible stimulants was persevered in, so as to rouse the nervous and vascular actions.

It seems admitted in actual practice, in all portions of the British Empire, and by the great body of the medical profession, that during the premonitory stage, or that of simple diarrhœa, opium is the sheet anchor of reliance. Some give this remedy alone—some with chalk and aromatics—some with calomel ; but all give opium in some form or combination, thus following still the original practice in India. Opium thus used acts at once as a cure of diarrhœa and of the earlier stage of cholera, and as a prevention of the coming and fatal collapse.

After all our experience, in all parts of the world, the treatment by calomel and opium at the commencement of the disease, and calomel with diffusible stimulants in its subsequent stages, as originally practised in the East, is that treatment which has been the most steadily and the longest approved by the profession.

In the Report on the results of different methods of treatment pursued in Epidemic Cholera, and addressed to the President of the General Board of Health by the Treatment Committee of the Medical Council, we find the following summary :—

" The evidence of these tables condemns the eliminant treatment altogether as a principle of practice.

" It testifies against the stimulant principle, excepting as a resource in extreme cases.

" It displays a decided advantage in the alterative principle, especially as carried out by calomel and opium ; and it shows a still superior advantage in the astringent principle as applied through the means of chalk and opium—the *general* per-centage of deaths following each plan of treatment being—

Of eliminants	71·7	per cent.
,, stimulants	54·	,,
,, alteratives, calomel and opium	36·2	,,
,, astringents, chalk and opium	20·3	,,

In order to judge correctly of the value of this evidence, it is necessary to examine, as far as may be possible, the degree of severity of the cases brought beneath this test. The only means at our command (on the present occasion, at least) to make this examination, is to consider the relative proportion which the cases of collapse bear to the number of deaths of their own classes respectively. Examining, therefore, the collapse cases with the number of deaths, we find that calomel and opium stands highest in the scale of success, and the order of preference appears as follows :—

Calomel and opium	59·2	per cent.
Calomel (larger doses)	60·9	,,
Salines	62·9	,,
Chalk and opium	63·2	,,
Calomel (small doses)	73·9	,,
Castor oil	77·6	,,
Sulphuric acid	78·9	,,

According to this result, the superior success of calomel and opium in severer cases appears a distinct fact elicited by the present inquiry. It is accompanied by other facts—viz., the relative advantages of those other modes of treatment which follow in their order of success. This order marks the use of calomel in small doses, of castor oil, and of sulphuric acid, as actually to be deprecated in severe cases.

" Chalk and opium, as shown above, stands at the head of the list, in the general per-centages, both in hospitals and in private practice ; but in the comparison of the collapse cases with the number of deaths, the average declines to the fourth rank."

The names appended to the report, of which the above is an extract, are :—John Ayrton Paris, President of the College of Physicians; James Alderson; Benjamin Guy Babington; Alex. Tweedie; Nathaniel Bagshaw Ward; all Fellows of the said College. In the " Report on the Treatment of Epidemic Cholera in the Provinces throughout England and Scotland, in 1854, being Supplementary to the Metropolitan Report, addressed to the President of the General Board of Health by the Treatment Committee," all the above facts are substantially corroborated.

I have only to state, in conclusion, that in cholera, in common with the last stages of violent fevers and dysenteries—as, in fact, in all diseases of great exhaustion—the patient will always owe much to the horizontal position, and to careful and unremitting nursing. The most careful nursing, and the most attentive watching of the patient, are both of the utmost importance in this disease ; and so easily is the balance of circulation fatally overturned, that a strict attention to the recumbent posture is absolutely necessary to success. In no other diseases are these simple matters of so great importance to be attended to ; and in the disease under special notice, I have seen many a life apparently lost from inattention to them.

For the following Tables I am indebted to my friend Dr. Balfour, of the War Office. They exhibit the average sickness and mortality from cholera in certain of our foreign possessions ; and show by how much more fatal epidemic cholera has proved in the country of its birth than in any other.

TABLE I.

Stations.	Periods of Observation.	Aggregate strength.	Admitted.	Died.	Ratio per 1000. Admitted.	Ratio per 1000. Died.
United Kingdom, Dragoon Guards and Dragoons	1830—46	98,985	171	54	1·7	·5
Gibraltar	1818—46	93,400	459	131	4·9	1·4
Malta	1817—46	61,998	209	47	3·4	·8
Ionian Islands	1817—46	26,494	None			
Bermuda and	,, ,,	22,945	None			
Newfoundland	1825—46	7,678	None			
Nova Scotia and New Brunswick	1817—46	43,248	210	59	4·8	1·4
ætla	,, ,,	154,736	356	127	2·3	·8
ape of Good Hope	1818—36	29,344	None			
Windward and Leeward Command	1817—36	86,661	None			
Jamaica	,, ,,	51,567	None			
St. Helena	1818—36	5,908	None			
Wern Africa	1819—36	1,843	None			
Mauritius	1818—36	30,515	268	32	8·8	1·1
eylon	1817—36	42,978	788	257	18·3	6·0
Mds, H.M.'s Regiments	1826—43	117,588	4195	1232	35·7	10·5
Europ. Tr. E.I.C. { Bengal	1825—44	88,380	...	1021	...	11·5
Bombay	,, ,,	50,987	...	288	...	5·6
Madras	,, ,,	101,210	...	432	...	4·3

TABLE II.

Stations.	Periods of observation.	Strength.	Cases of cholera.	Deaths.	Ratio per 1000 of strength. Cases.	Ratio per 1000 of strength. Deaths.	Proportion of deaths to cases.
United Kingdom. { Dragoon Guards and Dragoons	1832	6,408	114	29	17·8	4·5	10 in 39·3
,, ,, ,,	1833	6,379	32	14	5·	2·2	10 ,, 22·8
,, ,, ,,	1834	6,261	25	11	4·	1·7	10 ,, 22·7
Troops generally *	1832	45,583	886	233	19·4	5·1	10 ,, 38·
,, *	1833	42,614	223	71	5·2	1·7	10 ,, 31·4
,, *	1834	38,587	154	61	4·	1·6	10 ,, 25·2
Gibraltar	1834	3,034	459	131	151·3	43·2	10 ,, 35·
Malta	1837	2,159	209	47	96·8	21·8	10 ,, 44·5
Nova Scotia and New Brunswick	1834	2,071	210	59	101·4	28·5	10 ,, 35·6
Canada	1832	2,909	259	94	89·	32·3	10 ,, 27·5
,,	1834	2,588	97	33	37·5	12·7	10 ,, 29·4
Jamaica	1850	756	51	29	67·5	38·4	10 ,, 17·6
Mauritius	1819	1,652	113	20	68·5	12·1	10 ,, 56·5
,,	1820	1,395	155	12	111·1	8·6	10 ,, 129·1
Ceylon	1819	2,533	236	89	93·2	35·1	10 ,, 26·5
,,	1820	2,703	42	12	15·5	4·4	10 ,, 35·
,,	1825	1,448	111	31	76·7	21·4	10 ,, 35·8
,,	1829	2,279	48	14	21·1	6·1	10 ,, 34·3
,,	1832	2,056	344	107	167·3	52·	10 ,, 32·1

* Special Reports.

THE YELLOW OR HÆMOGASTRIC FEVER.

GENERAL AND TOPOGRAPHICAL OBSERVATIONS.

IN most, if not all European countries, we find that fevers of the continued, typhoid, remittent and intermittent characters prevail, with bilious remittents in the autumnal seasons. In Egypt and Turkey, again, we find the plague; on the West Coast of Africa and in the West Indies, along with remittents, we have occasional outbreaks of destructive epidemic yellow fever; in the East Indies, formidable bilious remittents.

All these fevers, while they take their origin from peculiarities of soil and general climate, have certain features of resemblance, and yet many wide and essential differences and distinctions : they all unite under the common generic FEVER—only to demonstrate to us, for the millionth time, the surpassing difficulties of this great subject.

"The yellow fever—" the hurricane of the human frame," as Blane terms it—would be as difficult to import into the climate of England, as would be the typhus, and the enteric typhus of our crowded cities into those of Jamaica or Bengal; such are the peculiar characters imparted by local circumstances to those pervading and dangerous diseases. The yellow fever, for instance, is altogether arrested by a moderate degree of cold, while plague is nipped by cold and dryness, as also by great heat and dryness of atmosphere. Indeed, yellow fever is arrested in its progress by extreme heat as well as by moderate cold. It is thus confined within a definite line determined by temperature; the elevation to a heat steadily above 90°, and a depression of the temperature to much below 65°, being well known generally to extinguish the disease—heavy rain and frost doing so at once.

Yellow fever is everywhere more prevalent and more severe along the low banks of rivers, in large towns, at their embouchures especially, in cities planted on the low seaboard, in low, marshy and heated plains, and in the harbours of low marshy countries. It is a disease essentially of tropical regions, or of countries having tropical or semi-tropical climates; and everywhere, whether the disease has been endemic or epidemic, the temperature in summer has averaged 80°; but on rare occasions, when it fell to 62°, the mortality has been the greatest. Jörg affirms also, from personal knowledge and the observation of others, that this fever never occurs in the open country or in small villages, but always in large cities or smaller towns with great trade.

On the other hand, it has been observed at the Hill Station of

Newcastle, Jamaica, of about 4000 feet in elevation, and nine miles from the seaboard, that sporadic cases "resembling" yellow fever occurred between the years 1842–48, and in 1856 yellow fever actually manifested itself there; "showing that though the high land stations may, in ordinary years, present a degree of health little inferior to Europe, yet when an epidemic constitution prevails, they are by no means exempt from its influence, and may even, as in the case of Newcastle on the late occasion, suffer severely, though to a far less extent probably than the lowland stations under similar circumstances."

William Fergusson, speaking of the expedition to St. Domingo, in 1796, " as one of the survivors of that war," says:—"Our head quarters were the town and its adjunct Brizoton, as pestiferous as any in the world; and here we had constant yellow fever in all its fury. At the distance of a mile or two, on the ascent up the country, stood our first post of Torgean, where the yellow fever appeared to break off into a milder type of remittent. Higher up was the post of Grenier, where concentrated remittent was rare, and milder intermittent with dysentery prevailed; and higher still was Fourmier, where remittent was unknown, intermittent uncommon, but phagedenic ulcers so frequent, as to constitute a most formidable type of disease; and higher still were the mountains above L'Arkahaye, of greater elevation than any of them; far off, but within sight, low down, in what was called the bight of Leogane, where a British detachment had always enjoyed absolute European health, only it might be called better, because the climate was more equable than in higher latitudes.

" Here were the separate regions or zones of intertropical health mapped out to our view as distinctly as if it had been done by the draughtsman. Taking Port au Prince for the point of departure, we could pass from one station to the other, and with a thermometer might have accurately noted the locale of disease according to the descending scale, without asking a question among the troops who held the posts. It was just as impossible, or more so, to carry a yellow fever up the hill to a post in sight, as it would have been to escape, had they been brought down and located amidst the swamps of Port au Prince." . . "Even here at home, in certain peculiar seasons of heat and drought, yellow fever may not have been entirely unknown. The year 1807 was one of those, when two soldiers of a militia regiment in the garrison of Sheerness, in Kent, died of a fever under my own inspection, whose cases might have passed muster for the endemic of St. Domingo." The opinion here suggested accords with that of Frank, who regarded yellow fever as an intense variety of the worst form of the autumnal bilious remittents of temperate regions. Dr. Dickson, speaking of the destructive epidemic yellow fever of Marié Galante, in 1808, says, that " the different types of fever were CONVERTED into each other, of the worst and most aggravated species he ever witnessed. Yellow fever, in the *continued form,* others with comatose *remittents* and *intermittents,* the exacerbations of which were so violent as to carry off a patient in two or three paroxysms, while others sunk into a low protracted character of fever resembling *typhus."* Here the question would appear to have been whether the differences were of a kind to justify separation.

The yellow fever, like the remittents and intermittents of hot climates, would seem to take its origin from terrestrial exhalations; with this further similarity, that yellow fever may, under certain favourable conditions, be propagated as remittents have occasionally been said to have been, by contagion. This manner of regarding the subject, as stated by Dr. Alison, of Edinburgh, is the only means of reconciling, not the conflicting and valueless opinions, but the apparently contradictory facts presented during the various epidemics of yellow fever recorded by so many able observers of those calamities. Differences of opinion, too, must have arisen from the circumstance that different forms of the disease existed in different places, and in different epidemic visitations; while authors too often insisted on regarding it as always of one uniform type. There is, as stated, reason to conclude, also, that remittents may, like the continued fevers of temperate climates, be occasionally propagated by contagion; and of all the accessories to such condition, crowding of the sick would appear the most efficient.

Another circumstance of preliminary importance and interest in the natural history of yellow fever is, that " whether it spreads by contagion within certain limits or not, it will in all probability be confined to a tainted district even in that climate; and that on careful inquiry, in almost every such case, it will appear that *there are* boundaries at no great distance from the spots first affected, beyond which the disease has not formerly spread, and need hardly now be apprehended."* As examples, the limits set in Philadelphia, half a century ago, and more recently, the Neutral Ground, Gibraltar, are adduced. In the recent Lisbon epidemic it was always noted that there were " most deaths where most dirt." These facts impress as a necessity the principle of immediately abandoning a place where yellow fever exists, and not returning to the locality originally occupied until the disease shall have for some time altogether disappeared.

But to continue the general comparison :—Robert Jackson " considers endemic fever, whether it appears in the torrid or the temperate zones of the earth, to be radically one disease."

" The forms of endemic fever are in fact so extremely diversified, the symptoms so opposite in their nature to each other on many occasions, as to produce the distinctions of inflammatory, putrid,

* " Brit. and For. Med.-Chir. Rev." for April, 1854.

nervous, bilious, simple, complicated, mild, malignant, &c., from the operation of a cause that is distinctly and demonstrably one." . . "The history of differences or distinctions constitutes what is called nosology, a study of much importance to medical science; but in so far as respects endemic fever, a study of more perplexity and loss than utility, as labouring to discriminate where there is no radical difference, or to bring the products of chance under a constituted law of nature."

Of the gastric or bilious remittent fever, this celebrated writer says :—" Bilious remittent fever is one of the most common, and one of the most important of the febrile forms which occur in armies, and even in civil communities. It belongs to all countries; and it is endemic in the West Indies at all seasons of the year, especially among native subjects, and those who have been so long resident as to be acclimated. It owes its origin to emanations from the soil, more generally or more partially diffused." Besides its own febrile mode of final termination, favourable or fatal as may be, "it is prone to assume a new form and to acquire a new quality so as to constitute a new disease which has its own law of movement. It thus assumes the contagious character, or is readily convertible into contagious fever in protracted campaigns in temperate latitudes."

The nosological confusion complained of by our great military physician has been commented on by many succeeding writers. " We can scarcely touch upon the subject of fever," says Sir Henry Holland, " particularly that which our present knowledge obliges us to consider of idiopathic kind, without finding in it a bond by which to associate together numerous forms of disease; but withal a knot so intricate, that no research has hitherto succeeded in unravelling it." Dr. Corrigan, of Dublin, states distinctly, that typhus, or maculated fever, may supervene on either inflammatory or bilious fever; and we are familiar with the epidemic association and concurrence of influenza, puerperal fever, and erysipelas. The relation of epidemic influenzas to other forms of disease, particularly to some of the exanthematous, intermittent, and continued fevers, has been remarked by Sir Henry Holland. " These connexions," he says, " though in no case sufficient to establish identity, yet are intimate enough to suggest some community of cause, and a closer correspondence in every part than is expressed in our nosological tables. The pathological and practical physician may both draw knowledge from this source."

The association of whooping-cough with the bowel disorders and remittent fevers of children has been noticed by the author above quoted, as has also that of dysentery with the aphthous ulcerations about the fauces and lips of young persons—all following upon influenza: again, the analogy of the milder forms of typhus and of intermittent with these epidemics is a most curious and interesting circumstance.

" I may repeat here," says Sir Henry Holland, " that the assured result of future inquiry will be to associate together, by common physical relations, diseases which have hitherto had separate and even remote places in our system of nosology." The opinion is in fact becoming more and more generally received that malarious and certain other fevers are not separate entities—that many of them have a more or less close affinity—that they occasionally replace each other, and that they frequently have a common cause.

The influence of varying meteorological agents on the nervous system, with their consequent elevations and depressions of the nervous functions, at different times, are important elements in this question ; but they have been too often overlooked.

Mr. Day, of Madras, after describing the several types of severe fevers, remittent and intermittent, in Mysore, concludes that " all the forms are so intimately mixed up, that it is difficult, if not impossible, to classify every case."

The doctrine held so long ago by Jackson and others, in respect of remittent and continued fevers, has recently been very ably expounded, as applicable to yellow fever also, by Dr. Alison, of Edinburgh, in the " British and Foreign Review."

In an article evincing an extended research and much ability, in this Review for January, 1848, and in which the author offers a just tribute to the profound knowledge of fever possessed by Robert Jackson, he says :—" It is to be remembered also that very considerable differences in type do not always disprove the existence of a single and common cause. We should have some difficulty in believing that the mild scarlatina simplex had any alliance with the malignant sore-throat with little or no eruption, if repeated observation had not demonstrated the transition stages. What more unlike than a mild quotidian and the pernicious intermittent which kills in a single paroxysm ; or a slight case of true cholera and the fatal and uncontrollable disease which devastates India. And if any one had seen only the milder forms of the remittent fever, and had had no opportunity of tracing up the several grades, he might well believe, when he saw suddenly the severest variety, that he had before him a distinct affection. A cause is not unalterable ; a morbid poison has not always the same concentration : it is ever varying in its intensity, and in the action it exerts on the system, more or less susceptible of it. And this has long been insisted on by writers on the endemic fevers of the tropics." After quoting Jackson's declaration that a malarious disease " is subject to changes at shorter or longer, but unascertained intervals, without any visible material change in the qualities of the localities or climate," the reviewer justly observes, that " in this absence of a malarious disease for a term of years, a resemblance is perceived with the absence of epidemics for a longer or shorter period."

Another remarkable and important fact is, that while the coloured population and acclimated Europeans suffer only from remittents, or from the very milder forms of yellow fever, the unacclimated European is everywhere and at all times the victim of the most virulent and fatal form of this epidemic.

It may be said, in addition, that a first attack of yellow fever gives a certain degree of immunity from a second, proving so far self-prophylactic; and likewise, that a previous residence in a warm climate greatly lessens the susceptibility to the disease.

Topographically, then, yellow fever may be defined—a disease not proved as yet to be a disease *sui generis*—endemic only in low districts on the sea-coast, but, under certain circumstances, sporadic in other places; rarely, if ever, appearing beyond 48° N. or 27° S. of latitude, and but seldom above the elevation of 2500 feet above the level of the sea, nor without a temperature of at least 72° promoting its production and propagation; depending, in part, on causes yet unknown, but in circumstances favourable to its extension, *capable of being propagated by infection.** It prevails in three different regions of the globe—America, the West Coast of Africa, and Spain.

Mason Good prefers the trivial name *yellow* to that of *paludal* fever, which is too limited to express its source in every instance.

Among the prominent points acting on the propagation of yellow fever, Hirsch dwells especially on the influence of acclimation. He maintains:—

1. That the susceptibility of individuals, not yet acclimated, is in proportion to the degree of geographical latitude under which they had previously lived.

2. That the susceptibility of strangers decreases in proportion as they prolong their sojourn in the yellow fever district.

3. That the residence within the tropics is not sufficient to remove the susceptibility.

4. That acclimation is only established by having gone through a severer epidemic without having been affected by the disease.

5. That the immunity is lost by several years' residence in colder latitudes, or in localities exempt from yellow fever, or even by the absence of the yellow fever from the place of residence during a long period.

6. That, however, perfect immunity is never produced, even by long acclimation.

7. That the immunity is greatest for that locality in which the acclimation has been obtained, that it is often lost by change of residence, even to a not more unhealthy place.

The following are the conclusions arrived at by Dr. Mühry, of

* *Vide* "Brit. and For. Med.-Chir. Rev." April, 1854.

Göttingen, in respect of miasmatic and contagious diseases, the distinction between them, and their geographical relations :—

1. *Miasmatic diseases* are specially dependent upon the influences of soil, humidity, temperature, and seasons, *like a vegetation.*

2. They generally manifest themselves and operate immediately after invasion, without any regular period of incubation—*like a poison.*

3. They may occur again and become chronic in the same individual, without any diminution of his susceptibility.

4. They do not regenerate themselves in the human organism.

1. *Contagious diseases* manifest themselves quite independently of soil, and also (with some particular exceptions) of temperature and seasons.

2. The attack always occurs after a longer or shorter, but regular period of incubation.

3. They generally occur only once in the same individual, and if they return it is after a long space of time.

4. They reproduce themselves solely in the human organism.

The relation of contagions to temperature, or the geographical distribution of such diseases, may be thus expressed. The majority of them are ubiquitous, *i.e.*, independent of temperature, and appearing in every zone of the world, irrespective of the period of the year. Examples of this truth are variola, scarlatina, rubeola, pertussis, cynanche parotidea, aphthæ, puerperal metritis, erysipelas, hospital gangrene, and malignant pustule. Those, on the other hand, which are influenced by temperature and the seasons, are divisible into three classes :—

1. Those which are confined to high temperatures, and are common in the tropics—lepra, frambœsia, dysentery, and aphthæ.

2. Those which are most common in the temperate zones—erysipelas, puerperal metritis, pertussis, and croup.

3. Those which are found in the regions between the tropical and polar zones—plague and typhus.—Henle's *Zeitsch. für Rationelle Medicin.*

SYMPTOMS AND PROGRESS.

The yellow, like all other fevers, makes its invasion with more or less severity according to age, sex, constitution, previous habits of life, and character of the prevailing epidemic ; but the following symptoms will be found to characterize the slighter, the severe, and the more fatal seizures :—

It is ushered in suddenly, and generally, as in cholera, in the night or early morning, by sense of coldness, a rigor, or actual shivering, followed by a vascular reaction proportionate to the amount and duration of the previous congestive cold stage ; heat and dryness of skin follow, with pain of the loins and limbs, headache, pain of the eye-balls, which are suffused, and of a glassy, drunken-like aspect ; the tongue is loaded, the edges red—there is nausea, with sense of rawness of the fauces and œsophagus, and uneasiness at the epigastrium. All the secretions are suppressed. As in the remittent fever, these symptoms may not extend beyond twenty-four or thirty-six hours, terminating then, under proper means of cure, in the restoration of health.

But this fair prospect of recovery too often proves only a deceptive lull before the coming storm : nausea, eructations, faintness, vomitings, epigastric distress set in, with the ejection from the stomach of a fluid at first clear, but soon to become dirty brown, and eventually the true black vomit. The complexion now becomes, more or less generally, of a lemon yellow, which, as the disease proceeds, extends rapidly over the entire surface of the body. All the symptoms proceed from bad to worse, accompanied by a bloated, desponding, anxious, and inquiring countenance, incessant and distressing jactitation—ending rapidly in exhaustion and death.

As with scarlatina, one person will get the fever in its milder, while another will, at the same time and place, contract it in its most grave form.

When again the epidemic is of a still more severe or fatal tendency, and where the subject is, from constitution or previous habits of life, peculiarly susceptible to the impression of the morbid cause, then all the symptoms enumerated become fearfully urgent; and the danger is imminent from the very onset of the fever.

In youthful and plethoric Europeans the symptoms are now of exceeding violence and danger. The heat is of a burning pungency, while the skin is dry and constricted—the headache intense —the countenance bloated, oppressed, or agitated by the most fearful apprehensions, or by approaching delirium ; the bowels are constipated, the tongue red, clean, and tremulous, indicating increase of gastric and intestinal irritation, and consequent increase of danger—the urine scanty and surcharged—all the secretions are suppressed ; there is distension of both hypochondria, with pain, burning heat, and anguish of the epigastrium—eructations, hiccough, and vomiting, at first of a clear, glairy fluid, presently altered to brown and dark matter like coffee-grounds—the quantity of fluid brought up far exceeding any that has been used in drink. In persons of a sanguine complexion especially, the countenance is apt to assume a livid, yellow, and putrid appearance, with black incrusted tongue, while, in most cases, the whole surface of the body becomes more or less yellow ; and in this, the most severe and dangerous form of the disease, the patient may be carried off, exhausted in all his functions, so early as the second, but more generally on the third day. The yellowness of the skin may be general or partial ; and even the black vomit may be said to be a very frequent, but by no means a constant occurrence.

In some instances, the ejections from the stomach do not commence until the fever has almost subsided, and then the retching and vomiting are uncontrollably urgent, while in others, oozing of black dissolved blood takes place from the mouth, throat, and rectum. The type of yellow fever is continued, though occasionally exhibiting a partial exacerbation towards night; remissions, in the ordinary sense, can therefore hardly be said to occur in this disease. But there is a deceptive calm of which the inexperienced should have warning; for too often it is followed by a fearful storm of black vomit—ushered in by faintness, sinking of the pulse and temperature. This nearly hopeless condition may appear on any day from the third to the seventh, and sometimes, though rarely, even later.

Stupor is found to vanish as the hæmorrhages increase. This was remarked as universal in the epidemic yellow fever of Peru in 1854. Bleeding of the gums is stated to have attended almost every case of the disease, not excepting the mildest forms of it; and stupor disappeared as the black vomit increased; in other words—cerebral congestion was relieved by the hæmorrhages.

But uniformity in the order and character of the symptoms must not be looked for in yellow fever; for all the best writers on the subject, whether recording their experiences in the West Indies, the west coast of Africa, or the south coast of Spain, are uniform and unanimous to the contrary effect; certain symptoms in certain epidemics varying in their nature and in the time of their accession, while others, common to former visitations, are generally wanting in this. It is, doubtless, this circumstance which has led to descriptions of "two or three, or even four forms of the disease." The French Commissioners state that " the Barcelona fever is the yellow fever of America, the same that we have in the Antilles and at Cadiz;" but they add—" it is a Proteus clothed with different forms, and which offers such strange anomalies, both in the slowness and rapidity of its march, in the combination, the succession, and the degree of its phenomena, that it is impossible to assign to it a fixed and invariable course."* One condition, however, would appear to be nearly uniform in the experience of British practitioners; bile is absent, or nearly so, from the intestinal and renal secretions.

Dr. Gillkrest states, that where neither yellowness nor hæmorrhage supervene, the fatal issue may occur in the shortest time. " The countenance of the patient may not indicate great danger; but he is observed to lie with his limbs uncovered, his head hanging over the bed; he becomes sensible when spoken to, and will assist to arrange the bed-clothes, which soon again become displaced." The symptoms in these cases, though wanting in the yellow complexion and black vomit, were all of the worst kind; often ending in· a "low, incessant, and monotonous wailing, ex-

* "Brit. and For. Med.-Chir. Rev." for January, 1848.

tremely distressing to all within hearing." This distinguished medical officer adds, that in the last epidemic in Gibraltar, " in these cases where copious hæmorrhage took place from any of the natural orifices, black vomit and suppression of urine were much less likely to occur."

Another deadly form of the fever, he says, was characterized from the commencement by a countenance shrunk and *decomposed* —the face having a mottled ash-coloured appearance—the look sullen—the eyes of a dull, red colour—the tongue red and raw— the temperature below the natural standard : the scene, he adds, is closed not unfrequently within forty-eight hours.

SEQUELÆ.

It is remarkable, considering the violence of this disease, that so few *sequelæ* are noted by authors on yellow fever ; and so trivial do they appear to Dr. Copland, that " he does not believe in their existence ;" while Dr. Gillkrest is silent on his own experiences, and quotes, with expressed doubts, the observations of others.

THE BLACK VOMIT.

" The vomitings at the beginning," says William Fergusson, " are always in themselves clear and clean," the white vomit of some writers ;—" presently they become somewhat ropy ; then brown, dark, and darker, till at last the attenuated blood, escaping from its vessels, and mixing with the gastric fluids, comes up under the form of black vomit."

Dr. R. La Roche, of Philadelphia, in his elaborate " Observations on the Black Vomit," says :—" 1. The black vomit, being recog- nised to be blood acted upon by the acid contents of the stomach, we have no difficulty in perceiving that much of the difference it presents, in regard to its physical appearance, will depend on the manner in which the blood is effused into the stomach, whether drop by drop, or in a stream, and on the degree of acidity of the gastric secretion, or the quantity of serous fluid it meets with in that organ.

" 2. It has been found, for example, that whenever blood is exhaled therein in a quantity proportionate to these secretions, it exhibits a black colour, while the aqueous portion is limpid, or clear green.

" 3. If there be a slight excess of blood, more than enough to neutralize the acid, instead of black, we have a nut-brown, a chocolate, or reddish matter ; and the watery portion, when filtered, is of a rum, brandy, or red colour.

" 4. If the hæmorrhage be great, the fluid presents all the cha- racteristic marks of blood, either with or without admixture of black vomit."

Dr. Hewson Bache, U.S., gives the following as the results of many microscopical examinations of the matter of black vomit:—

" 1. Amorphous masses of coagulated mucus or serum, and the debris of blood-corpuscles, which gave the mass a red or brown colour.

" 2. Numerous and irregular masses, sometimes presenting an imperfect crystalline form (probably altered hæmatin), which were of different shades, from a reddish-brown to a deep black colour.

" 3. Red blood-corpuscles, in different stages of alteration, which did not correspond to the degree of acidity of the vomit.

" 4. Various forms of epithelial cells, as the squamous and conoidal. In one specimen, a perfect mucous crypt was observed.

" 5. Brown oil globules, some of which bristled with fine crystals of margaric acid.

" 6. Besides these constant elements, there were some occasioual ones, such as the sarcina ventriculi, and the torula, the former more frequently than the latter, and some inflammation corpuscles."

DIAGNOSIS.

The black vomit has been regarded by some authors as the only true diagnostic sign of yellow fever, and in a large proportion of fatal cases it certainly is present; but vomiting of matters nearly resembling those ejected from the stomach in yellow fever, occurs as an occasional symptom in the fevers of other countries; hence the following conclusions may, I think, be deduced from the recorded observations of American and other authors —

1. That yellow fever may, and does occur without black vomit.

2. That black vomit is not so exclusive and universal a feature of yellow fever as some authors have supposed.

3. That black vomit, so called, has been witnessed occasionally in the course of fevers of the East Indies, of the Mediterranean, and even in fevers and other diseases within the British Isles; and it is stated to be " a usual symptom in the yellow fevers of America, which are incontestably of marshy origin."*

4. That to regard black vomit as an invariable, and altogether exclusive feature of yellow fever, would be almost equivalent to asserting that none have been affected with this disease but such as died in the stage of actual vomit.

5. That in many yellow fever epidemics, in various countries, numbers have died of this disease without the occurrence of black vomit.

6. With rare exceptions, those who have recovered from yellow fever have not presented the symptom of black vomit.

7. On the other hand, the matter of black vomit has very generally been found, on dissection, in the stomach and bowels of

* "Brit. and For. Med.-Chir. Rev." for January, 1848, p. 70.

subjects in whom no vomiting of black or other matter occurred during life.

8. Black vomit constitutes, in the prevalence of an epidemic fever, the most unmistakeable sign of its being the yellow fever— the black peculiar matter ejected during life, or discovered in the stomach and bowels after death, leaving no further doubt as to the nature of the disease.

9. On the other hand, black vomit was remarkably absent in the fever of the Niger Expedition, and in the Gibraltar epidemic of 1814 it was seldom seen.

Where, again, the disease is mild in its character and progress, the diagnosis becomes one of exceeding difficulty; the resemblances between certain forms of the yellow fever and the remittents of tropical climates being numerous. But there are distinctions which, on careful observation, mark the yellow fever; and of these, the following are held by Drs. Gillkrest and Copland to be the most prominent :—

1. Yellow fever makes its invasion more insidiously, but runs its course more rapidly than the remittent, the latter being more open and phlogistic.

2. The shock to the vitality of the body is manifested earlier in yellow fever, as is also the contamination of the circulating fluids and soft solids.

3. Jactitation, mental depression, apathy, or delirium, appear much earlier in yellow fever.

4. The lemon-yellow of the skin appears much earlier in the yellow than in the remittent fever.

5. Nausea and vomiting appear earlier in yellow fever—the latter symptom being marked by more distress, and by the ejection of a greater quantity of fluid, unmixed with bile, and being composed of some exudation from the stomach, or of the serum of the blood.

6. The vomitings in yellow fever are unaccompanied by retchings or apparent effort.

7. The character of the pulse in yellow fever is distinctive, being rapid in its rise, then soft and asthenic, proceeding on to weakness, inequality, irregularity, and lastly, slowness.

8. The suffused, red state of the conjunctivæ, with more or less brilliancy of the eye, according to constitution and age of the subjcet, and having sometimes a drunken-like appearance.

9. The lurid redness of the countenance in many cases, and the depressed and anxious expression in all.

10. The severe deep pain in the orbits.

11. The clean, red, raw, or bloody state of the tongue; the soreness of the throat, pharynx, and along the œsophagus; an acrid burning sensation at the stomach, the sense of constriction in the chest, and anguish at the præcordia.

12. The thick compacted feeling furnished by the skin, its diminished sensibility at the advanced stage, and the dingy tint of it, with livid or leaden patches at last.

13. The constipation, scanty secretion, complete suppression of urine, and absence of bile in the dejeetions.

14. The leucophlegmatic, flaccid, swollen, and pallid appearance of the soft solids, without any very evident emaciation in most instances.

15. The lemon-yellow of the skin is distinctive, and would seem to depend on a stagnation of dissolved blood in the capillaries, and not upon the colouring matter of bile, as in yellow remittent fever.

16. The *continued type* of the yellow fever in general—its origin, progress, and propagation, as compared to remittent fever.

PROGNOSIS.

The black vomit, although generally a fatal symptom, is far from being universally so—numerous recoveries after its occurrence having been observed in every recorded epidemic. But prognosis in yellow fever is declared by Robert Jackson to be difficult and treacherous in the extreme, whatever the locality or the prevalent character of the disease may have been. . Referring to this disease, as last observed by him on the South Coast of Spain, he records the following symptoms as indicating danger :—

1. A sudden invasion by the fever, with intense pain of the head and eye-balls, accompanied by sickness and vomiting.

2. The fever being ushered in by a fit, convulsions, apoplectic stupor, or outrageous delirium.

3. A torpid, heavy, or statue-like aspect of countenance gave strong suspicion of danger ; as did a shrunken, pinched, emaciated, and elongated countenance ; also a bloated, flabby, and inanimate aspect.

4. A dry, rough, milky white, or a swollen and red tongue indicated danger ; as did a sombre, leaden, greenish-yellow, or livid, hue, with red sunken eye and ecchymosed lids.

5. Distress and anguish at stomach, with pain at the epigastrium, forcible eructations, or explosions of flatus from the stomach, gave impression of much danger.

6. Obscure hiccough marked danger.

7. A ghastly appearance, with a faint nauseous odour from the body, indicated extreme danger.

8. Yellowness of the skin, with turgid veins on the conjunctivæ in the latter stage, " always decisive of a fatal issue."

9. Torpor of the skin—to such an extent as to be insensible to the stimulation of blisters and sinapisms—is ranked among dangerous signs. .

10. Extreme dampness, or extreme dryness of the skin, indicates great danger.

11. Petechiæ are suspicious : streaks, or patches, if livid, green, or violet-colour, are almost certain indications of approaching death.

> "The life of his blood
> Is touched corruptedly, and his pure brain
> (Which some suppose the soul's frail dwelling-house)
> Doth, by the idle comments that it makes,
> Foretel the ending of mortality."

12. Vomiting of black matter, like the grounds of coffee, is reported a sign of the highest danger.

13. Vomiting of bitter bile, whether green or yellow, even with straining or severe retching, affords a sign of comparative safety.

14. Black watery stools, with shreds, "are of the worst prognostic."

MORTALITY.

In common with cholera and other epidemics, the mortality from yellow fever has been observed to have generally been greatest at its onset, although exceptions to this rule have been known ; insomuch that, even at an advanced period of the epidemic, the disease has made, as it were, a fresh start, acquiring fresh power and virulence.

The violence of the disease, and its power of propagation, whether at sea or on land, have appeared to receive increase from a certain warmth, humidity, and stagnation of atmosphere—from crowded localities and crowded apartments—from absence of cleanliness and due ventilation—from intemperance, and from dread of the disease. The following statistical details, which might be greatly enlarged, will be sufficient to exhibit the average mortality of Europeans from this disease :—

1. " In a period of little more than four years," says William Fergusson, " nearly 700 commissioned British officers and 30,000 soldiers were swept away by the virulence of this disease." This was at St. Domingo, in 1795, where Fergusson served during the whole time. Referring to the fate of the French army in the same island, he says :—" Witness St. Domingo, where one of the finest armies of France perished, at least for all the purposes of an army, within the year." Sir William Pym, speaking of the epidemic yellow fever in the several islands in the West Indies in which he served during 1794-'95, says that there died, " in the course of a few months, not less than 6000 men."

2. Sir Gilbert Blane states that, " in 1804, out of a population, civil and military, in Gibraltar, consisting of 16,000 persons, there died " a proportion considerably above the usual devastation of the pestilence of the Levant," or nearly 6000 persons.

3. " Under the mild, or what has been called the French and Spanish treatment, the mortality of Malaga, in 1804, was 11,486, out of a population of 36,054. In the epidemic of the previous

year, in the same place, 6684 deaths occurred out of 16,517 persons attacked."

4. Dr. Rush admitted that "in the Civil Hospital of Philadelphia, where bleeding was sparingly used, the physician depending chiefly upon salivation, more than one-half died of all the patients who were admitted."

5. The yellow fever which broke out at Brimston Hill, St. Christopher's, in 1812, is described as having been of great severity. "The entire number of cases treated was 422, of which not fewer than 118 died, affording a mortality that treads closely upon the heels of that in the plague."

6. At Barcelona, in 1821, according to Gillkrest, "scarcely a patient survived in the wards given up to the distinguished members of the French Commission; and the mortality under French and Spanish physicians, in the establishment called Seminaria, was 1265 out of 1739 cases treated."

7. Dr. Townsend, of New York, states that, in 1822, the mortality in that city was in the proportion of three to four of those treated—the virulence of the disease being continued into the month of October.

8. During five visitations of yellow fever at Gibraltar, the mortality was as follows :—

Years of the epidemics	1804	1810	1813	1814	1828
Military and their families	869	6	391	114	507
Civil inhabitants	4864	17	508	132	1170
Total	5733	23	899	246	1677

9. On the island of Boa Vista, the ratio of mortality amongst the various races was as follows :—

Spaniards, Portuguese, and French	1 in 2·28
English and Americans	1 in 1·6
Native population, slaves	1 in 33·4
,, ,, free	1 in 14·6

10. In Lisbon, in 1857, the deaths of males were nearly as two to one to those of females; and the mean age of those who died was about thirty-three years. Few children under ten were attacked, and few old persons over seventy.

11. In the worst quarters of the town the mortality was forty-two to forty-three per cent., the mean mortality being about thirty-three per cent. of those attacked.

12. It is necessary to add, however, that epidemics are recorded in the West Indies and America as having been of a comparatively mild character; but it has been doubted whether some at least of these visitations were not in reality aggravated or unusual forms of autumnal remittents. But however this may have been, there were other instances in which the symptoms and the rate of mortality left no doubt as to the disease having been of the true yellow fever nature.

POST-MORTEM APPEARANCES.

" If ever there was a disease," says William Fergusson, " which the humoral pathologist might claim as his own, it is yellow fever. The crasis of the blood is as much broken down before death, and its vitality destroyed, as it would be by introduction of poison of the serpent's tooth; we may truly say it is killed by the poison, and in the language of John Hunter, that ' fatal yellow fever is the death of the blood.' It swells up in floods from the mucous surface of the stomach in the form of black vomit; and it escapes from the gums, the nostrils, the eyes, the ears, even from the skin itself, in any and every part; and after death it will be seen to have lost all the character and composition of blood, being found in its vessels like the lees of port wine and the grounds of coffee. But, as I know well from dire experience, the affection from the first must be essentially gastric."

Sir Gilbert Blane has " started a doubt whether the yellowness of the skin in this disease was owing to bile, but rather to some *error loci*, or depraved state of the red globules. 1st. This colour does not appear first in the eyes, as in jaundice. 2nd. Sir Isaac Newton observes, that the blood reduced to their *laminæ* assumed a yellow colour. 3rd. The colour appears in ecchymosis some time after a contusion, and the yellowness of the yellow fever sometimes does not come on till after death." In more recent investigations a considerable quantity of urea has been detected in the blood.

In common with the bilious remittents of all climates, the force of the disease under consideration is directed almost exclusively on the abdominal organs, while occasionally, as observed by Robert Jackson, the brain is primarily affected, and the abdominal viscera secondarily. In those who die within forty-eight hours, it is no uncommon circumstance to find the liver in a state of anæmic collapse, softened and friable, while during life its function had been suspended, in common with that of the kidneys—a serous discharge, indicative of anæmia, having taken the place of natural bile. In several invasions of yellow fever, in different countries, the liver has been found loaded with fat.

During the epidemic at Gibraltar, in 1828, portions of liver were washed and bruised by Dr. Gillkrest, but without yielding any colouring matter. The organ he described as being pale, like boxwood. "No trace of bile has been observed in the pores, and little or no blood exuded from the viscus when deep incisions were made."

The following summary of appearances after death from yellow fever is taken from Dr. Copland's great work, from Dr. Gillkrest, and others :—

In the most malignant and rapidly fatal epidemics, the body seldom suffers much diminution of bulk, while the abdomen appears tumid and enlarged—there is a yellow tint of the surface, with livid blotches—some parts becoming of a brown or dark hue. The muscles are of a dirty husky hue, and flabby in texture, or friable on pressure. The abdominal viscera are more or less congested, indicating a remarkably rapid loss of vital cohesion of the several textures. Where diminution of the bulk of the body is perceptible, on the other hand, owing to previous large loss of blood from the digestive mucous surface, the viscera will be pale, softened, and somewhat shrunk.

The *post-mortem* appearances in the liver, as in the other viscera, vary in proportion to the violence and duration of the fever; exhibiting at times congestion, softening, friability; at others, a pale olive hue: while the gall-bladder is generally shrunk, containing no bile, or else there is found in it a little tar-like fluid. The rhubarb colour of the liver has been remarked as characteristic of some of the most severe forms of epidemic yellow fever. The anatomical modification of the liver in yellow fever is considered by Professors Jackson and Jones (U.S.) to be amyloid, suspending and ultimately destroying its function. The spleen and pancreas have generally been found in a softened condition.

The œsophagus, stomach, and duodenum present patches of a dark livid hue, with the epithelium of the mucous digestive surface detached in many places, while the mucous membrane is separated from the adjacent tissues. The stomach and small intestines contain more or less of the matter of black vomit. This matter, as also a black jelly-like substance, is frequently found in the intestines, even where no black vomit existed during life. Less frequently there is found in the intestines a fluid of a reddish tint, more nearly resembling blood.

The appearances discoverable in the heart and lungs will depend on the amount of blood which has been discharged in the form of black vomit, or which has oozed from the mucous passages; and where death has occurred without such losses, both lungs and heart were found gorged and congested, the blood being more or less dark and grumous. False polypi are sometimes found in the cavities of the heart of persons who have died of the yellow fever; and it would be interesting to ascertain whether " the typhoid anæmic murmur" of Dr. Stokes, of Dublin, prevails in the yellow and in the malignant remittent and intermittent fevers of hot countries. It is well known that, as in the hæmogastric, so in typhus, fibrinous coagula have been found in the hearts of patients who have died of the latter fever. In a case of typhus recorded by Dr. Gordon, of Dublin, the first existence of the murmur was coincident with, and caused by the formation of the polypus in the right ventricle of the heart. That this cause was competent to produce it is proved by a case exhibited to the Pathological Society by Dr. Stokes some years ago.

Dr. Cartwright, of Natches (U.S.), found the membranes investing the semilunar ganglion and cœliac plexus highly inflamed, of a deep scarlet, and sometimes even black, the inflammation extending deep into the surrounding tissues.

Staff-Surgeon Collins, in his report on the yellow fever in Barbadoes, states that "in every case of decided yellow fever, he found the urine highly albuminous, a condition which it assumes about the second day, and maintains throughout, increasing as the disease advances, and in cases of protracted convalescence, continuing long after all symptoms but debility have left the patient."

PREDISPOSING CAUSES.

Of the causes or influences which are rather predisposing than determining, Dr. Copland enumerates the following as the more important:—Adult age, the male sex, constitutional peculiarities, mental emotions, &c. The influences of these causes are apparent in a greater or lesser degree in all epidemics in all countries; while certain of them he states to be *intrinsic*, or appertaining to the individual, and others are *extrinsic*, and applicable more or less to whole communities.

Besides the noted susceptibility of male adults, they are of necessity also more exposed, through their active habits and occupations, to the exciting causes of the disease, which Dr. Copland conceives to impress themselves upon the organic nervous system; " for," he says, " if this cause acted directly on the blood, the aged and debilitated, the susceptible and the non-susceptible, the protected and the unprotected, would be equally liable to the contamination;" a course of reasoning quite as applicable to fevers, remittent and intermittent, and to cholera. Whether owing to constitution, habits, social condition, or occupation, it is certain that females have generally been less frequently and less fatally affected by epidemic yellow fever.

This is essentially " *la fièvre Européenne*,"—afflicting by a preference almost exclusively the fair race, and being most severe in the natives of cold climates; the natives of the infected locality, and those of tropical regions generally, being but mildly, or very little affected by the epidemic.

Depressing passions, irregular habits and modes of living, prolonged abstinence, fatigue of mind or body, and absence of repose, excesses of every kind, act both as predisposing and determining causes.

In temperate climates, the summer and autumnal seasons, characterized by high temperature, humidity, and stagnant condition of atmosphere, have been observed to be most favourable to developing the effects of the cause; and these *extrinsic* influences have proved powerful in all countries.

ENDEMIC CAUSES.

The question as to the origin and mode of propagation of yellow fever is matter of evidence, and that evidence ought, by this time, to be sufficient to reconcile conflicting testimonies with each other, and with the truth. But without troubling the reader with a long retrospect, I think it may be fairly said in respect of this much vexed question, that to maintain the disease now under consideration to be at all times and places propagated by contagion only, would be quite as erroneous as to assert that it is never thus propagated, or *vice versâ*.

Yellow fever, then, appears to have two sources of extension—1st, a peculiar endemic malaria ; 2nd, an atmosphere infected by aggregation of the sick. In this order I purpose here to continue the subject.*

The operation of the causes will, according to Mason Good, "depend partly upon the state of the body at the time of attack, but chiefly upon some modification in the power or qualities of the febrile miasm itself, by the varying proportions of the co-operative agents of moisture, heat, stagnant air, and other auxiliaries which have not yet been detected, in their relation to each other in different places and seasons.

" How far the yellow fever is capable of *origination* from any other cause than febrile miasm from marshy lands, or places subject to like decompositions and plays of chemical affinity, we cannot at present determine. Such places, however, are numerous, as damp, unventilated stations, stagnant water, thick impenetrable jungles, and woods that arrest the miasm as it ascends ; even high, arid hills, after heat and rain ; but, above all, a foul state of the hold on board ships, whatever be the cause of such impurity.

. . Heat alone, however high the temperature, is not a cause of the fever before us : there must be moisture, and, as the result of both, a rapid decomposition and exhalation of organic remains. Provided the air is dry, even tropical climates are found salubrious. The burning province of Cumana, says Humboldt, the coast of Cora, and the plains of the Caraccas, prove that excessive heat alone is not unfavourable to human life.

"It has been observed, however, that even high and arid situations, after heat and rain, may also furnish, by chemical decomposition of their soil, the specific miasm of yellow fever ; and it may here be added that, if by the violence or redundancy of the rain, the swampy low grounds be at the same time overflowed, the latter will become an arena of health, while the heights are the seat of disease."

* " The Epidemic Constitution of Seasons," of Sydenham, is a subject of the utmost interest and importance, and one which he investigated through the ancient route of *pure observation*. It is a subject which, in our day, has not received the regard which is due to it.

This learned and accomplished physician, on a review of all the evidence before him, asserts that "the common remote cause of this fever is unquestionably marsh miasm." He further states that—"Whatever be the original source of the fever before us, when once it has established itself and rages with severity, it is now very generally admitted that the effluvium from the body of the affected 'is loaded with miasm of the same kind, completely deteriorated as it passes off,' and that the disorder is from this time capable of communicating itself by contagion."

"The true scientific point of view," says Dr. Alison, "in which we ought to regard the invisible cause of all such diseases, is simply as a part of the great science of Poisons—of those agents, inorganic, vegetable, and animal, which, by the mysterious dispensations of · Providence, are destined to exercise an injurious or destructive agency on living structures. Knowing as we now do that many such poisons are continually formed, both by vegetables and animals, the effects of which, taken into the bodies of living animals, are very various, some of them truly *morbific, i. e.*, exciting a long series of changes, constituting a true disease ; and that the function of excretion in animals, wherever carried on, is in fact the provision of Nature for the expulsion of matter which, having lost its vitality, has come under the influence, in all parts of the body, of 'destructive assimilation,' and, if not expelled, will speedily and surely act as a poison ;—knowing, also, that it is in the course of destructive assimilation and excretion that almost all animal, perhaps all organic poisons are formed, we cannot be surprised to find, and it is perfectly in accordance with what we have now stated to maintain, that although the chemical process of decomposition affords no explanation of febrile disease, yet, in the course of the decomposition continually going on in living bodies, in dead bodies, and in the excretions from living, under conditions not yet fully ascertained, compounds may be formed from time to time which will not only act as poisons, but exert peculiar *morbific* powers, and some of which may subsequently spread by contagion ; and that it is only by inductive study of the history of each of the peculiar diseases thus engendered, that we can learn, either what are the peculiar conditions essential to its development or propagation, or what other powers exist in nature by which it may be opposed. Accordingly, we can refer to various facts as to several of such diseases, known only by observation, but which constitute of themselves, if we make no attempt to resolve them into others, an important and most useful body of science.

"The principle we have already stated, as applicable, certainly to several, perhaps to all such diseases, has a practical importance which justifies our dwelling on it a little farther—that the poison exciting them may have, even at this day, more modes of origin than one ; and, therefore, that because we see such a disease spreading by contagion—*i. e.*, by intercourse of the sick with the healthy—at one time and place, we are not entitled to infer that it must do so in all, or can have no other mode of propagation, or, *vice versá*, to draw the opposite inference. Without recurring to the subject of cholera in illustration of this, we have already stated that we have been satisfied by repeated personal observation, that dysentery, commencing only in the usual way, from exposure to cold and wet, and independently of any intercourse with patients already affected with it, may in some seasons assume the character of a specific inflammation, and spread from the sick to the healthy, *e. g.*, from patients to nurses and attendants, long previously healthy, and exposed to no other cause, in an hospital. In such cases, there is nothing unreasonable in supposing that a specific poison is developed under our observation."

These observations—the suggestions of an extended experience, trained in scientific investigations—go far to explain, and to reconcile, many angry disputes and controversies of former times.

After stating his belief that the poison of cholera, although extending itself in ways not yet understood, independently of immediate intercourse of the sick with the healthy, in most parts of the world, does likewise in this country, and in others, spread at times distinctly by contagion, Dr. Alison says:—"In like manner, it is thus only that we can learn whether the malaria arising from the earth's surface, and producing only intermittent or remittent fevers in general, may or may not, in certain circumstances, and at certain times, excite fevers which may take the continued form, and may propagate their kind, as small-pox or measles do. It has been repeatedly stated in this journal, that this seems by far the most probable supposition as to the extension of the yellow fever at Boa Vista, in 1845-46. This doctrine is the very same as has been repeatedly proposed by those who have studied the history of the various epidemics of yellow fever, as the only means of reconciling, not the conflicting opinions (which is a matter of little consequence), but the apparently contradictory facts presented by those calamities."*

Quoting Sir Gilbert Blane's account of the progress of yellow fever in the Hussar, Dr. Alison concludes:—"In the face of such facts, it would be wrong to assert, on the breaking out of yellow fever, or unusually virulent remittent fever, in any climate known to be fitted for its extension, that it will not spread by contagion: but we are fully justified, by observation of that disease, in asserting on any such occasion, that whether it spreads by contagion within certain limits, or not, it will in all probability be confined to a *tainted district*, even in that country."

" What the yellow-fever poison may be," says Dr. Blair, " has never been demonstrated. Whatever it be, it is probable that in all localities within the yellow-fever zone, it is the same thing.

---

* "Brit. and For. Med.-Chir. Rev." loc. cit. p. 331.

The auxiliaries to it, however, may be different, as well as the
vehicle of communication ; and perhaps it may be generated in a
variety of soils."

"The cause of yellow fever," says Robert Jackson, "is one ;
the act assumes a variety of aspects according to contingent circumstances." The great majority of observers in our day seem to
regard yellow fever as of local or endemic origin, but as being
capable also, under certain conditions, of being propagated by
contagion.

Dr. McKinlay, R. N., speaking of the yellow fever of the
Brazil Coast, says :—"My own opinion is, that the disease was
not imported into Brazil ; on the contrary, that it was of endemic
origin. Whether it spread afterwards by contagion, or through
the atmosphere, I do not profess to determine, but I feel inclined
to adopt the latter view. Of this, however, I feel convinced, that
people arriving, more especially from a cold country, in a harbour
like Rio, Bahia, or Pernambuco, when the disease is prevalent
there, will almost to a certainty get the disease, even if they never
touch a human being or susceptible agent in those places. I may
add that this is infection, or indirect or modified contagion."

"We think we are justified in concluding," says the reviewer
already quoted, "that the presumed" hæmogastric pestilence "has
no pathognomonic signs, and presents no peculiarities which may
not be explained by supposing it to be the result of the most concentrated action of a particular cause. In other words, *the severe
fevers resulting from all the admitted causes are not distinguishable by
symptoms from each other.*"

In the report of the Sanitary Commissioners of New Orleans, on
the Origin and Spread of the Epidemic Yellow Fever of 1853, we
find the following resolutions :—

"1. That there is no just or tenable ground for the opinion that
our fever was imported.

"2. That to none of the sources to which general impression
ascribes its origin, have we been able to trace even colourable presumption of truth.

"3. That from analogous phenomena happening at the same
moment of time, and over an unlimited space in the city, and from
what we certainly know of contagion and its mode of action, the
inference is made inevitable that the fever was one of indigenous
origin, resulting from local influences developed and intensified
by peculiar atmospheric states."

The reporters, finally, arrived at the following conclusions :—

"1. That the late epidemic has not been derived from abroad,
but is of spontaneous origin.

"2. That there existed here, as attested by our records, very
peculiar meteorological conditions, known by general experience

to be capable of producing, in co-operation with local causes, fatal and malignant forms of fever.

" 3. That these conditions were present in an exaggerated degree, and impressed upon the prevalent type of disease, susceptibilities and habits of assimilating it to another and distinct form of fever.

" 4. That this showed in all the localities within the range of the meteorological state or influence, an infectiousness not necessary to or characteristic of the fever, but purely casual and accidental, the result of physical causes, and which it loses as soon as these causes are changed or disappear."

INFECTION.

To reconcile the extreme and opposite views entertained by so many able and honest writers, on the subject of the propagation, or otherwise, of this disease by effluvia from the sick crowded together, it is necessary, as already stated, to enter on a careful comparison of all the evidences as to the facts in each epidemic which rest on individual observation and experience, discarding all opinions.

It results, I think, from such a systematic inquiry, that those authors who, on their experience during a long life of active service, as Robert Jackson, William Fergusson, Gilkrest, and others, declared that they had not been able to discover any instance of propagation of yellow fever by infection, under the order, cleanliness, and freedom of ventilation of military hospitals, were as honest and truthful, and therefore as deserving of our consideration, as those others who, like Lind, Blane, Chisholm, Pym, and others, found that under other and opposite conditions of filth, crowding, and defective ventilation on board ships, and in other unfavourable situations, this fever assumed a different—an infectious character. Here, as it appears to me, each party spoke to the absolute truth, according to their observation and experience ; and they reported the facts which presented themselves in each epidemic as they occurred. It is at least but fair to say that we owe something to bygone discussions, however much we may lament their unnecessary acrimony ; for from them we learn that yellow fever is sometimes propagated by infection, but more generally not so.

The necessities of the question, as now understood, will not allow everything to be given up on the one side, nor everything to be maintained on the other. Truth demands an abatement of extreme opinions, and an adjustment according to the facts. In the history of yellow fever in various countries and at different times, we have numerous examples of contingent and created infection—of infection bred by ignorance and neglect of sanitary precautions, but not one instance of inevitable, unavoidable infection. In respect of yellow fever, as of other epidemics, it is generally places more than persons that become infected. In the autumn of 1860, yellow fever was introduced into Port Royal, Jamaica, by the crew of H.M. ship *Icarus*, in a manner hardly admitting of dispute ; and the disease was as certainly conveyed by the men of the *Icarus* to those of the *Imaum, Hydra,* and *Barracouta.* ` But again, in the epidemic of Oporto in 1856, and of Lisbon in 1857, the importation, the circumstance of importation, was altogether unsupported by any reliable evidence. The disease did not spread into the interior, nor was it conveyed even to Cintra from Lisbon. In H.M. ships *Highflyer* and *Dauntless*, in 1852, yellow fever was demonstrably infectious on board the vessels, yet on the landing of their crews, and their being placed respectively "in the airy, spacious naval hospital" of Port Royal, and the hospital of the 34th Regiment at Barbadoes, and "indiscriminately intermingled with the soldiers of that corps affected with various complaints, in no one instance has any individual been attacked, nor has any hospital attendant suffered."

Robert Jackson admits that, in respect of vessels "having a great number of persons ill of the yellow fever, a contagious fever will thus be produced, and carried to whatever port the ship may be destined to go ;" but he adds that, although the imported fever is contagious, "it is not the yellow fever, though the yellow fever may be the source whence it originally springs."

Speaking of infected ships, Dr. Wilson, of the navy, asserts, on the other hand, that "nearly every person who joins a ship in such a condition has the prevalent disease sooner or later ; but no number of persons from such a ship, labouring under the disease in any stage, or in any force, and placed in a situation where the disease does not exist, though in the centre of a mass of healthy people, can excite it in a single instance." The truth would appear to be, according to Sir Henry Holland, that "wherever human beings are brought and kept together in close contact—in prisons, barracks, ships, or besieged fortresses—there especially it would seem that the atmosphere becomes fitted for the reception, retention, and propagation of the *fomites* of disease."

There are situations and circumstances under which yellow fever has not been found to propagate from person to person, and they have generally been on land, where the sites have been favourable, and cleanliness and ventilation carefully secured; and there are other conditions which occasionally obtain on board ship, and in other unfavourable situations, under which it is certain that this disease has proved highly contagious. To understand the actual causes of these differences in effect, so as to enable us to anticipate and prevent the worst of them, is a subject deserving our most serious consideration. And, not to refer to the artificial embarrassments caused by vague and voluminous discussions, the natural difficulties of the subject—the anomalies of the disease itself; everywhere and at all times—have actually been great and perplexing to the inexperienced. We find, for instance, that not only have many of the symptoms of yellow fever varied in different epidemics at different times, but they have varied in the same epidemic, in the same localities or towns, nay, in the same ward of an hospital. The writers who have differed in their histories and descriptions of different epidemics, must not therefore be charged with inaccuracies.

The result, then, of the most extended inquiries leads to the conclusion that, in by far the greater number of epidemic yellow-fever visitations on shore, the disease has not been propagated by contagion; while on board ship, and occasionally on shore also, under circumstances of crowding, damp, and impure air, and neglect of general and personal cleanliness, it has proved otherwise, as in the well-known instances of her Majesty's ships *Bann* and *Eclair*.

The primary source of the pestilential fevers in the two ships named, is still matter of dispute; some contending that the original fever, in both instances, and as received into each ship, was but the endemic of the African coast; while others assert with equal confidence that the disease on shore and on board was, from first to last, the true yellow fever. The question is one of the highest interest and importance; but on reference to the official reports of Sir William Burnett and Dr. Bryson, the subject would appear to be settled in the estimation of those able and experienced officers.

Dr. Bryson, while introducing the subject of the fever on board the *Bann*, states that in 1823, " fever of an epidemic character began to manifest itself in the colony of Sierra Leone, and speedily extended to vessels in the harbour, in the river, or in the adjacent rivers or creeks, and to the different settlements along the coast. In the latter part of March it first assailed the crew of the *Bann*." Dr. Bryson goes on to say, that Sir W. Burnett was unable to account with certainty for the origin of the fever, either in the colony or in the *Bann*, " but distinctly proves that it was not, as had been supposed, imported by a vessel named *Caroline*."

Sir William expressly states, "that it was, in the first instance, merely the common endemic of the country, brought on by hard labour and exposure to the sun, not possessing, under these circumstances, any contagious properties, and continued so until after the middle of February; that it subsequently, by the state of the weather preventing ventilation, and from a great number of sick being confined in a small space, became contagious; and although it became impossible to trace the fever in question directly from the *Bann* to any individual of the garrison of Ascension, yet there is just reason to believe that the disease was introduced into the island by the ship."

Dr. Bryson, after enumerating the symptoms generally, including the black vomit, in the ships serving on the African coast during 1823-25, says, that "in almost every instance where the disease assumed a formidable character, its origin could be traced to one or more of the common well-known predisposing and exciting causes. He concludes that in none of the ships "does it appear to have assumed a contagious form but in the *Bann*."

In the second instance, her Majesty's steam-vessel *Eclair* quitted Plymouth on the 2nd of November, 1844, and after touching at Teneriffe, Ascension, and various other places on the African coast, she reached Sierra Leone on the 22nd of February, 1845. Here the crew was employed "variously"—fresh meat, vegetables, and fruits being served to them in abundance. "The general standard of health in the colony, as well as in the *Eclair*, was considered high; nothing in the form of endemic disease having yet made its appearance amongst the crew of the latter, nor any of that mental depression which subsequently affected them."

Between the 15th of February and the 16th of March the crew was employed along the coast, principally in boats, exploring creeks, and they were thus "exposed much to all the vicissitudes of the weather, to malarial exhalations from the muddy banks of the rivers, and from contagious mangrove swamps: they slept sometimes on shore, but generally in beds; they experienced much fatigue, disappointment, and mental depression. While this duty was being performed, diarrhœa affected many of the crew; and on the 3rd of April "the first case of fever occurred." Then followed, up to the 15th of June, twelve cases of fever, seven of which proved fatal; while of those who remained on board the ship, two fatal cases of fever occurred. "From these facts one important inference at least seems clearly deducible, namely, that the disease was contracted from local causes exterior to the ship; for although the two cases occurred in persons who had not been out of her, still, from her close proximity to the land, the whole crew must have been more or less exposed to the same malarious emanations as the men employed in the boats, although perhaps in a less concentrated form, while not having suffered from privation and fatigue, they were not so susceptible of the disease."

Notwithstanding the sufferings and death here recorded, the labour of the men was continued up to the 2nd of July, the *Eclair* returning on the 4th to Sierra Leone, with her crew "comparatively speaking healthy—the last case of fever advancing favourably to convalescence."

From the last named date till the 15th of August, the men were employed in surveying the stores of the *Albert*, and in clearing out her hold, in which was found "a strange collection of rubbish and dirt," which had remained in her hold since leaving England on the Niger expedition. Leave to go on shore at Sierra Leone was at this time given to the men, followed by all the exposures and irregularities common to such occasions; and thus, says the surgeon of the ship, "were our people, previously reduced in health by exposure in one of the worst situations on the coast, employed at an unhealthy period, and in the worst month of the year, in very disagreeable work, which they knew was quite thrown away, the vessel being worn out, and utterly useless for any purpose whatever."

Here, in this simple record, we perceive that the conduct of the officer in command was as reprehensible as it was without excuse; indeed, he was signally wanting in his first duty—that of care for the helpless men placed under his orders.

During the passage from Sierra Leone to the Gambia, fourteen persons were seized, of whom, including a gentleman passenger, seven died. "The fever," says the surgeon, "appears to have been" (*quære*, originally) "as distinctly remittent as that contracted at the Sherbro; and some of the men had" (*quære*, subsequently) "unequivocal black vomit; whilst several of the bodies, it is said, became yellow after death, although in the 'Medical Journal' the latter appearance is not mentioned." The report adds, that the obscure light on the deck, where the men were treated, must have rendered changes of complexion less obvious.

Between the 15th and 17th August, the fever continuing, and two more deaths having occurred, the *Eclair*, after taking in coals at Goree, stood across to Boa Vista, where she anchored on the 21st of the same month. It being the opinion of Dr. Kenny, a resident practitioner at Boa Vista, as well as of the medical officers of the *Eclair*, that the two or three cases of fever now on board the ship were "the common African fever," pratique was at once given by order of the authorities on the island.

On the 30th August, sixteen new cases being added to the list, and five deaths, since the ship anchored at Boa Vista, the commander had the crew, sick as well as healthy, removed on shore—the disease being still regarded by Dr. Kenny, the Portuguese colonial surgeon, and the medical officers of the ship, as "common African fever."

"A report, however, had gone abroad," says the surgeon, "that black vomit had occurred in some of the fever cases, and I mentioned the fact to Captain Estcourt, who assured me that he had heard nothing to cause foundation for such a report."

Dr. Bryson goes on to state that "from the day of landing the sick, until they were re-embarked, on the 13th September, 1837, additional cases of an aggravated type occurred, twenty-five of which proved fatal." It was now that, in the fatal seizure of Dr. M'Clure, who nobly volunteered to serve on board, it began to be suspected "that the disease had acquired contagious properties;" yet, even then, Dr. Bryson suggests that as Dr. M'Clure had but recently left Sierra Leone, he might have imbibed the poison there.

From the departure from Boa Vista to the 12th October at Stangate Creek quarantine station, to which the ignorant fears of the quarantine officers consigned this ill-fated ship, the record is one immense course of suffering and death, including that of the heroic young surgeon, Sidney Bernard.

Dr. Bryson, who considers the fever on board the *Eclair* to have been " merely of a typhoid character," concludes as follows :—

" Having thus traced the fever of the *Eclair* from its first appearance on board at the island of Sherbro, until it ceased previously to her arrival at Sierra Leone, and from its reappearance there in a more concentrated form, until it finally disappeared, some time after her arrival in England, it is impossible not to be struck with the close similarity it bore to that of the *Bann*. Both vessels contracted the disease at Sierra Leone, and apparently from the same cause or causes, and under similar circumstances. In both vessels, in the course of a few weeks, it assumed an epidemic character, if it did not acquire contagious properties ; the one vessel proceeded to the barren rocky island of Ascension, a few degrees south of the equator, where a disease of the same character made its appearance amongst the inhabitants, and committed great ravages ; the other proceeded to the nearly equally barren island of Boa Vista, a few degrees to the north of the equator, where, in like manner, a disease a short time afterwards broke out and raged with equal severity. This is not the place, however, to trace the progress of the fever on the island of Boa Vista, nor is it, perhaps, the time, considering that the subject is still under investigation."

The investigation here referred to was soon afterwards concluded by Dr. M'William, of the navy, in a manner alike honourable to his reputation, and satisfactory to the great body of the medical profession. Two points have been established by Dr. M'William; namely, that the fever on board the *Eclair* had become contagious ; and, secondly, that the disease was propagated from the ship to the inhabitants of Boa Vista. We thus find that the similarities between the case of the *Bann* and that of the *Eclair* are highly interesting and important.

" 1. In both instances the fever became increased in violence from the influence of the shore.

" 2. At Ascension, the mortality in the garrison was over 50 per cent. of those attacked, while it was but 16 per cent. in the crew of the *Bann*, although they were under the most unfavourable circumstances of ventilation, cleanliness, &c.

" 3. At Boa Vista, the sick list became rapidly augmented when the sick were landed.

" 4. In both cases, also, the coloured people on board escaped, or nearly so.

" 5. If these cases of the *Eclair* and the *Bann* be taken together, agreeing as they do in all their mean features, it is logically impossible to doubt the existence of a multiplying or contagious virus."

Thus far the able reviewer already quoted, who now arrives at the following conclusions from the whole course and tenor of the argument :—

" 1. That yellow fever is decidedly contagious on some occasions.

" 2. That the proofs of the universality of this property are defective. Importation can seldom be proved; inoculation is impossible, and the disease requires a peculiar susceptibility of condition in order to act.

" 3. That it is not safe to generalize from the first observation, and to conclude that yellow fever is at all times contagious, because it is undoubtedly so sometimes; for these reasons :—

" a. Because there are fevers undistinguishable by symptoms from contagious yellow fever, which certainly are not contagious.

" b. Because we are not sure how far contagion may not be an accidental property impressed on a poison by contingent circumstances, or may be only the development of a property of self-reproduction always possessed by the morbid poison, but generally in so slight a degree as to be unappreciable. If the former opinion be correct, yellow fever is both contagious and non-contagious; if the latter, it is also in the majority of cases non-contagious, in the conventional meaning of the term.

" 4. That contagion is only a property accidentally impressed on the yellow fever appears probable :—

" a. Because in no other way can we explain the extraordinary discrepancies and opposing statements of men whose honesty of purpose is undoubted.

" b. Because it is almost a necessary assumption, in order to explain certain facts in the history of yellow fever.

" c. Because it is in accordance with analogous phenomena manifested by other morbid poisons.

" d. Because there is really some direct proof of it in the apparent development of fever on board ships with clean holds, and removed from the influence of the land.

" 5. That if this conversion of a non-contagious into a contagious poison be denied, there is no alternative but to admit the existence of a specific contagious yellow fever.

" 6. That the doctrine of a specific contagious yellow fever is alone supported by the fact, that it destroys the necessity of admitting the convertibility of poisons, a circumstance considered by many observers as in the highest degree unlikely and unphilosophical."

The following is Dr. M'William's summary of the questions relating to the fever on board the *Eclair*, and that which prevailed subsequently at Boa Vista :—

" In my humble opinion, the history of the epidemy of Boa Vista comprehends every condition upon which the proofs of the infectiousness of a disease are supposed to rest, namely :—

" *The healthiness of the island before the arrival of the Eclair, with yellow fever on board.*

" *The outbreak of the same disease among the inhabitants of the island within a reasonable period afterwards.*

" *The immunity of distant villages for long periods until the arrival of infected persons, and the radiation of the disease in every district from infected foci.*

" *The comparative immunity from the disease obtained by persons who adopted common but partial precautionary measures against infection.*

" *The absolute immunity from the disease procured by persons who adopted strict measures of isolation and segregation.*"

On a careful review of this question, we receive the following additional authority in support:—

On the 31st December, 1850, the Royal College of Physicians of London delivered a Report to the Lords of Her Majesty's most Honourable Privy Council, respecting the Bulam, or yellow fever, which had been drawn up by the President and Fellows of the College, in consequence of a communication from their Lordships.

The points investigated by the College were as follow:—

" 1. As to the Bulam fever being *sui generis*, and distinct from remittent or the marsh fever of warm climates.

" 2. As to its being an infectious disease : that is, communicable from person to person, and likewise capable of being imported.

" 3. As to the non-liability of persons to a second attack of that disease.

" After a very careful consideration of all the facts and arguments adduced on both sides, with reference to the first question proposed, the College are of opinion, that sufficient grounds have not been laid for stating that ' yellow fever ' is a disease *sui generis*.

" With regard to the second question, it appears to the College to be sufficiently proved, that this disease is, under certain circumstances, infectious, and, consequently, that it may be imported.

" The principal circumstances under which the infectiousness of the disease is likely to be developed, would seem to be a high temperature and moisture of the atmosphere, particularly in unhealthy seasons, and when the influence of these causes is aggravated by local insalubrity of site, and by the absence of free ventilation.

" That the disease has been in some instances imported, the history of the epidemic fever which occurred in her Majesty's ship *Eclair*, and at Boa Vista, in 1845, affords conclusive evidence.

" The third question proposed respecting the non-liability of persons to second attacks, does not admit of being settled in a decided manner. Strictly speaking, there is no disease of which it can be affirmed, absolutely, that one attack renders a person insusceptible of a second.

" The College are unwilling to conclude their report without strongly recommending to their Lordships, that, on any future appearance of this formidable malady, persons should be sent out, thoroughly qualified by education and by habits of observation, to collect evidence on the important questions which have now been proposed to the College. This was done in the case of the *Eclair*, and most .valuable information was thus obtained."

PREVENTION.

Dr. Alison justly observes, that we may do more for the prevention of sickness and suffering among mankind, by studying the mode of propagation of epidemic diseases, even so far as yet known, and giving that advice by which they may be shunned, than we should do by the discovery of a new remedy, more powerful than any that is known in medicine. The truth of. this declaration ought to be deeply impressed on all who enter the medical departments of the public service; for it is with yellow fever, as with cholera, and other concentrated forms of disease;—whatever will prove most effective must rest on measures of prevention; and of these, the immediate removal from the place where the yellow fever may prevail, and the not returning to the locality, or to the ships, originally occupied by troops, inhabitants of towns, or seamen, constitute the first necessity of the case. The most eligible localities to choose will be found in elevated and well-drained situations, to windward of the infected spots.

Dr. Alison further states, that the most important principle ascertained in this department of medicine is—" that as to several of the most virulent of the epidemics which have been permitted to afflict mankind, the means of effectually restraining their diffusion are known, but cannot be carried into effect without both trouble and expense to the community that is to benefit by them; and that these means are *very considerably different* in the case of these different diseases—in the case, particularly of small pox, of erysipelas, of puerperal fever, of plague, of cholera, of continued fever, and of yellow fever.

As to yellow fever, regarding it as originating in an aggravated form of the remittent from malaria, and therefore affording illustrations of the natural history of that destructive agent in its most virulent form—we can go somewhat farther. Recollecting what has been stated of the very limited origin of the sausage poison, and of the cadaveric poison exciting erythematic inflammation— not in putrefaction generally, but in a certain stage of the decomposition of certain matters only—we shall be prepared to hope that a somewhat similar *limitation* may be ascertained for the development of this poison likewise; more particularly as we have already stated, that both in this climate, where it (in general at least) only excites ague, and in hot climates where, under a temperature

of 80° or more, of some duration, it excites so much more formidable diseases, all the conditions which we can as yet point out as
essential to its development may exist without its showing itself.

On this point the experience of the medical officers of the army
and navy, for the reasons already given, being the result of observations on organized masses of men, is the most valuable; and
facts are already known which may often be applied to practical
use, and promise to lead hereafter to more minute and more
uniformly applicable information. Not only is the general measure
of removing the population of a district known to be malarious
always to be recommended when the yellow fever shows itself, but
precise limits may sometimes be assigned. It seems certain that
the poison often originates in parts of the timber of certain ships,
and is long confined in them."*

That on board ship, as on shore, the limits of putrefaction or
other processes of decomposition are confined within *narrow limits
of space*, seems more than probable; and the special investigation
of such limits constitutes a branch of inquiry of the utmost importance, and one in which many facilities are afforded to the
medical officers of our fleets and armies.

The most speedy means of prevention, in respect of towns and
garrisons, will always be found in the removal of both the sick and
the healthy to a locality where the temperature is sufficiently low,
such as a neighbouring elevated range, or dry, well-ventilated
ground : the next most ready means is segregation.

1. In Gibraltar, in 1810, the infectious character of the prevailing yellow fever being suspected, " the infected were segregated
and removed to an airy locality, communication with them was
prevented, the healthy protected, and the mischief was very soon
arrested."

2. In 1813, this disease again made its appearance there, when
nearly 8000 persons left the garrison and encamped on the neutral
ground. The open nature of the ground, and the strong breezes,
arrested the progress of the epidemic, very few cases having occurred after this removal.

3. Upon a review of all the facts and circumstances observed at
different times, at Gibraltar, Dr. Hennen concludes, that they were
demonstrations of the value of " segregation and moderate quarantine."

4. " *The disease will stop*," says Dr. Copland, " *as soon as the
susceptible are separated from contaminated places, persons, and
things.*"

5. Let houses, barracks, and hospitals be purified by water and
air; but no attempt be made, *during the prevalence of the epidemic,*
to cleanse sewers, drains, or privies, for such measures have always
proved mischievous when practised at the time stated.

* " Brit. and For. Med.-Chir. Rev." April, 1854.

6. Tents, boarded sheds, and temporary hospitals should be so separated from each other as to admit of the most free circulation of air in every direction.

The prophylactic influence of bark or quinine has long been observed during service in unhealthy countries, and in our Continental wars; but nowhere more emphatically than on the West Coast of Africa. Donald Monro mentions the use of bark in Hungary, as a prophylactic against fevers, so far back as 1717; and it was so used by our army surgeons on the Continent in 1743.

"In the *North Star*," says Dr. Bryson, twenty men and one officer were employed on boat duties at Sierra Leone; they all took wine and bark with the exception of the officer; he was the only person who suffered an attack of fever. Two boats were detached from the *Hydra*, in 1844, to examine the Sherbro river; the whole of the men were supplied with bark and wine, and not one of them was taken ill, while the whole of the gig's crew, with the exception of the captain, who were similarly exposed for two days only without being supplied with either, contracted fever of a dangerous character. Facts like these are not to be mistaken."

Dr. Bryson suggests that a daily prophylactic dose be administered, and that its use should be continued for at least a fortnight after the return of the men on board their ship. He gives a decided preference to quinine over the bark.

Whenever fever of a formidable nature makes its appearance on board ship, she should at once proceed to sea, and run into the coolest atmosphere within reach.

1. With seamen, as with soldiers, the first and most immediate measures of prevention should obviate direct solar exposure, fatigue, and excesses in the use of spirituous and fermented liquors.

2. Seamen, when employed on unhealthy coasts, should be kept as remote from the shore as is consistent with duty, anchoring some miles out, during the night especially.

3. The duties in boats should be conducted as much as possible in the mornings and evenings—avoiding alike the noon-day heats, and the deadly emanations from the shores common to the night.

4. The labour in boats should be conducted with as much care to the men and absence from fatigue as possible, avoiding exhausting perspiration.

5. The seamen should not land, unless under urgent necessity; and then the more high and dry lands should be carefully selected for encampment.

6. The meals should be regularly served and carefully cooked, no more spirit-ration being issued than is customary.

7. Under necessary fatigue, cold, wet, and mental depression, the issue of extra necessary spirit-rations will be proper.

8. Coffee should be given early in the morning, as a habit.

9. One or two doses of quinine should be given daily as a pro-phylactic.

10. The rendezvous boat should have an ample tarpaulin for the protection of the men against night dews and noon-day heats.

11. Besides a complete set of blanket-clothing, each man should have a duck-dress and flannel waistcoat.

12. Where the nature of the service can admit of it, no boats' crews should be absent from the rendezvous boat or from the ship during the night. This would constitute, of itself, the greatest safeguard of all.

13. Dry-cleaning of the decks, attention to cleaning out the holds, and great attention to the personal cleanliness of the crew, should be carefully observed; also the application of antiseptic and disinfecting substances to all the discharges from the bodies of the patients.

14. The free ventilation of every part of the ship should be care-fully maintained.

15. The labour of the men should be sparingly used, and they should, when possible, not be exposed to wet or damp; and they should not be put to work till the sun shall have dissipated the early morning fogs, and till after the serving of coffee.

16. The holds of ships should not be cleansed on the spot where the fever has originated, or during its prevalence, but should be deferred till the arrival of the vessel in a colder latitude.

17. Green wood should not be placed on board ship in hot cli-mates. Wood for ship use should be stripped of the bark, cut into moderately sized pieces, and partly charred. These directions are chiefly taken from the admirable Report of Dr. Bryson, already quoted.

CURE.

Previously to entering on a consideration of the means of cure, the physician should determine, with the utmost care, both the type of the prevailing fever, and the age, constitution, and habits of life of the individual. There are, beyond question, pervading characters in every epidemic—one being of an adynamic, another of a somewhat sthenic, or phlogistic nature; and it is obvious that on the right determination of these preliminary questions very much must depend. But, with all the care which we can employ, it must be confessed that, as regards the essential nature, causes, and treatment of this terrible disease, the amount of our real know-ledge is lamentably defective. In the yellow fever, as it appeared on the coast of Spain, the brave Robert Jackson speaks hopelessly as to the influences of all means of cure; and he was in all things the very opposite of a despairing physician.

"From the wide range which the symptoms take," says Dr. Gilkrest,—"so wide that but for the *black vomit* being *liable* to occur as a connecting link, in the various forms during the prevalence of an epidemic, we should, from the symptoms, as well as from *post-mortem* appearances, often have reason to suppose that different remote causes were giving rise to different impressions. It is obvious that in no disease is it more difficult to lay down rules of practice, and in none can the medical officer's tact and attention be more needed."

"All medicine," says Rostan, "consists in diagnosis;" but he adds, as justly as emphatically, that "the medicine of symptoms is the worst of all medicines." We must, therefore, beware of a false diagnosis; and recollect also that, as regards the important question of treatment, it too often happens that "What is new is not true, and that what is true is not new." Holding in recollection these preliminary cautions, we shall be the better prepared to enter on the question of the little that is known, therapeutically, of yellow fever.

The history of the treatment of this disease, like that of the bilious remittents of hot climates generally, is found stamped with the characters of the doctrines taught in our medical schools, rather than on any ascertained etiology or pathology.

As in the remittents of the East, at different times, so in the Western epidemic yellow fever, emetics and purgatives formerly preceded a systematic course of Peruvian bark, wine and opium; blood-letting being used only where violent reaction, and conse· quent inflammation, were supposed to exist.

But this plan of treatment not proving satisfactory to Dr. Rush, of Philadelphia, he had recourse to repeated blood-lettings, seldom exceeding sixteen ounces at a time, pursued into the fifth and even the seventh day of the disease, or so long as the pulse retained any firmness. Calomel with jalap powder was freely administered throughout, as a purgative and cholagogue; and this course of treatment Dr. Rush declared to be the most successful in his time.

In the West Indies, Robert Jackson abstracted blood even more freely still, to the amount of thirty to forty ounces at a time, and repeated until a powerful impression was made on the disease. Then followed Dr. Chisholm, with "bleeding to the extent necessary, plentiful alvine evacuations, MERCURIAL PTYALISM, and cold affusion."

Different as such means of cure may appear, they were not in reality so different as they seemed, for the yellow fever epidemics, observed and described by so many able men, differed as to time, character, circumstances, and localities, so as very greatly to reconcile certain differences in their treatment. Such influences on health and on disease must ever be held in recollection in passing judgment on the conduct of those who have gone before us; otherwise we should be doing injustice to their memories.

Referring now only to the experiences of our own day, and of epidemic visitations such as we see them, it must be confessed that it is not here as in remittent fever : we must not have recourse to heroic measures of cure, whether by blood-letting or by quina ; for we cannot cut short the yellow fever.

In more recent times blood-letting has not proved needful or useful, whether in this epidemic as it prevails on the African coast, or that of Spain, or yet in the West Indies. As in cholera, the shock to the organic nervous system, and the injury to the blood, especially when the subjects of treatment are placed in low, damp, or crowded localities, induce so great a prostration of the nervous and vascular functions, even in the young, and in those apparently of a phlogistic habit, as to render any considerable abstraction of blood from the arm a more than questionable operation. Where general or local depletion promises relief, it will be found of advantage amongst the newly arrived and plethoric, and in those placed in favourable, open, and airy localities, and where the character of the epidemic fever is more of a phlogistic character than otherwise.

Having duly considered the individual circumstances of the patient—the stage of the disease, and its degree of severity—he should be placed in a position which secures a cool air and free ventilation—nothing being so prejudicial as the contrary states ; and he should be made to look with a confident hope to the result. The following means should then be put in practice :—

The warm bath will be found grateful and useful as a preliminary measure, having in view the objects of purifying the skin and promoting a determination to the surface of the body. The temperature should be such as to prove grateful to the patient, and gentle frictions with oil should follow the use of the bath.

Of internal remedies our list is necessarily limited ; for there is so much irritability of stomach, with such dangerous vomiting in prospect, that even the most useful and agreeable medicine may be rejected. With a view to anticipate and allay this distressing and dangerous disposition, effervescing drinks in moderate and repeated doses should be given—such as soda or seltzer water flavoured with champagne, spruce or ginger beer—all which are grateful to the stomach.

As in remittents, so in this disease, the bowels should be freely evacuated by means of jalap powder with calomel, or by calomel followed by senna and salts mixture. Throughout the progress of the fever, indeed, and whatever the degree of its severity, the depurative functions must be kept in activity by alterative doses of mercury, purgatives, and diuretics. In this manner, by mild means, and with the aid of farinaceous diet and demulcent drinks, the severer forms of the disease may be somewhat mitigated, while the milder degrees of it will in a few days be advanced into convalescence ; but too often we have to deal with more grave ills.

If, in the severe cases now contemplated, blood-letting be had recourse to, the blood should be abstracted from the epigastrium previously fomented, and by means of leeching or cupping, carefully avoiding the induction of vascular and nervous depression. We have now to regard black vomit and the death of the patient as probable contingencies in the progress and termination of the case; and we must, with such means as we know, proceed to anticipate and prevent them. Of these, turpentine exhibited by the stomach and in the form of enema, and applied to the whole abdomen as an epithem, has been for many years past recommended by Dr. Copland, as holding forth a favourable prospect—assisting its operation by wine, brandy, camphor, and opium, as diffusible stimulants.

In the epidemic yellow fever of Peru, described by Dr. Archibald Smith, and which took three years to attain to its full development, one attack formed no security against a second. From the very gradual manner in which this epidemic acquired maturity, so as at length to constitute unequivocal yellow fever, the Spanish physicians compared it to the tender cub which, as it grew up, became the voracious beast of prey.

The treatment found successful in this epidemic, after the failure of other remedies, was turpentine in one drachm doses by the mouth, or half-ounces in the form of enema, " several times daily" —using it also as an epithem to the abdomen. In this manner fifty per cent. of the Indian race are stated to have been saved, even " in the last stage with black vomit." This course of treatment was not so successful with the other coloured and mixed races, and it was the least successful with the European. Dr. Smith " can only recal to mind three decided instances of a white man having reached the stage of full homogeneous black vomit, and yet to have survived that danger."

On the decline of the febrile stage, the infusion of valerian with ether, camphor, and musk, was generally used, as were the carbonate of ammonia, opium with creasote, camphor and opium, and capsicum with opium, in form of pill. Two minims of creasote and half a grain of opium in pill, and administered every four or six hours, were very effective in preventing the accession of black vomit.

Very recently also this practice has been very favourably reported upon by Mr. Laird, of her Majesty's ship *Medea*, who exhibited the turpentine in doses of fifteen minims, with a little nitric ether and camphor mixture, every three or four hours, which course of treatment was pursued until a remission of symptoms ensued; when quinine and a nutritious diet concluded the treatment.

As adjuvants, occasional doses of blue pill followed by castoroil — sinapisms — cupping — blisters — evaporating lotions to the head, &c., were employed; and, out of sixty cases treated, only four deaths occurred. This was indeed a remarkable, and I believe an unique amount of success; and should it prove in other epidemic visitations of yellow fever equally true, we shall no longer approach this disease with hesitation, the result of dread.

Blood-letting Mr. Laird found to be "extremely hazardous," and an operation which, "except in some particular cases, might be safely dispensed with;" but local depletion by cupping, from the epigastrium and nape of the neck, appears to have been occasionally useful.

The action of the turpentine on the skin and kidneys is rated highly by Mr. Laird, who found the medicine seldom to disagree with the stomach, or induce strangury. Turpentine exhibited internally did not excite the pulse; and applied to the abdomen in friction, along with olive-oil, "seemed to act better than if it had been taken by the mouth," in the instance of "a sailor-lad, with black vomit and suppression of urine, who would not take the draught." The report of this interesting case goes on to say that "three hours after the frictions were applied, this patient made a pint of healthy-looking urine, and after an interval of eight hours, he passed a pint and a half more urine of the same character. Early next morning black vomit, which had been present for about thirty-six hours, entirely ceased, and the lad appeared otherwise much improved." The frictions were continued; but while struggling against the administration of a nutritive enema, he was seized with convulsion, and died.

"On dissection, no trace of black vomit could be detected, unless a little dark green matter found in the ileum might be considered as such. The mucous lining of the stomach was much congested, and discoloured dark-red, but its epithelium was perfectly intact; and although the liver presented the usual fawn colour, the skin was not tinged yellow, as was the case with the other patients who died with black vomit. This case, I might be excused saying, ought to have been a recovery from black vomit, had not the unlooked-for head affection come on.

"In another case of black vomit, I gave turpentine in doses of forty minims, combined with hydrocyanic acid, with the evident effect of controlling this fatal symptom, although the patient was carried off soon afterwards by profuse and uncontrollable hæmorrhage of fluid-looking blood from the mouth and nose."*

Dr. Blair, of British Guiana, another recent writer on yellow fever, was sparing in the use of blood-letting, even as a local mode of abstraction, having recourse to it only for the relief of severe and early cerebral and epigastric distress.

His treatment consisted in twenty-grain doses of calomel, with twenty-four of quinine, followed by castor oil. In severe cases he repeated the calomel and quinine every six hours; and never had occasion to exhibit more than six such doses to one patient; and ptyalism did not result from this treatment. "Emesis was fre-

* "Medical Gazette," April 14, 1855.

quently moderated or checked by the exhibition of drop doses of creasote made into a light emulsion with mucilage and sugar."

This gentleman used cold ablutions, sinapisms, and blisters; while he exhibited as adjuvants—Rhenish wine, chalk mixture, with essential oil, creasote, liquor potassæ, ammoniacal paste, musk, carbonate of ammonia, spirit of mindererus, magnesia, laxative enemata, lemonade. The diet consisted in barley-water, sago, arrowroot, tea, chicken-broth, beef-tea, and toasted bread.

The treatment of the epidemic yellow fever,. as described and treated by Dr. McKinlay, was as follows :—

Purgatives, calomel and antimony every three or four hours, cooling saline diaphoretics, sponging with vinegar and water, quinine and bitter infusions during convalescence, with barley and rice-water for drink. To alleviate and overcome vomiting, he used effervescing draughts, with tincture of opium, enemata containing turpentine, sinapisms and blisters to the epigastrium.

Such is a fair exposition of the most recent means of cure adopted in the treatment of yellow fever. That all or any of them may prove very generally effective to the cure of other epidemic visitations, is more than present experience will warrant us to conclude; but that they present subject-matter worthy the attention of the tropical practitioner, may, I think, be admitted.

Desiring to attract and to concentrate the attention of the reader to the little that appears to be practically ascertained respecting. the modes of treating yellow fever, I have purposely avoided the entanglement which might result from an enumeration of all the adjuvants which have at different times found a place in the lists of authors, and which are common to the treatment of yellow fever and to the remittents of tropical climates. The truth is, that many remedies have been recommended for the cure of both diseases— not on the ground of proved experience, but simply as unreasoned opinions. We have been oftener told what they were, than what they signified.

Postscript.—Were I to treat a case of yellow fever, I should, for the reasons given by Dr. Macrae, of Calcutta, page 564, apply the nitro-muriatic acid solution perseveringly, and from the accession of the disease, to the entire surface of the body; for here, as in epidemic cholera, we have to deal with a peculiar blood disease. The internal use of the same means might prove of advantage in aid of the swathing and other general remedies.

DELIRIUM TREMENS.

WITHOUT calling in question the occasional occurrence of acute delirium, as an affection connected with inflammatory irritation of the arachnoid membrane—the conjoined result of " a .drunken bout" and of insolation—I propose here to notice only the true delirium tremens, as it generally appears amongst European soldiers in the East Indies. It is usually seen, both in hospital and private practice, as the immediate result of hard, or of long-continned drinking; and occasionally also as the indirect result of the temporary withdrawal of the accustomed stimulating drink; or it arises, in a more or less subdued or masked form, when the soldier has for some days been subjected to the abstinence of the hospital system of discipline, on account of a shock to the nervous system, resulting from a wound or accident, or for the treatment of acute disease—as fever, dysentery, or hepatitis.

The importance and interest attaching to delirium tremens—the brain fever of drunkards, according to the older returns—will be rendered apparent by a reference to the numerical table at the end of this article, and with which I have been favoured by Sir Alexander Tulloch. The disease, as already suggested, is important also, as forming a very frequent complication with many of the acute diseases of tropical climates—a fact not sufficiently noticed by the generality of authors. The subject derives a terrible importance also from the fact that delirium tremens frequently ends in insanity —the *vesania ebriosorum* of scientific authors.

Dr. John Macpherson, of Bengal, in his recent admirable "Statistics of Delirium Tremens," from his experience in the General Hospital of Calcutta, divides this disease into three classes :—

" 1. Cases occurring after hard drinking for a short time— generally up to the date of admission.

" 2. Cases in which the system is chronically affected, but in which drinking has been kept up to the date of attack.

" 3. Cases in which the system is chronically affected, but in which the attack is consequent on the withdrawal of stimulants generally, along with impoverished diet, bad clothing, exposure to damps, and other depressing circumstances, the attack sometimes coming on when they are under treatment for other diseases."

It is too generally known how prevalent delirium tremens is in India, and how much Europeans are there addicted to intemperance. I believe I should not be far wrong in stating that an army of 18,000 strong in Bengal sends more than 600 cases of ebrietas to hospital in the year, slight cases not being sent; and that although the numbers of cases of delirium tremens is reduced more than one-half, " owing to a more correct system of returns, separating ebrietas from delirium tremens, yet even now it rarely falls short of 150 ; and the proportions in Madras and Bombay are not very different."

In Calcutta the vice of drunkenness is stated by the author to be " fearfully prevalent" amongst European soldiers, sailors, pensioners, and invalids, " who live a most reckless life"—the pensioners, unhappily for themselves, " leading a life of complete idleness."

SYMPTOMS AND PROGRESS.

Delirium tremens appears in forms more or less acute and com-plicated, as the disease may occur in the newly-arrived or in the old seasoned soldier. In the cases of young soldiers, we find that occasional courses of drinking, with insolation, will produce great perturbation and excitement of the nervous and vascular functions, amounting, in some instances, to maniacal fury—the most strange illusions, violence, and hurry of manner, with incessant muttering and general irritability, the face being flushed, and the head hot. There is great anxiety, with oppression of the præcordia, vomiting, spasmodic pains, and occasional headache; the urinary and intes-tinal excretions being scanty and depraved, the tongue foul and tremulous. While this earlier stage continues, the skin is harsh and dry, the pulse frequent; but if the disease proceed, symptoms of exhausted nervous and vascular energies take the place of the previous tumult and excitement, even in the youthful and newly-arrived soldier. The alcohol here seems to act through the blood in a cumulative and poisonous manner, operating eventually on the organic and cerebral nerves.

In the old soldier, again, habituated to the abuse of intoxicating liquors, every debilitating cause—even the withdrawal of the accustomed bane—is followed by collapse of the vital powers, as indicated by nervous depression, excessive gastric and intestinal irritation, a feeble pulse, sometimes frequent but more generally slow, a cold and clammy skin, a hurried and imperfect respiration. The manner, though wild, is more subdued, and the temper melancholy, the mind being in a perpetual anguish—haunted with imaginary alarms and illusions; but when the attention is aroused by a question, the answer is generally rational. The wretched sufferer, deprived of half his reason, is yet miserably conscious of his condition; in short, the moral and physical ills produced by habitual inebriety are here concentrated.

After a time sleep is entirely banished, with aggravation of all the symptoms; until at length, as the disease advances, and the energies sink, a complete exhaustion of the vital powers announces the immediate approach of danger. I have seen men walking about in a frenzied state, muttering and chattering, whose death took place within a few minutes, instantaneously, and as if struck by lightning; while, in other instances, death was preceded by aggravated tremor, ending in general enervation and convulsion.

Mr. Playfair, of Bengal, describes a soldier as insisting on being discharged from the hospital, because the guard had conspired against his life; or he saw his comrades attempting to shoot him through the windows. He then collected his bedding, and every-thing he could find, and piled them against the door, to guard against the supposed attack, crying aloud for justice or revenge. With the fury and strength of a madman, he then threw everything about the room ; after which he seated himself in the corner, and with eyes fixed on vacancy, he listened to and conversed with imaginary beings.   In this latter mood he would injure no one ; indeed, such is not the general desire, though there is usually some person of whom the patient complains.   As in ordinary insanity, so in this disease, *personal fear* predominates.

The patient often calms on finding himself under the restraint of the strait-waistcoat, and begins to relate his grievances ; and then only can he be prevailed on to take medicine ; at other times restraint only seems to increase the fury of the patient, who foams at the mouth with rage, blaspheming in the most horrible manner.

A patient supposed himself a messenger sent from Heaven to save the souls of those who sought his protection, and pointed to the heavenly hosts on the wall, with " the devil looking round the corner, afraid to advance."   Another soldier imagined himself charged with the most unnatural crimes, but asserted his inno- cence in the most pathetic manner ; while a third believed himself condemned to be shot for a crime he never committed.   But though he was to suffer innocently, he called for instant execution, and, placing his back to the wall, requested that a file of men might be ordered to despatch him.   A fourth complained that his wife's honour was in danger from the designs of villains ; and lifting up the corner of the quilt, pointed to Mr. Playfair the place of her imagined concealment.

A soldier of the Bengal Artillery is mentioned by Dr. Spry, who required six men to secure him in the strait-jacket.   He had stripped himself naked during the night, burst from the hospital into the adjoining dead-house, barricading the door with tables, on which the bodies of five deceased comrades were lying.   Here an appalling scene was presented—the raving drunkard being in close conflict with the dead, uttering at the same time the most dreadful imprecations that language can afford.   Such are some of the effects of excessive spirit-drinking on the European soldier.

In these terrible cases, if the patient did not sleep he speedily died.

CAUSES.

With soldiers habituated to excesses, the sudden privation of the accustomed drinks—the absence of sufficiently nourishing food —the debility caused by acute diseases, as fever, dysentery, diarrhœa, and cholera—active measures of depletion—these are all frequent causes ; as are the abuse of tobacco-smoking, the use of opium, and of drugged beverages.

But while it is admitted, that in young men, occasional courses of drunkenness, with or without solar exposure, constitute the most frequent causes of the more acute forms of delirium tremens, there can be no doubt that, with the older soldiers of protracted residence in tropical climates, the habitual tippling and tobacco-smoking, especially when, of a sudden, one or all of the long-used stimuli have been withdrawn—form by far the most general cause of the disease in its true and more frequent examples.

In no other disease have cause and effect been so much con-founded as in that now under consideration; in no class of observations of morbid events is it therefore more necessary to study well the natural history and observe the natural course of diseased action.

Stimulation of the brain, or over-excitement of its functions, whether by moral or physical agents, long or repeatedly applied, must have its limit of endurance, neither class of excitants being compatible with health beyond a certain time. Both the causes of delirium tremens are cumulative, and when the limit of endu-rance has arrived, the disease becomes manifest, exhaustion of the nervous energy then merging in a new form of disease, resulting from previous irritation. It is to the over-action of the cause rather than to its discontinuance or withdrawal, that we are gene-rally to refer the complicated series of events constituting true delirium tremens. But every surgeon who has treated soldiers in tropical climates has seen occasional instances of delirium tremens to arise, on the other hand, within a few days of admission into hospital, in hard drinkers, while being treated for acute diseases, wounds, or accidents; in other words, when the accustomed stimuli had been withdrawn, and a shock to the nervous system had been superadded. I here speak only of the disease as it appears in the East, where the nervous and vascular systems of European soldiers are already so influenced by heat, malaria, irre-gular habits of life, &c., as to constitute a disease aggravated beyond what is ordinary in temperate climates. The mild forms of delirium tremens do not in India "constitute by far the most numerous" class, as they are said to do at home.

The truth of these observations is seen in the relative statistics of the army and navy. In the latter, though delirium tremens is found to result from excessive debauches in harbour, the disease is neither of such frequent occurrence, nor so fatal in its results by many degrees, as in the army, and especially amongst soldiers who are paid daily; for with these last, in place of the periodical drunken bout following upon the receipt of the month's pay, after the olden custom, there is now prevalent a far more injurious course of excitement in the daily tippling of ardent spirits.

COMPLICATIONS.

The complications of delirium tremens would alone constitute this disease one of much importance in military practice; for not only is it, in this form, very prevalent, but it is both insidious and dangerous in the hands of the inexperienced.

In the soldier habituated to the use of ardent spirits, nervous symptoms arise as frequent complications in course of treating him for other diseases, and such symptoms will always be found, varying in degree, in persons of better condition who indulge freely in wine, spirituous liquors, and tobacco. After the free use of depletory means for the removal of fever, dysentery, or hepatitis, how often do we find the patient exhibit at first a latent or sub-dued nervousness, soon to be unmasked in all the illusory and real horrors of delirium tremens :* in other words, when febrile or inflammatory symptoms have yielded to the use of blood-letting, purgatives, sudorifics, and low diet, how often do we see the patient become low, desponding, tremulous, agitated, and sleepless ; symp-toms, which, if disregarded, become sources of aggravated suffer-ing and danger in the sequel : in short, life may here be sacrificed, if the enervated condition under consideration be mistaken for, or treated as, cerebral inflammation.

It is here, then, when, under the depressing influences of the measures of cure indicated, room has been afforded for the display of nervous irritability and exhaustion, that other quieting means of a special nature become really necessary to the successful treat-ment of the case ; and many a physician has found the safety and advantage of such means, under such circumstances, without having been sufficiently alive to the reason of his success.

PATHOLOGY.

Lesion of innervation is patent in this disease. We at once perceive over-excitement, great irritation, and consequent exhaus-tion of the functions of innervation :—with chronic poisoning by alcohol we have exhaustion of the sensorium. Alcohol, in com-mon with various other substances, is cumulative when used habi-tually ; and hence its effects on the brain and nervous system generally, ending in what is termed nervousness, excitability, and eventually in intoxication more or less acute, and in delirium tremens ;—the *dyscrasia potatorum* of authors. Congestion of all the secreting organs, and consequent arrest of all the depurative functions ; depravation of all the secretions of the body, whether recrementitious or excrementitious, would appear to constitute the most ordinary results of excessive spirit-drinking. When delirium tremens has actually set in, the urine is declared by Dr. Bence Jones to present an extraordinary diminution in the total amount of phosphatic salts excreted, as compared with the vast increase of the same in inflammation of the brain.

"Alcohol," says this physician, " hardens the skin when ap-plied locally. It hardens and thickens the stomach. When long

* Delirium tremens is always designated by the European soldiers as ''THE HORRORS.''

continued it thickens the cellular tissues of the liver. It passes off by the lungs and kidneys, and affects both organs. Ultimately it lessens the amount of carbonic acid expired, and hinders the removal of the products of decomposition by the urine. It changes the composition of the blood, and affects the nutrition of every organ and structure in the body. It has its own peculiar poisonous action on the muscles and nerves. As a poison it has been placed by its effect on nerves and muscles between ergot of rye and arsenic."

"Alcohol is the chief poisonous ingredient of unadulterated fermented liquids. Like all poisons, when not taken in too large a quantity, or too long continued, it has a medicinal action, on which its dietetic value depends. This action may be summed up in one word, stimulant."

Alcohol, according to Dr. Bocker, diminishes the excretion both of the solid and fluid constituents of the urine.

2. Alcohol does not increase the cutaneous perspiration.

3. Alcohol does not augment the fæcal excretion.

4. Alcohol diminishes not only the absolute quantity of carbonic acid exhaled by the lungs, but also the relative proportions of it in the products of respiration.

Dr. Marcet concludes his experimental inquiry into the action of alcohol on the nervous system as follows :—

"1. That alcohol acts through the circulation principally, though not exclusively, on the nervous centres by means of absorption.

"2. That alcohol exerts a slight but decided action on the nervous centres through the nerves, independently of the circulation.

"3. That the influence transmitted through the nerves may be of two kinds :—

"(a). It may give rise to a shock, or temporary complete suspension of sensation and of muscular motion (with the exception, perhaps, of that of the eyelids); although respiration continues.

"(b). It may produce no other visible effect than shortening life."

MM. Duroy, Lallemand, and Perrin have come to the following conclusions as to the action of alcohol on the economy :—

1. That alcohol is not an alimentary substance, it acts only as a modifier of the nervous system.

2. It is neither destroyed nor transformed in the economy.

3. It becomes especially concentrated in the liver and in the brain.

4. These facts explain the production of functional and organic changes in the liver, brain, and kidneys."

Dr. Ogston of Aberdeen, in his pathological observations on the bodies of known drunkards, gives the following results of the inspection of the bodies of 44 persons :—

1. *Cranium.*—Abnormal appearances within the cranium, in 43 cases, 97·7 per cent. of the whole.

2. *Chest.*—Abnormal appearances in the respiratory organs, in all, in 33 cases, or in 75 per cent. of the whole. Simultaneous abnormal appearances in the head and respiratory organs in 32 cases.

Abnormal appearances in the pericardium, heart, aorta, or pulmonary artery, in all, in 26 cases, or in 59 per cent. of the whole.

Abnormal appearances within the chest, in all, in 38 cases, or in 86·3 per cent. of the whole.

3. *Abdomen.*—Abnormal appearances in the stomach, in all, in 24 cases, or in 54·5 per cent. of the whole.

Intestines.—Abnormal appearances in the intestines, in all, in 8 cases, or in 18·18 per cent, of the whole.

Liver.—Abnormal appearances in the liver, in all, in 36 cases, or in 81·8 per cent. of the whole.

Spleen.—Abnormal appearances in the spleen, in all, in 18 cases, or in 40·9 per cent. of the whole.

Kidneys.—Abnormal appearances in the kidneys, in all, in 28 cases, or in 63·6 per cent. of the whole.

Entire absence of morbid appearances existed in none of the cases.*

Such have been the *post-mortem* appearances. But, during life, besides the contamination of the blood from the generally pent-up and vitiated state of the secretions—the result of universal congestion—there is reason to conclude that, as a direct consequence of spirit-drinking, the circulating fluid is dissolved, and otherwise depraved. The result altogether is, a severe irritation of the entire nervous system, followed by nervous and vascular collapse. The habitual use of alcohol, even when falling short of intoxication, arrests destructive assimilation, and thus causes at once a retention of effete tissue, and a diminished depuration. After death, likewise, we have the evidence of Dr. Macpherson that he "has seen rum very apparent in the lateral ventricles." Nervous exhaustion, with serous effusion into the sub-arachnoid cavity, is a frequent cause of death in all countries.

The influence of season is expressed by a very great increase of deaths during the hot months in Bengal; the mortality in the eight hot months being in the General Hospital "about three times what it is in the four cold ones; and in the Medical College, in the eight hot months, more than double what it is in the cold ones."

On the relative frequency of morbid changes in the viscera, as witnessed in Bengal, Dr. Macpherson observes :—

* "Brit. and For. Med.-Chir. Rev.," for Oct., 1854.

" 1. That the most constant were red patches in the stomach.
" 2. Opalescent appearances of the arachnoid.
" 3. Serous effusion.
" 4. Changes in the liver.
" 5.   ,,   ,,   heart.
" 6.   ,   spleen.
" 7.   . .   ,,   kidneys, not always examined."

PREVENTION.

Doses of two grains of emetic tartar, or half-drachm doses of powdered ipecacuanha, have been exhibited as means of prevention of habits of drunkenness ; some practitioners recommending that the emetic be given at the moment that craving for strong drinks comes on, while others add the medicine to the intoxicating potation with a view to excite nausea, or cause vomiting, and thus produce a feeling of disgust.

Dr. Gilbert, of Lurgan, administers tartar emetic " secretly, in occasional doses of from five to ten grains, as soon as convenient after the person commences drinking strong liquors, in tea or in any other proper vehicle. It generally produces such nausea, vomiting, and fear of death, as completely to frighten the person from going on in his drunken course of life, for that time at least ; and, much to the joy of friends, ultimately produces, in many instances, what nothing else would effect, a complete change of life, one from drunkenness to temperance."

Mr. Higginbottom, of Nottingham, considers the ipecacuanha more safe, and altogether preferable to tartar emetic ; and that from its " extraordinary power of stimulating the whole system, equalizing the circulation, promoting the various secretions, and indeed of assisting each organ of the body to perform its function, and to restore it to its normal state"—ipecacuanha should always have the preference. He gives the powder in half-drachm doses.

The inspector-general, Henry, on an extensive observation of delirium tremens as it appeared in Canada, says :—" As the diarrhœa, which so often warns of malignant cholera, may be readily cured by proper medicine, and the dangerous attack averted ; so in the premonitory stage of this malady, a manly effort, aided by a little medicine, may save both the reason and the life. When the tippling of the sot, or the outright intemperance of the drunkard, are about to end in this disgraceful disease, the poor slave of evil habits will sometimes be induced to make great efforts to break his chain ; but at first he will feel himself most miserable : relaxation and debility have succeeded artificial tension and strength, whilst the stomach craves its customary stimulus, and some substitute must be found.

According to my experience, gentian, as below, is the best medicine under these circumstances :—

  R Infus. gentianæ comp.. . . . . . . ℥xij.
   Tincturæ ejusdem . . . . ℥v.
   Magnesiæ sulphatis . . . . ℥iv.

A common wine-glassful the first thing in the morning, again at mid-day, and in the evening.

If the patient can be persuaded to take it regularly for a week, his morbid craving for stimulating drink will be abated, the tone of his stomach improved, his moral dejection lessened, and he will feel himself a new man. Of course this applies only to persons in whom organic mischief has not yet taken place."

The Asarum Europæum is constantly used in Russia as a cure and preventive of excessive and habitual drinking. By acting on the digestive organs it counteracts the irrepressible longing for alcohol which so frequently follows a sudden abstinence from drinking, and proves thus to some degree a prophylactic also. It is used in the form of decoction, with the addition of valerian and orange-peel.

TREATMENT.

The natural cure of a paroxysm of delirium tremens, whether induced by the toxic action of alcohol, or by overstraining of the mind, is sleep; and this termination we have to favour by every safe means within our reach; for by continuance of wakefulness the patient dies. A distinguished staff-officer, at home, of regular habits, after six weeks of anxious wakefulness, was reduced to a most dangerous condition. On my entering his room, he asked if I had come to place him in arrest, for that he had committed murder. But for timely sleep this valuable officer must speedily have sunk.

The first observation I would offer is, that the violence and frequency of this disease have considerably diminished of late in civil life, and presumptively also in the army, so as to diminish the vigour of treatment, which should be directed to the calming of nervous irritation, by mild anodynes and diaphoretics, while we guard against exhaustion by a light nutritious diet, placing the patient under the most proper hygienic conditions at the same time.

Before entering on the treatment of this dangerous disease, however, the medical officer must institute a rigid scrutiny into all the antecedent circumstances relating to the soldier's health;— such as, his constitution—age—length of residence in a tropical climate—previous diseases, and especially if the present be the first seizure of delirium;—habits of life—whether he is at the moment a sufferer from an actual drinking bout, or whether the intoxicating drink has been withdrawn for two or more days;— whether the patient is a habitual and confirmed drunkard. From a careful consideration of these circumstances, together with an examination of the abdominal regions—of the skin—pulse—tongue —condition of the nervous system—of the secretions—and of the

nature and degree of the delirium—the observer is enabled readily
to determine whether the condition of the patient be one of gastric
and vascular excitement, with congestive or inflammatory tendency
in the cerebral or abdominal cavity, or of nervous irritation and
exhaustion only.

Cases will occur in young and plethoric soldiers, during their
first excesses, in which febrile, congestive, and inflammatory complications are manifested. Here a moderate general blood-letting,
or leeches applied behind the ears, will prove a necessary preliminary measure of cure—the after part of the treatment, and especially the means for securing the critical sleep, being carefully
carried out. But when the case is not of this acute nature, the
subject being even young and plethoric, we may control the disease
by active purgatives, opiates with antimony, and by cold applied to
the head and face, while the body is immersed in a warm bath.
On removal from the bath, a full dose of calomel and opium should
be administered, followed in two hours by a powerful cathartic,
composed of compound decoction of aloes, infusion of senna, sulphate of magnesia, and tincture of senna. After the free action of
this purgative, or of croton-oil, which many prefer to every other
form, it will be necessary to quiet the nervous agitation ; and this
is best done, in the acute form of the disease, by a combination of
tincture of opium with antimonial wine, exhibited every two hours
until a tranquil sleep is secured. The union of antimony with
opium here yields a reciprocal efficacy. Dr. Graves, of Dublin,
gave a table-spoonful every two hours of the following mixture :—

> Antimon. tart. . . . . gr. iv.
> Tinct. opii . . . . ʒj.
> Aquæ . . . . ℥viij.*

But opium, given early and largely, with the view to overstep
the stage of excitement, and thus forcibly to induce sleep, is unsafe.
It should be given as suggested, in aid of the tendency of nature,
in as moderate doses as may be, consistently with the assuring of
sleep. To obtain repose for the brain by any means is the first
indication of cure ; and this cardinal object has been attempted by
opiates—by opiates with antimony—by chloroform—by chloroform
with opium—by chloroform by inhalation—by the Indian hemp—
by heroic doses of digitalis—by the expectant or placebo system.
Delirium tremens is doubtless, to a certain extent, of " the class of
self-limited disorders," and the fact ought not to be lost sight of in
its treatment ; but he who has to deal with this disease in India must
put a guarded limit to his expectations of the curative powers of
nature, and be careful to come to her assistance in time ; otherwise
the limit may be that of death. Doubtless the alcohol is eliminated

---

* The question whether ipecacuanha may not in most cases be substituted for the
emetic tartar is well worthy of consideration, the former being far less depressing in
its actions.

in due time from the blood and secretions, but with the limit of this process, as to time, we are unacquainted. Meanwhile, we must have special regard to the condition of the nervous system, and to the nature and extent of the complications in each individual case.

When the symptoms, as here supposed, are the direct and immediate results of a fit of drinking—no inflammatory action being present within the cerebral cavity—the course of treatment suggested will generally prove of speedy effect. In the true delirium tremens, however, or that resulting from the withdrawal of an accustomed stimulus, with exhaustion of the nervous and vascular systems, the treatment becomes at once more complex and difficult.

Here, as in the former instance, we should commence by the exhibition of a full dose of calomel and opium, followed by a powerful aromatic and stimulating cathartic, with a view to remove retained and vitiated intestinal accumulations, and to act as an energetic cholagogue. After the free operation of the cathartic, opium in moderate doses, conjoined, in healthy subjects, with antimony, and in old or anæmic subjects with camphor or ammonia, should be given every two hours, until evidence of abated nervous irritability and nervous exhaustion be made apparent, in a tranquil sleep. For the purpose of allaying nervous agitation and sleeplessness, very large and very unwarrantable doses of opium have been exhibited; but it should at all times be the object of the attentive physician to obtain his objects by a moderate use of direct narcotics; and happily, in the use of chloroform, internally exhibited, we possess a powerful and harmless means of commanding nervous perturbation and depression. Chloroform, in very severe cases, may be conjoined with small doses of laudanum, and so as to command sleep. Chloroform is thus valuable in itself, and as enabling us to dispense with large and repeated doses of opium.

As stated in the article on fever, Doctors Corrigan and Gordon, of Dublin, have, for some time past been in the habit of using chloroform in delirium tremens. One drachm is given by the stomach at first, and it is often increased to two drachms, or even larger doses. The dose is repeated every two or three hours, until sleep results; and, unlike opium, this medicine does not lock up the secretions. The moderate use of chloroform by inhalation has likewise been had recourse to with marked benefit in cases of extreme violence, the patient awaking refreshed and restored after several hours of sound sleep. In America the Indian hemp has been exhibited in large doses every hour, it is said, with similar results. Heroic doses of tincture of digitalis—half an ounce repeated in four hours, and in rare instances a third dose of two drachms—have been exhibited by various practitioners, in different times and places, and very recently by Mr. Jones, of Jersey; while he declares that smaller doses, in the earlier stages of the disease, are inefficient, if not injurious.

On the effects of half-ounce doses of tincture of digitalis in delirium tremens we may conclude with Dr. Peacock, of St. Thomas's Hospital—" 1st. That the drug, when exhibited in full doses, does not by any means produce the amount of depression which our previous experience of its action in small and frequently repeated doses would have led us to expect; and, 2nd. That the remedy, in conjunction with other means, may probably be more usefully employed in the treatment of certain cases of the disease, and especially when it occurs in young and robust persons, whose strength has not been broken down by prolonged habits of intemperance; and particularly when it arises as the immediate result of excessive spirit-drinking. Delirium tremens, like other acute diseases, occurs under varied and opposite conditions, and it would be alike opposed to sound theory and practice to extend the same treatment to all cases of the disease."

But to aid the actions of narcotics or calmatives, the use of active cholagogue purgatives, of warm baths, of spiced negus, and of well-made soups, will materially advance the solution of the symptoms; by such means we may emulge the depurative organs, while we support the depressed nervous energy. Articles of diet at once nutritious, light, and easy of digestion, should be carefully exhibited, in order to guard against exhaustion. Wine and porter I have always given in preference to alcoholic drinks, and these have been allowed only with soups or solid articles of diet.

Personal restraint and coercive measures are seldom called for, and should not be used without a necessity. The disposition of the patient is generally harmless; and by careful and constant attention on the part of the attendants, and by judicious management, he can be induced to comply with all the requisite orders of the hospital.

In the hands of exclusive practitioners, I have often seen means, apparently opposite in their nature and influences, followed by successful results :—for instance, a late friend of mine, a surgeon of the Bengal army, and one of the most able men whom I have ever known, entertained a positive dislike of opium, from its well-known quality of locking up the secretions. He treated delirium tremens with very large doses of calomel, followed by purgatives; and his success was, according to his impression, equal to that of his brother officers. But this instance only proves how much the use of cholagogue purgatives has to do with the treatment of this disease, and how necessary it is that they should always constitute a prominent part in its treatment.

It is here, as in other complicated diseases; it is not by one favourite remedy, or fancied specific, that disease is to be overcome, but by the proper application of all the known remedies.

To conclude :—For the just treatment of delirium tremens, then, there must be sundry means adapted to the various conditions of so formidable a disease;—cholagogues and purgatives, diuretics

and sudorifics, to elicit secretion and to discharge vitiated matters
—opiates to calm and promote sleep—diffusible stimulants to maintain the nervous, vascular, and respiratory forces, and suitable
means of nutrition. Narcotics alone will not fulfil the true indications.

*The following Table exhibits the Relative Prevalence and Mortality
from Delirium Tremens amongst the European Troops of Her
Majesty's Army in the several Commands mentioned :—*

Delirium Tremens.	Aggregate strength.	Admitted.	Died.	Proportion of deaths to admissions.
West Indies	86,661	1426	175	1 in 8
Jamaica	51,567	191	42	1 in 4½
Cape of Good Hope..............	22,714	13	3	1 in 4⅓
Mauritius	30,515	514	50	1 in 10¼
Ceylon	42,978	35	7	1 in 5
Bermudas	11,721	102	9	1 in 11
Nova Scotia and New Bruns-} wick .... }	46,442	207	18	1 in 12
Upper and Lower Canada	64,280	296	18	1 in 16
Gibraltar.........................	60,269	44	5	1 in 9
Malta	40,826	38	5	1 in 8
Ionian Islands	70,293	192	30	1 in 6½
United Kingdom	44,611	27	4	1 in 6¾
Bengal, 1836 to 1840	36,286	672	14	1 in 48
Madras, 1832 to 1836	31,267	496	21	1 in 24
Bombay, 1836 to 1840	18,073	113	15	1 in 7½
Tenasserim Provinces, 1836-37	7,000	34	5	1 in 7

The above table suggests many inquiries, but which cannot be
answered without entering into a variety of circumstances affecting
the moral and physical condition of the soldier.

Why the mortality by delirium tremens in Madras should be
double that of Bengal, for instance, and why that of Tenasserim
and of Bombay should so very far exceed that of both the sister
presidencies, are points of much interest. Again, so far as ordinary tropical influences are concerned, the colonies of the Cape of
Good Hope, Mauritius, and the provinces of Tenasserim, enjoy a
remarkable exemption, the deaths by fever, dysentery, and hepatitis being few in these colonies, as compared to the other British
possessions ; yet in these most favoured climates, delirium tremens
proves most fatal.

Even within the British islands, we find that, though delirium
tremens is comparatively a more mild and rare disease, the ratio
of deaths to cases treated is nearly eight times as great as in the
unhealthy countries under the Bengal presidency.

It may be that, as in the instance of mercury, a certain amount of injury is prevented by so much of the alcohol being removed from the system by the copious perspirations prevalent throughout India generally, and in Bengal especially, during so many months out of every year. That the excessive transudations which occur in the hot and rainy seasons have such a tendency, appears to me more than probable; for, in the instance of mercury, we have a demonstration of the fact.

Through the same channel of the skin, but by means of active exercise in the open air, the " three-bottle-men," the fox-hunting squires of old, " carried off" their port wine. The hunting during three days of every week kept the depurative functions in activity, and thus they lived on to a lusty old age, while, without such active habits, they must have died in youth and middle life from visceral disease and delirium tremens—the inevitable fate of the sedentary sot.

PART IV.

CHRONIC DISEASES OF EUROPEANS

ON THEIR

RETURN FROM TROPICAL CLIMATES, AND THEIR CURE.

NOTE.—In the following attempt to explain the physiological influences under which the balance of European health is disturbed in hot climates, as well as the counter effects of the climate of Europe, there are certain inevitable repetitions of matters which have already been set forth in the chapter on medical climate. But many persons will peruse this fourth part of the present work to whom the other parts will not possess the same interest ;—and it is better to repeat than to be misunderstood.

INTRODUCTORY CHAPTER.

IN the foregoing portion of this work, I have endeavoured to explain the origin of those formidable diseases which, under tropical influences, affect the stranger European, and to trace them to the altered physiological actions induced by an unnaturally high range of temperature and other causes which, during a residence generally protracted, disturb the various functions on whose just balance health must everywhere depend.

I purpose now to examine the converse of all this—the reverse of everything that holds under tropical influences—to describe the flow and ebb of excitement—the inertia, approaching to a collapse of the various functions of the body, which follows as a necessary consequence of the previous tumultuous action—and to describe both the condition and the treatment of the tropical invalid on his return to his native climate. I design, in short, to trace the peculiar physiological circumstances that have led to the state of ill-health common to tropical invalids, and also to explain the real or essential nature of their diseases ; and, finally, I shall detail the special conditions to be regarded in their treatment. As in the previous portion of this work, I venture with much diffidence to approach the subject by the high but difficult road of physiology.

The courses of investigation here spoken of are surrounded with the difficulties inherent in everything that relates to climate as a science; but fully impressed with these great disadvantages, I am nevertheless more and more persuaded, by every-day experience, of the necessity of prosecuting such inquiries in the manner here proposed. I believe it to promise a superior usefulness in result, whether we regard the advancement of the preventive or the curative departments of our profession.

A familiar acquaintance with the most concentrated forms of disease, as they prevail in tropical climates, assists materially towards a just appreciation of those that lie between, or of minor degrees of disease, as they prevail in more temperate regions. Observation of the nature and power of external causes in the production of disease within the tropics assists us also to form a more just estimate of the power of other and different circumstances of climate, whether morbific or sanative, in our native country. In other words—the antecedent circumstances being known, the consequents become more easy of being appreciated. This counter-experience, acquired in the observation of invalids on their return to Europe from hot climates, ought to be of much value by extending the circle of our acquaintance with the conditions of health resulting from the influences of tropical climates.

Without a knowledge of the antecedent circumstances which, under tropical heats, disturbed the functions of the stranger European, as well as a knowledge of the converse present conditions which, under the cold and damp of Europe, disturb his functions in a different and opposite manner, it is impossible to obtain a just or comprehensive view of the history of his health, to appreciate his actual condition, or to regulate his medical management. "To know the cause of disease," says Dr. Watson, "is sometimes to be able to *cure*, often to be able to prevent it." The subject is of great and of increasing importance also, seeing that the numbers are annually increasing, who, from choice or necessity, betake themselves to the intertropical possessions of this empire. This consideration, as well as the great difficulties above alluded to, render it a matter of serious regret to me, that in such an undertaking I am not aided by the experience and observations of other and more competent authorities.

With the exception of the admirable " Observations" of my late friend, Dr. James Johnson, the subject as here proposed to be treated is almost, if not altogether new. It is incumbent on me, therefore, to explain the grounds on which I pretend to undertake the discussion of it.

During a residence of two-and-twenty years in various parts of India, and in some of its worst climates, I had extended opportunities, in peace and in war, during seasons of prosperity and adversity, in hospital and in private practice, of witnessing the influences that affect the health of both Europeans and natives. For many years I was a severe sufferer from fevers, remittent and intermittent : in Gondwana, in Upper Ava, and in Calcutta, I nearly fell under the violence of malignant remittents. I have seen how the masses and how individuals were affected, how they lived and prospered, how they sickened, recovered, or died ; —the habits of life and the causes of death, in short, of the Asiatic and European races. I have had the further advantage of witnessing the influences that tend to produce like results in the native climate of the European on his return home; and it is this last circumstance that specially encourages me to make the present attempt, trusting that, ere long, I may be followed by other experienced and more competent observers from amongst my brother officers of the medical departments of the Indian army.

In proceeding to treat an European invalid just returned from India, it will be found that a consideration of all the antecedents, within the tropics, is quite as necessary to a just appreciation of his condition, as that of the present influences of an English climate. Both circumstances of climate have, in fact, so strict a relation one to the other, that a consideration of either, examined apart, must fail to lead to a thorough understanding of those important agencies and changes which modify and stamp the habit and constitution of the individual, so as to render him a special and peculiar subject of medical care. These truths, which can admit of no denial, will, it is hoped, be received in excuse of the following details. And let no one consider these subjects tedious or unimportant, but rather that the manner of their exposition may be so.*

It is necessary to hold in recollection, in reference to the subject-matter of the following Section, that of the sufferers from the diseases treated of, a large proportion always consists of young officers belonging to every branch of the Indian services, civil, military, and naval. They generally present in their persons, on their arrival in Europe, examples of the severer ravages of acute tropical disease, or of those which, from their original violence, from their frequent recurrence, or from the consequence of active treatment, have baffled alike the endeavours at immediate cure, and those intended to promote convalescence by recourse to the many changes of climate attainable by a removal to the Hill Ranges and the Seas of the East. None of the servants of the Government are sent home but such as have resisted all the known means of cure ; for none can, under existing regulations, obtain sick leave but through the most strict medical scrutiny, and through a succession of different checks ; there must be exhi-

---

* The object of these cursory remarks is to point out the injurious results following upon exposure to extremes of climate. Were it proposed here to speak of the *remedial* powers of climate, I should quote largely from the valuable work of Sir James Clark on "The Sanative Influence of Climate,"—a work deserving the careful consideration of all classes of the community.

bited in every case a proved and certified necessity for so pro-tracted an absence from duty as is involved in a return to Eng-land.

Of the other class of sufferers, or those who have retired from the public services of India, in middle or more advanced life, it may be said generally that, from their longer residence in India, and from their comparatively increased years, their ailments are of a more chronic character. The peculiar circumstances here mentioned render it evident that, in treating persons of either class in England, the duties and cares of the physician are increased and complicated in no ordinary degree.

The return of the tropical sojourner to the land of his fathers, strange as it may seem, is not unaccompanied by serious risks to his health, and by many moral considerations of a painful and dis-tressing character.

Since the day when, as a mere youth, he bade adieu to his sor-rowing relatives, quitted the protection of the paternal roof, and his native climate, he has undergone changes in his moral and physical nature but little considered or understood by his kinsmen and countrymen in general, amongst whom he now finds himself, in middle or more advanced life, differing in habits, associations, and pursuits from those around him—his nearest relatives departed, and he an invalid and a stranger in the land of his birth. This is a great and sad revolution in life, whether we regard it in a moral or a physical sense, and the medical officer who has observed its violently acute causes abroad, and its chronic and protracted consequences at home, can bear testimony to severe and compli-cated sufferings on the part of a highly intellectual portion of our community.

The youth, on his arrival in India, is at once placed in a society wherein the social affections and the domestic habits of our native country are cherished and cultivated with a luxuriance character-istic of the climate, and of which no other country, perhaps, has offered so distinguished an example.

At a distance of twelve thousand miles from the British shores, and separated for more than half our lives from all those who, in our early youth, were most cherished, it is but natural that in India we should cling together the closer that all feel in common —the old Indian and the new comer—the utter uncertainty of again revisiting the homes of our youth. Such is the state of feeling in the East; and throughout the whole period of an Indian's career, whatever his line of service, he lives in a society whose generous kindness in prosperity, and whose soothing attentions in adversity or in sickness, are unequalled in any other quarter of the world; and it may be said with truth that no one who deserved its consideration was ever otherwise treated by the community of the Indian presidencies.

If we look to the physical condition of the youth, it is at first,

under favourable circumstances, no less cheering. All the functions of life receive an impulse from the agency of heat, while the
susceptibility to impressions is increased in the like proportion.
The comforts, and even luxuries of life, are within his reach if he
will be but prudent; for want of any kind in India is unknown,
except to the heedless or the profligate. Disease, tropical disease,
too, is as yet a stranger to him; and should he be in the army,
and not have campaigned, or served in unhealthy countries, or
during the most unhealthy seasons, the equable determination to
the surface of the body, produced by an elevated range of temperature, tends, along with the increased excitability of the nervous
and vascular systems, to raise the animal spirits, and impart a feeling of invigoration and health delightful to the senses. But time
passes on, and even if, through the contingencies of service in
various regions, or through his own imprudence, disease has not
ensued, the lengthened application of these operations of climate,
which at first appeared beneficial, are sure to impair the health,
and that, too often, with a termination so suddenly dangerous or
fatal, as at once to shock and terrify all who behold it. Loss of
time in the climates of the East implies loss of opportunity to save
life; for an omission or a mistake in the treatment admits of no
future correction or remedy. As an example of the amount of
disease which may occur in India within a brief space of time, I
will quote the report on Ensign F., of the Bengal Army:—" Has
been in India only three years and a few months, and has already
had four separate attacks of hepatitis, two of dysentery, one of continued fever, and two severe tertian intermittent fevers, besides
numerous other illnesses." This officer bore the marks of his
stormy career of disease, being greatly shattered; but he was young,
and he recovered his health. In tropical climates the attentive
observation of the early stages of disease is of the utmost importance, for then we can both prevent and cure with ease; we now
can cure by mild remedies, while by such simple and easily applied
means of cure, we prevent severe ill-consequences. In the East,
diseases of every kind, when once established, proceed with a
tumultuously rapid course to the destruction of certain organs;
and exactly as may be the judgment and power with which remedies
are applied, so will the result prove a complete cure, with speedy
restoration of vigour, or a partial and imperfect cure, ending in
chronic disease.

The distinctive value of the two courses here indicated, is most
important to the welfare of fleets and armies; for by early and
just measures of cure, the men are restored to service, while by
feeble and inert courses, they are consigned to the hospitals, there
to linger and die, as I have mentioned, of chronic disease.

It will now be proper to look in some detail to the operation of
those causes which tend, by their protracted application, to deteriorate or destroy the best of European constitutions; because a

practical acquaintance with these causes, and with their modes of operation, is absolutely necessary to a right understanding of their effects. In India we find that no amount of talent, or of general and professional knowledge, can compensate for the absence of local experience in the treatment of its diseases; and it is hardly necessary to say that the same kind of experience is quite as necessary to the just management of their sequelæ in Europe. A careful consideration of all the influential circumstances, moral and physical, under which the European lived within the tropics, ("Whilst he did climate there," as Shakspeare expresses it), will go far, however, to supply the want here mentioned; and it is in the hope of contributing in some degree to this end that I venture to submit the following observations.

The most immediate of the tropical influences on European constitutions are evidenced in the excited conditions of the nervous and vascular systems, interfering as they do with the rhythmical action of the heart, more or less according to the term of exposure; while the most important are those affecting the functions of the skin, liver, lungs, and kidneys; and owing to the extraordinarily high range and rapid changes in the temperature, humidity, and other qualities of the atmosphere, all these important influences are exemplified in extreme degrees.

The transmission of the nervous influence, according to Eckhard, is more rapid when the temperature is higher.

During the hot and rainy seasons, which in Bengal extend from the beginning of March to the end of October, the determination of the fluids generally is to the surface, accompanied by an increase of the nervous excitability and animal heat; by an acceleration of pulse, and a prodigious increase of the pulmonary and cutaneous exhalations, the latter amounting, in the rainy season, to an exhausting discharge, as if the very serum of the blood were exuded. At this latter season, through the saturation of the atmosphere, its vivifying properties are diminished, while the excessive decomposition of animal and vegetable matter gives to the air in some of the most unhealthy localities the properties of a tainted vapour bath. The perspiration is not carried off by evaporation, while the transudation is enormously increased—thus, heat accumulates in the body, and the local action of cold produces serious consequences, rendering the system susceptible of the least impression from cold or malarious influences, with a strong tendency to congestion in all the abdominal organs.

When the atmosphere is saturated with moisture, there can be no cooling relief to the body by evaporation. The air, according to Professor Smith, of Edinburgh, expanding with the heat, while the lungs remain of the same capacity, they must take in a smaller quantity by *weight*, though the same by *measure*, of oxygen, the supporter of life. This, he adds, is one of the reasons of the lassitude felt in warm climates: "but if, in addition to the air being rarefied, it be also still further distended by the vapour of water being mixed with it, it is evident that a certain number of cubic inches by measure, or lungsful, will contain a less weight of oxygen than ever ; so little, indeed, that life can hardly be supported, and we need not wonder at persons lying down almost powerless in the hot and damp atmosphere, and gasping for breath." It has been supposed by some observers, indeed, that in hot climates both the volume and the weight of the lungs are diminished as compared to those properties in Europe.

The natives of India, of the higher classes, avoid all exertion during the rainy season ; while the working classes, at all seasons, are sparing of extra labour, and when compatible with the work in hand, sitting is ever the posture of the artisan in the East.

The excessive watery discharge from the skin during the rainy season must of necessity have the effect of rendering the venous blood unnaturally dense, and of thus causing the European to be more liable to congestive forms of disease. Dr. C. Williams refers the disposition to liver complaints, dysentery, and cholera, to the stimulating properties of the blood, deprived, as we have seen, of more than its usual amount of water, and of less of its hydrocarbon.

Such, briefly, are the hot and rainy seasons of tropical climates, and such are some of the reasons for their proverbial unhealthiness. The mind even seems to partake in the general relaxation and lassitude, being unfitted for vigorous or sustained efforts of any kind. During the eight months here under consideration, the sleep is seriously disturbed—a circumstance in itself sufficient to account for many of the attendant evils.

The "cutaneo-hepatic sympathy" of Dr. James Johnson is well known, and so is the theory which considers that, while respiration is less perfectly carried on, owing to the rarefaction of the air, a vicarious decarbonization of the blood is established by a great · increase of the biliary secretion. If, as supposed by Liebig, the function of the bile is " to support respiration and produce animal heat, by presenting carbon and hydrogen in a very subtile form to the oxygen of arterial blood," how greatly must the condition of the vital functions—respiration, the generation of heat, circulation, and secretion—be influenced by the palpably increased secretion of bile in tropical climates, followed as that excited action of the hot and rainy season is by a proportionately diminished action and consequent tendency to congestive disease in the cold season? Indeed, we are everywhere, in hot climates, thrown back on the observation of that acute and accurate pathological observer, Dr. John Clark, that of all the viscera in the human body the liver is the most subject to disease.

The condition of the atmosphere during the hot and rainy season produces in reality many of the results of an insufficient supply of air, or of air despoiled of a portion of its oxygen. The heated and rarefied states of the air produce a double result; for the introduction into the blood through respiration of a limited supply of vivifying property, impedes and retards the disengagement of putrescent effluvia from the lungs and skin; and thus the imperfect oxidation of the blood causes not only a correspondingly imperfect elimination of effete matters from the circulating fluids, but also the return of poisonous matters into the blood—all which circumstances predispose the system to the reception of malarious and epidemic poisons, and to their consequences. All these circumstances, however difficult of proof, are of vast importance to be well considered; and there seems at length some reason to hope that the vicarious nature of the relations existing between the depurative functions of the liver, kidneys, mucous surfaces, skin, and lungs, may receive demonstration from chemistry.

The blood being less arterialized in proportion to the elevation of temperature, it is evident that in tropical climates, according to Dr. Reid, the systemic circulation becomes decidedly venous and consequently unfit for carrying on the process of nutrition, and that it passes less freely through the capillaries into the veins. The lungs, too, are, in hot climates, relieved from some of the labour performed by them in temperate or cold regions; and thus it happens that many persons enjoy good health in hot climates, who, from tendency to pectoral disease, could not have lived in Europe; indeed, many persons in the curable stage of consumption—that is, labouring under the preceding stage, or that of "tuberculous cachexia," regain their health and survive their relatives at home. Those, on the other hand, who go to India with softened tubercles, or even in the stage approaching it, are only hurried into their graves.

Mr. Curtis states that in his time, 1782-83, "diseases of the thoracic viscera were exceedingly rare, or rather never appeared at all in India, under an idiopathic form. Pulmonary consumption was wholly unknown." The correctness of these observations is confirmed by modern statistics.

In the instance of Europeans desiring to proceed to India, or in those of officers wishing to return to their duties there, I always rest the question of their fitness to encounter the climate on the existence or otherwise of organic disease in any of the three cavities. Where, on careful examination, none such is discoverable, I determine at once that such person may proceed to a tropical climate with an average probability of enjoying health. When any considerable degree of functional disturbance is apparent, within the cerebral or abdominal cavities especially, I call for delay, and await its removal. As a general rule also, no one, whether ill or well, should be sent to a hot climate who bears the heats of European countries badly.

On the other hand, where there exists a hereditary or other disposition to morbid affections of the chest, I recommend such persons to proceed to India, as offering the best prospect of escape from a condition of disease which, in England, terminates too frequently in hopeless pulmonary consumption. Such, in a few words, are the principles on which I have been in the habit of resting this important question.

During the hot and rainy seasons here referred to, the function of the kidneys is always diminished, while at the same time the urine is surcharged with saline and other impregnations.

Unnatural and over-excited in all his functions as the European subject has hitherto been viewed, we soon find him, under the influence of the cold seasons, affected in a manner completely the reverse. The blood, owing to the larger proportion of oxygen used in respiration, now becomes more arterialized, while its consistence is rendered more viscid. In the cold season, a larger quantity of oxygen is consumed in maintaining the temperature of the body. The now altered balance of the circulation and nervous function; the entire drying-up of the surface, and the corresponding congestion of all the viscera; the consequent diminution of the biliary, and the enormous increase of the renal secretions; the oppressed state of the cerebral, thoracic, and abdominal functions, leading to the most formidable and complicated diseases, and to the suppression of chronic eruptions in a previous state of development; all these circumstances render the cold season of Bengal the reverse of healthy, except to those of sound constitution, or the newly-arrived European, or such as have not suffered from the previous unhealthy seasons.

The fevers of this season, unlike those of the hot weather and rains, approach gradually, insidiously, but not less dangerously, than those more ardent and concentrated types of fever last named. It will be seen that congestion has repeatedly been mentioned as participating in the most dangerous of our diseases. That climate has a principal share in producing this unfavourable state there can be no doubt; but admitting this, we must consider also that the absence of all exhilarating exercises of mind and body, with their animating, varied, and healthful influences, on all the functions, predisposes much, when aided by a too full and stimulating diet, to this end; unhappily, too, the European resident in tropical climates has no sufficient remedy against the evils of this double inaction, except moderation in diet, which many will not adopt; for during the hot and rainy seasons, the amount of exercise necessary to health in temperate regions would here be impossible, and would be hurtful even if possible. Those who would preserve their health, therefore, must be temperate—use such bodily exercise as each season admits of, and relieve their minds from the monotony of routine official duty by the inexhaustible resources of European literature, science, and elegant accomplishments. It is only thus that health, happiness, and reputation can be insured under the accumulated disadvantages of our position in India, where too commonly the whole time is given up to business.

I shall now enumerate the diseases peculiar to each season, pre-mising that it is to a long continuance of exposure to the various causes stated, more than to their intensity, that we must refer the greater portion of the injurious influences of tropical climate on European constitutions.

It has been seen that in hot climates the lungs are relieved of a portion of carbonic acid through the increased activity of the cutaneous exhalations, while the kidneys and mucous surfaces are similarly relieved of uric acid, urea, salts, and water. This state of activity, which holds during eight months of every year, will ex-plain how it is that in such climates diseases of the air-passages, lungs, and kidneys are of but rare occurrence, while, on returning to Europe, dangerous diseases of these organs are liable to occur.

In many persons, on their return home, the disturbed balance of function between the skin and kidneys gives much trouble, and requires an attentive medical care; for owing to the more or less partial arrest of the cuticular discharge, during the English winter and spring seasons especially, the urea and other salts, carried off in part through the skin in India, can only pass off through the kidneys in our native climate. The processes of accommodation and adjustment, under the cold of Europe, are of much difficulty to some constitutions, requiring alterative and sudorific medica-ments, aperients, warm baths, and warm clothing for their even-tual accomplishment.

Fever is by far the most common result of the high temperature of our hot season in the East, complicated with disturbance of the nervous centres and occasional determination to the liver. This fever is generally of the continued, occasionally of the remittent form, and of an ardent character. It demands experience and care in the treatment. Cholera is most prevalent and fatal in the hot months of April, May, and June.

In the succeeding rainy months, fever assumes a remittent cha-racter, with diminished vital action generally, and a dangerous abdominal congestion. In place of the burning dry skin and racking headache of the fever of the hot season, we have here a moist, cool surface, indicating a want of action in the sudatory vessels, an oppressed pulse, and a tendency to the most formidable collapse. As the season advances, dysenteries as well as fevers become more frequent, severe, and complicated, the former impli-cating the whole of the abdominal organs.

The diseases peculiar to the cold season are, congestive fever, of the continued form; intermittents, with the sequelæ of tumid or indurated spleen or liver; insidious, subacute, hepatic inflamma-tion, terminating rapidly in abscess; dysenteries, frequently com-plicated with hepatic disease,—all more or less acute, according to individual habit or length of service in India. Apoplexies of the most fatal form known in India occur at this season, as do the paralytic affections so commonly associated with them. Chronic eruptions, in active development during the two previous seasons, are now suddenly repelled, and are followed by congestion of some of the viscera.

Having exhibited in the rapid manner here sketched, the diseases to which the European stranger is liable in the East, and the powerfully deteriorating influences to which he is exposed during each year of residence, we shall now suppose him, after a sojourn of from twenty-five to forty years, returned to his native country. Here he enters at once, and without preparation, on a season of eight months' cold and moisture, in exchange for the same period of excessive tropical heat, and excessive moisture conjoined. I am here speaking of the English season from the beginning of October to the end of May. This is a great revolution in climate, and it at once induces a corresponding physiological change in the system, stamping the individual with a peculiar physical character. The exhalent organs of the skin, which for so long a succession of years had been called into the most violent action, now become sealed, as if with a coating of varnish; from the extreme of transudation he comes at once, under the rigour and vicissitude of an English winter, to constriction and dryness of the entire surface of the body. The result of such changes it is easy to perceive.

From the previous extensive, equable, and sometimes violent determination to the surface of the body, he is suddenly subjected to an opposite action—an extreme dryness of the surface, amounting, occasionally, to a furfuraceous desquamation of the cuticle, and at other times to a miliary eruption, accompanied by determination of the entire mass of the blood inwards; a loaded condition of the great venous trunks of the abdominal, thoracic, and cerebral cavities, with diminished power in the heart and arteries.

This is by far the most common result of exposure to the cold of an European winter and spring; but we occasionally find its opposite—a relaxation of the surface, inducing a copious and clammy sweat on the least exertion, accompanied by extreme languor of the circulation, with cold, damp extremities. This state, which is generally confined to persons of leucophlegmatic habit, is only to be removed by a complete restoration to health.

The nervous function, highly exalted during the earlier period of residence in the East, becomes now proportionately obtunded, depressed, and, in extreme cases, exhausted. These are great changes, and it is next to impossible that any man shall go through them with impunity; indeed, the first inspection of the Indian on his return home proves that he has been subjected to changes foreign to his original nature. He has now to undergo others which, through long acquired habit, have become almost equally foreign to him.

The effects of a long-continued application of heat, by promoting both the undue extrication and expenditure of the nervous energies, as evinced in the primary increase and subsequent diminution of their actions, must eventually disturb and debilitate the functions of the cerebro-spinal and organic systems, so as, sooner or later, to affect the integrity of every function of the body.

The children, again, of the upper classes of Europeans in India, and who remain there during the first five or six years of infancy only, exhibit a restlessness and mobility of the nervous system—a busy idleness—beyond their age, as compared to the habits of children of the same ages born and bred in England. This excited state of the nervous function is associated with a comparative incapacity for long-continued application to study, or for sustained effort of any kind; but this disadvantage, complained of to me by many schoolmasters in and around London, gradually yields to time and a temperate climate, until it finally disappears, between the ages of fourteen and eighteen. There is likewise a marked disposition to muscular relaxation, and to a loose relaxed state of the joints in such children, and to consequent lateral curvature of the spine, especially amongst girls; but I have seen several cases of the same nature even in boys. An acquaintance with these facts is of much importance, as bearing on the moral and intellectual training of such children.

Passive congestion is the condition most prevalent, under the circumstances of European cold; and no matter what his previous disease in India, the morbid condition now superadded proves a serious difficulty to the invalid. If the patient suffered from tropical dysentery, his distresses are greatly aggravated during the long English winter and spring. The sufferers from fever, hepatic or splenic disease, are similarly distressed by severe abdominal congestion; and if the tendency, through plethora or other cause, be towards the cerebral cavity, apoplexy is produced by exposure, or the absence of care, during the season of cold and damp in Europe. When the liver becomes the seat of congestion, this morbid condition may be confined to the venous trunks, or to the whole secreting parenchyma; or it may extend to both. In either case it is a serious state of disease.

I have seen many persons also, whose relatives at home were weak-chested and consumptive, become subject to severe chest diseases from the same cause. In short, if the sufferings were great under the long-continued exposure to the tropical heats, they are neither small nor unimportant under its opposite in Europe—especially under exposure to damp cold, which exercises a peculiarly baneful influence. My experience here in the last twenty years would lead me to conclude that, if there really be any such immunity from cold during the first year of residence in England as we hear spoken of so generally in India, it is enjoyed only by the healthy, the youthful, and the robust. Numberless examples have satisfied me as to the truth of this observation. A dry, or even frosty cold is well borne, comparatively, even by the enfeebled tropical invalid; but the *damp* cold produces sensations of inde-scribable distress and depression in persons possessed of consider-able powers of resistance. Many invalids, again, arriving in Eng-land in an enfeebled state, seek what they call "the bracing air" of Brighton and other such places during the winter and spring months, in forgetfulness, or in ignorance, that without a previous restoration to health, this said bracing is impossible of attainment. Many valuable lives are annually sacrificed in this vain endeavour. The truth is, that in general, the cold which a tropical invalid can bear without injury for a year or two after his return to Europe, is not of a low degree ; and in extreme cases of disease, the in-door temperature, carefully regulated during the winter and spring seasons, is that alone which is safe to him. He must now be treated with a climate very different from such as may in a year or two, and when health is restored, be suitable to him. Common sense points out that the delicate and the sick must be prepared for invigoration, and not forced into it. We cannot "comfort" such a person "with cold," as the Americans do their English customers with ice. In truth, the newly returned Indian invalid cannot bear exposure to cold, and he cannot bear exposure to heat. It depends, in fact, on the state of the health and constitution at the time whether cold is to prove salutary or injurious.

Certain moist winter and spring seasons are followed in tem-perate climates by increase of sickness and mortality in summer. "The proverb, 'a green yule makes a fat churchyard,'" says Dr. Farr, "probably expresses a scientific fact, notwithstanding the evident fatality of cold ; and we may hope that the population will escape some of the epidemics which germinate in mild winters, and burst out suddenly in summer." Referring, however, to the dangers arising from cold, the authority quoted adds, that "as age increases, the system rapidly loses the power of producing internal heat; and the resulting fatality by reduction of temperature is doubled every nine years after the age of twenty to forty."

In India all our numerous and excellent appliances are directed towards the counteracting of heat, while here, in England, they ought to be directed, especially in the case of the tropical invalid, so as to defy cold. The applications of the former to health and comfort are well known in the East; but amongst the returned Indians, the necessity for the last is not so generally nor so well understood.

More unfounded still is the prevalent notion amongst inexpe-rienced and thoughtless lay persons, that on returning to England from hot climates they are to take leave of all their ailments, at the same time that they need take no care whatever as to their habits. This is only another out of many examples of the facility with which the mass of men receive mere opinions as established facts. It is but the "It is true, they say it" of the Spaniards, and that is enough for the unreflecting many, who see only with their ears.

"A moderate acquaintance with mankind," says Dr. James Johnson, "is sufficient to stamp the truth of the remark, that experience seldom instructs the mass." This is quite as true as the observation of the older doctor of the same name, the moralist and lexicographer—viz., that there are some men who are incapable of acquiring experience. In nothing are both remarks so just as in all that popularly relates to health, whether private or public, personal or general.

A gentleman of the civil service came home after twenty years' residence in India, on private leave, not being considered sick. He arrived in October, and early in the following month he made a journey of four hours on a railway, with the window open. The lung next the window became that night completely engorged; and owing to the impoverished condition of the blood, and to the deficient powers of the system, the substance of the lung rapidly filled with serum. He died in a few days.

Engorgement of the lungs of a fatal character is no infrequent result of exposure to cold, in feeble and anæmic persons, on their arrival from hot climates, during the English winter especially, and three such instances have lately come under my observation—all modes of treatment proving vain. "It is really lamentable," says James Johnson, "to see men returned from a tropical climate, walking about the streets of London, or going to places of amusement, in the cold raw evenings of winter, while the hacking cough, emaciated figure, and variegated countenance, proclaim a condition of the lungs which ill comports with this exposure to the vicissitudes of a northern climate." Sir James Clark justly observes of the natives of tropical climates, and of children in this country, that owing to their habit of body being disposed to tuberculous affections—the most nearly allied to tuberculous cachexy—pulmonary diseases are prevalent and rapid with them in our "cold and humid atmosphere." The same may be said with truth of the tropical invalid in general, but of the anæmic class more especially. Catarrhal affections, more or less severe, are almost universal with tropical invalids on first coming to England; and many become thus affected on their passage through Egypt and the Mediterranean, weeks before their arrival at home.

A captain of cavalry, while in India, had discharged a large hepatic abscess through the bowels. He consulted me on account of aphthous diarrhœa, from which after a few weeks he seemed to recover rapidly. A drive through the streets of London on a cold, foggy November afternoon, in an open carriage, brought back the diarrhœa with great violence, and he died at Guernsey in a month. Major —— arrived in England in October, worn to the bones by diarrhœa of ten months' duration. By the end of November his health had greatly improved; but on the 27th of that month he went out in a hard frost. The result was remarkable. He passed some hours of the night deprived of the powers of speech and of

swallowing; and though the surface of the body and the extremities were warm, he felt all night " as if his inside had been filled
with ice." A dangerous recurrence of diarrhœa was the result. It
is needless to multiply instances.

If the temperature of the cold season of Bengal be such as to
prove unfavourable to the European invalid and to the old Indian
—to all, indeed, excepting the newly-arrived and the robust of
constitution—how careful ought all who have resided long in
warm latitudes to be on coming at once from a climate in which
they are annually exposed to eight months of great heat, to another where they are subjected to eight months of comparatively
great cold, in which the conjoined humidity is most injurious by
its more rapid abstraction of animal heat. Such persons should
recollect that, though the compensating powers of nature are great,
they have their limits. Referring to the unpleasant impression
produced by the cold season of Bengal on the skin of the older
residents, I would here mention that a dislike or horror of this
season I invariably observed to form the first indication that the
individual was " climate-struck ;" in other words, that the general
powers had become enfeebled, while the nervous and vascular
systems had become morbidly sensitive to all the changes of season,
but most so to the damp cold of the night. Truly has it been
observed that cold and damp together are noxiously sedative.
Cold indeed, as a chill, or night exposure after the day's heat, or
after fatigue, constitutes the most frequent cause of some of the
most formidable of our acute diseases within the tropics.

The medium temperature of the English summer and autumn is
favourable to the health of the general population, and it is especially so to that of persons arriving from tropical climates ; for,
even amongst resident Englishmen, the winter and spring seasons
cause a rapid increase of sickness and mortality from those diseases
which contribute most to the ordinary annual mortality of the
climate—congestive and inflammatory diseases being most prevalent also in the seasons last mentioned. These are obvious circumstances, but I see them continually disregarded by invalids from
India.

A gentleman in the second year of his residence in Calcutta
suffered from acute inflammation of the liver, but came home soon
afterwards in what he deemed perfect health. On getting into the
English Channel he was exposed to a cold easterly wind, which
caused violent congestion of the liver and right lung, from which
he nearly lost his life.

A friend of mine who had resided twenty-six years in India, on
being asked how he got through the winter and spring seasons at
home, replied :—" A tight band drawn round the head, and another
round the belly, with indescribable sensations in the skin of the
whole body, represent my feelings during the cold weather."

There is another influence, though seldom of a serious nature, which often proves injurious to the returned Indian; I mean over-exertion of the muscular powers. Men who for years used no other exercise in India than an evening and morning ride of a few miles, at a gentle pace, will, under the counter-influence of cold, make great and prolonged exertions at home in riding and walking. The exhaustion of the nervous and muscular energies, resulting from such imprudence, is very injurious, and weakly persons do not recover from it for months subsequently. I have seen permanent disturbance of the heart's action follow upon such over-exertion.

An Indian officer of a stout habit, but of previously good health, ran, he said, for a quarter of a mile only, to overtake a railway train. From the time of making this exertion he never enjoyed an hour's comfort, both the circulation and respiration being now permanently disturbed. His death, which took place two years afterwards, was one of unusual suffering.

We have seen that in hot climates the lungs are relieved of a portion of carbonic acid through the increased activity of the cutaneous exhalations, while the kidneys and mucous surfaces are in like manner relieved of uric acid, urea, salts, and water. These conditions, which hold during eight months, or more, of every year in Bengal, will explain how it is that, in such climates, diseases of the lungs, air-passages, and kidneys are of but rare occurrence; and how, on returning to Europe when the complete converse of all the above-named physiological actions is taking place, or has been established, dangerous diseases of the lungs, bronchi, liver, kidneys, and mucous surfaces generally, are so liable to occur.

It is but natural to conclude, also, that both in India and in Europe material and opposite changes take place in the chemical constituents of the blood, as well as in those of all the excreted fluids. I entertain no doubt on this head, but we must look to animal chemistry for the demonstration of the facts.

If in hot climates the animal heat rises from $2°·7$ to $3°·6$ above that of temperate climates: if for years the functions of the system are adapted to this increased temperature, what disorder must be produced when circumstances render the stimulus of this temperature impossible—when the tropical invalid, or the old Indian, returns to his native climate?

The process of respiration under the tropical rarefaction of the air, and under the condensing cold of an English winter and spring, must also be materially affected, so as to cause corresponding changes in the amount of oxygen absorbed, and in that of carbonic acid expired. The increase of the animal temperature in hot climates is dependent, to a certain extent, on the more rapid circulation and metamorphosis of the blood, for less oxygen is inspired in hot than in temperate regions, owing to the rarefied state of the air in the former.

The relation between the functions of the lungs and liver, unnaturally disturbed in hot climates, becomes again on a sudden disturbed in a direction towards the restoration of the balance of health, on our return to temperate climates. This is a difficult process to the tropical invalid, and one that is attended with risk to both health and life. In addition to these hazardous circumstances, the dangers from excesses in diet, from close and overheated rooms, and from subsequent exposure to night-cold, are not to be overlooked.

Anæmia is common to a very large proportion of tropical invalids on their return to Europe. In this morbid state, the paucity of blood corpuscles causes a diminished absorption of oxygen, a quicker circulation, and consequently a diminished animal heat. I have no doubt, that by long-continued exposure to tropical heats and to malaria, the nervous and muscular systems of the heart and uterus are relaxed and weakened, becoming thus irritable, and defective in contractile power. I believe that to these circumstances we must, in a great measure, refer the diminished power of the forces that circulate the blood, and the intermitting character of the pulse so common to old Indians; also the frequency of uterine hæmorrhage in females who have been long in India.

We have now viewed the European from his arrival in India, during his career of active service in the tropics, to the termination of his public life and his return home. How vast the range of the physical and moral influences to which he has been exposed, and how changed does he find himself on his return, which is, in fact, his first settlement in life; how altered are those of his nearest relatives who remain to greet him, and how many more of them have been gathered to their fathers!

The depressing influence of the great and long-continued flux and reflux of the functions—of all the causes, in short, just enumerated—will go far to account for the hypochondriasis and other disorders, not to speak of the graver ills to which our countrymen are prone on their return to Europe. If the returned Indian be the father of a family, he has seen his children removed from the care of a mother and his own control, at the tender age of five years or earlier, their education, moral and intellectual, being consigned to relatives in England, perhaps to utter strangers; and thus we occasionally find that the children of the absent grow up without that deep instinct of filial reverence, those family affections, and that self-respect, which are so necessary to preserve youth in the trying passages and ordeals of life. He has again seen these children return to India, the land of their birth, at the age of eighteen, knowing their parents only by name, their natural affections being fixed on those at home who had the care of them, the domestic ties having been broken in infancy, never to be repaired. Truly has the Hindu poet said, "There is no remedy for a soul wounded by the sharp sword of separation." The sons have been rendered strangers in the house of their father, the daughters have never known the care of a mother ; and it may so happen, that before either has been allowed time to cultivate the acquaintance even of their children, they are again doomed to separate, the father being driven home to repair the shattered constitution, while the sons and married daughters remain in India. No wonder that, under such unnatural circumstances, the home of his youth should be to him cheerless.

It has been seen that all the conditions of life, in the instance of the European resident in tropical climates, tend to ultimate depression of the constitutional powers, whether we regard the influences of an unnatural climate, aggravated by an unsuitable regimen, or the moral circumstances. In warm regions, moreover, there is a precoce development and maturation of the European constitution, while, unhappily, the tendency to decay is, in proportion, unnaturally and prematurely accelerated.

Curtis says that " persons returning from either India often bring home with them a constitution wasted and debilitated by the diseases of those climates, from which they recover with difficulty, or not at all :"—in other words, those Europeans who have been injured in constitution by heat and malaria are, for a longer or shorter time, rendered incapable of resisting the rigour of an English winter and spring ; and the disabilities are greatly increased when visceral disease is superadded. In truth, the great majority of those who come home from India on account of ill health adopt a course of conduct directly at variance with justice to themselves. They " trust to climate," as they call it, without adapting their habits to the altered circumstances of their healths and constitutions; and after passing some twelve or eighteen months in doing nothing, or very little, towards the restoration of health, they apply to a physician for relief, only when within four or six months of the expiration of their leave, when they are expected to be on the way to the East. What ought to be done in all cases is—to proceed to the removal of organic disease, or to the restoration of disordered function, immediately on arrival from India—so that the remaining, latter, time may be advantageously made use of, to mature and confirm the health in the pure atmosphere of the country, under proper regulation as to diet and exercise. It is not enough to cure the disease—a margin being in every case necessary to the assuring of health.

Let it not be supposed that I here present an exaggerated view of those disorders and diseases, or of the social and moral disadvantages to which an European is subject, during a residence, more or less protracted, in a tropical climate ; nor yet of such as may visit him at home. I do not relate a mere description ; for I have personally, largely, and repeatedly shared in the sufferings I detail—both in India and in this country. Mine is not a picture drawn from the imagination.

It must be recollected that I am not speaking of the healthy old

T T

Indian—a select life in any country—nor of the youthful and
healthy officer on furlough; for to both the cold of an English
winter may prove tonic and agreeable. Such men may control,
through their superior power of resistance and of accommodation,
the influences of one law of nature by the operations of another.
These observations refer to such only as have suffered from protracted residence in hot countries, and to those who have laboured
under the diseases incident thereto. And here I must bear testimony to the manly fortitude and cheerful resignation of the Indian
officer under suffering. We find in him no peevish, fretful, or
presumptuous intolerance of sickness. He does not expect an
instant cure of all his diseases : and failing of this, he does not
flee in ignorant fancy to the empiric. He has generally seen and
suffered so much as to render him considerate at once of what is
rightly due to himself and to others. He is therefore, and under
all circumstances, an object of interest to his physician and
surgeon. The highest surgical authority in this country has often
spoken to me emphatically on this remarkable characteristic of the
Indian officer, and on this account, as well as on that of the great
intelligence of the Indian officers generally, he designated them a
" PECULIAR CLASS." The Highland chief who said—" Doctor, I
want to be cured immediately"—gave expression to a natural
feeling; but thus speedily to realize the expectations, in the sequelæ
to tropical diseases, is rarely indeed practicable.

I know not a better test of good sense, or of a well-regulated
mind, than that furnished by our conduct in sickness. Under suffering are exhibited in the most marked manner the results of a
sound education, religious, moral, and intellectual. The practised
physician detects at once the sensible, firm, and well-trained mind;
and with the same speed he discovers the senseless, frivolous, and
ill-regulated tendencies of his patient's disposition. I have everywhere observed that the same absence of principle which leads
weak minds into extravagances in religion, renders the same
persons also prone to follow quackeries of every other kind, moral
and medical, as well as religious.

We come now, in conclusion, to the practical issue as to the
medical treatment of the European in the Eastern and Western
hemispheres. In the first, we have had to overcome, by the most
powerful remedial means known in medicine, the most acute and
dangerous forms of disease, and that under the continuous disadvantages of a high range of temperature, and other injurious influences; while in the latter instance, we have to deal with the
sequelæ of these formidable diseases, in a temperate climate, and
under the sedative influence of cold.

It is obvious that under these opposite circumstances of climate
and of disease, our means of cure must have corresponding differences. Inasmuch, however, as the injurious influences of tropical climates, in the great majority of instances, have an exact

relation to their duration, so also do those favourable operations of temperate climates require time for the demonstration of their results. The sick furlough, which allows of but two years' actual residence in Europe, is not sufficient to numbers of those who seek relief from it; and I have strong reason for concluding that the remarkable proportion of casualties amongst officers on their return to the East and West Indies, is not referable so much to their second process of acclimation, as to the circumstance that many are forced to return too soon, and before their diseases have been effectually removed. If we could be furnished with the statistical results of lengthened residences in the West Indies, under the old rules, and with the then difficulties of obtaining leave of absence, as compared to the now existing short residence, with facilities for procuring leave, we should have, I am sure, a demonstration of the justice of the observation here offered.

It must be obvious, that with a large proportion of invalids from the East Indies, nothing but care in diet, clothing, and in all the habits of life, along with a judicious use of medicines calculated to restore the healthy balance of function, and thus to assist the influence of their native climate, can avail to their recovery.

With all these aids, too, the object in view must be a work of time. I seldom see those who have suffered much restored to health under the two years of furlough; and I have in many instances been constrained to postpone the return to India to the utmost limit; but such cases have been examples of extraordinary suffering and danger. It is an old observation in the British Army that the "East Indies takes more out of a man than the West;" but the observation is true only because of the long residence of the European in the former countries. In the olden times even, European regiments were seldom kept in the West Indian Islands above half the time they served on the Indian continent: and of late the time of service in the former countries has been further shortened; hence the real cause of the difference in the comparative injury to constitution in the two hemispheres.

When British regiments are ordered home from the East Indies, those soldiers who have served above seven or eight years, generally volunteer to other corps serving in India, in the hope of completing their time there. They have become domesticated in the East, and prefer the ease and comfort of their position in that country, and the luxury of having native servants, to the rough chances of service in Europe, or in our other colonies.

Comparatively few return with regiments except those who have only been exposed for a short period to the climate, or men who are what is termed, in military language, "worn out," having completed the usual period of service exacted from soldiers. Yet even amongst the youngest of these subjects, there is an excess of mortality over that of soldiers serving in the United Kingdom, of three per thousand annually during the first three years after their return from India! If this be so with the youthful and comparatively healthy soldier, what must be the influence of the variable climate of England on the exhausted and more aged invalid during what may be termed his probationary residence in it, and how insufficient must be the ordinary sick furlough of two years for the restoration of health in all cases of tropical diseases, and how dangerous must be the cold of our winter and spring to the broken-down tropical invalid?

British soldiers who have served in India entertain an extreme aversion to home service, especially during the winter and spring seasons; and pensioners who have served in hot climates volunteer cheerfully to settle in the Australian possessions. The very deprivation of the accustomed sensations derivable from heat, will account for many of the discomforts and personal sufferings complained of by every healthy European during their probationary acclimation on return to their native climate; but the Indian invalid finds in the homeward voyage round the Cape of Good Hope, and nowhere else, that equable temperature, to quote the words of Lord Halifax, between "the climate in which men are roasted and the climate in which they are frozen," which is alike agreeable and necessary to him.

Among the older soldiers who return home, the excess of mortality beyond that of the same class in the United Kingdom of the same age, does not much exceed three or four per thousand annually, notwithstanding their longer service in the East; but they are the survivors of hundreds who have sunk under the same course of service, and must obviously have possessed uncommon vigour of constitution originally, to have stood the trial of tropical service for the greater part of twenty-one years.

Referring finally to the influence of protracted residence in tropical climates, it has always been remarked in the East Indies that Europeans are frequently carried off in what is there termed —"the one year more"—the last year of residence; after the stamina has begun to give way, and, too often, after the ties which bound them to home are broken. It is a peculiarly melancholy event; for the deceased has all but completed his term of years, and all but accomplished the object of his hopes and of his long-cherished ambition. With a view to insure comfort at home, he remains a year or two longer in India; and with the goal in sight, he is cut off, and all his fond anticipations end but in death. All statistical evidence goes to prove the increase both of sickness and mortality in relation to length of residence; yet with these proofs before them, we see in India that every season brings with it instances of Europeans, broken down by long residence, and who fall victims to the unnatural struggle against the fatal "one year more."

The Dutch, who are not given to jesting, appear, nevertheless, to have been aware of the uncertainties and dangers of deferring the departure from the East till "next year;" for in one of their older settlements there was found an inscription over the grave of a Dutchman to the following effect :—

> " Here lies ————— Minheer,
> Who was to have gone home next year."

In Mr. Neison's Report on the Bengal Military Fund, and referring to the mortality of retired officers of the Indian army, as given by Mr. Christie, it appears, that as compared to the mortality of England, that of retired officers is uniformly in excess, age for age, being for the ages of forty-eight and under sixty about one-third more. After the age of sixty, the mortality of both retired officers and soldiers but little exceeds that which prevails even in civil life amongst persons of the same age, who have never left this country. But while the mortality amongst retired officers is proved to be as stated, that of the widows of deceased officers, on their return to Europe, is found to differ so little from the mortality of females of like ages in England and Wales as to be hardly appreciable. This fact can, as I conceive, only be attributed to the circumstances, that—firstly, the European female is not subjected to the hardships and direct solar and other exposures to which military officers are liable; and secondly, to the perfectly temperate habits of ladies in India, which save them from many of those formidable diseases which there deteriorate the health and destroy the lives of their husbands. Thus the widows of our officers come to England in the enjoyment of health, and they live as well and as long as those who have never been absent from their native country.*

I would urge, in conclusion, one other important consideration, which should be held in recollection, before entering on the medical treatment of the retired Indian—viz., that though not old in years, or, least of all, in mental character or habit, he has become prematurely aged in his physical constitution. The general principles of medical management must therefore be carefully modified and specially adapted to this condition of the system.

Under no circumstances of disease can such a man be treated with the vigour that may be safe, or even proper, in persons of the same age, but who have passed their lives in England. Indeed, no contrasts can be greater than such as are exhibited in the moral and physical constitution of the European newly arrived within the tropics, and in the same person on his return to his native climate after an absence of thirty years.

In the first case we have a youth, buoyant with health and

* For these interesting and important statistical facts in corroboration of my views, I am indebted to Major-General Sir A. Tulloch and Mr. Neison. They were obtained long after this article was written.

animal spirits, with all his functions exalted through the stimulus of heat, and with the mind eager for employment and for distinction; while in the last we perceive but too often premature age, with obtunded sensibilities and depressed functions, coupled with profound mental depression, amounting in some cases to the most severe form of hypochondriasis—all resulting from the opposite states of the nervous, vascular, hepatic, and other excretory functions, brought about at first by an unnaturally high and continned range of temperature, and now by the sudden application and sedative influence of cold.

It is true that the Indian, coming home at the middle or more advanced stage of life, approaches the land of his fathers with hopes and expectations quite as exalted, though by no means possessing the same glow of enthusiasm and buoyancy, as when a mere youth he quitted the paternal roof—

> "And from the dregs of life hopes to receive
> What the first sprightly running could not give."

Lord Clive, though but forty-two years of age on his final retirement from India, writes to his friends whom he left in the East :— " I have suffered so much ever since my arrival in England, that I have not been able to interfere so much with public affairs as I could wish. Parliamentary concerns have embroiled me more than is good for my health, and I really begin to grow tired of them." He then exhorts his friends to be satisfied with a moderate competency, and return to England while they have youth to enjoy it, rather than by staying longer lose that youth, and sacrifice that constitution which no riches can possibly compensate for. Clive's disease is spoken of by his biographer, Sir John Malcolm, as " a severe bilious complaint, attended with spasms from gall-stones, loss of appetite, and indigestion; a continuation or consequence of that derangement of the liver from which he has already suffered so much in Bengal." This great commander, in a letter to his friend George Granville, describes his personal sufferings as " very distressing to the mind and to the body ;" and on hearing of Granville's death, he expresses " his indifference, not only to the world's politics, but to the world in general."

To give a more concentrated view of the physical circumstances above related, it may be said, that in hot climates, the air being expanded, less oxygen is taken in at each inspiration. The necessity for hydrocarbonaceous food is therefore lessened. Less of the " elements of respiration" ought to be taken in the food than would be taken in colder climates. In consequence of the external increase of temperature, less internal heat is required.

Exercise increases the heat of the body by increasing the rate of circulation and respiration. In a very hot climate, all increase of heat is undesirable. Moreover, the excessive heat renders muscular action impossible, because the circulation is chiefly directed (in consequence of the activity of the skin) to the surface, in order that fluid may be furnished for evaporation, to keep down the heat of the body, and to prevent the parching of the surface which must otherwise ensue.

In consequence of the lessened muscular action, less of the albuminous constituents of the food are required to supply the waste of the muscles. Hence, in hot climates, less of both kinds of food should be taken, and Nature points this out in the absence of appetite; to force an appetite, stimulants are taken, and then the system is loaded with nourishment. The excessive perspiration requires an excess of liquids; but instead of water alone, sugar and spirit, the elements of respiration, are taken with the water, in the form of beer, and the spirit, by its stimulating properties, is doubly injurious.

The excessive flow of blood to the surface—the consequence of the high temperature—no doubt prevents, for a time, the evils resulting from an excess of the two kinds of food. The chemical changes and evaporation going on in the skin draw the circulation to the surface of the body, just as the flame of the lamp draws the oil up the wick. Whilst the high temperature lasts, this increased action of a flow to the surface is kept up. It is probable that the action of the heart is thereby made feeble by the excessive suction of the skin, as we see it frequently is, temporarily, by the perspiration bath. As soon as the temperature falls the blood ceases to flow in excess through the skin. According to the degree of cold, it is almost driven from the surface. It accumulates within, and congestions and inflammations are produced. Free action on the inner or outer surface of the body for a time relieves the congestions and enables the circulation to proceed.

After such alternations for years, the resident in the hot climate returns to a far colder home. There no heat leads the blood to the surface; it accumulates in the vessels and capillaries of the internal viscera. The outward appearance is that of anæmia, whilst in reality an internal plethora frequently exists.

The more frequent and severe the temporary congestions of the viscera have been whilst in the hot climate, the more permanent does the internal congestion become when the surface is constantly exposed to cold. Though the face and extremities may look void of blood, the capillaries of the liver and spleen will often be full, and the engorgement of the venous trunks, which was the effect of previous congestion for years, becomes permanent when the coldness of the atmosphere leaves the blood to be circulated by the enfeebled heart alone.

If the nervous influence be the power which regulates the contraction and relaxation of the capillaries, how much must this important part of the circulation be affected—first, by the long-continued heat of the tropics—and secondly, by the cold and damp of the climate of Europe, so as, under both agencies, to disturb alternately, and conversely, this great function?

Tropical heat has had the effect of exalting for a time, and then diminishing the nervous energy, and thus of eventually relaxing and diminishing the circulating power of the capillaries; while cold, on coming to England, will have the contrary effect of con-stringing the capillaries, and thus of determining the great mass of the circulating fluid upon the internal organs :—such power, acting on the enfeebled European on his return from tropical climates, must prove of extremely injurious effects.

Dr. Billing concludes his admirable " Principles of Medicine " by stating that they " have been deduced from physiology ; and for the explanation of the pathological phenomena he has referred to the action of the capillaries and nerves—nerves and capillaries together, not artificially separated, but as they exist in nature— ramifying and supporting each other throughout; for by their combined action upon the blood sent to them by the heart, they produce the phenomena of health—in their deranged actions they originate disease."

Dr. James Johnson justly observes, that " The powers of the constitution, however plastic, cannot immediately accommodate themselves to great and sudden changes of climate, even when the translation is from a bad to a good one ; and the tropical invalid requires full as much caution and prudence in approaching the shores of England, as he did in landing at the former period on the banks of the Ganges." Speaking of the beneficial influences of the voyage home round the Cape of Good Hope, the same autho-rity states, that " When the European has become much debili-tated by liver affection, dysentery, or fever, and its consequences, the main hope of recovery rests on change of climate, and, under such circumstances, the sea-voyage often effects a cure. Indeed, the instances are not few where more benefit is obtained by the voyage home than by the subsequent residence in England." But this voyage, with its uniformity and salubrity of the sea air, aided by the mental exhilaration of a *home anticipation*, producing as it often does, " surprising effects on the animal economy," is not now nearly so much resorted to as it ought to be.

The overland journey, as it is termed, subjects the invalid to numerous discomforts, both by sea and land—often to insufficient accommodation, always to a more or less hurried meal—to a, hurried and uncomfortable journey through Egypt ; and if, un-happily, he arrives in England in the winter or spring, he has to encounter their rigours within six weeks, with very imperfect, or with no preparation, instead of the four months' voyage round the Cape of Good Hope, with its rest, ease, and comforts, and with its unequalled climate.

The clothing with which invalids are supplied in India is altogether insufficient to protect them against the cold of an easterly wind in the English Channel; and hence the frequency of chest affections, diarrhœa, and abdominal congestions, even before they set foot on shore.

In a moral and physical point of view, and more through the agency of moral and physical influences of an extraneous character than through age, no two persons could present contrasts greater than may every day be recognised in the very individual under our consideration, as compared to the youth of five-and-twenty years back.

The average age at which the Indian, whether civil or military, retires, may be taken at fifty to fifty-five years. A certain proportion of those who thus return home are, to all public purposes, worn-out men; and but few of those even who are equal to the exertion make any effort to enter upon public duties in England— duties for which their official aptitude, their administrative experience, and their varied abilities so eminently qualify many of them. Of old men there are none in India—the members of the civil service averaging thirty-five years of residence, on the average, with fifty-five years of age—the general of forty years' service being but a year or two older.

I may here mention that, of all the mental occupations, the mathematical have proved, in my experience, the most injurious to the mental faculties; engineer officers, accountants, and persons devoted to statistical pursuits, having, in course of my observation and practice, broken up in mind to a most remarkable extent. Some have lived for years in a state of nervous distress and incapacity, while others have lingered in insensibility on the water-bed, the victims of overwrought nervous system, and eventual softening of the nervous masses.

Several causes present themselves as efficient to such morbid results, as the necessary intensity of the mental application in all matters of calculation, the severe sameness of the pursuit, the sedentary habit, and the absence of that salutary variation in mental labour and employment which seems as necessary to mental integrity as variety in diet to the bodily health. It has been nobly said by Cowper that—

" A want of occupation is not rest,
A mind quite vacant is a mind distressed."

I would now refer to a question of great importance, and one in which I have often had to interfere. Officers of all classes frequently leave India in such a state of ill-health and exhaustion as to feel hopeless of recovery within the time allowed by regulation for ordinary leave of absence. In this state of moral and physical depression, despairing of health, they often express their purpose to retire from public service and enter into private life. The advice I have almost invariably given in such cases has been to the following effect :—"You have at least two years' absolute leave, at the expiration of which come to me and I will then tell you what you had better do.   At present, borne down by mental and bodily suffering, you are altogether unequal to the determining of any important question in life ; and, for the rest, your case is not so hopeless as you suppose."   Often have I been warmly thanked in aftertimes for this counsel, and that not seldom before the expiration of the two years ; many declaring with much feeling that " I had saved them from ruin."

However desperate the case may appear, provided there is youth on the side of the patient, we ought not to despair—a circumstance which I would strenuously urge on the attention of all medical officers throughout India, as well as on that of the profession at home when dealing with this description of patients. Resignations, under the circumstances mentioned, ought seldom to obtain the sanction of the physician, whether civil or military.

The series of converse actions and reactions is thus far completed. We have seen that up to a certain stage, for a limited period, and under temperate habits, the functions of the body, as well as the mental energies of the stranger European, are exalted in the intertropical heats, to be again seriously depressed by disease, or by a protracted exposure to the same influences which at first proved stimulating. But on his return to his native climate all the functions, mental and corporeal, of the tropical invalid are about to be subjected to new trials—to depressing moral influences, and to the sedative influences of cold ; and this state of double depression continues to afflict him, until, through the restoration of health, this same cold shall become to him a powerful tonic, bracing the mind and the body—proving a source alike of vigour and of enjoyment.

Such, in brief, are the widely-extended successions of changes and of profound impressions of which but a sketch is here presented. That so happy a termination as health—that to accommodate the system to the last of its numerous changes—that to restore the long-lost balance of the functions—should, for its consummation, require time, much care and management, must be sufficiently evident.   In truth, a more important subject, whether regarded in a physiological, pathological, or therapeutic sense, can hardly engage the attention of the physician.

ANÆMIA.

OF all the conditions incident to tropical invalids, that morbid decrease of the blood which we term anæmia is the most general. It presents the sequel most common to fevers, whether remittent, intermittent, or continued; indeed, whatever may have been the nature of his previous acute disease—whether it was fever, dysentery, diarrhœa, hepatitis, or cholera—we are pretty sure to find, in the tropical invalid, that ill state of the general habit termed cachexia. All the diseases just mentioned tend, directly or indirectly, to spoil the blood.

Where organic lesions are present, as the results of previously acute disease, or of a long residence in hot climates, they will generally be found associated with an anæmic condition of the system, so as seriously to complicate the case, and add to the difficulties of treatment. These considerations have induced me to select ANÆMIA as the first subject for attention; for the cachectic state now referred to must be very generally kept in view in the treatment of the European invalid on his return from tropical climates. It has an important bearing on much that relates to the history, nature, and treatment of most of his disorders and diseases. The depraved state of the blood in diseases of the spleen has been noticed in the first part of this work, and there the subject has received a separate and special consideration.

. Anæmia is frequently produced by long residence in the malarions districts and stations of tropical climates, even in persons who have not been sufferers from other actual disease, acute or chronic, such as the fevers and fluxes of their more unhealthy localities. This is what may be termed the *cachexia loci*—etiolation; or more properly, paludal cachexia. It is, in truth, a chronic marsh poisoning in a large proportion of persons. European females of the better class, though far less subject to the more formidable of the tropical diseases than males, are yet, through long-continued disturbance of the nervous, vascular, and secreting functions, very liable to become anæmic. The excessive perspiration will of itself produce anæmia in weakly constitutions. The very treatment necessary to the cure of acute disease, especially blood-letting, mercury, and drastic purgatives, along with the most rigid abstinence, tends powerfully, even in young persons, to produce a deficiency of red particles; while the same course of treatment in persons of more advanced age, along with their more protracted exposure to malarious influences, are sure to diminish the old blood-globules, and to prevent the formation of new. The "debility" spoken of by all writers who have noticed the condition of tropical invalids, as one of their main characteristics, will be found, in the great majority of cases, to be none other than the debility of the cachectic habit—of anæmia, in fact.

Owing to this impoverished state of the circulating fluid, all the functions of the body are enfeebled, all the secretions defective, diluted, and depraved; the patient is wanting in the power to repair any serious injury. I often find severe and protracted anæmia to result from the unguarded application of leeches. Three hundred leeches, and in one instance five hundred, were mentioned to me as having been applied to the abdomen in remittent fevers, attended with gastric or hepatic complications, and in dysenteries.

Mr. E——, then a youth of sixteen, fell into the hold of a ship upon his loins. He writes:—" I was bled three times; hot fomentations were used for ten days, and I had seventeen dozen leeches on (204), and was bled once more."

Lieutenant S—— says:—" I had three different times sixty leeches applied, and I think twenty more afterwards, making in all two hundred in less than ten days." This officer was tall, slender, and of delicate frame, and only nineteen years of age. If, as generally believed, the Indian leech abstracts an ounce of blood—nay, if it be allowed to abstract but half the quantity, how large must be the aggregate amount of depletion in these cases?

Annesley ascertained that the Indian leech abstracts, on the average, one ounce and a quarter, " besides what flows from the bites." This simple fact should prove a warning not to apply leeches in the careless or indiscriminate manner witnessed by me in its results, a few more examples of which I will adduce.

Mr. ——, a mercantile gentleman from one of the Indian Presidencies, states, January 3rd, 1855, that after a fall from his horse he had twenty-two dozen of leeches applied at once, by order of Dr. ——, while Lieutenant —— states, that in the course of two months he had thirty-six dozen of leeches applied to the abdomen while suffering from fever.

Lieutenant —— was seized in August, 1849, with diarrhœa, followed by intermittent fever and enlargement of both liver and spleen. By order of his regimental surgeon " he was bled to twenty ounces, and about a hundred leeches were applied during the subsequent five days." This officer is described in the Medical Report of his surgeon as " of weak constitution." The patient went to another station, where another surgeon states that he subjected him to " depletion, keeping up a drain from the organ" (the liver), and occasionally a large number of leeches have been applied, as indicated by symptoms. Lieutenant —— concludes: —" I had altogether applied to my side, from December, 1849, to January, 1851, fully one thousand two hundred, at the very least."

But all wonders must cease regarding the leechings of lay persons, when we come to the following case of a medical officer:— " When I went to India, my constitution was excellent, and I was able to withstand any amount of fatigue; but within three months of my arrival, I suffered from an attack of Bengal remittent fever, with great determination to the liver and colon, accompanied by spasms of the stomach and gall-duct; and the treatment of the early stages of the disease having been inactive and inert, it was the opinion of the late Mr. Twining that I would remain a martyr to the ill effects of the climate of Bengal for life. This opinion has been fully verified—disorders of the liver, spleen, mucous digestive surface and bronchial tubes being the result. Early in my illness, organized lymph tubes were voided from the bowels; and this state being regarded as purely inflammatory, leeches were applied in vast numbers. Occasionally fifty leeches were applied in the twenty-four hours; and for weeks in succession the number of leeches expended amounted to upwards of one hundred and fifty per week. Great exhaustion followed, with a high degree of anasarca of the body and limbs. I came home on sick leave, and I was told by Dr. Marshall Hall, and your friend, the late Dr. James Johnson, to whom, under the providence of God, I owe my life, that there was not on record a case of such extreme depletion—an opinion in which Dr. Abercrombie, of Edinburgh, fully concurred. I rather resembled a model of wax than a being endued with life. On summing up the extent of local depletion which was employed in my case, to the best of my judgment and belief, I am under the mark when I state that the number of leeches which were applied within the space of six years amounted to three thousand." It is almost unnecessary to say that this excellent officer was constrained to abandon the service early in life.

Mr. Twining, speaking of the congestive fever of the cold season in Bengal, observes:—"The altered appearance of the blood, in many of those fevers which arise from exposure to the malaria of the jungles, is very remarkable, and merits careful investigation. Connected with this morbid condition of the blood there appears, occasionally, some corresponding disorder of the solids, and particularly of the vascular system, which favours prolonged and profuse oozing of blood from leech-bites." The condition of the blood here mentioned is the anæmic; and without stopping to inquire as to the author's meaning on the other points of pathology here only hinted at, it may be questioned whether, in such a condition of the system, blood-letting ought at all to be practised. Certainly no one can doubt the unhappy consequences of the " prolonged and profuse oozing of blood from leech-bites" in such cases. Some men never recover from the effects produced on the blood, and on all the functions, nervous and vascular.

The anæmic patient generally presents a pale, sallow, or dingy, bloated, and exsanguine complexion, the eye being of a morbid, pearly whiteness, the pupil relaxed, irritable, and often much dilated; the expression dull and inert; the mind being irresolute, feeble, and despondent, the memory impaired; in extreme cases, the mind is fatuous, but more generally we perceive a peculiar and characteristic peevishness. The abdomen is tumid, inelastic, and congested; the skin harsh and constricted to the touch, and of a temperature generally below the natural standard.

The digestion is feeble and depraved; the processes of depuration are imperfectly performed; the feet swell. In anæmic patients, I have found the temperature in the mouth to be generally below the natural standard. The mean of eighteen observations, by insertion of the thermometer in the mouth of an anæmic patient, during the months of November and December, afforded a temperature of 90°. On four days the temperature was taken before he left home, and after his return from a walk; the mean temperature was 85° before going out, and 88° on his return. After a journey to Scotland, the temperature remained at 98° for two days, on the two following days it fell, and was observed at 97°. The patient was an officer of engineers, a man of high scientific and practical attainments.

How and to what extent an anæmic condition of the brain, spinal cord, and nervous central ganglia may affect the functions of the nervous system generally, the present state of our knowledge does not enable us to determine; but that such a condition of the blood must have an extensive influence no one can doubt. I have seen an instance of what could only be termed nervous apoplexy from anæmia of the brain.

Neuralgic pains of the abdomen are very commonly to be found on exploration of that cavity; and when they are present in the epigastric, or in either or both the hypochondriac regions, there is a risk of their deceiving the inexperienced as to their cause; thus leading to very grave errors in treatment. The pains here spoken of, when of a neuralgic character, will always be found to disappear on the return of health; and I would seriously urge the necessity of care in explorations, lest the pains in question be mistaken for those produced by organic disease in either liver or spleen. These abdominal neuralgic pains are common to chlorotic females in all countries, and they seem to depend on a morbid sensibility of the nervous system induced by depravation of the blood, which in its normal condition is the natural support of the nervous system. Here, in Europe, the patient presents the complete reverse of the order of his original acute state of disease under the sun of the tropics—to the acute disturbance of all the functions of life, torpor and feebleness of corresponding extent have succeeded.

There is now a general cachexia, with atony of all the vital functions. The motions of the heart, along with those of respiration, are feeble and perturbed on the least exertion, and a blowing murmur in the direction of the pulmonary artery, and frequently a loud venous murmur in the neck, can be discovered. Palpitations and throbbings in the head are common, accompanied by giddiness and *tinnitus aurium*. The voluntary muscles are attenuated, feeble, and relaxed, and there is a disinclination from all exertion.

The excretory functions are imperfectly performed; the bowels are torpid, the tongue being coated and exsanguine. It is evident that here, owing principally to an altered condition of the organic constituents of the blood, a corresponding alteration has taken place in the nutrition of the various tissues of the body. We find, in short, that the functions of the stomach, bowels, kidneys, liver, lungs, organic nerves, and brain, are seriously disordered, through deficiency of blood, or through blood of a depraved quality, or both. I have frequently seen a temporary fatuity to result from anæmia, general and cerebral; but it occurs more generally in that form of the disease which follows upon malignant fevers, remittent and intermittent. The fevers of the Indian taràis, of the provinces of Aracan and Gondwana, and of the Crimea, have been observed to terminate in mental enfeeblement, which looks as if the malarious influences had much to do with the nervous depression, as well as with the anæmic condition.

> " We're not ourselves
> When Nature, being opprest, commands the mind
> To suffer with the body."

Anæmic patients, especially if advanced in life, are prone to hæmorrhages and to passive congestions of a serious nature in the abdominal or thoracic cavities, according to individually acquired or to hereditary tendencies. The state of disease here under consideration demands much care in the treatment. The heroic remedies, originally required to save life, are no longer possible to the cure. In their place must now come those agents calculated to restore enfeebled functions to a healthy vigour, and then we have to rebuild the sunken and shattered frame. We have to impart tone to the organs of supply, by attention to diet, air, exercise, the various habits of life, and by the proper use of medicines, while we have a due regard, by these various means, to the regulation of the excretory functions of the skin, liver, bowels, and kidneys. Such are the conditions that hold in the instances of vast numbers of persons arriving from our intertropical possessions, and such I conceive to be the indications, which, for a longer or shorter period, according to the duration and severity of symptoms, should be followed in their treatment. Without such care, the climate of England will do but little for them. When a young man presents the conditions here mentioned, I am never satisfied with merely prescribing medicines for him. I advise his passing as much of his time as possible in the open air, under the most gentle exercise, and far from the temptations and from the atmosphere of our great towns. I recommend " the best of tonics, relaxation of mind, with exercise in good air"—that is to say, not a London life. The patient must be taught that time is as essential to his cure as medical treatment, and that the attempt to forestall the one is to lose the other, and thus sacrifice the health which it is our endeavour to restore.

There are many considerations which will suggest themselves to the medical observer why invalids should not be kept within the atmosphere of great cities. Everything within them tends to retard convalescence; and there are even districts in England which appear unfavourable to the restoration to health of tropical invalids—especially those whose atmosphere is humid.

"The health of different parts of the country differs widely," says Dr. Farr, " and the difference is greatest in summer. In the summers of 1841-50, the mortality in 506 districts, comprising, when the census was taken, 10,126,886 people, was at the rate of 18·15 in a thousand *annually;* while in 117 districts, comprising the chief towns, and 7,795,882 people, the mortality was at the rate of 25 in a thousand *annually.* Thus at least 7 in every 25 deaths which occur in towns are the result of artificial causes."

Ever since my return from India, I have remarked that the most rapid, as well as effective restoratives to health, have resulted from a visit to the Highlands of Scotland. Doubtless the moorland exercises of walking and riding, with the cheering accompaniment of sport, and the general prevalence of temperance in diet, have, in this instance, contributed largely to the benefits derivable from inspiring pure air. But the peculiar local properties of the air have appeared to me to aid likewise in the beneficial results;—I mean the union of the ocean air to that of the mountains, such as we everywhere find it in the Highlands. A pure mountain air we appreciate in many countries; but the proximity of the Atlantic and German Oceans to the mountains of Scotland cannot fail to constitute a powerful and peculiar accessory.

Those who have to remark on the difficult and tedious convales-cence of invalids in certain unfavourable localities, will require no arguments as to the importance of this subject; " but few have a clear conception," says Liebig, " of the influence of air and tem-perature on the health of the human frame." I seriously impress on the anæmic patient the necessity of avoiding all occasion for the use of mercury. If benefit does not accrue within a given time, I recommend travel, and it is surprising what an impetus this simple measure gives to the flagging functions, and to the restora-tion of the blood. With no class of invalids is the *medicina mentis* of more importance than here—the benefits to be derived from a well-regulated course of " dietetics of the mind" being second only to a proper adjustment of the ordinary medical appliances. " A journey," says Sir James Clark, " may indeed be regarded as a continuous change of climate, as well as of scene, and constitutes a remedy of unequalled power in some of those morbid states of the system in which the mind suffers as well as the body." For the morbid business-imagination—for your worn-out, steady, moping business-man—the old heathen poet's remedy was wine: the

Christian poet's remedy is a more moral and philosophic one—a resolute mental holiday—" a wise vacancy."

With the aids to be derived from a temperate climate, the medical management of these cases is generally easy : that is, when the patient is not advanced in life, and the anæmic condition is not complicated with organic disease. The various salts of iron may almost deserve to be termed specifics : this is so much the case, that we can hardly go wrong in prescribing the citrate of iron, the citrate of iron and quinine, the compound iron mixture, the prot-oxide and sesquioxide of iron, the old wine of iron, with or without the addition of tincture of the sesquichloride, the ammonio-citrate of iron, &c., while the regulation of the bowels may be effectively promoted by the use of the aloetic pill with myrrh, or aloes with iron. By these means we promote the development of the blood.

To obviate the tendencies to headache, and to excitement of the heart's action, often arising from the use of chálybeates, I am in the habit of ordering the sesquioxide of iron in the first instance, and as a preparation for the other stronger salts. When carefully prepared, it is an admirable tonic and sedative. A few cases will best illustrate this portion of the subject.

CASE 1.—Capt. T——, aged thirty-two, originally of plethoric habit, has resided fourteen years in the Presidency of Bengal. Four years ago he had a severe attack of remittent fever, followed ever since by annually recurring attacks of intermittent fever. During the first illness he was bled from the arm, and by leeches to the temples and the epigastric region ; he used calomel to slight salivation, with a continuous course of powerful purgatives, the diet consisting of sago and arrowroot. From this violent seizure he recovered but slowly, and only after a residence of six months in the mountain ranges of the Himalayahs. On his return to his corps in the plains, however, he soon became subject to tertian ague. For this last disease, Captain T—— took mild mercurials, purgatives, and quinine. He was occasionally, and for months together, able to perform his duty ; but in the rainy and cold seasons his fevèr recurred, and he was at length, and after much suffering and emaciation, ordered home. He is now in a state of complete anæmia, with a pale, bloated, and lemon complexion ; and mossy, dry, and scanty hair. There is no enlargement of the spleen or liver ; the abdomen is doughy and inelastic ; the skin harsh, dry, and constricted ; the pulse feeble and slow ; the tongue pale and flaccid ; the bowels are constipated. His appetite is good, but he feels distressingly inflated after meals, and he is unable to bear the slightest pressure on the abdomen after food. There is great debility and emaciation. He was ordered to take two pills of watery extract of aloes, with sulphate of quinine and iron, every night. These had the effect of regulating the bowels, and of im-parting tone to the digestive organs, while, as a general tonic, he used the old wine of iron with the tincture of the sesquichloride three times a day. He was allowed a light but generous diet, with bitter ale at dinner. He was directed to use warm baths at 96°, three times a week, just before going to bed, and to use friction to the skin night and morning, when dressing and undressing. He improved rapidly in health even while in London; and by communications from him I learned that, in the country, he became so much improved in health that in eight months he was enabled to discontinue all medicine. During eighteen months that I was in occasional communication with this officer, he continued to report favourably of his health and strength; and at the end of two years he returned to India.

Remarks.—This is an example of simple uncomplicated anæmia, resulting from remittent and intermittent fevers, and their necessary treatment by blood-letting, mercury, purgatives, and low diet. The patient had been under able and experienced medical management, but the malarious influences proved too powerful to be resisted even by his robust European constitution. By a careful attention to his habits of life, and to the simple rules of medical treatment mentioned, Capt. T—— left England in perfect health.

CASE II.—Lieut. M——, aged twenty-six, of vigorous frame, served nine years in India, and latterly in Sindh, where he contracted severe intermittent fever. He was leeched largely and repeatedly, and took calomel, purgatives, and quinine. After ten months' residence in this unhealthy province he became so enfeebled by repeated accessions of fever, that a return to Europe was at length considered necessary to his recovery. He is now in the pale and bloated state characteristic of the diseased condition of the blood under consideration, being in what may be termed an *acute* state of anæmia. The pulse is hurried and feeble; the abdomen hard, full, and tense; but I cannot discover, on the most careful exploration, that there exists any enlargement of either liver or spleen. He had two attacks of ague on the way home— one in Egypt and the other at Southampton. The complexion is very pale and bloodless; the mind feeble and desponding; the appetite is wanting, and the bowels constipated; the entire surface is harsh, dry, and heated. He is a cigar-smoker, and I attribute much of the disturbance of the heart's action to this circumstance, having observed the same result in hundreds of instances in India. To regulate the bowels, he was directed to take, every morning, a solution of the sulphate of magnesia and quinine, with dilute sulphuric acid; and as a general tonic he took, twice a day, two ounces of a mixture containing the sulphates of quinine and iron, with dilute sulphuric acid. When by these means the tendency to fever had been subdued, the frequency of the circulation moderated, and the bowels brought into regularity, the more simple chalybeates were employed. He was then ordered a light diet, with a little wine, or bitter ale, and no cigars. He used warm baths, with powerful friction to the entire surface of the body night and morning. In a few weeks he was able to proceed into the country.

Remarks.—This officer recovered but slowly, being subject to aguish attacks whenever exposed to cold or damp. He owed much to his own good sense, for he carefully avoided everything that he perceived to be injurious. By persisting in the use of chalybeates, by travelling, and by regulated exercise, he at length completely recovered his health, and was enabled to return to his duty in India at the expiration of his furlough.

ON THE TREATMENT OF INVALIDS SUFFER-ING FROM THE SEQUELÆ TO THE FEVERS OF TROPICAL CLIMATES.

FEVERS, remittent, intermittent, and continued, are the diseases most frequently seen amongst Europeans in India. Next to fevers stand the formidable bowel complaints, as dysentery, diarrhœa, and cholera. These, together with diseases of the liver, form the chief scourges of our Indian armies, European and Native. There is not a district, station, or cantonment, in the vast extent of Hindustan and the dependencies to the eastward, or in Ceylon, in which malarious fever in some form, dependent as to type and intensity on local circumstances, will not be found to prevail, either as an occasional epidemic, or as the endemic of the soil. Of the better classes of Europeans, many escape attacks of dysentery, diarrhœa, cholera, and hepatitis during even a long residence in the East Indies; but there are very few who do not at some time suffer from some form or other of fever.

Out of an aggregate European force of 25,431 men of Her Majesty's army serving in periods of eight and ten years respectively, between 1823 and 1836, in the stations of Calcutta, Chinsurah, and Berhampore, for instance, all in Bengal Proper, there occurred, according to Colonel Tulloch, 13,596 cases of fever; and though the climate of Lower Bengal is very inimical to European health, comparatively to that of many parts of India, and though the years included within this return were subsequent to the first Burmese war, still the proportion of fever cases is enormous, making every allowance for such unfavourable and contingent influences during one or two years of the period under consideration. It must not be forgotten, that of the soldiers engaged in the Burmese war, seventy-three per cent. perished at Rangoon and Upper Ava, and that in Arakan " three-fifths of the whole perished in the course of eight months;" so that, of the few survivors, the admissions into the hospitals of the three named stations could not materially affect the results. In the Mysore division of the Madras native army alone, out of an aggregate force of 194,170 men serving there during twenty-four years, there occurred 63,810 cases of fever; and out of an aggregate British force of 82,342, serving in the Presidency of Madras generally, from 1842 to 1848, there occurred 22,923 cases of fever. Amongst officers and the better classes of Europeans, who, from their better habits of life, are not so subject to hepatitis and dysentery as soldiers, it will very generally be found that fever in some form has been the first disturbing cause of illness, and that to recurrences of fever are to be referred many of their subsequent more local diseases on their return to Europe, whether these last be seated in the liver or in the bowels.

The experience of the West Indies confirms the statistics of fevers in the Eastern hemisphere. Out of that portion of the inhabitants of George Town, Demerara, who are likely to resort to public institutions—the total population of the town amounting only to 20,000—there were admitted into the colonial hospital, from June, 1846, to June, 1847, 2938 cases of remittent and intermittent fever; and the annual consumption of quinine in Demerara and Essiquibo—countries somewhat resembling Lower Bengal in medical topography and climate—averages 3000 ounces!

If we look to the embouchures of the Mississippi, we shall find a state of public health, and a prevalence of fever especially, not less remarkable. The New Orleans Charity Hospital is one of the most extensive fever hospitals in the world. It appears from the records that, in a period of nine years, from the 1st of January, 1841, to the 1st of January, 1850, there were admitted into this hospital 73,216 patients; of which number were admitted, for all the different forms of fever, 33,381; and among these last, for intermittent fevers, 17,217.

Great as are the advantages possessed in India by the officer over the common soldier as to habits of life, accommodation, &c., it is still matter of every-day observation, that even amongst the better classes of Europeans there, civil and military, the sequelæ to malarious fevers are both severe and frequent. Some of these I have already noticed; but here I shall confine my observations to the slighter forms of organic diseases, and to the functional disturbances and ill-health which follow on tropical fevers, remittent, intermittent, and continued: those conditions, in fact, which are common to the three types, and which are most frequently observed in England as the results of tropical fevers. It should be held in recollection, also, in reference to the subject of this article, that most of our tropical remittent fevers are in a great degree, and very generally, of a gastric character, one of the prominent conditions consisting in acute congestion of the mucous digestive surface; so much so as to cause Robert Jackson to designate the bilious remittent fevers of the West Indian Islands by the term "gastric, or bilious remittent fever." This profound observer considers the fevers of all countries to be more or less of this nature; and practically, although the thoracic and cerebral viscera are occasionally affected in a serious degree, and although the cerebral and spinal systems are always disturbed in their functions, still we find, in tropical fevers at least, that almost all the symptoms exhibited during life, and almost all the lesions discoverable after death, are to be referred to, and centre in, the organs of the abdominal cavity. The importance of a constant and due regard to these considerations, as bearing on the condition of persons who have suffered from the fevers of the East and West Indies, must be manifest.

The liability to the recurrence of fever on exposure to slight causes, is also an important and very distressing consideration. I have known many young officers, originally of strong constitution, so harassed with fever, recurring again and again, that after coming to England two or three times for the recovery of health, they have, on repeated and desperate trials of Indian climate, been compelled to resign the service. Some of them have never regained sound health at home, and of those who strive on, many fall a sacrifice to relapses on their return to the tropics.

Patients who come to England for the recovery of health, after having suffered from tropical fevers, present morbid appearances varying according to form and constitution of body, or as the fevers may have been of long continuance, and more or less concentrated, and according to the severity of treatment. Some are puffed and bloated, having a leaden, yellow, or copper-yellow complexion, while others are emaciated and lemon-coloured; presenting the very type of the marsh cachexy. Many present the purely anæmic condition described in the last article. In fact, the distressing state of broken health which follows on protracted tropical fevers, appears under separate and distinct specification, according to the special organs affected, and to the degree of anæmia which may be present. But whatever the configuration or complexion may be, we are sure to find the pathological condition centred in the abdominal organs, so as sometimes to involve their structure, but at all times to disturb their functions. When the patient has been a sufferer from intermittent fever, we find that, owing to the repeated and violent congestions attendant on the frequent recurrences of ague, with its severe and protracted cold stages, the vessels of the abdomen, but especially the venous trunks, become dilated, and the blood, already spoiled by use, is detained in them, so as to be still further deteriorated. The vital energy and vascular tone of all the abdominal viscera are more or less impaired in cases of this nature, according as the previous fever has been of longer or shorter duration; in other words, the nervous centres, and all the organs depending on them, share in the general injury and depression. The obstructed and depraved state of the blood, and consequent depravation of all the secretions and excretions, and of assimilation also, must not be overlooked.* We sometimes find the heart impaired in its functions, through long-continued and often-repeated engorgements of the great venous trunks during the cold or congestive stages of remittent and intermittent fevers, and from the violence of the subsequent bounding reactions. Through the operation of these causes, associated, as they often are, with an anæmic condition of the system, the heart is occasionally found to be flaccid in its texture, and dilated in its cavities, while its action is feeble and irregular. In every form of malarious fever, but more especially in " the tremendous remittents of hot climates," it is manifest that the sensibility and energy of the entire nervous system are blunted and enfeebled, and that the muscular system, voluntary and involuntary, is relaxed and enfeebled also, in consequence both of the lesion of the nervous system and of the altered condition of the blood, so common to tropical fevers, and as resulting from their treatment.

These disturbances, repeated during years, in a climate moreover which, of itself, and without the intervention of actual disease, disturbs greatly the functions of the nervous, vascular, and muscular systems, will go far, I think, to account for the *intermitting* state of the heart's action, so often noticed in these essays as characteristic of a large proportion of returned Indians. A long residence in the East, without the intervention of fever, may alone induce the irregular state of the pulse now under consideration; but a lengthened stay in India, together with repeated fevers, is almost certain to cause it.

From many of the symptoms indicative of disturbed function of the heart's action, witnessed in malarious countries, and from the periodical nature of some of them, I have long entertained no doubt that they often have their origin in the efficient cause of fevers, remittent and intermittent. A cause which operates so seriously to the disturbance of the nervous and vascular functions generally, which induces paroxysmal fevers of the most deadly nature, visceral congestions, and neuralgic affections; a cause which produces most serious disturbances of the cerebral and organic nervous functions, may well be believed to aid at least, along with the general enervation and muscular relaxation, in occasioning the feeble and intermitting states of the heart's action, the epigastric pulsation, and the other nervous and vascular disturbances so frequently observable in the persons of returned Indians.

Sufficient attention has not been given to the lesions discover-

---

* To such as would inquire more at large into the causes and consequences of tropical fevers, I would recommend the perusal of the admirable articles in Dr. Copland's " Dictionary of Medicine,"—a great work that should be placed, by authority, in the hands of all naval and military surgeons.

able in the heart and great vessels in persons who have died of the concentrated fevers of hot climates. The observations of Maillot, of Antonini, and Monard would show that softening of the heart is a frequent accompaniment and sequel of algid fevers, and the *post-mortem* examinations of the French surgeons in Algeria tend to the same conclusion as to the result of malarious fevers there. The importance of the subject demands a more careful attention than it has hitherto obtained.

Dr. Barlow states (Guy's Hospital Reports) that a very feeble state of the ventricular parietes may, by causing delay in the circulation, give rise to irregular or intermittent pulse; also that dyspepsia and other diseases associated with irritation or with lesions of the brain and upper part of the spinal cord, will materially affect the action of the heart, so as to render that action feeble or irregular. The conditions requisite for the regularity of the pulse he describes to be—a regular supply of blood to the left ventricle, and a due supply of nervous influence ; and, on the other hand, the chief, if not the only cause of intermittent pulse is a want of due supply of blood to the left ventricle.

I have all my life been familiar with this disturbance of the circulation, and suffered very severely from it in person, as the result of numerous malarious fevers, and of overwrought nervous system during my residence in Calcutta. One of the first instances that came under my notice, on my return to England, was that of an aged general officer of the Bengal army. On remarking to him that his pulse intermitted very much, he said, " Yes, I know it does, and it has done so for about fifty years." This gentleman died at the age of ninety-three.

Another officer of plethoric habit, who had resided long in India, and in whom a distressing irregularity of pulse existed, was largely bled at his country residence on account of cerebral congestion ; and from that day, 1840, to the present time, the intermissions have entirely disappeared, and his health has in all respects been good.

Complicated with all these morbid conditions, alterations in the structure and functions of the mucous digestive surfaces are frequently observable, with their train of irritable dyspepsias and constipations.

In the great majority of persons suffering from the sequelæ of tropical fevers, we find that the whole abdomen is tumid, doughy, and inelastic, with evident venous congestion of all its viscera, while the action of the heart and arteries is feeble. There is, in fact, such a stagnation of the venous blood as to weaken the functions and spoil the secretions of the stomach, liver, bowels, and functions of the spleen, while the general circulation, and the functions of the skin in particular, are oppressed and enfeebled.

All these conditions become aggravated when the sufferer from tropical fever arrives in England in the winter or spring seasons.

In other instances we find congestive enlargèment, with the commencement of interstitial deposits, more or less chronic, of the liver, spleen, and mesentery, accompanied, as in the former case of simple abdominal congestion, by torpor of the digestive powers, depravation of all the secretions, a feeble and oppressed circulation, and morbid derangement of the cuticular functions. In both instances there is great sensitiveness to the impression of cold; the regular periodicity of malarious countries now giving place to the smouldering, dumb, or bastard forms of remittent and intermittent fevers, resulting from the change to the climate of England. The medical management of such cases, whether functionally or structurally affected, is always a matter requiring care, and the cure may occasionally, in persons greatly debilitated by fever, or by long residence in India, be protracted. We have to emulge with one hand, while we impart tone with the other. We have to maintain a gentle but persistent action in all the depurative organs, at the same time that by medicine, proper diet, free exposure to the air, and by exercise, we improve the quality and augment the quantity of the blood.

Case I.—A gentleman of robust frame and short stature, aged thirty-eight, had resided sixteen years in India as an indigo planter, and during that time he had been continually, and in all seasons, much exposed to direct solar heats, to excessive rains, and to cold. His habits of life had been moderate, and for fourteen years his health had been excellent. Two years ago, while exposed to cold and damp weather, he was seized with severe intermittent fever, the stage of rigor lasting frequently for three hours. Medical aid was obtained from a distance, and but irregularly. Calomel and antimony, followed by brisk purgatives and by quinine, overcame the immediate violence of the fever, but he has ever since been out of health. The least exposure to the sun, to damp or cold—circumstances never considered when in health—now excited him to fever, especially if such exposure occurred about the full and change of the moon. His fever by degrees, and under the influence of quinine, lost the severity of the rigor, until that symptom entirely ceased, and on the accession of the cold season it assumed the continued form. At length he became worn out by repeated irregular attacks of fever. His muscular system, which had been powerful, fell away, while the abdomen became large, full, and tense. In this state he was recommended to return to England, where he arrived in the month of March.

He now presents the true physconia, or parabysma, of systematic writers, in the sense of " morbid congestion."

Among the causes of this state of stagnation, Dr. Mason Good justly considers the absence of valves in the abdominal veins as prominent, owing to that want of support to the returning column of blood which belongs to the veins distributed to more superficial parts. That the cold stage of severe intermittent fever, or the stage of congestion, must, when often repeated, tend powerfully to produce, and to maintain, stagnation in the abdominal venous trunks, seems evident. It proved so in this case. The abdomen is now full, hard, and round as a barrel, but percussion affords no evidence of enlargement of either liver or spleen. The complexion is of a copper-yellow hue. The skin is harsh, dry, and cool, and when the integument is pressed between the finger and thumb, the marks are long in regaining the colour of the surrounding parts, owing to the feebleness of the capillary circulation. The sublingual and conjunctival surfaces look pale, and exhibit a deficiency of red particles in the blood; there seems to be an entire suspension of the exhalent and absorbing functions; the pulse is feeble, slow, and oppressed; the respiration hurried on the least exertion, and impeded by the fulness and tension of the abdomen. Abdominal congestion would seem to be the sole cause of his weakness and his sufferings. The bowels never act without the aid of medicine; the intestinal secretions are pale and scanty; the urine natural in appearance. The muscular frame is so enfeebled that he cannot walk a hundred yards without fatigue. His sleep is broken, uneasy, and unrefreshing.

The patient was directed to take a tablespoonful of the following mixture every morning in a small tumbler of cold water, or so much as should produce two evacuations daily :—Saturated solution of sulphate of magnesia, seven ounces and a half; dilute sulphuric acid, half an ounce; sulphate of iron, sulphate of quinine, of each a drachm. He was directed at the same time to use two doses daily of a mixture composed of fluid extract of taraxacum with bitartrate of potash. These medicines after a time acted freely on the bowels and kidneys, while the functions of the skin were promoted by warm baths twice a week, immediately before going to bed. Frictions to the surface were prescribed; and horse exercise advised. The diet was ordered to be light and spare; and as all food produced a sense of weight and oppression, he was allowed to take a small tumbler of weak brandy-and-water at dinner. On this plan the patient improved steadily, though slowly, during six weeks, when he wrote to me from the country that he could walk for an hour without fatigue or hurried respiration, his waist being now reduced by seven inches. The biliary secretion became abundant, and the appetite and digestion had greatly improved. The taraxacum was now exchanged for a pure chalybeate, and the purgative was directed to be used every other day only. When the weather became warm in May, the convalescence was rapid; and in the following month he proceeded on a tour to the continent. He used the waters of Homburg; but in his own opinion the change of air and the continued exercise were of most effect. He returned to England in September, in perfect health.

Remarks.—This was a case of excessive 'abdominal congestion resulting from fever, accompanied by anæmia. This state of the blood was doubtless maintained by the stagnation of so large a portion of the circulating fluid in the abdominal venous trunks. The whole machinery of life was clogged. By the removal of intense abdominal congestion the general circulation was liberated, the quality of the blood improved, while the nervous system was thereby invigorated. Perspiration, digestion, and secretion were also set free towards the restoration of the general health. Youth, a robust constitution, and temperate habits of life, favoured the patient and aided his recovery. His treatment was simple but effective. In a case such as this, a persistent course of tonic purgatives is always necessary; and I believe that purgative medicines, when conjoined with tonics and chalybeates, as in the present instance, do not injure the functions of the colon, as they are too apt to do when given singly in large or repeated doses, or where given with or after calomel.

When this gentleman arrived in England, it was supposed by his medical attendant in the country, that effusion had taken place within the abdominal cavity; but this I was unable to verify, owing to the extreme fulness and tension of the entire region. Certainly the case wore a very unfavourable aspect, and dropsy, general or local, might well have been apprehended.

Case II.—Major ——, of the Indian army, aged forty, had served twenty-two years in India. For the first sixteen years his health had been good; but during the last six years he was employed in field-surveying, the duties of which necessarily exposed him to great variations in temperature and humidity, as well as to the malarious influences. His constitution, originally delicate, appeared indeed to have been improved and invigorated during the first ten years of residence in India. After that his health remained stationary till six years ago, when he was seized, in the month of May, with the ardent remittent fever of the hot dry season. Violent determination to the head, with tumidness and pain of the right hypochondrium, took place immediately, accompanied by delirium. He was freely bled, generally and locally, and took calomel, sudorifics, and purgatives in large doses. His recovery was rapid, and apparently complete. By the month of August he had regained his usual health, when acute bilious diarrhœa came on, rendering mild mercurials, with ipecacuanha, laxatives, and low diet necessary. Again he recovered rapidly, and in the end of October proceeded on his duties of surveying.

The country was jungly, and the soil remained moist and marshy from the previous annual rain. His public establishment and private servants contracted intermittent fevers, but by the aid of small doses of quinine, and by selecting elevated grounds of encampment, Major —— hoped to escape. He did escape until the end of January, when he was attacked with severe fever of the continued form, accompanied by jaundice. He was again bled moderately, and used calomel, antimony, purgatives, and low diet; but his recovery was slow. From this time to the present he has never been in good health. Every year he has been more or less harassed by fevers, sometimes continued in type, at others intermittent, and his health and strength have been gradually reduced. He was urged to go to sea, or to return to Europe, but circumstances of a private nature prevented his doing either. At length, and after years of distress and suffering, he came home in the month of February, worn out with fever. He was now greatly exhausted in all the functions of the body and mind, and in a state of great emaciation. The abdomen was hard and flattened, the abdominal muscles being in a state of extreme tension all over, and this state, owing to neuralgic pains, was rather increased by tactile examination and percussion. All seemed hard beneath, but I could not perceive that any one region was more indurated than another, and there was no tumidness in either hypochondrium. The pulse and respiration were slow and feeble, the heart flaccid, and sluggish in its movements; there was a frequent hacking, dry cough. The complexion was of a dingy parchment hue, the skin being extremely harsh and dry to the touch; the hair was of a mossy dryness, its growth being imperceptibly slow; the nails were exfoliated and crumbling off—all indicating that nutrition was at the lowest ebb. The intestinal secretions were scanty, pale, and fœtid; the urine of a natural appearance, occasionally limpid. For years the bowels had not acted without the aid of medicine. He had no appetite, and experienced great oppression, with sense of distension, after the smallest meal. The sleep was disturbed and unrefreshing; the general habit was anæmic, and the mind greatly depressed.

To promote the functions of depuration, and to impart tone to the digestive organs, Major —— was directed to use the nitro-muriatic acid bath three times a week, just before going to bed, while a combination of the nitro-muriatic acid with tincture of sesquichloride of iron was taken in water, three times a day. The gentle action of the bowels was promoted by the *pilula aloes et ferri* of the Edinburgh Pharmacopœia. Animal food was used but sparingly, while fruits and vegetables were allowed; also weak brandy-and-water at dinner. He took gentle exercise on horse-back daily, or whenever the weather admitted; but the cold easterly winds of March he could not face. Such days were passed, huddled up in coats and blankets, by the fireside. Yet, with care and attention, his health amended, though very slowly, so that by the end of June he was able to ride ten miles on end, the appetite and power of digestion having greatly improved. By this time he had gained eleven pounds in weight, while his mind had become cheerful and hopeful. The medical treatment

was continued till the end of August, by which time the major acquired seventeen pounds in weight, along with considerable increase
of vigour in all his functions. · The bowels now acted without
medicine, the biliary secretion being abundant. By the middle
of September he proceeded to the Highlands of Scotland, where,
with the aid of a pony, he was enabled to ascend the mountains,
and enjoy grouse shooting; but he was incapable of any sustained
muscular exertion. With little further aid from medicine, Major
—— continued to regain health and strength during two years
that I was in occasional communication with him, and he returned
to India at the end of three years " as well as ever he was."

Remarks.—A torpid discharge of all the functions of the body
was the character of Major ——'s case on his arrival in England.
To the previous excitation, within the tropics, of the various
functions, and to the tumult and disturbance of tropical fever, had
then succeeded a torpor and impaired tonicity of the circulation,
respiration, and of the nervous functions, with interrupted and
depraved secretion and excretion. The gastric and intestinal digestion appeared paralysed, with characteristic dryness of the
mucous surfaces, and atony of the muscular layer of the stomach
and bowels. He did not appear to labour under any organic disease
of the liver or spleen, nor could I discover through exploration, or
through the symptoms, that any anatomical changes existed in the
other abdominal viscera.

Major —— was so exhausted on his first arrival at home,
that, viewing his recovery as hopeless within the time allowed by
the regulations of the Indian army, he desired to resign his commission and retire into private life. I objected to this resolution,
urging that his mind was enfeebled, and that he was consequently
not in a fitting frame for coming to the determination of that or
of any other important step in life. He yielded to my reasoning,
and thus a valuable appointment, useful to himself and his family,
has been preserved. By similar advice, given in India and at
home, to officers both civil and military, I have saved many a
valuable public servant from the commission of a hasty and irre-
trievable mistake.

The cases just related furnish fair examples of the average results of tropical fevers. The first presented pure abdominal congestion of the passive form, and the last a general torpor and loss
of power in all the abdominal functions. Many more examples
might be added; but those now furnished appear to me, together
with the two cases about to be briefly noticed, sufficient to illustrate the subject under consideration.

Case III.—While writing this article, the following cases came
under my care; and as they represent a state of disease not infrequent, owing to the present rapid transit to Europe from India,
I here present them.

"Lieutenant ——, Madras cavalry, aged twenty-three, had served four years in India, during which he enjoyed good health, with the exception of occasional headache and an irregular state of the bowels. Towards the end of November, 1850, he obtained a year's leave of absence to visit his family in England, and marched to Bombay for that purpose. When half way, he was seized with jungle (remittent) fever. In nine days, though feeble and exhansted, he was enabled to resume his march, and arrived in Bombay in the end of December. Here he was attacked with tertian intermittent fever, the cold stages being severe and long-continued, and followed by an imperfect reaction. As in the first seizure, Lieutenant —— was treated with calomel, purgatives, and quinine. On board the steamer, both in the Red Sea and Mediterranean, he suffered from repeated attacks of ague, and when the day was in the least degree cool, he was obliged to take to his bed. He is now (February 9th) in London, in an extremely emaciated and enfeebled state, and though five feet ten inches in height, he weighs but nine stone and three pounds. The liver and spleen are greatly engorged and tumid, their regions bulging out perceptibly, and feeling tender on the least pressure. The complexion is of a dull leaden yellow; pulse, 112; bowels constipated; urine madder-coloured; tongue clean; skin warm, moist, and relaxed. The little food he is able to take causes great oppression and distension at the stomach, and he is unable to bear the pressure of his dress over the abdomen. The cold is most distressing to his feelings, and he shivers whenever he quits the fireside. There is complete and general anæmia, and the circulation is distressingly hurried in ascending the stairs.

He was ordered to take of the saturated solution of sulphate of magnesia, combined with dilute sulphuric acid, the sulphates of quinine and iron, so much every morning as should procure two free evacuations from the bowels; while he used two doses in the day of the sulphates of iron and quinine, with dilute sulphuric acid, as a tonic and febrifuge. His diet to be carefully regulated, using animal food to dinner, but sparingly; no wine or fermented liquor allowed. Warm baths were directed to be used twice a week at bedtime.

Feb. 15th.—Great improvement has already taken place; the bowels and kidneys act freely, and he is not so much distressed by the cold nor by gastric oppression; pulse 94.

26th.—Bowels violently moved in the night, when enormous quantities of frothy, fœtid matter were voided. This discharge has afforded great abdominal relief, and his waist is reduced four inches. Urine copious and less charged, the complexion clearing, while the shiverings have nearly disappeared.

Hitherto the bowels have acted but twice a day, under the influence of the tonic purgative, and the present discharge is viewed as the liberation of pent-up bile rather than an ordinary purgative effect. The medicines and diet as before.

28th.—Continues to improve in all respects, and is able to walk a little in the open air on dry days; pulse 78. The appetite is becoming keen, and requires restraint. Urine copious, and nearly natural; bowels freely moved twice a day. Treatment continued,

March 4th.—Has acquired nine pounds in weight, while the tumidness of the abdomen is greatly reduced. Pulse 76; urine copious and natural in appearance. The bowels continue to act freely twice a day.

12.—Getting well; complexion nearly natural and the waist of the usual dimensions. He is now able to wear his former clothes, buttoned, with ease. He takes long walks in the open air and increases daily in strength. The tonic aperient to be taken every other day, then every third and fourth day, so as to be gradually discontinued, while a pure chalybeate is substituted for the quinine and iron mixture.

Remarks.—The case just related affords an example of the acute and immediate consequences of malarious fever. The rapid transition to Europe, by steam, brought the sufferer home with his tropical ills fresh upon him, with the addition that his fever had now assumed a low continued form. " Visceral disease," says Dr. Billing, " converts ague into continued pyrexia;" and in further illustration of this principle, the same authority adduces the hectic fever of pulmonary consumption, and the irritative fever of surgical cases, which latter he considers " a mixture of morbid sensibility and pyrexia from inflammation." It has appeared to me both in India and England, that quinine, when given in large doses, and for a continuance, has occasionally had this same effect—namely, the conversion of ague into continued fever. Blood-letting in the cold stage of intermittent fever has been found to produce a like result. This young officer had been altogether ill but little more than two months, yet the powers of the constitution were completely subdued by malarious fever and abdominal congestion. But the duration of his illness having been but brief, his recovery was rapid. No mercury was exhibited in this case, the general anæmia and splenic engorgement prohibiting the use of that mineral.

CASE IV.—Lieutenant ——, of the Bombay army, aged twenty-nine, had served eight years in India. The medical report of his case by the surgeon of his corps represents him to be "of a naturally delicate constitution, with a predisposition to liver complaint." In November, 1849, after two years of "bad health, suffering constantly from fever and hepatic derangement," in Guzerat, Scinde, and Moultan, he quitted the latter station for Kurrachee. "Deriving no benefit at this place, he was sent to Bombay, and eventually to Mahabaleshwar," a mountain station for sick and convalescents. " He rejoined his regiment at ——, in February, 1850, apparently in improved health ; but soon after he suffered another attack of fever, which has since returned regularly at the spring tides, and been invariably attended with congestions of the liver and incessant bilious vomitings." Calomel and opium, saline purgatives, quinine, and tonics procured relief " for a few days," but " the obstinacy with which the complaint returns has greatly debilitated the constitution."——" The influence of the moon, too, is very remarkable." In another statement, dated in May, Lieut. —— is reported to be continually harassed with fever, while " quinine has lost its power." He was then ordered to return to Europe for the recovery of his health, and arrived in England in July, 1850.

Feb. 26th, 1851.—The patient states that ever since his arrival he has resided in the north of England, but that his health has in no way improved ; fever, accompanied by a dull heavy pain in both hypochondria, having recurred about the full and change of the moon every month since July last. There is now pain and some slight fulness of both liver and spleen, with a hard tumid state of the whole abdomen ; the bowels are constipated, and the urine generally high-coloured ; the pulse is feeble and slow ; the surface relaxed, cool, and damp to the touch ; the tongue is loaded with a thick white fur. He is much distressed by aguish feelings in cold and damp days. The general condition is anæmic.

On the plan of treatment prescribed in the last case this officer recovered rapidly ; and from the time when the bowels were made to act freely, his disposition to fever daily subsided. In a month he returned to the country, greatly improved in health and strength, using only the tonic and febrifuge treatment.

Remarks.—In both the cases just described the tendency to fever disappeared in remarkable coincidence with the subsidence of abdominal congestion, through the use of gentle but persistent evacuants, combined with tonics. That a temperate climate and the absence of malaria may have materially aided in these results, I entertain no doubt, although in the last recorded very obstinate instance, climate alone proved insufficient ; and so it proved also in the case of a gentleman from the south of Spain, whom I lately treated, and who was much distressed by ague, until brought under the influence of the emulgent treatment here described. He had taken enormous quantities of quinine without effect.

Every one has seen intermittents, on the other hand, which resisted the influence of ordinary purgatives, and of every anti-periodic remedy, until mercurial purgatives were exhibited ; in other words, until the necessary degree of freedom was given to the abdominal circulation, through powerfully emulgent means. In Zeeland, the biliary functions are said to suffer so much during the intermittents of the country, that they are called by the inhabitants *gall-fevers.*

I frequently find, in the instances of persons returning home from hot climates, that the bastard or dumb ague resists the influence of quinine and all forms and varieties of tonics and anti-periodics, even when the use of these last have been preceded by emulgents ; while the same difficulties are encountered in the cure of the neuralgic affections which are so often associated with, or which follow upon intermittents. In such cases, the preliminary depuration through the channel of the kidneys, mentioned in pages 192-3, followed by a ten or twelve days' course of the arsenical solution, will often produce surprising results. I see cases of this nature in which I have reason to believe that the inertness of quinine has been the result of over-dosing with it, and of undue persistence in the use of it.

That the partial stagnation of the venous and arterial circulation in the liver, spleen, and other abdominal viscera tends, by the detention of the blood, to unfit it for the purposes of the general circulation, and to dispose also to attacks of intermittent fever, would appear highly probable. Dr. Proud goes so far as to declare that the blood in the portal system is deprived of a portion of its vitality. A condition of the blood exists in the cases here under consideration similar to that in varicose veins ; and it has been observed by Mr. Bransby Cooper that the discharge of such blood by puncture of the diseased vessels "does not produce any constitutional effect, the blood contained within the varicose veins, being to a certain extent thrown out of the general mass of the circulation, and retained in a half-stagnant state within them."

CHRONIC DIARRHŒA.

The late Dr. Matthew Baillie, who had seen much of the diseases of tropical invalids, describes a diarrhœa, of an " almost constantly fatal" character, in persons of a sallow complexion, " who have resided for a considerable time in warm climates." It consists " of an evacuation of a matter resembling in its appearance a mixture of water and lime, which is generally frothy on its surface. When this kind of purging has once taken place, it is hardly ever radically removed, although it may for some time be occasionally suspended." Dr. Baillie, who was rather of a despairing disposi-tion, as a physician had " no opportunity of examining the con-dition of the liver and bowels in such patients after death ;" and his treatment consisted of very small doses of mercury, with astrin-gents and bitters, and great care in diet. My object in the present paper is to exhibit the pathology and set forth the treatment of this complicated and dangerous disease.

In tropical invalids, suffering, on their return to Europe, from chronic diarrhœa, we perceive, along with the cachexia so generally characteristic of the class, an excessive irritability of the mind and body, an anxious countenance, and a blanched condition of the entire surface, conveying an impression that the patients have been drained of all their fluids, and thus become dried up and attenuated. The *vis vitæ* appears in such cases to be absolutely washed out of the body.

The abdomen is generally tumid, but occasionally, in common with the muscles and integuments of the entire frame, it is shrunk and shrivelled. Pain, other than neuralgia, I have seldom been able to trace in this cavity, on the most careful exploration of its various regions by tactile examination and percussion.

The skin will generally be found dry, cool, and sometimes harsh to the touch; occasionally of a soft, velvety character; all indicating a diminished vitality—diminished exhaling. and absorbing power—the secreting function being suspended through dryness. The state of the system, as already stated, is usually anæmic. There is much restlessness, the little sleep that is obtained being unrefreshing. The intestinal secretions are sometimes of the appearance and consistence of pea-soup, and at others serous or watery, or, as some patients describe them, like soap-and-water, or semi-fluid and yeast-like, with little or no colouring matter. The evacuations are generally voided without any pain. They are always copious and exhausting, especially during the night or in the early morning.

The disease occurs occasionally in paroxysms, and is sometimes preceded by distinct feverishness—the paroxysms of diarrhœa and of fever recurring once or twice a month. The urine, in all the instances in which I have examined it, contained oxalate of lime in greater or less quantity. The appetite is sometimes voracious, at others defective and capricious.

The secondary or chronic diarrhœas of Europeans who have resided long in hot climates are always difficult of cure; and when of long standing, they constitute a class of disease dangerous and intractable beyond most others.

Whether the disease under consideration presents itself in the form of diarrhœa originally contracted as such in India, or as one of the sequelæ to acute tropical dysentery, as the result of hepatic disease, fevers, cholera, malaria, the abuse of mercury and purgatives, or from errors in diet and habits of life, we seldom find the disease simple in its pathological nature—that is, confined to the mucous digestive surface alone. On the contrary, a careful exploration of the abdominal regions, coupled with an attentive consideration of all the antecedent and attendant circumstances, will generally show that diarrhœa, in a large proportion of instances, is complicated with, if not mainly dependent on, chronic disorders and diseases of the liver. And here it is worthy of remark, that in India diarrhœa is a frequent and immediate evidence of dangerous congestion, or of inflammation of the parenchyma of the liver, and sometimes it results both in India and in Europe from abscess of that organ. The first approach of congestion or of inflammation of the liver suspends its secreting power, and diarrhœa is the result. An entire suspension, or its converse, an excessive flow of the biliary excretion, will generally produce diarrhœa.* That there are in India, on the other hand, diarrhœas of a simple and uncomplicated nature, is a fact well known; but they are mostly acute and comparatively easy of cure, the subjects of them recovering on the spot; so that in effect none are sent home but the most severe, protracted, and complicated cases.

Although chronic diarrhœa generally follows on previous tropical disease, I have seen it affect persons on their return to England, who, during their residence in India, had never suffered from any of the diseases of that country. The health of such patients, however, had been enfeebled, and they were thus rendered susceptible to the influence of cold or damp, or to what is always more injurious to the returned Indian—to both conjoined. The returning Indian is often seized with diarrhœa from exposure to cold on board ship, especially if exposed to the spring easterly winds. The cold of the English winter and spring proves very adverse to the cure of this disease, and I have constantly to send patients suffering from it to the sheltered places on the coast, as Hastings, Bournemouth, Ventnor, &c. Fatigue is almost as injurious as cold. An officer whom I sent to Bournemouth missed his way home, and had to walk beyond his powers. The result was a relapse which nearly proved fatal.

Diarrhœas of course vary in their nature with their causes, and these last constitute the most necessary points for primary consideration in practice. One will depend on disorder or disease of the liver; another will result from fever; a third from dysentery; a fourth has for its cause a hyperæmia of the mucous digestive surfaces; while a fifth is associated with anæmia of the same textures, as well as of all the abdominal organs. I have seen cases in which the abuse of purgative medicines appeared to produce chronic diarrhœa, and others in which the same effect seemed to result from the large or the protracted use of calomel.

A morbid state of the biliary secretion, and its injurious influence in producing and maintaining the chronic bowel complaint here noticed, have been mentioned emphatically by some writers on the diseases of tropical climates, as a fact of most frequent occurrence; and so also, with more justice, has the total absence of hepatic secretion, constituting what is termed the *white flux*. This latter form of diarrhœa, whether associated with intermittent

---

* Dr. James Lind, describing hepatitis in Calcutta in 1762, says—"The cure of inflammation of the liver proved uncertain and tedious, as it was frequently followed by colliquative diarrhœa, which speedily put an end to the patient's life;" so that, whether hepatic disease may be more immediately or more remotely antecedent, diarrhœa is frequently found to be its result.

fever or not, often recurs in paroxysms, more or less distant. On such occasions it is common to find the tongue assume a more or less red, abraded, or even ulcerated state; but it is worthy of careful remark that, on the restoration of the hepatic function, all these indications of mucous-intestinal irritation gradually subside. The intermittent fever, so generally the antecedent of chronic diarrhœa, would appear to stamp its character of periodicity and of paroxysm upon its consequent, and thus to render it more or less paroxysmal or periodical, according to the severity of the original ague; in other words, according to the intensity of the primary malaria. A periodical excoriation, or else an aphthous state, of the mouth, tongue, and fauces is also a frequent occurrence in this disease; and when either of these morbid states is present, there is usually, and for the time, a mitigation of diarrhœa. But when the abraded or ulcerated mucous surface heals, then the disorder of the bowels recurs with more or less severity.

Those who have visited Simla, and some of the stations near it on the hill ranges of the Himalayas, have very generally observed a change to a pale, colourless state of the intestinal secretions soon after their ascent into those regions, resulting, it is presumed, from the comparative cold and damp of the mountain air. Diarrhœa is, in fact, a frequent result of this change of climate; so much so, indeed, as to have received from the British residents there the name of "the hill trot." Exposure upon active field service, or during the night and the early morning marches in India, especially during the cold season, often produces the same result. Both the conditions here mentioned, the pale secretion and the diarrhœa, would appear to result from hepatic congestion, the consequence of the sudden application of cold and damp to the surface of the body, previously relaxed by the heat of the plains. The result is, a diminished or suspended secretion of bile, and a consequent disorder in the entire process of digestion, the matters voided from the bowels being colourless, acrid, and irritating.* Officers of the Bengal army who marched from Sindh, where the thermometer rose to 135°, to Cabul, where it fell below 75°, have stated to me that, soon after exposure to this relative cold, they all became more or less jaundiced: some were seized with diarrhœa, but all were jaundiced. By some very observant patients, I have been told, on the other hand, that in their instances diarrhœa commenced in India by enormous and long-continued "discharges of pure bile," which would appear to have exhausted the functions of the liver: then came the "white flux," with its complete suspension of the nutritive processes; the anæmia of all the organs and

---

* In that excellent periodical, "The Indian Annals of Medical Science," will be found (vol. i.) admirable Remarks on Hill Diarrhœa and Dysentery, by Mr. Alexander Grant, of the Bengal army, to which I would refer the reader who desires to be informed on this subject, and on the influence of the climates of the "Himalayan Sanataria" generally.

tissues of the body; the anæmic ulcerations (chronic aphthæ) of the mucous digestive surface; and all the attendant difficulties and dangers, so as to call into trying exercise the toilsome and difficult requirements of the physician.

In his admirable " Remarks," Mr. Grant characterizes the Hill Diarrhœa and Dysentery as "peculiar and often inveterate" forms of disease; and he does not hesitate to pronounce them " endemic of the group of Hill Sanataria that includes Kussoula, Simlah, Sabathoo, and the new station of Dugshai." Mr. Grant states that it is this " peculiar class of diseases which occasions nearly all the mortality, and has, in some instances, been a serious source of inefficiency and loss to regiments for years after their return to the plains." He adds, however, as deserving of particular notice, that "no healthy corps has as yet been sent to any of the Hill Stations: on the contrary, almost all the regiments were in an inefficient condition—the constitutions of the men being more or less broken down, or tainted with malaria, and numbers of them suffering from intermittent fever and its sequelæ, enlarged liver and spleen." These facts corroborate in the strongest manner my early observations on the climates of the mountain stations hitherto occupied by British troops in the East Indies;—namely, that they may be made of the utmost and most extended value in PRESERVING THE SOLDIER'S HEALTH, but that for the cure of his diseases, contracted in the hot and pestilential plains, they are of very subordinate value.

As an example of diarrhœa very formidable in its nature, and of very frequent occurrence, I adduce the following:—

Colonel ——, aged sixty-three, served forty-three years in India, where during many years he enjoyed an average share of good health. In 1840 he came home intending to resign the service, being possessed of a competent fortune; but the call made by the Indian government in 1842, on all military officers then on furlough to return to their duty in India in consequence of the disaster at Cabul, induced Col. ——, out of pure military zeal, to proceed to join his corps, despite of a certificate from myself, and from the late Mr. Turner, to the effect that he was not fit to serve in India. An accomplished and distinguished officer, he was soon placed in positions of varied and important trust, and he served in the campaigns of the Sutlej in 1845-46, and in that of the Punjab in 1849.

Colonel —— had previously been twice on sick leave to England, and by the recent exposures and exertions he began again to feel the exhausting influences of severe and unremitting duty, as well as those of climate, when, in January, 1850, he was unfortunately induced to accept a mission into a malarious district. Here he was seized with an acute attack of intermittent fever, from which he recovered but slowly, and he arrived in Calcutta from the

N. W. provinces in April, 1850, weak and exhausted. The season and the opportunities for departure to England being considered unfavourable, Colonel —— was induced to remain in Bengal, making an occasional trip to sea; but the climate still proved inimical. In August, that being the height of the rainy season, he was seized with a wasting diarrhœa, which harassed him even after his embarkation for England, by the Cape route, in the end of January, 1851.

During a four months' voyage no improvement took place, notwithstanding the most prudent care in diet. He was, on the average, purged eight times every twenty-four hours after leaving Calcutta; and on reaching lat. 30° north, a great aggravation of purging, accompanied by vomiting, took place. The cold to which he had looked as a friendly and bracing agent, "penetrated into his bowels," as he described it, and he landed in the middle of May, 1851, at Torquay, in a state of great exhaustion. He passed a night at Exeter, during which he was purged twelve times, and from Clifton he wrote me :—" My nerves are dreadfully shattered ; indeed, at this instant, I am a sad wreck."

May 24th.—Visited Colonel —— on his arrival in London, when he presented me with a brief statement of his case from Mr. ——, of Calcutta, who died of fever a few days after the date of his addressing me. This was the second time within the year that the same melancholy circumstance had occurred to me; and in both instances the patients presented their letters in ignorance of the death of their medical friends.

The following are my notes of the present case :—

Colonel —— is reduced to the bones. The exterior appearance is completely blanched, the integument having a velvet-like character, while the mouth, throat, and conjunctivæ exhibit a better condition of the blood than could have been anticipated. It is my practice, in such cases, to evert the lower eyelid, and to examine the mouth and fauces, as affording the truest indices to the condition of the blood. The edges and tip of the tongue are red and irritable, but there are no aphthæ. The patient describes the evacuations as copious, thin, "and of that colour," pointing to a white marble chimney-piece. The abdomen is flabby and yielding in all its regions, and the liver is found on exploration to be smaller than natural. Pulse 72, jerking and irritable. There is, as he believes, a febrile movement about the full and change of the moon, which he says is perceptible only to himself, and it is always attended with aggravation of the diarrhœa. The urine first voided had a green hue, and being desirous to know whether it contained bile, I requested a friend, an eminent physician and chemist, to examine it. Next day he reported to me as follows :—" I consider it certain that your patient has Bright's disease in a very quiescent state, or else he is very near death. I am not sure of bile; it may be there in a small quantity." Colonel —— was treated with the vegetable and mineral astringents, conjoined with opium, with a view to restrain the discharges; he was directed to use a bland, unirritating diet, and to be very careful at all times to avoid quantity. By the 28th June the number of motions in the twenty-four hours had been thus reduced from six and eight to one, but the matter voided remained as colourless as ever. Two grains of mercury and chalk, with one of opium, were now given night and morning, with a view to elicit biliary secretion, over-action of the bowels being restrained by the use of astringents at the same time. In about twelve days this course of treatment produced the desired effect, the bowels becoming tranquil; the skin being now perspirable for the first time since he left India, and much desquamation of the cuticle having taken place under friction with the Indian hair glove, while the pulse, from being hard and jerking, became soft and natural.

By the 18th of July, when Col. —— left London for the country, the secretions had become quite natural in appearance; the appe-tite, digestive power, and strength having greatly improved. Within a month from his departure he wrote me :—" I have not, after the manner of snuff-takers, rapped at the lid of a pill-box since I saw you, and I am almost persuaded I advance in convalescence daily, and that I gain strength, at least I feel that I walk more at ease, as the pilgrim said who boiled his peas." But convalescence did not continue to advance at this rate. On the 4th of November he wrote—" I am tolerably well, but I have not quite attained the point I could wish. There are but few things I can do with impunity. Over-exercise prostrates me; a deviation in diet and beverages from strict regimen upsets me; and I cannot venture upon wine out of my own house, and then not daily, so that my customary strong drink is brandy-and-water. Pickles, preserves, and even honey disturb me. I have no pain or uneasiness of any kind, but just a sense of a delicate state of the stomach and bowels. It is most sensible about the pit of the stomach—that is, the lower orifice of the stomach, on indulging in any kinds of acids. I take only two meals daily—a full though plain breakfast at half-past eight, and a spare dinner at five." Referring to the distressing irritability of temper so common in cases of this nature, Col. —— says :—" Whilst I was nervous, wayward, and irritable, it was a great relief to me to sit down and pen a few lines to a friend or re-lative. Now, however, that I have become composed, and some-what settled and at ease, it is an effort to me to place myself before a writing-desk, and forego the pleasure of whiling my time with books or wandering about."

In the beginning of December, Col. —— came to London on private business, when I was glad to find him of quite his ordinary appearance of condition and of health. The bowels now acted but once in twenty-four hours, and the secretions were healthy. Being desirous to know the state of the urine, I had it again examined by my friend, Dr. ——, who was so kind as to send me the following very satisfactory report:—" I find nothing excepting the excess of urate of ammonia, and possibly the very slightest trace of albumen. But I am not sure of this, there is so little present." Col. —— returned immediately to the country, where he was directed to use the fluid extract of Bael, with a view to give tone to the stomach and bowels.

On the 26th January, 1852, the Colonel writes :—" Some time ago, owing to imprudent exposure and very cold feet, my bowels became affected. As they did not of themselves return to their natural state, I had recourse to the Bael. For a day or two I took a dessert-spoonful three times a day. Thinking this too much, I reduced the quantity to twice a day. The taste was rather mawkish at first, but afterwards became agreeable. It has produced the beneficial effect of removing the laxity of the bowels. My appetite is much better than it was before I had this slight return of complaint, and I can venture on both beverage and diet that I dared not touch previously."

This gentleman is now (October, 1852,) quite well as regards diarrhœa, but is affected with chronic gout in the hands as an hereditary complaint.

Remarks.—Colonel ——'s case affords a good illustration of the fact that chronic diarrhœa of the most formidable character may, and often does, depend on suspended function of the liver. The danger of the case, also, was extreme; and I believe that, but for the action of mercury, this valuable and accomplished officer must have died; indeed, he very nearly died on landing in England. This kind of diarrhœa, like some forms of ague, cannot be cured without mercury, or without nitro-muriatic acid, the action of which is similar; but the latter requires time to establish its influence, and here we had none to spare, the danger being imminent. Referring to the gradual subsidence of albumen in the urine, I may here mention that in several instances in which diseased states of the liver or spleen, or of both, existed, I have found albumen in the urine as a functional affection, and it always disappeared on the restoration of health; in other words, on the removal of the visceral affections.

Astringents, it will be observed, were of no radical avail in this instance, nor was anything more expected from their use than to arrest excessive serous discharges, and thus obtain time for the introduction of the appropriate remedy, which in event proved radical of cure.

In the next case a wasting diarrhœa was associated with a great enlargement of the liver of many years' standing.

—— Esq., originally of a powerful constitution, but a *bon vivant*, had resided twenty-seven years in India; and till August, 1840, had enjoyed good health. At this time, torpor of the liver, with distressing dyspepsia, harassed him, and these disorders were speedily followed by diarrhœa. "Mercurials had always removed these symptoms for a time, but they invariably returned after a few days. Slight ptyalism had been induced, but without rendering convalescence in the least degree more satisfactory."

Mr. —— sailed for the Cape of Good Hope in January, 1841, and returned to Bombay in January, 1842. At the Cape he had been treated with "direct astringents, in various forms and of various kinds," but change of climate and medical treatment left him much altered for the worse, being greatly attenuated, with considerable œdema of the lower extremities—the discharges from the bowels being "copious, frequent, watery, and of a light buff colour." Alteratives and astringents, with opium, having failed of doing any good, Mr. —— was sent to England in the end of 1842.

Here he consulted the late Dr. James Johnson; but though receiving benefit from treatment, he has never, during more than six years, passed a day without astringent and opiate medicine. He was therefore compelled to resign the service.

In April, 1849, I found Mr. —— worn to the bones with diarrhœa, and with an immense enlargement of the liver. Dr. M'Lennan, from whose experienced and able direction the patient had derived much benefit while in India, being now in England, I felt desirous to have the advantage of his concurrence in the treatment by the nitro-muriatic acid bath, by immersion of the whole body. Dr. M'Lennan writes:—"When I first saw him the whole appearance was so cachæmic as fully to bear out the description of one of his friends, that he was dropping into his grave; or, to use the very words of another friend, that he seemed like one who had been interred and exhumed again." He was emaciated to a great degree, with cheeks and eyes sunken, voice hollow, and debility so great, that I fully expected from that cause to find the presence of anasarca or ascites;—the former only was present to a slight degree. His complexion was of an ashy colour, deeply tinged with green; skin yellow, dry, and harsh; digestion greatly impaired; appetite gone. Bowels harassed by incessant purging, which was only kept in check by vegetable and mineral astringents, aided by large doses of opium. The liver extended from the seventh to considerably below the margin of the false ribs, particularly in front.

In this state he commenced the use of the nitro-muriatic acid bath to the whole body—i.e., to the trunk and extremities; and by a steady perseverance therein for several months, he very greatly improved. The enlargement of the liver steadily and progressively decreased; fulness and weight of the body increased; complexion became clear, and at length even pinkish; skin soft, of natural colour, and perspirable. Subcutaneous veins showed the presence of blood in sufficient quantity. He became cheerful and even active;

and in this state of improvement embarked for Malta, whence I have just heard from him to the following effect:—" I have been examined thoroughly by my medical man, and he says all enlargement of the liver has disappeared, and that my secretions are in every respect natural and healthy. I am increased considerably in size, and have got a plump rosy face, such as I have not had for these many years past."

"There can be no question," adds Dr. M'Lennan, "that in this case the improvement was solely attributable to the bath; for the other medicines taken were palliatives to arrest the course of the ingesta, for such time as to afford opportunity for some nutriment to be given to the system; and one of them at least, the opium, was antagonistic of improvement of the secretion, and thus of the hepatic recovery."

Remarks.—Whether we consider the duration of disease in this instance, or the severity of the symptoms, the case is remarkable, as proving the remedial powers of the nitro-muriatic acid. When the patient first came under its influence, he was all that Dr. M'Lennan describes him—a man in an apparently hopeless state of exhaustion. Beyond six feet in height, and largely proportioned, he weighed but ten stone two pounds. In six months his weight had increased to twelve stone seven pounds; and when he last wrote to me, he said "that he was still getting stouter." The rapid improvement in the condition of the blood was no less convincing. Here, also, as observed by Dr. M'Lennan, the counteracting astringent influences of opium were overcome by the superior emulgent power of the acids. In this respect their eliminating actions are shown to be superior to those of any other medicine, mercurials not excepted; but, as often stated in the present Essays, these last mineral preparations were contraindicated, owing to the cachectic state of the patient's constitution. In this interesting case the nitro-muriatic acid removed the diarrhœa, by reducing the hepatic enlargement and restoring the integrity of the functions of the liver.

Recurring now to the general subject, I may observe that the pathology of chronic diarrhœa, whether simple or complicated, is but ill-understood. Sir James Annesley states that where chronic diarrhœa and dysentery were, during life, associated with organic disease of the liver, this last was usually found " of a slow nature, and most frequently implicating the internal structure of the viscus;" while Mr. Twining, in his *post-mortem* examination of such cases, found " the liver of a grayish colour, occasionally approaching to drab; its size decreased; its structure soft and friable, but tough; and when cut, the section was almost bloodless, unless some of the veins were divided." Here we perceive an anæmic state of the liver.

Chronic dysentery is, in all cases, the result of an inflammation, more or less extensive, of the mucous surface of the large intestine, with ulceration, more or less extensive, of this texture, and of the solitary glands, frequently associated with inflammatory and congestive states of the liver, spleen, and other abdominal organs; whereas chronic diarrhœa generally, as it is seen in the cases of Indian officers on their return to Europe, presents no appreciable inflammation of any portion of the mucous digestive surfaces; indeed, when diarrhœa has existed for any length of time, we find an opposite state of the general system, and of the bowels, to that of inflammation—an atony of the system, and consequent atony of the digestive functions, and a specially atonic condition of the discharges from the whole of the secreting organs of the abdomen, including those of the mucous membranes. The brain and nervous centres are likewise in a state of complete anæmia. These circumstances have not been sufficiently considered either in the pathology or in the treatment of the disease.

I have observed, both in India and in England, that a very severe form of chronic diarrhœa frequently followed upon intermittent forms of malarious fever, and it was found in the general hospital of Calcutta, that amongst the European soldiers who had served in China, the diarrhœa, which was then always a sequel to the agues of the country, proved very generally fatal. Out of one detachment of twenty-eight cases of chronic diarrhœa admitted into the above-mentioned hospital from China, and of whose cases I have received reports, twenty-five men were noted as having previously suffered from intermittent fever, and eleven men were noted as suffering from pain in the epigastric region, and that of the liver. These poor soldiers were in the last stages of chronic diarrhœa of the worst kind, and but few of them could have survived to reach their native country, fourteen out of the twenty-eight admitted into the Calcutta General Hospital having died there; in truth, their complicated state of disease left little or no chance of recovery.

The following *post-mortem* appearances are recorded in the hospital reports :—Excessive emaciation of the whole body ; anasarca more or less general ; serous effusion occasionally found in the cavities of the pleura and pericardium; a flaccid, flabby state of the heart; omentum " perfectly transparent, without a particle of fat ;" in other cases, " omentum absorbed and shrivelled up ;" pylorus and commencement of the duodenum abraded and granular; "pancreas hard and gritty;" the liver large, soft, and flabby, sometimes blue, together with occasional enlargement of the spleen, this organ being " softened like grumous blood," while in other cases it was " small and indurated." A pale, attenuated, " diaphanous" condition of the small intestines was generally observed; cæcum frequently ulcerated and thickened, exhibiting marks of former disease; colon sometimes attenuated, but more generally thickened, occasionally " cartilaginous," its mucous membrane being often found ulcerated in many places ; mesenteric glands generally much enlarged, mesentery sometimes containing calcareous deposits " as large as peas."

If we refer to European writers for a more intimate pathology of this chronic form of diarrhœa, our knowledge is but little extended. But however defective our appreciation of the more intimate and essential lesions observable after death in the liver, stomach, intestines, spleen, and mesentery, there is abundant evidence during life that, added to other morbid conditions, the circulating fluid is depraved, and that consequently there is a depravation of all the secretions and excretions of the body. I have known instances of chronic diarrhœa which ensued upon large losses of blood, as in the parturient state; and also from superlactation, in the case of a lady who nursed twins. Both instances occurred in persons of a previously constipated habit. These circumstances of depravation of the blood, together with an irritated and an occasionally ulcerated state of the mucous membrane of the bowels, and also an irritated and perverted state of the nervous functions, constitute important and appreciable characteristics of chronic diarrhœa. To the contamination of the blood caused by visceral disease, and the consequent passive venous congestions within the abdomen, we have superadded occasional congestion of the mucous membrane of the bowels, and an imperfect performance of the assimilative and depurative functions. Altogether this is a dangerous and often an intractable disease.

Such patients are rarely allowed to die in India, a change to sea, or to Europe, being sought long before the advent of imminent danger. But with all the dangers confessedly attendant upon chronic diarrhœa, it is surprising how some cases, apparently hopeless in their nature, will recover in England; and those, on the other hand, who ultimately sink from the disease pass their last days with their families, out of notice of the medical men who originally treated them on their arrival at home. This is the explanation why Dr. Baillie had never seen a *post-mortem* examination of this kind. Since my return to England I have witnessed several deaths from this disease, opportunity for examination of the body having been allowed in eight instances.

There can be no doubt, I think, from many of the symptoms presented to us during the treatment of the cases here contemplated, that in a large proportion of those who recover, the mucous surfaces have been throughout in the blanched and anæmic condition mentioned by some authors who have had opportunities of making *post-mortem* examinations, and that the mucous follicles were enlarged, patulous, and excoriated or ulcerated. When to these states of disease we have so often superadded the antecedents of structural alterations, or severe disorders of the liver, or enlargements of the spleen and mesentery—all inducing general anæmia—it must be evident that the case is one of a grave character. It is, in fact, in many instances, but the last inevitable stage, or symptom, in the progress of complicated tropical disease. The great emaciation in many cases warns us at once of the impending danger, and of the injuries, more or less irreparable, done to the mucous structures and their glands.

Anæmia in its most aggravated form exists as the result, but certainly as the concomitant also of nearly all chronic diarrhœas of tropical invalids; and this attenuated and depraved state of the blood, and of all the secretions derived from it, tends greatly to keep up diarrhœa—the serum of the blood appearing to transude through the intestine. The enormous fluid discharges passed from the bowels are here referable not alone to the softened condition of the mucous membranes and follicles, but also to the absence of natural absorption, and to the impairment or suppression of the bile-secreting function of the liver. This is what has been termed the "*sweating of the bowels.*" The diminution of the general mass of the blood, and its depravation in quality, must also produce an anæmic condition of the mucous membrane of the bowels, with occasional gelatinous softening of its texture, either or both of which conditions offer serious impediments to our curative endeavours,—impediments often increased by hepatic and other complications. In the instance of an officer of the Indian army, who had been brought to the verge of the grave by diarrhœa of long standing, recovery appeared to be materially promoted by his living in the open air during summer and autumn. Could we in these cases impart oxygen to the blood, and thus impart to that fluid more life and consistency, we should, I think, assist the cure in a very material degree; and I make it an invariable rule with all such patients that they occupy a chair or couch, during temperate weather, in the open air, taking care that they are well-clothed at the same time. Where, as here, the blood-forming processes are suspended; where spanæmia is superadded to the existing anæmia, no means should be neglected which can tend to vivify the circulating fluid.

In considering the best means of cure, it is absolutely necessary—first, to ascertain minutely the previous states of health and the habits of the patient; and, secondly, whether the diarrhœa be simple in its nature, or associated with hepatic or splenic disease. Along with these considerations, a careful examination of the matters voided is always requisite. Much will depend on the judgment and care given to these preliminaries, for much of the perplexity, differences of opinion and of practice, result from inattention to them. But of all the difficulties encountered in the treatment of chronic diarrhœa, one of the greatest is that which relates to the due regulation of the diet, especially when the patient is of the male sex. In this most simple and all-important matter it is truly astonishing how unreasonable and unreasoning we often find the most able and excellent men. With females I have rarely known much difficulty, on the contrary; while with men I have often noticed a morbid craving amounting to fatal infatuation, requiring the active and vigilant guidance of others to counteract; for here the mind is greatly enfeebled, the power of self-control lost. In these unhappy instances men may in truth be said to "pepper themselves into appetite, that they may eat and drink and die." The climax of devotion to the luxuries of the table, related of an old Indian, is believed to be suppositious; but, however this may be, it is characteristic of certain individuals everywhere to be seen:—"True, I have lost my health in India, my liver is gone, and I have nothing before me but a few years of suffering; but I have eaten mango fish." This would realize the picture of Hogarth's voluptuary, who dies with an oyster on his fork. The state of the mind in these unhappy cases amounts indeed at times to complete insanity on matters relating to diet, while in others we perceive the most uncontrollable irritability and morbid sensitiveness about the merest domestic trifles. I have known men of the most amiable and placable disposition to fly into a fury of rage, and to threaten their wives with everything short of personal violence and ill-treatment, when they have ventured the gentlest remonstrance against irregularities at table. The circumstances of the death by chronic diarrhœa, at the Cape of Good Hope, of a gentleman whom I had known well in India, were related to me by a common friend; and one of these was that up to the last day of existence the deceased continued to eat enormously of everything which he could bribe his servants to procure. He actually concealed mutton-pies under his bed-pillows, where they were found after death! A gentleman from India, naturally of a good temper, but afflicted with chronic diarrhœa, got into a paroxysm of rage with his native valet, and the result was apoplexy, and consequent incurable hemiplegia. It would seem that in these cases the morbid sensibility of the organic system of nerves supplying the mucous surfaces extended by irritation to the brain, and this the more readily in persons from India, in whom the previous exaltation of the nervous function within the tropics, coupled as that often is with anæmia, may render them more liable to such dangerous sympathies and complications.

I have known two persons who, on discontinuing the use of opium, fell into an epileptic condition. The first was a surgeon of the Indian army, who, for a time, conducted his own treatment; the other was a distinguished general, who had been treated with opiates for the cure of his diarrhœa on the voyage homewards by the Cape of Good Hope.

I am anxious to impress the fact that, in the disease now under consideration, the first step in the treatment is the enforcement of the strictest rule of diet, for without that all else is useless. This rule of rigid strictness applies to all stages of diarrhœa, and so satisfied am I of its justice, that I believe most cases of the disease, in India, of the simple and uncomplicated nature, would require but little treatment, other than rigid abstemiousness, provided it were applied at the very commencement of the disease. But, in the instances of tropical invalids on their return to Europe, we are necessarily called to the treatment when the diarrhœa has existed long and made great progress; and even here how often do we see patients sliding into their graves through their own negligence, or that of relatives, whom we feel assured that we might save if they could but be placed within the systematic control of an hospital? It is here no paradox to say that the less we put into the stomach the more it will digest.

In matters that relate to the conduct of the patient the circumstance next in importance to rigid care in diet is attention to the clothing, and the avoidance of all active exercise; and here his sensations and wants will generally be found on the side of safety. The sufferer should be incased in flannel in all weathers, sometimes with the addition of a silk or chamois leather covering, and a double layer of flannel should invariably cover the abdomen, the apartments being maintained of a high and equable warmth, especially in the winter season. In every form and variety of chronic diarrhœa, warm baths, used occasionally at bed-time, will be found of much service; indeed, every means which determine to the surface of the body is most efficacious. In the instance of two officers under my care, who contracted diarrhœa in England, and who were forced to return to India when but half-cured, I predicted that the equable determination to the skin, resulting from external heat in India, would restore their healths, and so it proved in both cases.

In determining the strictly medical treatment of chronic diarrhœa we ought to be guided by our knowledge of its nature and cause, for without this our measures are apt to become variable and uncertain in their aim and result. For practical purposes we shall do well to ascertain, by the most careful and minute examination whether the disease be confined to the mucous membrane of the bowel, or whether, with or without anatomical changes in the intestine, there be disordered function, or actual disease, in the liver. This is indeed a matter of the first importance, as regards the selection of remedies and the safety of the patient. Where the case is mild, simple, and uncomplicated in its nature; that is, confined to the mucous surfaces, we shall find it advantageous to begin our treatment by means calculated to allay general irritability and irritation of the mucous membranes. For these purposes the combination of mild opiates with alkalies will be found both grateful and useful. I sometimes found the liquor taraxaci, with soda or potash, and a sufficiency of opium to restrain over-action of the bowels, very beneficial; while, in other instances, the cretaceous preparations, combined with astringents and sudorifics, with opium in larger proportions, and with aromatics, succeed better. In this, as in other morbid affections where acidity and rancidity of the stomach and bowels are so liable to exist together, it is remarkable how often we find the mineral acids fulfil all the indications ordinarily accomplished by alkalies. So much is this the case that nothing but observation and experience can enable us to decide on the remedy most suitable to each case.

While these means are being used, it is generally necessary at the same time to repress excessive secretion from, and excessive action of, the bowels; and here the mineral and vegetable astringents are most powerful towards the cure, combined, as above recommended, with more or less opium, according to the urgency of the symptoms. The sulphates of copper, of iron, and of quina, combined with opium; the nitrate and oxide of silver, alone, or with opium in the form of pill, in solution, with nitric acid and laudanum; the nitric and nitro-muriatic acids, the solution of pernitrate of iron, the sulphuric acid, acetate of lead, bismuth, kino, catechu, krameria, simaruba, hæmatoxylon, tannic and gallic acids, nux-vomica, when combined with opium or with Dover's powder, will each in its place be found of value in the cure of chronic diarrhœa in its simple form. Independently of its calming and constringing influences, opium has another valuable effect;—it obtunds the voracious appetite so common to this disease.

The value of lead, in my experience, has proved superior to all other minerals; and cases wearing the most mournful aspect have been brought to a happy conclusion by its means. In several such cases I have given lead up to the point of inducing lead colic; and from that moment convalescence has set in.

Much of the indiscriminate disparagement thrown by some authors on the mineral and vegetable astringents has arisen, I think, from exclusive views respecting the pathology and consequent treatment of chronic diarrhœa, the pathology being too exclusively hepatic, and the treatment too exclusively mercurial; for there are cases of chronic diarrhœa in which mercury proves extremely mischievous, and others in which this mineral, or else the nitro-muriatic acid bath, will be found the chief or only means of cure. Astringents, again, even where they cannot cure, are of great use by moderating or arresting serous discharges, thus saving the powers of the constitution, and giving time for assimilation and for the operation of the more special remedies, such, for instance, as address themselves to diseased states of the liver, in diarrhœa with hepatic complication. Where the seat of diarrhœa is confined to the mucous intestinal surfaces, astringents and tonics are indeed the chief remedies proper to the case, aided by a well-regulated diet. When, by restraining serous discharges from the bowels, through the constringing influence of the proper mineral or vegetable astringent, we see the number of evacuations reduced to one or two formed motions in the twenty-four hours, instead of ten or twelve fluid discharges, while the patient regains flesh and strength apace, we are surely warranted in believing that the means are tending to the end.* I have, in fact, seen very many cases wearing the most hopeless aspect conducted to safety by the persistent use of astringents, often varied, but never discontinued, until the favourable result was assured. This circumstance I would urge on the attention of the inexperienced ; for I have often seen that both patient and physician, wearied, the one by protracted suffering, the other despairing of success, have felt disposed "to leave the case to nature," a fatal alternative in chronic diarrhœa.

The operation and power of astringents with opiates in conducing towards the cure of chronic diarrhœa are not rightly understood. In default of such combination, perseveringly used, diarrhœa goes on to a destructive extent—nutrition is reduced to nothing, the blood becoming poorer and thinner—until at length the patient voids only serum and the undigested irritating aliment : he is thus literally drained of nutrition, and scoured into his grave. Through the simple tonic action of astringents and opiates, strenuously persevered in, the irritable patulous condition of the mucous membrane is exchanged for constriction and tone ; and time—an important element in the treatment of all forms of chronic disease—is gained ; and thus cases apparently beyond cure eventually recover ; or they are thus prepared for the reception and benefit of other means which were at first inapplicable. The patient must indeed be perseveringly encouraged in this course of firmness in steady treatment, and be taught that constipation, even to a painful extent, is health to him ; otherwise he may be induced, through ignorance, despondency, or impatience, to abandon the only course which can save his life. We must, in short, do all in our power to bring the patient to tide over the disease.

Where marked periodicity occurs, I have long been in the habit

---

* Dr. W. Lemprière, physician to the army depôt, and who had served in the West Indies, in his report on the Aluminous Chalybeate Spring at Sandrock, Isle of Wight, 1812, states that he has used the chalybeate and astringent in chronic dysentery and diarrhœa, in general debility, especially in the cases of invalids from tropical climates, in hypochondriasis and dyspepsia, and it was used by Dr. William Saunders, of London, and others, in uterine and vaginal discharges. Dr. Lemprière exhibited this water also as a tonic and chalybeate to numerous soldiers from Walcheren, suffering from anæmia and visceral congestions, with marked and beneficial results. In the cases of soldiers from Trinidad, prostrated by aggravated malarious anæmia, with dropsical effusions, this same water effected a cure where all previous means had failed. "It should be understood," says this officer, "that iron, under its various preparations, not only increases the tone of the muscular fibre, but also the action of the circulating vessels, even to their remotest ramifications, and that when combined with alum, as is the case with the Sandrock water, this property is very considerably augmented."

In the fashion for continental waters I have no doubt that many of the valuable properties, and much of the important results, of our home waters have been overlooked by the profession, and consequently by the public. A water that should combine at once astringency with good chalybeate properties, is a desideratum in the cases of many of the greatest sufferers from tropical diseases.

of adding quinine to astringents and opiates, or to astringents with Dover's powder.

Astringents, in certain appropriate cases, constringe the relaxed vessels and mucous surfaces, and heal the aphthous ulcerations of these structures, in much the same manner, and apparently as efficaciously, as when applied in similar states of the mouth and fauces in the infant, provided always (I would repeat over and over again) that the diet be carefully regulated. The same may emphatically be said of the mineral acids. I have no doubt that the nitric acid, for instance, given freely with opiates, has a most beneficial effect on irritable and on ulcerated mucous surfaces; and there seems no reason to question that similar benefits result from the free use of the sub-acid fruits.

We endeavour, by such means, to restrain the morbid action of the bowels, which hurries the half-digested or undigested aliment through the duodenum, by the various astringents aided by opium. We thus obtain time for the process of nutrition; while, by the use of the mildest alteratives, and by tonics, we elicit the natural actions of the liver and bowels, and restore the activity of the absorbent functions. By these means, and by a light and appropriate diet, we conduce to the cure of the disease, and restrain the waste of the tissues.

A gentleman who had resided long in India suffered from severe diarrhœa on his return to England, first in the winter of 1842, and secondly, in the winter of 1846. On both occasions the discharges were fluid and enormous in amount and frequency, the entire mouth and fauces being one mass of aphthous ulceration. Alkalies with opiates were used night and morning, while three or four doses were given during the day of the compound powder of kino and ipecacuanha, with a grain of sulphate of iron, and one-fourth of a grain of sulphate of copper. The recovery was in both instances complete and rapid; but had the liver been diseased, the medicines here exhibited would have proved but palliative.

When structural disease of the liver exists, or when its function is defective or depraved, provided anæmia be not excessive, mercury in minute doses, conjoined with opium or Dover's powder, will be found valuable towards the cure. The anæmic condition of the system may, however, preclude the use of mercury, or it may cause mercury to disagree; and this last is more likely to occur when aphthæ are present. Under such untoward circumstances I am in the habit of prescribing the internal use of nitric acid, with or without the infusion of simaruba, and shielded by opium. Where an immediate and powerful effect on the function of the liver is desired, I use the nitro-muriatic acid in the form of a bath, as detailed in a subsequent essay. "The sulphuric, nitro-muriatic, and other acids," says Dr. Billing, "have been recommended by many experienced practitioners in fevers as well as for gargles; and I may observe that their utility, when applied to the mucous membrane

Y Y

within view, as in the fauces, will explain the efficacy of the vegetable or mineral lemonades in relieving the tenesmus, griping,
nausea, &c., of bilious diarrhœa, more quickly in the first instance
than opiates alone, as they not merely constringe and relieve the
congested or inflamed capillaries of the mucous membrane, but
help to wash away the acrid bile."
. But in this capricious disease, so difficult of cure, the mineral
acids may in their turn prove ineffective. We shall then do well
to have recourse to the vegetable acids, which often exercise a signal
power over chronic diarrhœa and dysentery. The subacid fruits
have long been used in such cases in the south of Europe, in the
East and West Indies, and the grapes of the Cape of Good Hope,
where the husk is swallowed as well as the fruit, have during many
years been celebrated for their efficacy in the chronic bowel disorders of the numerous invalids who annually resort to that colony
from the Indian presidencies.

"The prejudice," says Tissot, "against fruits in dysentery is
erroneous and pernicious." He adds :—" Ripe fruits of every sort,
but particularly summer fruits, are a preservative against this
disease." This writer then states that a Swiss regiment in the
south of France being attacked with the dysentery, " the officers
purchased the produce of several acres of a vineyard, and gave the
soldiers the grapes, which cured all those that were ill, and prevented any of the others from being attacked." Curtis states of
the European hospitals of Madras, in 1782-83, that the medical
officers never forbade the use of fruits in the chronic stages of dysentery and diarrhœa, and especially of such fruits as were astringents, as the mango, guava, and pomegranate, and a portion of
the rind was always directed to be eaten along with them, doubtless with the view to include the astringent property, tannin, contained in the rind, along with the acid of these fruits. Curtis adds,
that when personally as reduced by chronic bowel complaint " as
ever any European in India, the first turn towards recovery was
found by him at the hospitable tables of Vizagapatam, where all
the tropical fruits were in plenty." They were, he says, " grateful
and useful antiseptics."

Within these few years the Bale, or Bael fruit of Bengal, has
been held to be very efficacious in the treatment of chronic dysentery and diarrhœa. This fruit, incorrectly termed the Bengal
quince, for in reality it is of the orange tribe, is imported into
England in its unripe dried state, and, also, in the state of sugared
preserve made of the ripe fruit. The bark of the root, and the
stems of the fresh leaves, are all said to contain medicinal properties. " As to the Bael fruit," says a professional friend in Calcutta,
" I consider it the most certain remedy we possess for chronic
dysentery and diarrhœa. I have frequently seen it arrest the progress of these diseases in twenty-four hours, after all other medical
treatment had failed. On what the curative property of the fruit

depends I know not ; it is certainly not astringent to the taste, or, at all events, very slightly so. I am inclined to believe that much of its efficacy may reside in the thick mucilage which surrounds the seeds of the fruit. A singular property of the fruit is this, that it does not merely restrain undue action of the bowels, as in diarrhœa and dysentery, but also in cases of obstinate habitual constipation acts as a mild and certain laxative. It may be said in all cases to regulate the bowels." On the other hand, another brother officer and friend, who went from Calcutta to Egypt, suffering from chronic dysentery, writes me :—" The figs and grapes of Egypt have done more for me than ever the Bael fruit of Bengal ;" but here, doubtless, the climate of Egypt proved a powerful agent in aid of the fruits, which are everywhere confessedly beneficial in such cases.

I am indebted to Mr. Henry Pollock for the following account of his examination of the preserved ripe fruit, as imported in its dried and preserved forms from Calcutta, by several of our best chemists :—" The pulp and the dried shell of the fruit do not appear to me to differ chemically in any respect, except as to quantity. They both contain—1, tannic acid ; 2, a concrete essential oil ; 3, a bitter principle, which is not precipitated by tribasic acetate of lead, and a vegetable acid. The pulp, as I received it, also contained a considerable quantity of sugar, in which it was preserved. All three of the substances I have mentioned exist in the largest quantity in the dry rind. There is most acid in the pulp."

A practical chemist has stated to me that in the fruit, as imported by him, the mucilage exists in about the proportion of twenty per cent.

Galen is said to have represented the practice of his art as a conflict in which three parties are engaged—the patient, the disease, and the physician. The best state of things is when the patient and doctor are leagued against the complaint; the worst when the complaint and the doctor are in a confederacy against the patient. But this description overlooks the very frequent instances in which the patient and the disease are in conspiracy against the physician; and I know of no example in which so unnatural a league proves so certainly fatal to the subject. When the patient will eat voraciously he conspires against himself: he defeats the doctor, assuredly, but kills himself at the same time.

The preceding observations contain all that appears to the writer to be necessary towards establishing the principles of treatment in the chronic diarrhœa of tropical invalids. But as each individual case will present its special peculiarities, so it will require, also, special modifications of remedies in its treatment. I proceed now to another branch of this interesting subject.

The following cases are here presented with a view to illustrate the pathology of chronic diarrhœa :—

CASE I.—Mrs. ——, the subject of the following case, was seen by me about six weeks previously to her death. She was twenty-nine years of age, and had resided seven years in India. Very soon after her arrival there, she was seized with intermittent fever, which disordered her health, disturbing the functions of the stomach and bowels especially. She married in her fifth year of residence, and had then no ailment, other than an irregular state of the bowels, which were alternately constipated and relaxed.

Soon after marriage she went into a district of a very jungly and malarious character, and there her intermittent fever recurred with diarrhœa. She miscarried in the fifth month of her first gestation. From this time ague and diarrhœa never left her; and after contending with both during nearly two years, she was sent home, and arrived in England eighteen months ago. She was visited by several of the most able physicians of this country, and resorted to many of the provincial towns both for advice and change of air, but in all respects her disease became worse than ever, and her emaciation extreme. There was now severe diarrhœa, with feverishness towards evening, and cold, clammy sweat towards three A.M.; the liver was much enlarged; but, with the exception of a good deal of mucus, occasionally streaked with blood, the appearance of the intestinal discharges was natural. There was a sufficient appearance of bile. I suggested my suspicion that chronic abscess existed in the liver. No treatment afforded relief, and the patient died in six weeks.

For the following statement I am indebted to her able and attentive medical attendant, Mr. J. H. Hutchins, of Trinity Square, Tower Hill:—

" External appearances:—The body much emaciated; the cuticle of a pale lemon colour, and some slight bulging noticeable of the ribs on the right side. Thorax: The cavity very small, the diaphragm being high up, reaching to the fourth rib on the right side, the enormous size of the liver having encroached upon the usual position of the lungs and heart. The lungs were collapsed, crepitant, and healthy in structure, but pale and almost bloodless. There were no tubercles in the apices; the heart very small, and almost bloodless: its walls thin, and without any coagulable blood. Abdomen: The peritoneum slightly thickened, containing about six ounces of serum. Directly it was divided, the liver came into view, stretching four inches below the margin of the ribs, the entire right lobe adhering to their edges, and having two-thirds of its structure merging into a large abscess, containing two pints of purulent matter. This was protected by a firm sac, formed by adhesions of the peritonæum, which was entire. The remaining portion of the right lobe was much increased in weight and bulk, and its texture was very soft. The spleen was pale and soft; kidneys small and healthy; the stomach having slight patches of a dark colour, especially the mucous membrane. The intestines had slight patches of inflammatory appearance on their peritonæal surface; the large, especially the cæcum, having some plastic lymph on its exterior surface, the colon and rectum abounding with ulcerations on their mucous coats. The gall-bladder was empty; the mesenteric glands free from tubercle or other disease."

Remarks.—The conduct of this lady, under great and protracted suffering, excited the anxious interest of every one who approached her. She expressed " a wish that her remains should be examined," it is believed from a desire that her husband in India might know the actual cause of her death. The case itself is remarkable, as illustrating the pathology of chronic diarrhœa, in which, I believe, chronic abscess of the liver to be a not infrequent cause of death. Here I venture to conclude, that the hepatic abscess was of about two years' existence; in other words, that it had been formed in India, and had existed during twenty months of residence in England. The anæmic condition was adverse to all progress in the abscess, and the "firm sac" was all that nature was capable of performing in its conservative endeavour to bring about absorption.

CASE II.—The subject of the following notice survived but nine days from his landing in England, and his case, like the preceding, is placed in the front rank, in order to exhibit the pathology of the disease under consideration. ——, Esq., aged forty-six, resided twenty-eight years in India, eighteen of which were passed at sea, and the rest in Calcutta, in mercantile business. He states that in 1826 he suffered from a severe dysentery of Bengal, from which his convalescence was but slow, the bowels being irregular, sometimes constipated, and at other times loose, for a long time afterwards; but looseness ultimately became the dominant condition. Twelve years ago he had a severe attack of diarrhœa, and four years ago he suffered from a still more severe attack, after which he made a voyage to the Isle of France for the recovery of his health. For two years after his return to Bengal from this last-mentioned voyage, his health remained comparatively good; but in July, 1850, he was seized with the remittent fever of Bengal, since which his general health gradually declined, while the bowels became much relaxed, accompanied by extreme prostration of strength and anæmic giddiness. He struggled on for months, in the vain hope that a once powerful constitution would serve him; but tropical disease pays no respect to European vigour of body, and he was in the end constrained to come home.

He is now (August 23rd, 1851) in the last stage of emaciation and exhaustion from chronic diarrhœa. The entire skin is of a dirty mahogany colour, dry, and cold; the tongue is pale and bloodless, with ulcerated edges; the pulse extremely feeble and slow. The erect posture occasions faintness, and for months he has had increasing deafness. The intestinal discharges are frequent, copious, serous, and yellow-coloured, apparently well tinged with bile; no mucus or blood. There is no enlargement of the spleen or liver; the urine is natural. It is needless to detail the attempts at relief, for all such failed of any real benefit, and the patient expired, as stated, on the ninth day from his landing at Southampton.

From Mr. Newberry, the medical gentleman in attendance on the family, and whom I met in consultation on this case, I received the following statement of *post-mortem* appearances :—" Nothing abnormal in the thoracic viscera. In the abdomen the stomach and duodenum were healthy; jejunum in patches, highly vascular, but no ulceration in the mucous coat. In the lower part of the ileum the peritoneal coat was studded with ash-coloured spots, and in parts highly congested, the internal coat being of a chocolate colour, and in many places deeply ulcerated, but this was more particularly the case in the colon. In the descending portion of the colon there appeared to be old disease; the coats were much thickened, and for about three inches the calibre was not more than that of the small intestines, with numerous ulcerations. There was a large quantity of mucus secreted, and the follicles appeared much elongated, in many places containing pus. The rectum was also diseased, though not to such an extent as the cæcum and colon; the mesenteric glands were enlarged, and harder than usual; the liver, spleen, and bladder were of natural appearance."

Remarks.—Here, as in a large proportion of cases of chronic diarrhœa, fever had its prominent original share, but dysentery had its greatest share. Functional disorder, and then structural disease of the small and larger intestines, resulting from the original dysentery, and both subsequently aggravated by fever, all terminated in that form of chronic diarrhœa which so often proves fatal. Extensive and irremediable disease of the mucous surfaces was here the cause of death; and it would appear clearly that it had its origin in the severe inflammatory dysentery of 1826, aggravated, no doubt, by more recent fever.

Here, in all the stages of the diarrhœa, mercurial treatment would have been injurious, for the structure and function of the liver were unimpaired.

CASE III.—Mrs. ——, aged thirty-four, of a fair complexion and delicate appearance, resided fourteen years in India, and states that her mother, and a brother aged twenty-four, both died of hepatic disease. She married within two years of her arrival in India, and has but one child, now ten years of age.

In 1845, her husband's health being much impaired, she accompanied him during a long sea voyage, and on her return to India she was, for the first time, seized with fever, which, however, lasted but a few days. After this she enjoyed very good health in

all respects until July, 1848, when she contracted tertian intermittent fever, which, in the September following, was succeeded by
what was considered erysipelas of the throat, face, and scalp. During
eight days in which this disease continued, she writes that " one
thousand leeches were applied, a lady at the station having taken
the trouble of counting them." It resulted from all this that Mrs.
—— suffered from the usual consequences of large depletion,
including violent palpitations of the heart, and she recovered but
slowly, and with difficulty, a sufficiency of strength to enable her
to undertake a journey to Simlah, in the Himalayah mountains;
and here she arrived for the benefit of climate and change of air
in February, 1849. The anticipations of an improved state of
health from the mountain air were not destined to be accomplished; for ague recurred severely, accompanied by diarrhœa, of
which she had had a slight attack along with the original intermittent, and during a heavy fall of snow which took place soon
after her arrival, the diarrhœa assumed a dysenteric character,
and it has ever since become aggravated under the influence of
cold weather.

During more than a year that Mrs. —— remained at this
mountain station she made no progress towards recovery, ague
and diarrhœa, with occasional severe vomiting, continuing to harass
her, so that during the whole period of her residence in the hills,
she was capable of leaving her house but twice. A medical report
of her case, written at this time by an able and attentive observer,
concludes as follows :—" At times she progresses pretty satisfactorily for a few days; but an attack of fever, however partial,
invariably brings back again all her ailments—aches, pains, diarrhœa, sickness, leucorrhœa, &c." She quitted Simlah in November, 1850, in company with her still very sickly husband, travelling as best she could over more than a thousand miles, to the
port of Calcutta, whence she took passage for England in January,
1851, by the Cape of Good Hope, and arrived in London in June
of the same year.

During the homeward voyage her disease did not abate; for
she says that, besides much suffering from continued sea-sickness,
she was purged, on the average, from six to eight times in the
twenty-four hours, in a passage of four months, the matter ejected
being fluid, copious, frothy, and generally devoid of colour. Here,
for the first time during her protracted illness, she ceased to menstruate.*

Night-sweats were also occasionally distressing to her, both in
India and during the passage home, and they occurred chiefly at
the feverish and at the menstrual periods. The purging has

* The frequency with which women cease to menstruate during the voyage to India
and back to Europe is a remarkable circumstance, and one that continually presented
itself to me when in Calcutta. I observed that this temporary suspension and suppression of the uterine function was common alike to the married and the unmarried.

always been most severe during the night and in the early morning. She complains much of irritability of temper, and of want of self-control. For instance, she will sometimes eat of things which she knows to be injurious, and says she cannot help doing so. During a year or more, there has been an occasional hacking dry cough.

Since her arrival in England, Mrs. —— has resided sometimes in the country, and then returned to London, her health receiving no benefit from change of air, and as yet but very little from various measures of treatment. Once, and sometimes twice in every month, she is seized with sense of cold followed by feverishness, and accompanied by vomiting, and much increase of diarrhœa, while her emaciation increases. The pulse, usually natural, rises to 100 during the paroxysms, and the urine becomes much loaded, being of a deep red-and-yellow colour.

On these occasions, when, after long-continued and distressing retching, the smallest quantity of bile is ejected from the stomach, the febrile movement, diarrhœa, and vomiting cease, and a partial and imperfect convalescence sets in. It would seem as if the vomiting were an effort of nature to elicit a flow of bile, and thus restore the lost balance of the hepatic function. The liver is enlarged, and extends far into the right cavity of the chest.

The case of this lady is a sad one, for she has had to contend during two years, not only with most severe and distressing personal illnesses, but she has besides had to guide and to tend an invalid husband, suffering from the results of remittent fever, coup-de-soleil, and now from diarrhœa of a very severe nature.

November 22nd, 1851.—The patient is returned from a month's visit in the country, where she was most dangerously ill, and now she is suffering from one of her periodical attacks of feverishness, with sense of cold, but no rigor, vomiting, and diarrhœa. On one of my casual visits, two months ago, I ordered a nightly dose of blue pill and opium; but as Mrs. —— quitted London soon afterwards, this medicine was discontinued. In consultation with Dr. Billing to-day, it was determined to resume the use of mercury very sparingly every other night, omitting the opium, and exhibiting three times during the day the decoction of the bark of the pomegranate root.

From this time to the 4th of March, 1852, when she died, her sufferings were great and varied. Attacks of feverishness, with aphthæ of the mouth and throat, vomitings, occasional pain in the regions of the liver and of the cæcum, and excessive diarrhœa, occurred twice in every month, and latterly even more frequently. Thus she became gradually wasted and exhausted.

On these distressing occasions, one circumstance always excited the attention of the patient; viz., that after many hours of retching and vomiting, if even the most minute streak of bile was perceptible on the side of the basin, an immediate remission of fever, vomiting, and diarrhœa took place, followed by a few days of comparative ease. But no real amendment resulted from any plan of treatment. Everything failed in succession, and at length she sank, emaciated and worn out. The following report of the *post-mortem* appearances was recorded by my friend, Mr. Pollock, of St. George's Hospital :—

"The body was extremely emaciated. Abdomen : The liver was not much enlarged; its colour was very different from the natural healthy condition, and instead of the dark red appearance, it was of a yellowish red colour ; the peritonæal coat peeled off its surface most readily, and the structure was soft, fatty, and easily lacerated, as if rotten. The vessels were not unusually filled. The gall bladder was not distended, but was filled with bile ; the peri-tonæal membrane covering it was much thickened, and of a pearly whiteness, and the sensation given to the finger when the bladder was pressed upon was that of a thick india-rubber ball, elastic, as if its contents were not capable of escaping. On cutting into it, some dark fluid bile escaped, also a large number of gall-stones about the size of the common pea, and granular on their surfaces. Under the blowpipe they were entirely consumed. On examining the cystic duct, it was found contracted and thickened externally, and at the point of junction with the hepatic duct, where the two unite to form the common duct, one of these calculi was so firmly impacted, that it appeared as if very little bile would pass into the intestine. The stomach was contracted, contained very little fluid, and was apparently healthy. The small intestines were also rather empty ; their muscular walls were attenuated. The lower portion of the ileum was laid open ; the mucous membrane was thickened, but the glands were not affected. A darkish-red appearance pre-sented itself in the inner surface, which was partly occasioned by the vascular condition of the lining membrane, and partly by its being covered with tenacious mucus tinged with blood. The cæcum and ascending portion of the colon were much distended with most offensive and *acrid* flatus, and also contained some dark fluid fæces ; small isolated patches of congestion were observed on the mucous membrane, but no vestige of ulceration. The trans-verse and descending colon was contracted, and the small quantity of solid fæces contained in the bowel was of a light clay colour. The spleen was small and healthy. The kidneys rather large, and somewhat coarse in structure. The bladder was nearly filled with urine. The uterus and ovaries were healthy."

Remarks.—Here, as in a large proportion of cases of chronic diarrhœa that have come under my observation, intermittent fever was the first disturbing cause ; hepatic disease was the concluding or final event. Referring to the history of Mrs. ——'s case, and to the whole train of symptoms during two years of great suffering, it would appear that impaction of the biliary ducts had constituted the first permanent hepatic lesion. The ducts once impervious, or nearly so, the circulation and the secreting power of the liver became in a manner obstructed and locked up, and disease of its entire texture rapidly supervened, until, through fatty degeneration, the organ became null. The common duct having been completely closed, or nearly so, for so long a time, the hepatic cells must have been more or less destroyed, and the secreting power of the liver was thus interfered with, and ultimately destroyed also. Fatty degeneration was the result. In this lady's case there never had been any appearance of jaundice. Regarded in this manner, it seems as if fatty degeneration, which ultimately destroyed life, became for a time the means of protracting existence; for had the power of secretion continued, the ducts must have yielded to distension, and the patient must have died speedily from extravasation into the peritonæal cavity. We now perceive also how it was in this distressing case that vomiting and purging resulted periodically as an effort of nature to overcome hepatic and tubular obstruction and disease, and how it was that enormous congestion of the mucous surfaces was produced.

Postscript.—It is worthy of remark here, that the husband of the lady whose case has just been described, nearly fell a sacrifice to the same disease which proved fatal to his wife. He suffered from chronic diarrhœa most extremely during three years, and to the extent of being reduced to a mere skeleton. He had suffered also severely from intermittent fever, and his diarrhœa recurred in paroxysms, accompanied by an excoriated and aphthous state of the mouth and fauces.

By a persevering use, during many weeks, of minute doses of blue pill, added to Dover's powder and gallic acid, the function of the liver was restored, and he became in the course of three months stouter than he had been at any period of his life, no vestige of his diarrhœa remaining. This officer's health was restored by the use of alterative doses of mercury ; but the gentleman whose case is related at pages 679-81, who suffered during several years from diarrhœa, the result of an enlarged liver, received no benefit from mercury, given repeatedly and for a long time under direction of the most able physicians in this country. He was eventually cured by the nitro-muriatic acid bath. Such are some of the exceeding difficulties in treating so complicated a disease as that under consideration.

CASE IV.—The result of the following *post-mortem* examination, by Mr. Pollock, was exhibited in the case of the wife of a surgeon of the Indian army. As in the majority of the other instances, this lady's first illness was intermittent fever ; after which, hepatic enlargement, distressing and irregular feverish attacks, general anæmia, aphthæ, and excessive wasting of the entire frame, at length wore her out.

Mrs. ——, aged thirty-two. Examination of the body forty-eight hours after death : The body was extremely emaciated, and decomposition rapidly advancing.—Thorax : The cavities of the pleuræ contained a small quantity of fluid. The apex of the left lung was adherent to the walls of the thorax, and in its substance were a few crude tubercles. The remainder of the lungs was healthy. The cavity of the pericardium contained a small quantity of fluid. The heart was pale and flabby, but healthy.— Abdomen : A small quantity of turgid fluid was contained in the cavity of the peritonæum, especially observed in the pelvis. The liver was flattened and spread over a large surface. It was much less red than natural, and mottled on its surface by numerous pale spots and marks. On cutting across these marks, they were found to consist of deposits of lymph and pus, some of them being situated in deeper portions, but for the most part confined to the surface immediately under the peritonæal covering. The gall-bladder was distended with dark thick bile. Some old and very firm adhesions existed between the surface of the liver and the walls of the abdomen on the right side. The stomach was contracted and healthy. The spleen was dark-coloured, and its surface and its substance studded with deposits of lymph and pus, in size varying from a pea to a pin's head. The surface of the lower portion of the small intestine showed increased vascularity of the peritonæal coat in patches, and also was marked by dark-blue spots every here and there, as if from some mischief to the interior of the bowel. On laying open the small intestine, these discoloured spots were found to correspond to ulcerations of the mucous membrane, some being the size of a sixpence, others much smaller ; some healing, others quite cicatrized ; while some had nearly perforated the peritonæum. The ulcers were all smooth on the surface, and the edges not raised, and confined to the lower portion of the small intestine. The large intestine was healthy.

CASE V.— ——, a surgeon of eminence in the Indian army, aged fifty-eight, had served thirty-eight years in India, during which time he suffered from various tropical diseases, and the latter years he laboured through with difficulty. His first illness, in 1822, was a severe attack of epidemic cholera, from which, being then young and healthy, he recovered rapidly. In 1824 he was seized with violent remittent (jungle) fever, and this was soon followed by intermittent fever, which latter continued to trouble him, at longer or shorter intervals, during the ten following years. In 1832 he had again an attack of epidemic cholera, followed by severe pain in the hepatic region, for which leeches and blisters were repeatedly and largely applied; he also used mercury and purgatives. From 1842 to 1848 he suffered from dysenteric attacks, of more or less violence ; and in November of the latter year (1848) he came to England on sick leave, suffering at that time from general anæmia and tendency to diarrhœa. There was the usual anæmic murmur loudly perceptible in the heart and large venous trunks, with much debility and muscular relaxation. He was treated by me with chalybeates, and was seen by Dr. Watson, who concurred with me in my view of his case.

Circumstances, unfortunately, obliged Mr. —— to return to India, in October, 1849, still in the ill state of health described; and he served in the higher grades of the administrative medical staff during 1849-1850, returning to England in April, 1851. He was now extremely emaciated from actual diarrhœa, irregular attacks of intermittent fever, and aggravated anæmia. He resided on the Continent until March, 1852, when he came to England, reduced to the last stage of exhaustion from aphthous diarrhœa and anæmia, the discharges being large, colourless, and serous. There was slight enlargement of the liver, and anasarca of the lower extremities. Minute doses of blue pill were ordered night and morning, and under this treatment the function of the liver was completely restored in about a fortnight, the dejections being charged with healthy bile; but nevertheless diarrhœa, though now bilious in character, went on to great exhaustion, and there were occasional rigors, followed by feverish reaction. Quinine, with sulphate of copper and opium, were used; but after a time they failed to produce any result, and then I ordered salicin, with nitric acid and laudanum, which checked the diarrhœa and feverishness completely, the motions being now limited to one in twenty-four, sometimes to one in forty-eight hours. The diet all this time was composed of milk and farinaceous articles, soups, and the occasional use of weak brandy-and-water; but nutrition did not take place to the extent that might have been hoped for, and months passed without any real amendment. In August, 1852, the bowels being in a perfectly tranquil state, all medicine was discontinued at his own urgent request. The mildest chalybeates appeared to him to disagree, and he was thus left to the influence of diet. Still no disposition to an improved nutrition manifested itself, and in the middle of October he contracted a severe bronchial cold, followed by copious viscid expectoration, some slight oppression, and gradual increase of debility. In the first week of November, there was a slight recurrence of diarrhœa, and on the 5th of that month he sank from utter exhaustion.

The following *post-mortem* appearances are recorded by Mr. Pollock :—" The body was extremely pale, exsanguine and emaciated.—Thorax : Each of the cavities of the pleuræ contained rather more than a pint of serum. The structure of the lungs was perfectly healthy and crepitant, except that they were slightly emphysematous at their margins. The pericardium contained a small quantity of serum. The heart was rather large, and its surface somewhat covered with fat; the latter structure was infiltrated with serum to a very great extent. The muscular structure of the heart was pale-coloured (exsanguine), but firm. The right ventriele was somewhat dilated. The left ventricle was much hyper-trophied; its lining membrane was somewhat thickened and whitish ; the aortic valves were thickened, opaque, and contained spots of atheroma ; their edges were slightly contracted. The root of the aorta was roughened by deposit of atheroma, as also other parts of that artery to its bifurcation. The blood was ex-tremely thin, and perfectly fluid, no trace of coagula or stain being perceived in the heart's cavities.—Abdomen: The liver was rather large, of a healthy colour, and smooth on its surface, its structure presenting the natural conditions. The gall-bladder was much distended; its coats were very thin; its contents were simply serum, with two or three small particles of inspissated bile. The spleen was healthy. The stomach was natural. The coats of the intestines were extremely thin, and their contents fluid, and like yeast in consistence and colour. There were no indications of recent ulceration of the large or small intestines ; the mucous membrane of the cæcum was rather more congested than in health, and more so than the rest of the large intestine. The kidneys were very exsanguine, but not unhealthy in structure.

Remarks.—A long succession of severe tropical diseases—anæmia of several years' duration, chronic anæmic diarrhœa, defect of nutrition—inanition, in fact, destroyed this excellent officer. Could circumstances have admitted of his remaining at home in 1849, so as not to return any more to India, a valuable life might have been saved to his family; but two additional years of tropical service, in his then miserable state of health, left no hope on his last return to England, either from his native climate or from any other remedial means.

General Remarks.—The *post-mortem* appearances above recorded, while they exhibit the irremediable lesions of structure frequently existing as the cause of chronic diarrhœa, and thus establish the justice of the character of danger so often attaching to this disease, still afford no information which could have led to the effective treatment of the subjects. All the cases had been of an incurable nature for a long time previously to dissolution, and so far patho-logical investigation led to no practical results. I must here repeat, that in many of the cases sent home from hot climates diarrhœa is but, in fact, the last stage in the progress of compli-cated abdominal disease. We are, in medicine, always disparaging theory, pure observation, and opinion, and aiming at exactness. In pathology we hope to find this last, on the principle that the value of all observation or opinion ends where demonstration begins. But how difficult—often how impossible—is this demon-stration which we justly aim at; for it does not at all follow that because we see and examine we therefore understand. In anatomy, natural or morbid, in physiology, in general pathology, in thera-peutics, where are we to find mathematical demonstrations? We can, with great exactness, it is said, ascertain every alteration in the function of the kidneys, through chemical analysis; but no one has as yet determined the actual nature of granular degeneration of those organs. Notwithstanding these discouraging circum-stances, I venture to hope that something has here been done to exhibit the true pathology and the just treatment of such cases of diarrhœa as are of a curable nature. It will be seen that in four out of the five fatal cases of this disease here detailed, the liver was more or less seriously involved. In the case of Colonel ——, and in several of those successfully treated by me, this organ was evidently the principal seat of morbid action. Whether the ante-cedent may have been the cold and damp of the Himalayahs, or the protracted cold stages of intermittent fever, the morbid results have generally been the same—viz., congested, or permanently diseased liver, and consequent diarrhœa.

The circumstance that intermittent fever, and not remittent, has been so generally the antecedent—the most pervading or the most frequently recurring disease—prior to the advent of diarrhœa, with complicated abdominal disease, cannot fail to have attracted the reader's notice. But why intermittent fevers, which at their onset are incomparably less dangerous to life than remittents, should in after years found abdominal disease so much more fre-quently and dangerously, can only be referred to the greater seve-rity and the longer duration of the cold, congestive stage of the former, disturbing very frequently, and during a succession of years, the functions of the liver, spleen, stomach, bowels, and kid-neys. I am here speaking of the ordinary malarious intermittents, and not of the malignant types.

Congestion of a chronic nature I have long regarded as one of the conditions most certainly conducive to the destruction of an organ; for if the mere retardation or detention of the blood in the larger venous trunks be sufficient to spoil the circulating fluid, and render it unsuitable for admission into the general mass, and a source of its contamination, what must be the consequences, both general and local, of a protracted state of congestion of so large and of such important organs as the liver and spleen?

Postscript.—After this essay was written, the following confir-mation of many of the facts and views here contained was received from an unexpected quarter:—

Dr. Stillman, of New York, writing of the diseases of California, says of the chronic diarrhœa of that region:—"Many cases of Californian diarrhœa were preceded by intermittents; and although many do not appear to have suffered in that way, still it must be admitted that all were exposed to the intermittent malaria. The discharges," he says, "were copious, liquid, and voided without pain, or but momentary griping. The appetite was so insatiable that no opportunity of devouring whatever food could be obtained was neglected. By nothing was this affection more distinguished than by its fatality. Of twenty-five cases of chronic diarrhœa fourteen died before the 1st of April (in three months), and most of those remaining are known to have died since. Before death, emaciation and anæmia became extreme, and the mind, which in most cases had been cheerful and hopeful, at last gave way to the most childish imbecility."

Dr. Schulhof, writing of the diseases of the Delta of the Danube, says justly :—" Where there is ague, *dysentery* is not far off, the former predisposing for the latter by the disorders which it produces in the abdominal organs. . . . That ague on the one hand, and dysentery on the other, will leave behind them tokens of their visits by liver affections, every one will readily believe." That ague predisposes to diarrhœa even more immediately, would seem to be established.

CHRONIC DYSENTERY.

CURTIS, writing on the diseases of India in 1782-3, says :—" The stomach and intestines, the liver and mesentery, are here the grand sources of almost every disease; or, what amounts nearly to the same thing, in every standing complaint, if the radical affection does not lie in these organs, they are sure to become the principal sufferers in the issue." The justice of this observation is confirmed by modern statistics; for we find that there occurred, according to Sir Alexander Tulloch, out of an aggregate European force of 25,433 men of Her Majesty's army serving in periods of eight and ten years respectively, between 1823 and 1836, in the stations of Calcutta, Chinsurah, and Berhampore, all in Bengal Proper, 8499 cases of dysentery and diarrhœa; and though the years included within this return were, as formerly stated, subsequent to the first Burmese war, still the proportion of dysenteric cases is excessive, making every proper allowance for such unfavourable influence. The climate of Lower Bengal is, and has always been, very unfavourable to European health also, as compared to other portions of our Indian empire; but making every allowance for all circumstances, including the soldier's ill habits of life, the amount of sickness from dysentery and diarrhœa here exhibited is enormous.

In the Madras Presidency, out of an aggregate British force of 82,342 men serving there, from 1842 to 1848, there occurred 10,531 cases of dysentery, and 9189 cases of diarrhœa, making a total of 19,720 cases of bowel diseases, exclusive of cholera. It thus appears that next to the malarious fevers of India, bowel complaints are there the most prevalent diseases, while the dangers to health and to life from these last are even greater than from fevers.

Robert Jackson justly regards dysentery as "one of the most important of the maladies that occur amongst troops, particularly in the West Indies, where," he says, "that in some of the islands it amounts to one-half, even to more than half of all the forms of acute disease which appear in the hospital return of sick." This great physician adds :—"It is dangerous in itself—more fatal, in fact, amongst the military in the West Indies, either primarily or secondarily, than any other, the concentrated fever, as incident to strangers, excepted."

I am now to consider the sequela of acute tropical dysentery, as it is exhibited in the European returned from hot climates. It differs materially from the results of tropical fevers, inasmuch as the former involves structural disease, or the most severe disorder along the cæcum, colon, and rectum, and occasionally involves even the whole or greater part of the mucous digestive surfaces, and ulcerations and thickenings of these structures are much more common to chronic dysentery than to the disease last considered— viz., chronic diarrhœa.

I regard chronic dysentery to be, in fact, the special and proper sequela to the acute stage of that disease, and as consisting of an irritated state, an imperfectly cicatrized or ulcerated condition, more or less extensive, of the mucous surface of the cæcum, colon, or rectum, sometimes of all three. The state of irritation, partial cicatrization, or remaining ulceration of the mucous membrane of the large bowel constitutes what I believe to be the essential nature of chronic dysentery, as contra-distinguished from chronic diarrhœa, which latter is proved to be the sequela of fevers more frequently than of any other disease. As seen in Europe, chronic dysentery has ceased to possess any inflammatory character, even of the most chronic nature.

It may sometimes be difficult to assign the reason, but chronic dysentery, whether complicated or otherwise, has always appeared to me to be a more manageable disease in this country than chronic diarrhœa. I find that the process of healing an ulcerated bowel in chronic dysentery is much more readily brought about than is the restoration of the hepatic function in cases of chronic diarrhœa. The history of this latter disease given in the last article will in some measure explain the different degrees of difficulty and danger to be apprehended in the treatment of the two diseases. I have certainly not seen chronic dysentery the sequela to the acute forms of the disease, so frequently associated with incurable diseases of the liver as is the chronic diarrhœa, notwithstanding the great frequency of the hepatic complication in the former disease. But though I state this fact as the result of my personal experience of the chronic dysentery as it appears amongst the returned Indians, I am very far from desiring to underrate its occasional dangers here in England.

In order to exhibit the relations of the dysentery of India to diseases of the liver, I need only quote the following important facts from the statistics of Dr. Macpherson, of the General Hospital, Calcutta:—

	ACUTE DYSENTERY OF BENGAL.	CHRONIC DYSENTERY.
	Observation in the cases of 160 Europeans.	Observation in the cases of 55 Europeans.
	Cases.	Cases.
Liver found to be altered in	84	31
,, ,, contain abscess in . .	21	6
,, ,, be enlarged in . . .	40	5
,, ,, be gorged and turgid in	4	...
,, ,, be small in	7	8
,, ,, be pale in	26	11
,, ,, be granular in . . .	22	...
,, ,, be softened in . . .	12	1
,, ,, be indurated in . . .	5	4
,, ,, contain cicatrices in .	3	1
,, ,, contain hydatids in. .	...	1
,, ,, be nutmeg in . . .		6
,, ,, be cirrhosed in . . .	...	1

Dr. Macpherson is doubtful whether the cicatrices were the sequelæ of hepatic abscess. This able officer adds that, on a comparison of acute with chronic dysentery, it appears " the liver is most frequently altered in the latter; that abscess is about equally frequent in either form; that in acute dysentery the liver is frequently enlarged and soft, while in the chronic it is more generally small and indurated."

The stomach and small intestines also suffer more frequently in the chronic form, and the mesenteric glands are more frequently altered in it.

Referring to the complications of hepatic disease with dysentery at the other Presidencies, Dr. Macpherson finds as follows:—

In Madras, out of 51 cases, there were found 26 hepatic abscesses; and in Bombay, out of 30 cases, there were found 12.

In New Orleans, hepatic abscess was found by Dr. Robertson " the common cause of death in dysentery."

Sir James Annesley observes that, " Although both chronic dysentery and chronic diarrhœa are, in India, occasionally met with in simple and uncomplicated forms, and even terminate fatally without any appearance of disease being detected in the liver, yet such complications are much more frequent than simple forms of these diseases; and not only is disease of the liver associated with organic changes in the large and small intestines, but the mesenteric glands, pancreas, spleen, and omentum, frequently also present signs of altered structure."

" It is worthy of remark," says Dr. Macpherson, " that the liver

z z

has been found, in the General Hospital of Calcutta, to have been altered in 111 out of 215 cases; in the Medical College Hospital, in 13 out of 30 cases; while Sir James M'Grigor found it, in India, altered 16 times in 21 cases; and in Egypt, as in India, he found it diseased." If it be thus, upon examination after death in India, in respect of an organ so large as the liver, and generally so unmistakeable in the morbid appearances which it presents, what proportion of hepatic disorder and of disease also may we not expect to find in the living sufferers from fevers, chronic dysentery and diarrhœa on their return to Europe. That the liver is largely involved in such persons there is not, and never has been, any doubt in my mind; and every day's observation and practical experience proves its truth. It should be noted of chronic dysentery as of chronic diarrhœa, that none but the worst cases are sent to England—those which have resisted every means of cure within the tropics, including voyages to sea and other climatic changes.

It is necessary now to look to the lesions of the intestinal canal and other organs; and we find that, in the 160 cases of acute dysentery already mentioned, the following facts are recorded:—

	Cases.
The ileum is noted as over-vascular or congested in . . .	21
Slight ulceration and abrasion are seen in	3
In a state of sphacelus in	1
Mucous coat of the stomach over-vascular or softened in . .	4
Mucous coat of the stomach ulcerated in	1
Large intestine, chiefly cæcum, sigmoid flexure, and rectum ulcerated in all the cases.	
Cæcum, transverse and descending colon, free from ulceration in .	3 only
Large intestine, but generally the cæcum, perforated in . . .	8
Ileo-cæcal valve ulcerated and destroyed in	3
Suppuration of appendix vermiformis not uncommon, recorded in .	1 only
Thickening and stricture of intestine	4
Dilatation	1
Mesenteric glands enlarged or inflamed in	17
Spleen enlarged in	6
Kidneys diseased in	2

In the 55 cases of chronic dysentery, the following facts are recorded :—

	Cases.
Large intestines were ulcerated in	50
Colon contracted in	3
Cæcum nearly closed in	1
Colon perforated in	1
Stomach noted as unhealthy in	6
Chronic inflammation and softening in	2
Increased vascularity in	2
Pylorus in a state of abrasion in	3
,, ,, cancer in	1
Small intestines noted as unhealthy in	12
Ulceration or abrasion of the ileum in	2
Mesenteric glands enlarged in	16
Spleen enlarged	4

After this summary, we shall be prepared to learn, that out

of 2044 admissions from dysentery into the General Hospital of Calcutta, from 1830 to 1850, there occurred, according to Dr. Macpherson, 457 deaths, or 22·3 per cent.; and "the extremes of mortality have been 14·8 in 1833, and 34 in 1845."

Having shown so much of the antecedents of the cases of European sufferers from tropical dysentery, we have now to contemplate their condition as they present themselves in England. But I would again observe, in a prefatory way, that how dangerous soever acute tropical dysentery may be (and few have witnessed more of its dangers and complications than the writer of this work), still its sequelæ in the chronic form, as they present themselves in Europe, are neither so difficult of cure, nor so fatal by many degrees, as the chronic diarrhœa of the same class of persons—viz., the returned Indians. In my personal experience, and speaking of all the cases of chronic dysentery that I have treated in England, I should say that some have recovered slowly, and with much trouble, some recovered rapidly, but, excepting the very complicated cases, and those which eventuated in chronic diarrhœa, few died. But it must be remembered that many of the cases of severer hepatic complication die speedily in India; for they are not often seen in England, even in the persons of those who come home by the more expeditious route through Egypt.

The sufferer from chronic dysentery presents himself in a state of impaired nutrition; there is emaciation, dryness and harshness of skin, with an anxious or irritable expression of countenance, and pallor or sallowness of complexion. The hair, as in fevers of long standing, and in chronic diarrhœa, is scanty, dry, and mossy. The tongue is generally coated, the edges being red and irritable. The pulse is feeble, and sometimes frequent; the respiration natural. Where no enlargement of the liver or spleen exists, the abdomen will generally be found flattened, and free from tenderness; but the conditions of this cavity, on exploration, will necessarily depend on the existence, or otherwise, of structural disease, or of severe disorder or irritation in any or all the organs contained in it, and on the duration of the illness. In short, we must be prepared to witness, in the returned Indian, the consequences of previously acute disease more or less violent and extensive; the stages of fever and of inflammation having long passed away, we have now to deal with their more or less severe remote results. Sometimes we see young men whose cases have been of short duration, and who arrive quickly from the tropics, in whom subacute inflammatory symptoms are manifest; but such cases are exceptional.

The symptoms of chronic dysentery vary only in degree from those of the acute disease. The motions, in the former disease, will be voided with tormina and tenesmus, and will contain mucus with blood, and purulent matter with blood, according as the mucous membrane of the large intestine is more or less injured in its structure; but when the motions are passed without tormina or tenesmus, and only contain mucus, the condition will be found one more of irritation than of a serious character. When, on the other hand, we find chronic enlargement of the liver associated with chronic dysentery, the anatomical changes, and consequent disturbances of various important functions already described, will prepare us for much increase of severity in the symptoms, with corresponding difficulty in the treatment. We have here to deal, not only with disease of the larger bowel, but with actual disease also, or great disturbance in the functions, of all the associated organs. As in chronic diarrhœa, the discharges are most frequent in the night and early morning.

A knowledge of the functional and structural changes existing during life is of the greatest importance, and these last are best ascertained in their nature, extent, seat, and complication by a careful examination of the abdominal regions, and an inspection of the matters voided. Without such examinations we can neither arrive at a just diagnosis, nor at a treatment proper to each case.

A more or less extensively ulcerated state of the mucous membrane and glands of the large intestine, with thickening of its coats, and narrowing of the bore of the bowel through deposit of fibrin between its coats, with or without complication; these constitute the essential conditions of chronic dysentery, and the restoration to health can only be effected by cicatrization and absorption; and that these favourable processes are in progress is best ascertained by observation of the more natural appearance of the evacuated matters.

In considering the means of cure in chronic dysentery, there is no one consideration of more serious importance than the diet—a diet which barely sustains the system, and which is bland and unirritating, being all that ought, in the earlier stage of treatment, to be allowed. Neglect of proper diet not only retards the progress of cicatrization, but it tends to reproduce and to extend ulceration, and thus to cause dangerous and even fatal relapse. A deprivation which the patient may regard as the verge of starvation would, in many cases, prove salutary, by calming peristaltic irritation, and thus affording time for the healing of ulcerated or abraded surfaces. Robert Jackson forcibly condemns "a form of diet termed generous, where the intestinal canal is ulcerated, its coats thickened, the mesenteric system obstructed, and other of the abdominal organs contingently diseased." But while we have rigid regard to the *quantity* of food to be allowed in all the stages of this disease, we must not neglect care also in its *quality*. The justice of the remark by Graves, that "*meat is far too much refrained from*," has generally been verified in my experience, especially in its latter and protracted stage—the moderate use of animal food being almost always well borne in this disease as in the diarrhœa; but the meat must be of the best and most tender kind—spare in quantity, thoroughly masticated. Well prepared broths are very valuable articles of diet likewise; and where a scorbutic taint is present, they should be rich in both animal and vegetable properties. We must, in fact, adapt the diet as we do the medicine to the nature and progress of the disease.

Next to diet, we should enjoin care in clothing, and in abstaining from exercise. The clothing should, in all cases, be such as to ensure an equable determination to the skin, and, in bad cases, the rest should be absolute.

Having to deal with relaxation, with thickening, or with actual ulceration of the mucous surface of the large intestine, along with various complications, our medical appliances must be apportioned accordingly. In illustration of this part of the subject, I would adduce the following cases:—

CASE I.—December 29th, 1848.—Lieut. ——, of the Indian Army, aged twenty-one, is stated in the report of the regimental surgeon to have resided but two years in India, and to have been of regular and temperate habits. But, shortly after his arrival in India, in March, 1846, he was seized with acute dysentery; and from that date to February, 1847, he experienced three several attacks of the same disease. The second attack was of a dangerous acute nature, "and he passed a large sphacelus on the seventh day of the disease. During the period between these grave attacks, he has never passed a week without recourse to the aid of medicine, in some shape or another, for uneasiness and derangement of the bowels. His liver is subject to constant great functional irregularities; and I have sometimes observed a fulness of the right hypochondrium; but this organ has never been the subject of the patient's complaint. He appears to have a constitutional scorbutic tendency; for when in his best health, his gums and teeth are invariably coated with blood on first waking in the morning." These official details extend from the 26th of August to the 8th of October, 1848. The attacks of dysentery commenced at the former date, with severe griping and cutting pains across the belly; and during the day he voided several offensive frothy stools, with mucus and some blood; "there was likewise frequent vomiting and much tenesmus." The treatment consisted of leeches to the abdomen, fomentations, blue pill with ipecacuanha and opium, and occasional doses of castor oil. This course of treatment, varied only by the occasional use of a drastic purgative, was continued up to the 2nd of October, when the bowels are described as "excessively torpid," the matters voided being tinged with "muco-purulent matter, but otherwise the evacuations are healthy."

On the 29th of December, 1848, I first saw the patient in London. His manner indicated great nervous excitement; the complexion was dark and muddy, and there was much emaciation;

the skin was perspirable; the pulse natural; the tongue clean. The bowels were still lax, the motions numbering from three to five in the twenty-four hours, and were voided principally during the night and early morning. He voided much ropy colourless mucus, but without griping or straining. There was no tenderness on pressure in any part of the abdomen; no enlargement of the liver or spleen. He was ordered to take an ounce three times a day of a mixture of infusion of simaruba, with dilute nitro-muriatic acid and laudanum; while the diet was directed to be very spare, and to consist of farinaceous articles with milk; he was directed to use warm clothing, the warm bath occasionally on going to bed, and to avoid all exercise.

February 5th, 1849.—The lax state of the bowels continues, but there is much less mucus voided. Ordered a fourth of a grain of sulphate of copper, with half a grain of opium, mixed with extract of gentian, in the form of a pill, three times a day.

March 9th.—Much improved. Has but two motions in the twenty-four hours. Thinks the pills cause nausea, and I therefore substituted two grains of gallic acid for the sulphate of copper. The complexion and general condition are improved, and he is allowed solid animal food.

May 19th.—He says he feels quite well, with the exception of " a sensation of cold in the bowels, and of a feeling that they would be moved by the use of cold drinks." Has but one consistent motion in the twenty-four hours. Ordered four grains of pow- dered nux vomica three times a day in pill, and allowed a tumbler of bitter ale at dinner.

June 5th.—He declares himself now " really well in all respects, and that he has acquired his ordinary condition and weight;" com- plexion much improved. Ordered a vinous solution of quinine and citrate of iron twice a day; and in the event of the bowels becoming constipated, he was directed to use an enema of cold water; when a more effective aperient became necessary, he was ordered to take a mild dose of magnesia and rhubarb with ipecacuanha.

Remarks.—The case of this young officer had in India been of a dangerous character, for he voided exudation-tubes of the croup- ous character, and frequently also shreds or dark-coloured flakes of dead mucous membrane. The nervous temperament and the seor- butic complication also added greatly to the difficulties of early treatment. But on arrival in England the health had somewhat improved. There were then but slight traces or remains of ulcera- tion of the mucous surface of the larger bowel, and there was no he- patic or scorbutic complication. The treatment was therefore simple and freed from difficulty. I believe that the formula originally prescribed would have conducted his case to a successful and safe conclusion; but such were his terrors of what he would desig- nate " dysentery," that I felt constrained to use active mineral and vegetable astringents in order to appease his fears. The powdered nux vomica appeared to act very beneficially, and I generally find it so in the irritable state of the colon which so frequently follows the ulcerative dysentery of tropical climates.

In the instance of this young officer, as in so large a proportion of all who come home sick from India, the appropriate winding-up to the treatment consisted of chalybeates, given with a view to remove the anæmic condition; but in this completion, as in the curative endeavour, the salutary effect was greatly retarded by the temptations of the London clubs.

Case II.—October 18th, 1849.—Assistant-Surgeon ——, of the Indian Army, aged thirty-eight, had resided eight years in India. His complexion was naturally sallow, temperament phlegmatic, habit abstemious. "From childhood," he says, "until shortly previous to the present dysenteric attack, he had been subject to occasional bilious vomitings, and in 1840, while with his regiment in Singapore, he was seized with hemiplegia of the left side, from the effects of which he almost, but never quite recovered. In 1847, he was stationed at Masulipatam, and in May was seized with slight diarrhœa, to which sufficient attention was not paid. Dysentery supervened, from which, in spite of all treatment, he has, with the exception of an interval of seven months, been suffering ever since, more or less." During this interval he took no medicine, the purging stopping and returning in the same sudden and unaccountable way. The acute symptoms had lasted three months, during which leeches to the abdomen and anus, fomentations, blue pill with ipecacuanha, and mild aperients were used: then, as acute disease subsided, the mineral acids with opium, nitrate of silver and acetate of lead with opium, in the form of pill and enema, and change of air, were successively had recourse to, but the patient was "gradually losing ground," and in October, 1847, he embarked for England; having at the time "twelve motions in the twenty-four hours, watery, with a little blood." Opiates and astringents were used during the voyage home, by the Cape of Good Hope, and he arrived in England in February, 1848. From this date he consulted various medical gentlemen, and, amongst others, "a practitioner who devoted his attention more particularly to the diseases of that region," i. e., the rectum. No real benefit having resulted from any of the various courses of treatment, the patient was recommended by his friends to consult me, and he did so on the 18th of October, 1849. At this time he describes the "calls to stool as very frequent, particularly in the morning," the discharge consisting "of a thin, watery-looking fluid, often tinged with more or less blood." The stools amounted to six or eight daily, and were voided with "griping and attended with scalding of the anus." The liver was apparently free from disease, and there was little or no pain on pressure in any of the abdominal regions. From the date of his consulting me to the 30th May, 1850, the patient experienced occasional but never complete relief. He used the nux vomica, bismuth, gallic acid, the mineral acids with opium in bitter infusion, chalybeates with opium, &c.; but all without further result than moderating the symptoms.

At the date last mentioned, the patient came under the observation of Mr. Bottomley, of Croydon, whose kindness and attention were unremitting. This gentleman now recommended the use of mercury and chalk, with Dover's powder, of each three grains at bed-time. This treatment was persisted in till the 6th of June, when, feeling more weakly, being much griped, and passing "gelatinous-looking motions," cascarilla infusion was ordered.

June 20th.—At my desire the patient this day consulted Dr. Watson, of London, who regarded the case "as Mr. Martin had always done, as one of the larger bowel only, uncomplicated with any serious organic change in the liver, or other viscus." Dr. Watson ordered nitro-muriatic acid, conjoined to gallic acid, the use of which he continued until the 30th of August, when there was very copious purging of thin, watery, and bloody fluid, which was "squirted out with violence."

Towards the end of December, not having derived benefit from any treatment, the patient went to Hastings, where the late Dr. Mackness directed him to take bismuth, logwood, opiates, &c.; but no improvement resulting, he returned to Croydon at the end of March, 1851, in a very feeble and exhausted condition, from the constant drain of large fluid bloody motions. By the 20th of April, he was actually sinking, and could not turn in bed without assistance. I now visited him at Croydon, and found him voiding enormous quantities of bloody serum. In consultation with Mr. Bottomley, a pill, composed of diacetate of lead and opium, with a solution of the same medicines in the form of enema after each motion, were ordered. On the 23rd of April Mr. B. reported to me that the patient was "living only from hour to hour," and certainly neither of us looked upon his recovery as at all probable; so far from it, indeed, that we spoke of the desirableness of a *post-mortem* examination. The patient had deliberately made up his mind to death, and he took what he thought to be a final leave of me. The means last used, however, were strictly persevered in against all disadvantages; and the result was remarkable. Recovery took place from this hour. On May 13th the patient states, in his notes of the case, that "the remedies last ordered seemed at once to check the purging, and the injection was only used twice or thrice, and retained for a short time. The bowels had now become so costive that tepid-water enemata were requisite in order to relieve them." On the 9th of July the patient visited me in London, when I ordered twenty minims of the pernitrate of iron to be taken in water three times a day, and which was afterwards changed for the sesquioxide.

Under this treatment, aided by a nightly anodyne, the anæmic condition of the system was gradually overcome; the bowels were moved by enemata, sleep was secured, and the anæmic state of the pulse disappeared. By the 24th of March, 1852, the patient had increased in weight from eight to twelve stone, while he and his family declared his then condition of health better than it had been for years. His necessities, as well as his inclinations, pointed to his return to India, "where," he said, "I flatter myself I know my duties as surgeon in the service; and I feel sure that I am at any rate much better qualified to discharge them than I am for private practice in this country, of which I have seen little and like less." He proceeded to India, and enjoyed good health for a year or more, when he was cut off by epidemic cholera.

Remarks.—This officer passed through years of suffering of every kind, moral and physical, and he bore all with admirable fortitude. The character of the dysentery was severe from its commencement; but towards its termination it assumed a deadly form and appearance. The cure, too, was retarded by an ill condition of the general habit, of which anæmia formed but a part. With the utmost possible care on the part of the patient (an officer of great intelligence), all remedies failed in succession; and in April, 1851, he appeared absolutely to be dying. From this apparently hopeless state of disease, voiding enormous quantities of a fluid resembling the washings of raw meat, he recovered under the use of lead and opium, exhibited in the manner described—remedies which had been administered in India without effect. But such are the everyday incertitudes, the difficulties, and the dangers of medicine.

It will be seen that mercury had no share in the treatment of the cases quoted; indeed, it is seldom that I have recourse to it in the treatment of the chronic form of dysentery as it appears in Europe. When there is recent congestion of the liver, from the application of cold, for instance, a few mild doses of mercury with sudorifics and purgatives, aided by the warm bath at bed-time, will be found useful; but such cases are exceptional.

"In the more advanced stage of the disease," says Sir James M'Grigor, "particularly where there is hectic fever, with extensive ulceration of the intestine, mercury is invariably found to hurry on the fatal termination." Where there is ulceration of the mucous surfaces, mercury is extremely mischievous when persisted in, or when used to the extent of affecting the salivary glands. Of the evil consequences of such treatment I have seen many instances. Where a more continuous use of mercury, with a view to its specific influence on the liver, is called for, I find the following formula useful :—Compound ipecacuanha powder, gallic acid, mercurial pill, of each one scruple; oil of cinnamon, four drops : make into twelve pills. One or two of these may be given at bed-time for so many days as may be necessary, while tonics and astringents may be exhibited during the day. When, on the other hand, chronic enlargement of the liver is associated with chronic dysentery, *the condition of the system being anæmic*, I always have recourse to the nitro-muriatic acid bath in preference to mercurials, and of its effects in such instances many striking examples will be found in this part of the work. The hepatic and splenic complication have each its peculiar danger. In the hepatic we have a direct and immediate interference with the functions of the stomach and bowels, through circumstances of vascular, nervous, secretory actions and associations; and in the splenic complication we perceive the peculiar cachectic influence, affecting all the fluids and tissues, so as to prove a serious detriment and hindrance to cicatrization. Thus we perceive how both the complications here noticed must be attended with dangers and difficulties.

. Whether the condition of the mucous membrane of the intestine be that of relaxation, thickening, or ulceration, we shall find our best means of cure in the mineral or vegetable astringents and tonics, with or without opium.

Robert Jackson says, that where ulcerated surfaces are healed, or in a healing state, the foundations of congestion having been removed, and where purging continues from relaxation or irritability, kino, catechu, and simaruba have appeared to him " the most useful." But he found it necessary " to vary the form of tonic," as the effect, " often considerable for a few days at the first trial, is soon lost." . . " It is to this condition of disease that the arsenical solution particularly applies; and it is here a remedy of the greatest value." In the great majority of instances, I find it necessary, in order to secure the full effects of both astringents and tonics, to conjoin them with opiates, in more or less minute proportions, according to the urgency of the symptoms.

Whether we employ the mineral astringents—such as the diacetate of lead, sulphate of copper, nitrate of silver, or quinine, arsenic, or mercury, the mineral acids, the vegetable tonics or astringents, the rule of shielding them with one or other of the preparations of opium is equally applicable.*

In every stage of dysentery, whether acute or chronic, we must endeavour, by every means, to quiet irritation and movement of the bowels, as by such quieting means we most certainly guide the patient towards the healing of abrasions or ulceration of the intestinal mucous membrane. I repeat, that astringents and tonics, mischievous in the inflammatory stage, are here much to be relied upon. A bland and spare diet, proper medicaments, including warm clothing and warm baths, mental and bodily rest, with the careful observance of the recumbent posture—these are the rational

* The " Red Gum " of Western Australia—an exudation from a tree common to the forests of that country—a species of Eucalyptus—has proved an excellent tonic and astringent in several cases. I was favoured with the drug by Staff-Surgeon H. H. Jones, who made many successful trials of the medicine while serving at Kurrachee.

means found on experience to secure the end in view. But though this principle and these means ought never to be lost sight of, we shall have occasionally, in the management of chronic dysentery, to use gentle aperients, with a view to remove accumulations of matters in the cæcum and colon, organs often thickened, narrowed, and weakened by previous disease.

These last means will be more specially necessary as we approach the period of cure; and I have found castor-oil, in small doses, very useful. Occasionally, however, the oil produces griping and tenesmus, and thus proves very mischievous; so that the question of the agreement or disagreement should always be ascertained beforehand. The aperient which I have found most generally to agree, is a combination of rhubarb powder and magnesia, with those of columba and ipecacuanha, and bicarbonate of soda; a combination of magnesia, sulphur, and ipecacuanha, with some aromatic tonic, is likewise useful; and so is the washed sulphur, made into pills, with balsam of copaiba; but even such mild means as these should be exhibited but seldom, and active cathartics should never be employed. The inflammatory and congestive irritations of the larger bowel during acute dysentery cause the rapid and frequent expulsion of all the contained matters; whereas in the chronic stage there exists a diminution of both the irritative and natural muscular actions; and hence the necessity for the occasional removal of matters retained through torpor and inaction of the larger bowel.

Sudorifics, so powerful in the acute disease, I have seldom been able to use with the emaciated and exhausted patients who come home from hot climates suffering from chronic dysentery, the enfeebled mucous membrane and skin of such persons being unable to bear any medicine producing nausea and cuticular discharge.

An irritable state of the sigmoid flexure of the colon is common to both diarrhœa and dysentery in their chronic forms. This condition is caused by the frequent draining of vitiated, and there-fore irritating matters through the angle of the bowel. It is a painful and distressing affection, and requires much attention in the way of mild aperients and soothing enemata. Thickening of this portion of the bowel, and a consequent narrowing, more or less partial, is no unfrequent occurrence in persons who have suffered long from such ailments. Here, as in similar conditions of the rectum, enemata of acetate of lead, of nitrate of silver, of copaiba balsam, all conjoined with opium, will be found of much service. The value of finely-powdered charcoal, exhibited by the mouth, and in the form of an enema, was very favourably spoken of by the army medical officers during the late war, both in the Mediterranean and West Indian commands. It was used by Dr. Borland and others in the remittent and intermittent fevers of those countries as well; but its best effects were manifested in the acute and chronic forms of dysentery. Robert Jackson gave the

charcoal in scruple doses by the mouth, adding a few grains of
rhubarb and ipecacuanha powder, and in drachm doses, in rice-
water or arrow-root, as an enema, and that with signal effect.
One case is here recorded, in which the charcoal acted most
beneficially in the form of an enema. Under every form of treatment, warm baths, used at bed-time, and continued for half an
hour or an hour, will prove powerful in aid of internal remedies.
I would here add, that when the dysentery is ascertained to be
confined to the rectum, the chief medicaments, and those most
frequently to be repeated, should be of a local nature.

Owing to the muscular relaxation, so common to persons who
have resided long in tropical climates, and to tropical invalids,
hæmorrhoidal tumours, relaxation, and descent of the mucous
membrane of the rectum are very liable to occur ; and when to
this condition of the muscular system we add the general and local
results of chronic diarrhœa or dysentery, with their anæmic states,
and the tenesmus of months, or even years, no wonder that the
sphincter and the entire perinæum should prove inordinately flaccid.
This state of perinæal relaxation causes very distressing uterine
descent likewise, even in very young females. The pain and
irritation from hæmorrhoidal tumours keep up a disposition to
void the contents of the bowels, and to ineffectual straining, while
the loss of blood so frequently attendant on these affections greatly
aggravates the concomitant anæmia. Along with relaxation and
anæmia there exist here immediate mechanical sources of injury :
the descending mucous lining, or the tumours, as may be, from
within or without the bowel, and the hypertrophied integument
external to the sphincter, keep that muscle in a permanently
relaxed or half-closed state, impairing its tone ; and the hæmorrhoids, whether blind or bleeding, proceed from bad to worse.
In general, it will be found proper to wait for some improvement
in the general health before any kind of operation is had recourse
to; but where the bleeding from the hæmorrhoid is depressing,
the application of nitric acid to the bleeding point or points is
advisable. In other cases, and where the habit is in a better condition, I recommend the operation of Hey and of Abernethy—that
preferred also by Liston and Mr. Fergusson. This operation,
always safe, and generally successful, consists, first, in replacing the
obtruded internal pile, or relaxed mucous membrane, with the
oiled finger ; and secondly, in drawing out the loose hypertrophied
external integument with a common vulsellum, and in clipping off
portions of it with strong scissors, the directions of the excisions
corresponding with that of the bowel—the blades of the scissors,
according to Mr. Syme, of Edinburgh, being directed from the
circumference towards the centre of the anus. This operation at
once removes the mechanical external impediment to the natural
contractile action of the sphincter, while the cicatrices resulting
from the wounds afford permanent buttresses to support both the

sphincter and perinæum, or parts immediately external to and around the anus.

In cases where the relaxed, thickened, or otherwise altered mucous membrane, with or without condylomata, protrudes, the application of nitric acid, as first recommended by Dr. Houston of Dublin, or else the galvanic cautery, should be made. Like every operation for the cure of hæmorrhoids, the galvanic cautery and the nitric acid require care in the application;—and so does the ligature, which some operators still prefer. It should be remembered that the acid and the cautery do all which the ligature can do of good, and that without anything like the amount of risk attendant on the use of the latter, such as phlebitis, purulent deposit, &c. The acid should be of the strongest, so as utterly and at once to destroy the vitality of the parts to which it is applied; and it is better to repeat the application to small points at a time than to cover too large a surface at once with the acid. The same rule applies to the use of the actual cautery, likewise a safe remedy when used in the manner recommended by Mr. Henry Lee, of St. George's Hospital. Mr. Lloyd, at St. Bartholomew's Hospital, has for years been in the habit of smearing the whole surface of protruded membrane, and likewise the congested hæmorrhoidal tumours, with solid lunar caustic, it is said with uniform success; and he rarely finds it necessary to repeat the application above three or four times.

But whatever operation may be preferred for the removal of hæmorrhoids, condylomata, or altered and prolapsed mucous membrane, the clipping of the hypertrophied loose folds of integument around and external to the anus is a measure of absolute necessity to the cure. It should constitute the first and earliest operation, too, whatever else may be ultimately required in respect of morbid conditions within the sphincter. The clipping external operation, by restoring the free action of the sphincter, is very often curative of what are termed internal piles, and this circumstance should of itself secure for it a priority and a preference; but where it happens otherwise, the early removal of loose and thickened folds of integument, impeding the contractile action of the sphincter, is necessary to the eventual success of any and every means of cure directed to within the anus.

I state these circumstances upon observations of an extended nature, both in India and at home. But I would observe further of these cases, and, indeed, of all cases of returned Indians requiring surgical operations, that to treat them with justice requires a careful regard to their peculiar habit—care beforehand and care in the after-treatment being necessary. The nervous system of the returned Indian is excitable, and, if but recently from the East, he is often anæmic—conditions of the system which obviously require much attention. I saw a lady, but recently arrived in England, in whom the opening of a small encysted.

tumour nearly proved fatal; and in the case of a gentleman, the same dangerous symptoms resulted from the removal of a small internal hæmorrhoidal tumour by ligature.

The benefits derivable from horse exercise, in the prevention and cure of hæmorrhoidal affections, are not generally understood; yet they are very great. Riding on horseback acts beneficially by accelerating the course of circulation along the veins, while it brings the sphincter and adjoining muscles into alternate action, thus contributing, the one action with the other, to prevent venous engorgement, and to impart tone to the relaxed muscles.

I propose now to conclude with the histories of some cases of interest, with a view further to illustrate the treatment of chronic dysentery.

CASE III.—April, 1854.—Captain ——, aged thirty, had served in India six years, enjoying excellent health. In April, 1852, his corps was ordered to Rangoon, where he underwent much exposure and fatigue, being indifferently fed at times. In September, 1853, while serving at Prome, he was seized with acute dysentery. He was actively treated, with mitigation of suffering; but purging continuing, he was ordered home, and arrived in England in February, 1854. Purging still continued to distress him, and he obtained leave to reside with his relatives. Here he took calomel to salivation, with apparent benefit at first; but after three weeks all his distresses returned, and he came to London on the 18th of April, 1854.

He was then pale and anæmic, and much emaciated; skin cool and damp; pulse feeble and slow; tongue clean. He was purged from eight to ten times in the twenty-four hours, with much straining, voiding quantities of mucus streaked with blood. There was no hepatic complication, but he had tenderness on exploration along the cæcum and colon, with feeling of soreness in the course of the rectum. Ordered the following mixture, of which two table-spoonfuls were used three times a day, and five grains of Dover's powder, with two of gallic acid, at bed-time:—Infusion of sima-ruba, seven ounces and a half; extract of logwood and tincture of krameria, of each two drachms; dilute nitric acid and dilute hydrochloric acid, of each one drachm; tincture of opium, one drachm and a half. The patient was at the same time enjoined to avoid all exercise, to observe great caution in diet, especially as to quantity, and the use of warm clothing and the warm bath at bed-time.

April 28th.—Had a visit from the patient, stating, that though he had walked out daily during cold weather, he felt then "quite well," and that after the fourth day he had discontinued the night pills, contenting himself with the mixture. He added, that he had but one formed motion in the twenty-four hours, and that unattended by either blood or mucus in the discharges, and that straining and all uneasiness had disappeared. Ordered the continuance of the mixture twice a day, with a view to obviate any tendency to relapse.

July 18th.—Says he has been living in the country, and that by exposure to cold while fishing, and by irregularities in diet, he has brought back " looseness of the bowels on several occasions, but no dysenteric feelings." He then had recourse to his mixture, and always with complete success. He was again ordered to take five grains of Dover's powder, with two of gallic acid, every night, and urged to use temperance in diet. This course of medicine he continued for a month, with how much temperance, however, I know not; but he became well.

Remarks.—It were unsafe to conclude that, in a case such as this, because it yielded so readily to treatment, it was therefore free from ulceration, and from the more grave dangers of secondary purulent deposit in the liver. The appearance of the intestinal discharges, together with the feeling of soreness along the course of the large intestine, gave me the impression that ulceration did exist, and in such cases there is always a certain amount of contingent danger. That the symptoms gave way so rapidly was more than, under the circumstances, could have been expected, and the cure was effected, not by the employment of any specific, but by means suggested by experience.

Case IV.—April, 1854.—Major ——, aged forty-six, went to India in 1828, his actual residence there being twenty-five years. He enjoyed good health till 1832, when he had a severe attack of intermittent fever, which has recurred at intervals ever since. While in Calcutta, in 1839, he was seized with a diarrhœa, which resisted treatment during eight months, but he regained health in the heats of April, 1840.

In November, 1843, while serving at Delhi, he was seized with a low form of remittent fever, which emaciated and enfeebled him much, and for the cure of which he was sent to the Himalayah mountains, where he recovered. In the statement of Major ——'s case by the surgeon of his regiment, it is reported, that " in 1844 he had a severe attack of acute hepatitis, for which he was then actively treated, and subsequently sent to Simlah. He has since, at irregular intervals, been under treatment for dysentery, and on account of attacks of fever attended with much disposition to visceral congestion."

In 1847-48, while serving at Lahore, he had a recurrence of diarrhœa during two cold seasons, but which disappeared in the hot season of the latter year.

In May, 1851, in consequence of repeatedly recurring febrile attacks, he was recommended to proceed to the hills again, where he regained good health.

In November, 1852, Major —— rejoined his regiment, and

continued well till February, 1853, when dysenteric symptoms recurring with severity, he was, after. a time, ordered home, and arrived in England in April, 1854.

He was now in a state of extreme emaciation and distress; the complexion dark and sallow; the spirits prostrated; much pain along the colon and rectum, with severe tenesmus; pulse feeble, and 82 in the minute. The tongue and fauces are described by the medical gentleman in attendance as "red and angry, as if stripped of epithelium;" the motions white, fluid, and frothy, containing muco-purulent matter.

From April to the middle of August I saw the patient at intervals of two or three weeks; and Dr. Billing visited him occasionally in consultation. The treatment was obliged to be varied about every ten days; those medicines which appeared to agree best losing all effect, each in succession. Most of the vegetable and mineral astringents were used in conjunction with Dover's powders, morphia, simple opium, and bitter tonics, including the nitro-muriatic acid with opium and quinine,—all apparently with no other result than arresting the progress of the disease. On two occasions a grain of blue pill with morphia, given at bed-time, appeared to promote the function of the liver, to improve the secretions, and to correct the irritable condition of the mucous membrane; but at length extreme rectal distress supervened, with straining and inability to retain the contents of the bowels for an instant, when once the disposition to void arose; the matters discharged being extremely offensive, and containing mucus and pus. A drachm of finely-powdered charcoal in barley-water was now exhibited night and morning in the form of enema, with a remarkably soothing effect, while gallic acid and morphia in pill were continued three times a day. The effect of the charcoal was the most marked of all, the relief being very decisively evident; and by the middle of August the patient was sent into the country for change of air.

In February, 1855, Major —— called on me to ask my opinion as to his fitness to accept a command in Turkey. I then found that for some time previously his bowel complaint had been changed for constipation, and that he had gained considerably in flesh and strength, although not to the extent to permit of his entering on the active duties of his profession.

Remarks.—The case of Major —— is remarkable for the severity of succeeding tropical diseases during two-and-twenty years, and for the severity of the eventual dysentery. Originally of a powerful constitution, he went through an enormous amount of illnesses, one after another, without sinking. On arrival in England, and for months subsequently, his case appeared hopeless; but by a persevering course of treatment, frequently changed to meet the altering circumstances of the case, by home nursing, and by the utmost attention to diet, clothing, &c., this excellent officer eventually recovered.

CASE V.—June, 1847.—Lieutenant-General —— had served in India about forty years, and had enjoyed more than an average share of good health. In 1825-26, he suffered from occasional attacks of diarrhœa, but I had personal knowledge that he passed through the two campaigns in Ava, during the first Burmese war, without any material aggravation of his disorder.

In 1827 he came to England, ailing, and returned to India in 1830, restored to health. He served in the Affghan war of 1842-43, and returned thence to India in the enjoyment of good health. On being removed to Calcutta, however, in 1844, he was speedily seized with dysentery. Two short voyages to sea "did him some good;" but a voyage to the Cape of Good Hope being determined on, he went to that colony early in 1846. Here he states that "several relapses, and one of a serious nature, having occurred," he returned to Bengal merely to arrange his affairs, and embarked again for England, where he arrived in June, 1847. During the voyage, he says, "I had several attacks; but latterly I became so much worse that I don't think I could have survived another month on board ship." He adds, that "the treatment pursued during the voyage, which consisted of lead and other astringents, with opium, was entirely changed after landing, and that his recovery was from that time very rapid." It was so; but the symptoms at first wore an unfavourable aspect. There were frequent discharges, with much distress, referred to the rectum, especially in the early morning, all containing pus and blood, the latter being sometimes voided in considerable quantities. There was much emaciation and debility—indeed, great exhaustion, whenever three or four motions were voided in rapid succession. The treatment consisted in the use of the nitro-muriatic acid and laudanum, in infusion of simaruba—adding great care as to diet and clothing, and the rigid observance of the recumbent posture.

On this plan, General —— improved so rapidly that in a fortnight he was allowed the use of animal food, after which time the progress towards recovery was uninterrupted; and during some months, when any appearance of recurrence was manifested, his medicine, which he carried about with him, always arrested morbid progress, until at length his health was completely restored.

Remarks.—The favourable issue in this instance was more speedy and permanent than I could have anticipated, for the disease had been of two and a half years' duration, and had resisted all medical means, both in India and at the Cape of Good Hope, aided by two voyages to sea. The Bael fruit of Bengal did some good; but neither this, nor the grapes of the Cape, proved of avail to the cure, and mercury, whenever used on board ship, did perceptible injury. This case, in fact, looked unfavourable, for ulceration of the rectum was evident, and perhaps this state of disease extended higher up the intestine; but the course of treatment agreed at once, resulting in speedy and permanent recovery of health. It proved, unhappily, otherwise in the instance now to be recorded in conclusion.

CASE VI.—Lieutenant-General ——, aged seventy, had served much in hot climates, and had an attack of jaundice at the age of twenty-six. He served twice in the East Indies, suffering, on the first occasion, from slight attacks of intermittent fever, one severe attack of coup-de-soleil, and latterly from chronic dysentery, but which speedily gave way on coming to England. After two years' residence at home, he returned to India, and arrived there in the height of the hot season, making a long journey into the interior without injury to his health, which continued good for about fifteen months under various exposures. At the end of the period last named, General —— having experienced a slight recurrence of dysenteric symptoms, such as he had formerly suffered from, he returned to England, and I saw him in the end of spring. His symptoms were then far from urgent: he had lost flesh, and was much depressed in spirits; but in so far as the affection of the bowels was concerned, appearances promised a speedy recovery. He used to say that "he had never felt like the same man since the coup-de-soleil."

I saw the patient, in all, five or six times only, in the early summer of his arrival. The bowels were at this time irregular—sometimes relaxed, and again constipated, blood and mucus being occasionally observed mixed with the contents of the bowel; but there was neither pain nor straining in the act of defecation. The skin and pulse were natural; the tongue clean; the appetite good; the intestinal and renal excretions were natural. There was no tenderness on pressure in any of the abdominal regions—no enlargement of the spleen or liver; and the disorder, slight as it appeared, was confined to the rectum.

Great care in diet and clothing was enjoined, avoiding all exercise, other than a gentle drive in a carriage; and in the way of medicine, he was directed to take compound powder of kino in infusion of simaruba, confection of senna, with sulphur and bitartrate of potash, being used when the bowels required aid. An enema, to be retained in the bowel, was directed to be used at bedtime, composed of alum in decoction of oak-bark.

It was six months from this time that I next saw General ——, by accident, when he told me that he had been residing in the country, and been there "treated for the liver, by means of calomel, which had done him much good."

The greater part of the following year was passed in barely tolerable health, interrupted every six weeks or two months by actual recurrences of his disorder, for which calomel or blue-pill was always used in the country. Supposing that there was something hæmorrhoidal in his case, General —— now consulted a person who advertised to cure such diseases "without operation." From whatever means were here used, no benefit resulted, bowel complaint, on the contrary, becoming more troublesome.

He now consulted an eminent physician in London, under whose care "he rallied much during the winter of 1852-53." In the spring of the latter year the patient was attended in the country by another practitioner, who, on careful examination, found him at first in a feeble, broken state of constitution—depressed, anæmic, dyspeptic, suffering from chronic dysentery, fæcal matter being retained, and the evacuations being very offensive, and accompanied by muco-purulent matter and blood. There was no tenderness or enlargement of the liver, some tenderness with slight enlargement of the spleen, tenderness with tympanitic distension along the whole course of the colon, especially at its sigmoid flexure. Examination of the rectum disclosed congestion of the mucous membrane, with ulceration; no hæmorrhoidal tumour.

The treatment consisted at first of rhubarb, hyoscyamus, and alterative doses of blue-pill, followed by mild aperients; then nitrate of silver, with opium and quinine, were administered with excellent effect, followed by enemata containing oil of turpentine. Under this treatment, General —— appeared for a time to improve much, but the amendment was not of long duration.

In the early summer the patient returned to London, and consulted his former physician there. This gentleman reports General —— as "much thinner; much tenesmus, with extreme pain at times in the rectum." The condition of the patient was now such as to excite much alarm; the motions were dark and fœtid, and contained shreds of decayed mucous membrane; there were occasional rigors, and towards evening marked accessions of fever. In a month the symptoms greatly increased, with much pain across the lower belly, the motions being putrid and mixed with blood and pus. Towards the end of summer the pain in the rectum became excruciating, with total loss of appetite, and feeling of sickness and exhaustion, the patient declaring that "it was all up with him." Towards the middle of autumn, feeling "infinitely better," he quitted London for the country, and came a second time under the care of his former medical friend. General —— complained now, for the first time, of pain in the right side, which increased towards night; and, on examination, there was found considerable swelling in the hepatic region, with bulging of the ribs of that side, and dry cough. "These were new symptoms, and the patient became anxious for me to explain the cause of them. I told him that I thought hepatic abscess was forming during the last week. There was constant and excessive expectoration, purulent and bloody." Mercurial inunction was now recommended by the medical gentleman who had originally prescribed this mineral, and it was "carried to the extent of producing ptyalism." The patient expired in a fortnight, or about two years and a half from the date of his return to England.

On examination after death, the mucous membrane of the colon, sigmoid flexure, and rectum was found softened and ulcerated; the spleen dark, indurated, and enlarged; the liver containing a large abscess. The physician who saw most of this case in London gives it as his opinion, that "the suppurative action in the liver was, in a great measure, if not entirely, secondary to the ulceration of the lower bowel;" while the other physician, who was consulted early, gives the following summary :—

"1st.—Injury to the intestinal surface, from tropical influences of long standing.

"2nd.—Injured surface ulcerating in the last attack.

"3rd.—Abscess of the liver derived from absorption of pus from the ulcerated intestine."

This gentleman adds, that when he was consulted, he could, "on a careful examination, detect no sign whatever of liver abscess;" nor was there indeed, at the time of my first seeing him, any indication of hepatic disease, functional or structural.

Remarks.—The two cases here last recorded present a remarkable contrast—the first being immeasurably the severer of the two. The patient was in the last stage of exhaustion—bedridden; and when he stood erect, there was an instant call to void by stool.

In the last case, on the contrary, the symptoms, on arrival in England, were so trifling as to constitute to all appearance but a slight indisposition, the patient having been in London a fortnight before he thought of consulting me respecting his state of health; yet his disease proved eventually fatal. Here we perceive, in one out of many cases, the dangers attaching to chronic dysentery, even when it appears to be of the mildest character.

Suppurative phlebitis, and consequent purulent deposit—to use the ordinary but unsatisfactory expressions — may here be inferred, but what the actual morbid process consists in does not, as yet, appear to be demonstrated. Purulent secondary deposits are mentioned by many surgeons as resulting from the application of ligatures to hæmorrhoidal tumours; and this is but another instance of the so-termed purulent deposit from ulceration of the mucous membrane of the large intestine. Nor are such abscesses in the liver limited to cases in which ulceration exists in the mucous digestive surface; for they are observed to result from other lesions as well, and to affect the lungs as well as the liver, both organs being otherwise healthy. On the 15th of March, 1854, a stableman, aged forty-four, died in St. George's Hospital, of "phagedæna of the great toe; secondary deposits in the liver, and pleurisy."

On questions relating to the medical treatment of the case of General ——, I shall offer no opinion, as the patient came under my personal observation in the very earlier stage of his disease only, and at a time when his condition promised a speedy recovery. I perceived, however, from his frequent visits to London, that rest was wanting to this case, and rest in chronic dysentery is a most necessary means of cure—the neglect of it being productive of great mischief, sometimes of danger.

CONGESTION OF THE LIVER.

CONGESTION of the liver, whether of an acute or chronic nature, and regarded as it occurs in practice, is but an intermediate condition, or state of transition, between mere functional disorder and organic disease ; for, in general, and under appropriate treatment, all cases of hepatic congestion, whether active or passive, will end in the restoration of health. For instance, we continually see in India that tumidness of both liver and spleen occurs during the cold stage of intermittent fever, and that this form of congestion even recurs for weeks and months together ; and yet, under proper measures of cure, the patient ultimately escapes from organic disease of either organ. In these cases, the blood is still presumed to be in a healthy condition ; that is, uncontaminated by the protracted stagnation of passive congestions in the great abdominal viscera. But, on the return of the tropical invalid to his native country, we have seen that all the natural and physical circumstances constituting climate are greatly altered, and, moreover, that the blood is, through these very passive congestions, and the other causes stated, frequently and materially degraded in quality. The anæmic depravation of the circulating fluid is here, as in every other disease, a source of embarrassment and of difficulty in the treatment. In India, acute congestion passes on rapidly to inflammation : but of this transition I have not seen one instance in England. The passive form of congestion, however, is very frequent amongst Europeans, on their return to their native climate ; and one such, presently to be related, proceeded into acute congestion, and thence into inflammation and its results. That in these cases there is congestion of the duodenum as well, cannot be doubted ; the distended state of the portal vein rendering this complication a condition of necessity.

In this disease the complexion will be of a muddy-sallow, or lemon-yellow hue, livid or venous, according to the age and powers of the constitution, temperament, and length of residence in hot climates, of the individual. Congestion of the liver is generally produced by the application of cold to the surface of the body, and not unfrequently by errors in diet. Cold thus applied to the skin of persons who have resided long in hot climates, and in whom the fluids had for so long been derived to the surface of the body, and in whom therefore a determination of the fluids inwards, by cold, is peculiarly liable to take place, must necessarily prove a powerfully exciting cause. This disposition to congestion, through the agency of cold, is also much increased where the individual has suffered from malarious fevers, and from consequent disturbance of the balance of circulation. The feeling of the patient is one of epigastric fulness, uneasiness, and oppression, rather than of pain, of the region of the liver. The organ is oppressed by an accumulation and stagnation of blood, while its function is paralysed. With all this we have frequently a weakened condition of the heart and arteries, and a diminished power of reaction, consequently. It is only, however, when the hepatic congestion is associated with a similar condition of the cerebral organs, or of the lungs, that danger to life need, under careful management, be apprehended. In the cerebral, and in the thoracic complication, there is indeed a pressing and immediate danger, even under the best remedial means known to us.

I find that in the first part of this work, when speaking of the congestive fever of the cold season in Bengal, the following observations occur ; and I here quote them, to show how prevailing must be the liability to hepatic congestion in European invalids coming at once from hot climates into the winter and spring seasons of England :—" It is believed, that in animals whose pulmonary system is less perfect, there is a greatly increased quantity of blood transmitted through the liver. In hot climates, then, where respiration is less perfectly carried on than in cold ones, owing, according to Tiedemann and Gmelin, to the greater rarefaction of the air in warm regions, a vicarious decarbonization of the blood is established by an increased flow of bile ; and hence it is that the liver, weakened in its function, and torpid, in proportion to the excitement of the hot and rainy seasons, becomes disposed to congestion, or inflammation of its parenchyma, during the cold season : and thus are produced the dangerous states of disease noticed. An irritable or inflamed state of the mucous digestive surface is also a frequent complication ; and these two together constitute the great dangers of our congestive fevers of the cold season, as well as of those of the autumnal fevers of the more unhealthy countries of Europe."

There is no more efficient cause of congestion of the liver than antecedent torpor of its function — especially where this last disorder has been of long duration. To the tumult of the nervous, vascular, and secreting functions, within the tropics, has now succeeded an exhausted condition of all three. The system at large, and the organ now principally at fault, have lost their power of resisting the cold and damp atmosphere of Europe. To be more precise, the circulation through the skin, and also its function, which had been raised to the greatest degree by the high temperature of the tropics, are reduced to the opposite extreme by the cold and damp atmosphere of our northern climate. The blood which had long been drawn to the periphery, is now driven to the centre. Vascular reaction seldom ensuing, the congestion is of a passive nature. There is stagnation of the portal circulation, and a consequent contamination of the blood, with languor and oppression of all the abdominal functions.

When hepatic congestion is recent, the stagnation of the venous circulation is confined principally to the special organ, but it must be evident that a duration of no great extent will engorge the whole of the abdominal viscera as well—thus causing impairment of function in each and all of them—but more particularly in the original seat of disease—the liver. In truth, most of the diseases of persons who have resided long in hot climates should be carefully observed in connexion with the distribution, functions, and disorders of the portal system—a due regard to which, says Sir Henry Holland, will aid us much in interpreting many obscure points in pathology.

CASE I.— ——, Esq., of fair complexion and slender frame, thirty-five years of age, has served sixteen years in India, and during the first twelve years his health was good. Five years ago, while on official duty in an unhealthy district, and living in tents, he was seized with severe intermittent fever, in which the cold stages were oppressively distressing, lasting at first for two hours and upwards, accompanied by fulness and dull pain in the regions of the spleen and liver. He got well in three weeks, under the use of mild mercurials, active purgatives, and quinine. His fever recurred every cold season since his first seizure, his general health and digestive power becoming annually more enfeebled, and at last he was ordered home on sick leave. He arrived in England in the month of March, as he thought, much improved in health by the sea voyage. The state of the general habit was anæmic.

April 3rd.—He states that six days ago, while standing in an easterly wind, in a race-stand, he felt chilled, but had no rigor; he has been much indisposed ever since. The surface of the body is now pale, cold, and harsh to the touch; the pulse feeble, slow, and oppressed; the bowels are constipated, and the urine scanty and turbid. The hypochondrium is seen to bulge out; the left lobe of the liver is found, on exploration, to extend three inches beyond the margin of the ribs, the organ being enlarged in all directions. There is no pain on the most free pressure, and all that he complains of in reference to the hepatic region is a sense of weight and uneasiness.

Calomel in small doses was given every night for a week, in combination with compound extract of colocynth, the acetous extract of colchicum and ipecacuanha, followed in the morning by a purgative draught of compound decoction of aloes, infusion of senna, and jalap powder, with aromatics. After the third exhibition, these medicines produced copious biliary discharges, so as rapidly to diminish the volume of the liver. This plan of treatment was accompanied from the beginning by sinapisms to the hepatic region, warm baths every other night, and friction to the entire surface of the body. On the ninth day congestion had so far subsided, through copious excretion, that the treatment was concluded by the nitro-muriatic acid, in combination with fluid extract of taraxacum, given three times a day, and purgative pills were continued at bedtime, composed of compound extract of colocynth, compound galbanum pill, each half a drachm, with two minims of croton oil, made into twelve pills. Of these, two were given at first, and then one, until they were gradually discontinued. Warm baths and friction were used at longer intervals, till every symptom had vanished, when exercise in the open air, and mild chalybeates, concluded the treatment. The diet at first consisted of farinaceous articles, with thin soup, vegetables, and fruit; but, as health improved, animal food with diluted wine was allowed.

CASE II.—Lieutenant ———, of the Indian cavalry, states that soon after parting with his wife and child, who were obliged to leave India on account of ill health, he became depressed in spirits, and lost his appetite and flesh rapidly. Pain and tumour in the right side soon indicated inflammation of the liver, for which he was very largely bled, followed by a course of calomel purgatives, and blisters. Abscess, however, resulted, and the matter was discharged into the colon. He arrived in England in the month of April, in a very enfeebled and emaciated state, having slight cough, with little appetite, the digestion being much impaired, and the bowels constipated. There was no fever, the pulse being languid, the skin cool, dry, and harsh to the touch. The general condition was anæmic.

I ordered the decoction of taraxacum with dilute nitro-muriatic acid, mild aperient pills devoid of mercury, warm baths, and powerful friction to the skin; the diet to be spare, light, and nutritious, with a little bitter ale to dinner. Strict injunctions were given to avoid exposure to cold.

On this plan he rapidly recovered flesh, and by September his appearance indicated returning health.

I was requested to visit Lieutenant —— in the January following, in consultation with Mr. Squibb, of Montague-place. I then learned that, three weeks previously, the patient had taken a long walk, after which, while still heated, he went to hear the afternoon service in a neighbouring church. Here he felt chilled, and the result was an attack of bronchitis, from which I found him recovering. The object of the consultation was to determine the state of the liver, and here there existed passive congestion, with all its concomitants.

Lieut. —— was now ordered every night to take pills composed of three grains each of calomel and compound extract of colocynth, and a grain each of the acetous extract of colchicum and ipecacuanha powder, while warm baths and fomentations to the side were used daily. The effect of the pills was to cause copious discharges of black vitiated bile, great reduction of the previous bulging of the hepatic region, and great general relief. After a few days the quantity of calomel was diminished, and a quarter grain of morphia substituted for the colchicum. Presently, and as the secretions became healthy, all mercurial preparations were omitted, and the nitro-muriatic acid with fluid extract of taraxacum was substituted. Under this latter plan, which was continued for two months, Lieut. —— recovered condition. His cough, which had been constant, accompanied by coloured expectoration, ceased, and, after a residence of two months at Hastings, he returned to London, looking stout, and feeling well.

Case III.—Major ——, a distinguished staff officer, aged forty-two, served upwards of twenty years in India. About twelve years ago he suffered from intermittent fever; but a furlough to Europe completely restored his health. Had lately been much exposed to alternate heat by day and severe cold at night in the campaigns on the Sutlej, but did not suffer from fever. At Bombay, however, while living in tents, he was severely chilled, and this was followed by a sense of weight in the right side and epigastrium, which did not leave him till he got to Alexandria. He arrived in England in April, in apparently good health, so as to be able to use violent country exercises. In the end of May, after a long day's riding and cricketing, he was exposed to night cold, and this was followed by symptoms similar to those he experienced when at Bombay. There was a sense of weight and oppression in the epigastric region, with loss of appetite and constipation of the bowels. A fortnight passed in this state of indisposition, during which he was treated for ordinary dyspepsia. Severe rigors followed by reactive fever now came on. This fever was treated as ague, by large doses of quinine, of which he took twenty grains for days together. This treatment arrested the rigors, but fever, with hot dry skin, continued, and the abdomen began to enlarge, with oppression and uneasiness in the right side and epigastrium. He now removed to a provincial town, where his disease was still pronounced to be intermittent fever. Quinine was there continued, with occasional aperients, and latterly he used tonics and chalybeates, the diet having all along been but little restricted. For the last month he has been residing near London, suffering greatly from pain of the right side and shoulder. His days have been passed sitting by the fireside, supporting his head on his hands, while his elbows rested on his knees. His nights have passed in a burning fever, but he has had neither rigors nor perspirations.

He drove to my house on the 16th of September, and walked with the body bent forward on the pelvis, sitting in the same attitude, and breathing rapidly. His complexion was of a leaden yellow hue; the skin dry, and of a pungent heat; the pulse feeble, and at 108; the abdomen was tense, round, and hard as a barrel, with an enormous bulging of the right hypochondrium; the liver extending four inches downwards from the margin of the false ribs, and pushing up into the right cavity of the chest. Percussion and exploration of every kind gave no pain, but only a slight uneasiness. He complained of headache, the eyes being suffused, yellow, and muddy; the tongue deeply coated, and red at the edges; the urine was of a madder colour; the bowels constipated. The nature of his case was explained to Major ——, and he was urged to remain in bed, to which he seemed averse. He was ordered to take two pills composed of extract of colocynth, calomel, and ipecacuanha, with a quarter of a grain of morphia at bedtime, followed by a purgative draught, using a warm bath every other night; the diet to be purely farinaceous.

On the 19th September the patient again visited me, expressing himself as being much relieved. For the first time during months past he had had refreshing sleep; the skin was somewhat relaxed; the pulse 94; pain of the liver, head, and shoulder somewhat diminished. The medicines had acted powerfully on the bowels, the urine remaining as before. Major —— was now informed that his treatment could not be safely or effectively conducted abroad; and that in such cold weather it was dangerous to leave his house, or even his bed. The former medicines were directed to be continued.

Sept. 21st.—Called to see Major —— at his residence, where I requested a consultation with two medical officers who had lately been in attendance on him. It was here agreed that mild mercurials, with sudorifics, and small doses of morphia, should be exhibited over-night, followed by active purgatives in the morning, while warm baths were used at night, with frequent hot fomentations to the side during the day. The rapid and feeble state of the circulation, and the general exhaustion, precluded bloodletting in any form, either general or local.

27th.—On this plan of treatment great relief of symptoms ensued; the complexion improved; the skin became soft; the pulse was reduced to 80; while the tumid and tense state of the abdomen subsided apace, exposing the full extent of the hepatic enlargement and induration. But night fever recurred, accompanied by pain in the shoulder, as before. There were no rigors or night perspirations; the urine exhibited no change, being almost blood-red. The course of treatment already described was continued, gradually diminishing the amount of calomel, until, in the tender state of the gums, and the odour of the breath, the gentle influence of mercury was apparent. The tumidity of the abdomen and enlargement of the liver had now subsided greatly; the tongue had cleaned, and the pulse was reduced to 84; yet no healthy secretion passed from the bowel, and the urine remained unchanged. The nightly exacerbations of fever continued to recur, though much diminished in duration and force; no rigors or night-sweats. The gums were retracted, white, and disposed to ulcerate at their edges. Under these unfavourable circumstances, as regards the anticipated results of the mercurial treatment, mercury was discontinued, and immersion of the whole body, night and morning, in the nitro-muriatic acid bath, was substituted, continuing the daily exhibition of purgatives. The diet, which had hitherto consisted of farinaceous articles and soup, was further improved by the addition of a little solid meat, game, &c., the appetite having greatly improved.

Under this treatment the tumidness of the abdomen and liver still further diminished, so that the latter could no longer be felt under the margin of the ribs, though still considerably enlarged on its convex surface towards the chest; the night-fever was reduced to an hour's duration, and the sleep was refreshing; the tongue clean, but no improvement in the intestinal or renal secretions. With the exceptions stated, general improvement continued; when of a sudden, diarrhœa, with a furred, dry tongue, hot and parched skin, feverishness, and absence of rest came on, accompanied by great and rapid emaciation, a sunken countenance, and great anxiety. In this condition Major —— was seen by Dr. Watson in consultation; and though I had previously expressed a suspicion of hepatic suppuration, it was agreed, that even now, though highly probable, the direct evidence of this was wanting. Ten days from this time, November 13th, Major —— died, in great suffering from pain and oppression of the right chest, and in the act of coughing up a thick, greenish pus, mixed with blood, of which some spoonfuls were exhibited next morning. There was no *post-mortem* examination.

Remarks.—I have placed the case of Major —— in the present article, because I believe congestion, on two occasions, constituted the original disorder, proceeding, in the last instance, into acute congestion or subacute inflammation of the liver, and terminating in abscess of that organ. The congestive state at Bombay was overcome by the warm and equable temperature, and by the gestation of the sea-voyage, aided, perhaps, by nausea and sea-sickness. But in the second congestive attack no such favourable influences existed. I have confined my narrative of this interesting and instructive case to a bare recital of facts, such as they were reported by the patient, and to a detail of the symptoms, which I personally witnessed, avoiding all comment on antecedent circum-stances; but I feel bound to state, that I received the most candid co-operation and able assistance from the two medical men with whom I consulted in the treatment of this distinguished but unfortunate officer. Up to the time when the mild influence of mercury was evidenced by the action on the gums, and by the mercurial fœtor, so much improvement had taken place as to warrant the balance of opinion to lean towards a favourable result; and so, also, with respect to the action of the nitro-muriatic acid bath, up to the fourteenth day before death, the unfavourable circumstances being, that by none of the means used was a healthy secretion obtained either from the liver or kidneys. This was the result anxiously looked for, and never obtained. The important practical question here was, When did the suppurative process commence? My own impression was, first, that the formation of abscess had taken place within the fortnight before death; and secondly, that the abscess was of but small extent; for in India, in the instances of large hepatic abscesses, I have never seen one case in which rigors, colliquative sweat, and a permanently furred tongue, were all absent, as in this instance. The pain of the right shoulder amounting, during several weeks of July and August, to agony, indicated the seat of the active inflammation to have been centred in the upper convex surface of the liver, involving its peritonæal covering; for there is seldom much pain, and very often none at all, when the parenchyma alone is the seat of the inflammation. In general, these circumstances point to the actual seat of the subsequent abscess.

CASE IV.—Major-General ——, aged seventy-one, served thirty-six years in Bengal, and has resided fifteen years in England. Eight or ten years ago he is reported to have suffered from repeated attacks of intermittent fever, for the cure of which quinine was administered largely. These attacks were finally overcome by the use of calomel and purgatives, quinine having proved of no avail. His habit is spare but muscular, and in diet he has been through life abstemious to an extreme degree, having avoided wine and malt liquors altogether for years, and used animal food during the last two years but sparingly, once in twenty-four hours. He has been used to active walking exercise all his life; but during the last year official duties have interfered much with this salutary habit, while they have agitated and over-excited his mind. Within the last month he has been often exposed to severe cold at night, when returning from dinner-parties. He relates that his habit has always been to use cold ablution in the morning; but owing to the severity of the last winter and spring, and to the cold water proving ungrateful to his feelings, he has for some months substituted ablution with warm water.

On getting out of bed this morning, April 4th, he felt giddy to staggering, with nausea, and some degree of faintness; and, as the weather was warmer than of late, he bathed in cold water, took his usual breakfast, and drove to his office, where, during the last two days, his mind was unusually excited and agitated. To add to this distress he states, that for more than an hour of the forenoon he was persecuted by solicitations with which he could not comply. At noon he was seized with a violent rigor, accompanied by extreme pallor, and shrinking of the surface of the body, which was soon followed by vomiting. In this state he drove to my house. Violent shivering, with sense of extreme cold, lasted for two hours; but by warm drinks, and warmth applied externally, imperfect reaction was established, accompanied by moisture of the surface. The tongue is loaded with a thick white fur; urine for some time past scanty and surcharged; bowels habitually regular, but of late the excretions have been scanty and clay-coloured.

On examination of the abdomen, the region of the liver was found tumid, bulging, and very painful on pressure, so much so, that he started when it was touched, the abdomen throughout being puffed and inelastic. He felt no pain anywhere else. A full dose of calomel, with James's powder, was given immediately. At 7 P.M., reaction still continued moderate, with a warm gentle perspiration. Ordered two pills, composed of compound extract of colocynth and calomel, to be taken at bedtime, and a purgative draught for the early morning.

At midnight I was summoned to the patient, and found that, on getting out of bed, he had fallen on the floor without the power to recover himself. The face and neck were of a reddish livid hue, with deep somnolency, and difficulty of being roused; skin hot and dry; pulse full, but easily compressed. I found that another medical gentleman had been summoned at the same time with me, and we agreed at once that the patient should be cupped from the neck, while a blister was applied to the right hypochondrium. The cupping abstracted twelve ounces, with marked relief from cerebral oppression; but it was not till copious and repeated discharges of vitiated bilious evacuations from the bowels, that the patient was so far restored as to reply to questions.

April 5th, 10 A.M.—General —— is now perfectly restored to consciousness, and expresses himself as much relieved, especially from the sense of pain and weight in the side. No headache; skin moist and warm; pulse 90; secretion of urine copious, but of a deep porter colour. Ordered a pill, composed of two grains each of calomel and colocynth, to be given every two hours. Diet farinaceous.

9 P.M.—General —— was seized with a violent rigor, accompanied by stupor, but both speedily gave way to diffusible stimuli, ammonia, and the use of warm drinks. The following reaction was but trifling, and it now became apparent that ultimate recovery might be regarded as more than ever doubtful. In consultation with Drs. Chambers and Watson, simple calomel was ordered to be given frequently during the night, while a blister was applied to the nape of the neck.

April 6th.—After midnight, relaxation of the surface with flagging circulation rendered the use of wine and soup necessary.
The powers of life are now (10 A.M.) sinking, and he is dependent
on the frequent use of stimulants ; consciousness but partial.
Died at 6 P.M.

Remarks.—Here we perceive hepatic congestion of the most
severe character, followed by a congestive metastasis to the brain,
and accompanied by diminished power in the heart and arteries,
all taking place fifteen years after the return to the native climate
of the patient.   The organ primarily affected was the liver—that
which, during youth and manhood, had been most excited in its
function—and that, too, in a person of unusually abstemious and
active habits of life.   It would seem that with some persons no
amount of care will prove a sufficient protection against hepatic
disease.   All the circumstances of constitution, and of habit of
life, mental and bodily, were in favour of this gentleman's living
in health to an advanced age ; yet were they all frustrated by the
antecedent circumstances of service, and of long exposure to the
influence of a tropical sun.   In these respects, and in respect of
the influence of mental excitement on a nervous system very im-
pressible in its nature, the case is most interesting.   From the
time that General —— experienced discomfort in the use of the
cold bath, it may be inferred that hepatic congestion and functional
disturbance were present; and there can be no doubt that the
great and repeated mental excitements of the past year laid the
foundation of the cerebral complication which proved fatal, and
but for which the hepatic disease would easily have been overcome.   It is remarkable how often we find, towards the decline of
life, and when the vigour and the balance of the functions have
been impaired, that the liver—the organ most excited in hot
climates—assumes disease, and that in persons who had not previously suffered from actual disease of that organ, either while
residing in hot climates, or during a protracted residence at home.
Numerous such instances have come under my observation, and
have been reported to me by various medical men since my return
to England.   In March, 1851, an old gentleman who had resided
long in the East Indies, and enjoyed excellent health there, died
in London of influenza.   He had resided in England since 1814,
and till lately he carried his age well ; but during his last illness
the liver became enlarged, and for the last ten days of his life the
whole body was deeply jaundiced.

TORPOR OF THE LIVER.

Torpor of the hepatic function, under the intropulsive action of the united cold and damp of an European climate, would seem, *primâ facie*, and naturally, to follow on the former frequent disturbance and general over-excitement of that function under tropical heats; and so we find it, in fact, hepatic torpor being a very frequent disorder, both in its idiopathic and complicated states, especially amongst those who have resided many years in the East Indies, who have undergone much direct solar exposure, and who have been neglectful of the habits of life proper to the climate.

To the increased biliary secretion of the hot and rainy seasons in India, followed by proportionate diminution òf the hepatic function in each succeeding cold season—alternations extending over many years—a more enduring impairment of function has now succeeded, accompanied generally by great reduction in the reparative powers of the constitution.

The violent and repeated congestions resulting from the recurring fevers of many years' duration, and following on those of the remittent and intermittent types especially, seldom fail to produce functional disorders or structural alterations of the liver, spleen, or bowels—almost all the complications in the fevers of India, and almost all their sequelæ in Europe, being abdominal. The milder results, in young persons, generally consist in congested states, more or less acute, of the abdominal circulation, but more especially of the portal circulation, giving a tumid, inelastic, or doughy impression to the explorer. The opposite or converse influences of the climates of India and of Europe, and the converse disorders resulting from them, must be held in constant recollection in examining and prescribing for the tropical invalid, for they explain much that is common to each.

It may here be observed of the disorder under consideration, as, indeed, of all the ailments, functional and structural, to which this class of invalids is liable, that the season for most effective treatment, in so far as the influences of medicinal and external agents are concerned, is that of moderate warmth, or during our English summer and autumn. It is then that medical management may be carried out with the best results, because of the more equable determination of the fluids to the surface of the body, because of the naturally increased development of the hepatic function, and because of the diminished tendency to abdominal congestion during those seasons. I continually find that the treatment which proves but slow in its results, or but palliative, in the winter and spring seasons, becomes effective and curative in June, July, and August. This is especially true of the nitro-muriatic acid bath.

It is during the English winter that the Indian suffers most severely from torpidity of the liver, and it is in summer or autumn that he obtains the most sure relief.

In persons who have passed many years in hot climates, the evidence of torpidity of the liver is generally found in the more or less emaciated figure, sallow complexion, and constricted skin of the patient. He will be found of a "sallow, miasmatic, melancholy aspect." According to the physiological couplet of Dryden—

> "The yellow gall that in your stomach floats
> Engenders all these Visionary thoughts."

There is, in some persons, a remarkable and peculiarly offensive bilious odour issuing from the skin and lungs, which no amount of attention to personal cleanliness can overcome. Others, again, in addition to these unpleasant exhalations, see every object through a yellow medium;—the so-called yellow sight. The patient is harassed with dyspeptic ailments, varying in degree according to circumstances of constitution, previous habits of life, and length of residence in hot climates. There is in all cases a reluctance to exertion, mental or bodily, and frequently we find the mental faculties depressed to an extent that is truly distressing. The patient generally complains of headache or vertigo, accompanied by coldness of the lower extremities, the headache being sometimes severe, and occasionally paroxysmal. The sleep is dreamful, disturbed, and unrefreshing; the temper capricious, peevish. Occasionally there is a short hacking cough, and the bowels are always irregular, the functions of the cæcum and colon being much disturbed, the excretions being depraved, ash-coloured, and scanty; while the urine, in all the instances in which I have examined it, contained an excess of urea, uric acid, or phosphate of lime, but most frequently of all, the oxalate of lime in considerable quantities. The lithic, phosphatic, or mulberry diathesis may predominate, but some renal disturbance is almost invariably met with in this class of cases. Bile is sometimes present in the urine of such patients. Indeed, nature seems, in all forms of hepatic disease, in all climates, to establish a vicarious action in the kidneys, in compensation of the defective powers of the liver. This interchange of function also affords an important indication in treating the various hepatic derangements, by directing our attention to the use and value of diuretics, and to the judicious selection of them. In truth, we require, in the management of the cases under consideration, continually to hold in recollection the relative dependence and the compensating powers of the skin, lungs, liver, bowels, and kidneys, in reference to the constant relations and interchanges of their actions, one upon the other. In this disease too little bile is secreted, and the blood is consequently in a habitual state of impurity. There is acidity of the stomach and bowels, with a vitiated state of the digestion and assimilation. Prout thought he could discover in these cases an excessive acidity of the cæcum. There was always intense headache ; but on the restoration of the biliary secretion, and on its reaching the cæcum, " the headache vanished." More than twenty years ago, in the General Hospital of Calcutta, I observed and recorded the fact of morbid action being co-existent in the liver and cæcum.

An anæmic state of the general habit is common to patients suffering from torpor of the liver; so much is this the case, that anæmia of the liver might possibly be a more proper term than that chosen for the head of this article. If, according to Rokitansky, anæmia of the liver takes place in European climates, " accompanied by a diminution of its consistency," as " the result of hæmorrhages, exhaustion, or a reduction of the mass of the blood by extensive exudatory processes," how much more readily must such conditions hold in the instance of tropical invalids, taking into view the many deteriorating influences to which they have been exposed ?

The frequency of anæmia, and of its complication with general atony, amongst this class, I have had ample means of verifying. The vulgar expression, " He is a white-livered fellow," conveys a real significance beyond what might at first appear to attach to it, both as regards the depressed condition of the bodily and mental powers. Shakspeare's idea of the anæmic liver is perfect :—" For Andrew" (Sir Andrew Aguecheek), " if he were opened, and you found so much blood in his liver as will clog the foot of a flea, I'll eat the rest of the anatomy." Elsewhere Shakspeare asks why a man should " creep into the jaundice by being peevish."˙ Napoleon at St. Helena made use of the following remarkable expression :— "Nouveau Prométhée, le léopard d'Angleterre me ronge le foie sur mon rocher. J'ai voulu dérober le feu du Ciel pour en doter la France ; j'en suis cruellement puni."

" The liver," according to a popular writer, " is the seat of the affections throughout Hindustan. My liver is bursting (in grief) ; or, my liver is burning (in love), are the usual expressions." Fabian, when he suggests that Olivia only desires to rouse the dormant valour of Sir Andrew Aguecheek, says, she " put fire in your heart, and brimstone in your liver." " The ancients," says Mr. Wallace, " believed that the liver was the organ of sanguification, the source of animal heat, and the seat of the natural faculties."

" From whatever point of view we look at the physiology of bloodmaking," says Dr. T. K. Chambers, " the liver always forms a portion of the prospect. If we are considering the preparation of substances, for absorption or solution, its secretion plays an important part ; in the further fitting of these substances for forming constituents of the nutrient treasure, we find it lying between the place of their first reception and the mass of the blood ; if our attention is directed to the retention of the healthy condition, we

find it removing noxious or foreign substances both from the in-
coming nutriment and from that already in the circulation.   It
melts the metal, stamps the coin, and keeps it bright; whilst, as
respects the circulation of water with its burdens in and out of the
body, it furnishes a large supply to be afterwards taken up."

Anæmia, and consequent torpor of the liver, often follow on long-
continued hyperæmia of that organ.

In all cases of torpor of the hepatic function we find the process
of digestion and assimilation much impaired.   Owing to defective
quantity and quality of the gastric, biliary, and pancreatic fluids,
the nutritive functions are manifestly impaired.   The arrest of the
cuticular discharge, so abundant within the tropics—so powerful,
too, in carrying off acids and other redundancies from the blood—
occasions in many persons, on their return to Europe, an excessive acidity of the stomach, not to speak of the other more important alterations of functions already referred to.

It may be said, truly, that most of the influences of climate—
that most of the diseases resulting from these influences—and that
many of the habits of life of Europeans in India and other hot
climates, tend powerfully to disturb the functions of the liver, and
thus lead ultimately to serious disorders, and to actual disease of
that organ.   The summary offered by way of introduction to this portion of the work will have furnished the reader with examples of numerous climatorial causes of hepatic disorders and diseases; but
there is one other efficient cause, much overlooked, but which, on the
score of extensive influence, must not here be omitted—viz., mercury,
internally exhibited.   It has been observed in Europe that persons
who have used mercury, either in the liberal or rapid manner, or
as a protracted alterative course, have frequently been afflicted
subsequently with severe forms of hepatic disease.   There can be
no doubt that, through the repeated use of this mineral, even when
necessarily exhibited, the hepatic function is inordinately stimulated, to be proportionately enfeebled thereafter.   The action of
mercury on the liver may be viewed as having a close analogy to
the primary excitement, and subsequent exhaustion, of the functions of the stomach produced by dram-drinking.

Since my return from India I have frequently seen miserably
broken health, and permanent derangement of the functions of the
liver, as the results of yellow fever.   I have seen that the naval
and military officer when thus afflicted has never proved efficient
for active service thereafter.

In referring to the treatment of the troublesome and obscure
affection now under consideration, we must recollect, not only that
we have to deal with torpor of the secreting and excreting power,
but with viscidity and adhesiveness of the secreted fluid, and also
with diminished power in the gall-bladder and ducts to eliminate
their contents, with the addition, perhaps, of thickening of the
parietes of the vesicle and its canals—thus affording additional

and mechanical obstruction to the discharge of the bile. In some persons this torpor of function is so great, and the case proves so little amenable to treatment, that we are forced to suspect some alteration, more or less extensive, or some permanent injury to the elementary secreting structures of the liver.

The slightest reflection on the physiological and pathological changes, here but hinted at, will show the great difficulties that meet us in our endeavours at effective treatment. What little bile is secreted being vitiated, our indications of treatment should be directed to the production of a more abundant and more healthy action, and to the attenuation and elimination of the fluid secreted. A favourite remedy of this class has of late been found in the fluid extract of taraxacum. I believe it to be an alterative of some efficacy, especially when combined with the bicarbonate of soda, as exercising a solvent power on viscid bile, on fatty and other animal substances, while it supplies one of the declared offices of bile—the correction of the acidity of the chyme. This combination, but more certainly that with the bicarbonate or the bitartrate of potash, affects the excretion from the kidneys, increasing it in quantity and modifying it in quality. When I have recourse to this plan of treatment I direct its continuance for a month or six weeks, diminishing or omitting the alkalies after a time, but using the vegetable alterative in increasing quantities; and where I desire to increase the diuretic effect, I prescribe the acetate or the bitartrate of potash along with the taraxacum.

Alkalies, given singly, or combined with tonics, have long been in esteem for their solvent power over interstitial deposits. Formerly natron, subcarbonate of soda, was prescribed with the Peruvian bark, and the success of this treatment has given rise, in our own time, to the more general exhibition of alkalies in combination with the numerous bitter tonics. Alkalies and chalybeates exist in finer, because natural chemical union, in the mineral springs of various countries, and this union tends, by its combined effects, to produce the favourable results we now everywhere witness from the use of these waters.

Dr. Budd states that the soluble alkalies, potash and soda, have more remote effects than as mere antacids, by increasing the secretions of the liver and the kidneys, and perhaps by otherwise modifying the processes of nutrition. The effect of soda is different from that of potash, the latter acting more especially on the kidney. "The salts of soda, on the contrary, act more especially on the liver, increasing the secretion of bile, of which soda is a natural constituent, and are little esteemed as diuretics. In indigestion soda is more generally useful than potash, probably from its more direct effect on the liver." Dr. Budd concludes by stating that in common forms of indigestion, in which there exists "a furred tongue, defective action of the liver, and costive bowels, no remedy is more effectual than the bicarbonate of soda, in doses of fifteen grains three times a day, before meals, in conjunction with an occasional small dose of blue pill, to increase further the secretion of the liver, and with colocynth or aloes to keep up a regular action of the large intestine."

When alkalies prove cold or ungrateful to the stomach, I am in the habit of substituting the dilute nitric and hydrochloric acids. This addition to the dandelion proves in many cases powerful in effect as regards the function of the liver, and generally tonic to the digestive organs. The addition of the acids proves specially useful in cases where tropical dysentery or diarrhœa has previously existed, or where an irritable state of the mucous membrane is present. In this latter instance, however, its use is not borne long, and, in many persons, not at all, without the addition of the tincture of opium or of nux vomica. Such means, though slow in their effects, are infinitely more appropriate and safe than mereurials in these chronic forms of disease. They slowly but safely promote increase of secretion, while they impart tone to the functions of digestion. So much is this understood to be the case, that some physicians are in the habit of ordering the dilute hydrochloric acid before, and alkalies after meals. Of the latter class of remedies I have found a combination of the bicarbonate and nitrate of potash with a full dose of the extract of taraxacum, given three times a day for weeks together, to prove very effective in exciting the liver and bowels, both having been previously in a state of extreme torpor. Changes of treatment are indeed necessary in these chronic diseases, so difficult to treat; and the alternate use of alkalies and acids proves successful where neither, taken singly, would aecomplish our objects.

M. Trousseau has for years exhibited the hydrochloric acid after meals, he says, with much advantage. In an anæmic patient afflicted with obstinate chronic diarrhœa, he gave chalk at the commencement of the meals and hydrochloric acid after them, with the result of a complete cure. "I do not wish to go beyond the fact," he says, "and only repeat that in the different forms of dyspepsia connected with chronic affections, whether of the thorax or abdomen, hydrochloric acid, taken after meals, may lead to therapeutic results deserving attention."

In treating torpor of the liver, with its complications, it must be borne in mind that our purpose is to solicit rather than to urge the restoration of the impaired functions, and that such can only be effected with safety by gentle and persistent means, always holding in view the improvement in the nutritive qualities of the blood. We must here be content to look to the actions resulting from the means in use, however gradually brought about, rather than to specific operations; and we must even be careful not to push remedies too far. An over-sanguine and confident estimate of the influence of drugs leads to their grievous abuse; while, on the other hand, diffidence and despair of the action of remedies cause men to trifle with our science. True science will always be found between such extremes.

Whether exhibited as an aperient, or in purgative doses, I have found aloes in its several forms, superior to other purgatives. We are familiar with its irritant effects on the mucous surface of the rectum, and it is my opinion that such a drug cannot be other than active in the duodenum. In effect it is so, and it will be found, when given with ox-gall, taraxacum, the alkalies, the salts of iron, and ipecacuanha with colchicum, that its exhibition is at all times useful in stimulating and evacuating the duodenum, and that it thereby excites the secretion, and facilitates the discharge of bile.

Anæmia is uniformly productive of torpidity of the liver, the biliary secretion being depraved in common with its source, and having, in some cases, more of the character of serum than of bile. It ought here to be evident, that the endeavour to elicit a more abundant and healthy secretion, by mercurials and drastic purgatives, while the nutritive functions are impaired, and the blood remains impoverished, must be alike vain and injurious. In regard to the action of the bowels, it is well to recollect that constipation is a relative term, and that such a condition can only be termed morbid when it is attended with ill consequences. Constitution and habit make all the difference between one person and another; and the attempt to reduce all to one common level of regularity, by means of irritating or drastic purgatives, would be both irrational and injurious.

The most cursory inspection of a patient suffering from hepatic torpor and anæmia, the most superficial examination into the history of his case, ought at once to satisfy the medical observer that with mercury especially, he should in this instance, have nothing to do. The tropical invalid will generally be found to have had quite enough of that mineral during the acute stage of his disease, and when it was to a certain extent necessary to his cure. The true remedies in the anæmic complication are,—the alteratives already mentioned, bitter tonics, chalybeates, mild aperients conjoined to chalybeates, great attention to the diet, to the enjoyment of pure air, and to the habits of life—so as gradually to invigorate the system.

"It cannot be too often repeated," says Dr. Billing, "that persons frequently give much too large doses of remedies in chronic diseases and thereby fail. Medicine and dietetic directions fail merely from being too energetic:"—in other words, where in chronic disease remedies and diet fail, we should consider whether they may have been used too freely. It is impossible indeed to be too much on our guard against such errors in the treatment of tropical invalids.

It is not here as in convalescence from acute disease. Where debility has been of long duration, the beneficial results of tonic treatment can only be obtained by gentle and slow degrees. This is not a case for heroic remedies, nor is the cure to be effected by a *coup de main*. So much for the medical management of these obstinate disorders.*

When, on the other hand, I have reason to conclude that organic changes have taken place in the liver, or that its torpor is associated with induration or enlargement of the spleen, I have recourse at once to the nitro-muriatic acid bath. It is a very powerful remedy; it acts powerfully in promoting the depurative functions of the liver, kidneys, bowels, and skin. I have, therefore, during more than twenty years, in India and in England, used it in many of the chronic affections of the liver, functional and structural, believing it, on the ground of my experience, to be an agent of the first order of importance.

The chlorine bath I have also used of late years in London, with a more speedy effect in cure, and I hope to see both means brought into more general, because deserved, use. The acid and water bath can be prepared and used in the patient's house with perfect ease, and with eventual happy results; while the chlorine and vapour bath can only be obtained in establishments practised to their careful preparation. To secure the more rapid and effective action of bath means, I am in the habit of premising a few vapour or Turkish baths, with a view to open the pores and purify the skin; and where the latter can be procured, it is by far the best.

The form and manner of preparing and using the acid bath are as follow :—

Take of pure concentrated hydrochloric acid, by measure, three parts; strong nitric acid, two parts; mix the two acids very carefully and slowly, so as to avoid any evolution of heat, and then, having waited for twenty minutes, add of distilled water five parts, and mix the whole carefully.

I.—FOR THE GENERAL BATH, WHEN IT IS NECESSARY TO IMMERSE THE WHOLE BODY.

1. Pour into the bath about five pailfuls of cold water : add two quart bottles, containing sixty-four fluid ounces of the prepared dilute nitro-muriatic acid, and then sufficient boiling water to raise the temperature to 96° or 98°.

2. The patient should remain in the bath from fifteen to twenty minutes, a can of hot water being kept at hand and added in small quantities at a time to maintain the temperature.

3. While the patient is in the bath, hot and dry towels should

* When in the very act of writing, I received the following note from a seafaring gentleman in Cornwall :—"My dear Sir,—The source of all my misery arises from a hot climate—liver complaint—perfectly torpid. Mercurials serve only to increase the disease. If you can think of anything that will relieve the aforesaid state of inaction, I shall be very grateful."

be provided, in order that immediately he leaves it, the body may be quickly and thoroughly dried; after which the patient should at once retire to a well-aired and warmed bed. To prepare the second and the following baths, remove on each occasion about one-third of the liquid, then add one quart bottle of the dilute acid, and sufficient hot and cold water to raise the temperature to the proper degree. Should the bath excite too much irritation of the skin, less than one bottle of acid may be employed on each succeeding occasion.

II.—THE FOOT AND SPONGING BATH.

1. Two gallons of water are generally sufficient for an ordinary foot and sponging bath, which should be kept by frequent addition of hot water at a temperature of from 98° to 100°. To the two gallons of water, six ounces by measure of the prepared dilute acid are to be added and thoroughly mixed. While the feet are immersed, a warm sheet or some other suitable covering to protect the patient from draughts should be thrown over the shoulders. By means of a large soft sponge, the insides of the thighs, the right side over the ribs (the region of the liver), and the arm-pits, should be constantly bathed; at the same time, several folds of flannel may be immersed in the hot acid bath, and wrapped round the body. These baths should be used from fifteen to twenty minutes, night and morning, and on each occasion it is necessary to attend to the usual precautions of thoroughly drying the body and legs with hot towels before dressing or retiring to bed.

2. It must be remarked that earthenware or wooden baths should be employed, as all other materials destroy the efficacy of the prepared acid. The sponges and towels should after each bath be thoroughly washed in cold water to prevent their being destroyed by the acid.

I have been so much in the practice of prescribing this remedy, that, in order to save trouble to the patient and to myself, I have had the above directions printed; and I invariably place a copy in the hands of such as are to be treated. A course of two months of this bath is found generally to restore the healthy action of the liver; nor does it interfere with the use of bitter tonics, or even with mild chalybeates, but, on the contrary, it rather gives effect to their operations. In the severer instances, hereafter to be considered, I have continually to use this means for a much longer period. The use of the bath should be discontinued whenever tenderness of the gums, or general malaise occurs; and the same rule should be observed in regard to the internal use of the mineral acids.

The varying and relative influences of the nitro-muriatic acid bath, like the results of mercurial and other fumigations and inunctions, will depend on the more or less active condition of the cuticular functions in different persons. There is no greater constitutional difference in different persons than that which relates to the functions of the skin; and this circumstance will naturally account for the varying effects of remedies employed in the dermic manner. But the greater power and more uniform effect of this remedy on persons in health have in a vast number of cases been manifested. Servants both male and female have complained of bilious diarrhœa from the immersion of the right forearm merely in the bath; and others have requested to be relieved from attendance on patients while using it—declaring that the inhaling of the steam issuing from the heated mixture has purged them actively. The acids would appear to be absorbed through the skin, and perhaps more through the lungs. It has continually happened that servants, after stooping over the bath, and inhaling its steam, have been purged within twelve hours thereafter; while others have apparently been similarly affected by the immersion of the right hand. The effect has been so general that a wooden ladle has been used by them for agitating the bath.

The cuticular irritation—the chlorine rash of Mr. Wallace—which is occasionally seen in persons who are using this means, has generally appeared to me to retard rather than promote and advance the cure; and when the irritation has been severe, it has been found necessary to suspend the use of the baths for a time; even when moderate in degree, the papular irritation has appeared to me to counteract absorption, on which the virtues of the bath seem principally to depend. I am aware that the great benefactor of mankind, Jenner, ascribed much virtue to counter-irritants—to tartar-emetic especially—in chronic diseases of the liver, and that Mr. Wallace, of Dublin, was of the same opinion in respect to "*permanent* cutaneous irritation;*"* but in a long course of observation of the effects of nitro-muriatic acid in emulging the liver, and as a general alterative, the curative result has appeared to depend principally on absorption, and independently of any cutaneous irritation. But the chronic rash, although a hindrance to absorption, is by no means a permanent impediment to the cure; for in some persons who were distressed in this way, evidence of the most powerful emulgent action was eventually manifested in biliary vomiting and purging.

In treating torpor of the liver, after the cessation of other means of cure, I recommend warm and tepid baths, and especially those of sea-water, in aid of other tonic medical treatment, reducing the temperature as the patient approaches health. I may here add, however, that the most cursory view of the changes which take place in the volume and weight of the liver, and in the several processes of digestion, must make it evident that to strict diet we should look for a powerful aid in the treatment of all forms of hepatic disease, whether acute or chronic. The free use of green vegetables and fruits should in all cases be enjoined.

The neglect of nitro-muriatic-acid treatment in cases of the nature here treated of, and in which mercury, in every form, proves not only insufficient but pernicious, is much to be regretted.

Dr. C. J. B. Williams, who considers nitric acid the best medicine he knows for the state of convalescence from inflammation, and in the various cachectic states following on acute disease, or on habits of intemperance, offers the suggestion that its beneficial influences may be referred to its possessing a large proportion of oxygen in loose combination, and that it thus promotes a more free circulation through diseased parts, or through effused solids, by further oxygenating them. This distinguished physician, speaking of the nitro-muriatic acid and chlorate of potash, says:— " It seems most probable that these agents are chiefly useful in supplying to the blood the oxygen necessary for the formation of fibrin or deutoxide of protein ; the respiration in its weakened state being unable to furnish a due amount." It seems to me, likewise, that nitric acid could never have attained to so great a reputation amongst surgeons in the cure of secondary and tertiary forms of syphilis, if its actions had not been found by them analogous to those of mercury, and that without the disadvantages of mercury. A " correspondence in the effect of the two remedies" was observed by Dr. Helenus Scott, of the Bombay army, the original author of this plan of treatment. The nitro-muriatic acid is found to act powerfully, though slowly, on all the secretory and depurative functions, and on that of the liver especially ; and it can only be thus, and through the other influences ascribed to the acids, that they and mercury operate in curing syphilis and other chronic diseases.

Another valuable quality of the nitro-muriatic acid is this—that, whether exhibited internally or externally, its influence in promoting the secretions is not in any sensible degree counteracted by opium, even when exhibited in the largest doses. Of this fact I continually receive examples in treating chronic diarrhœa complicated with disease of the liver. We obtain, in short, from the use of the mineral acids in the treatment of chronic disease, all the remedial aids which can be obtained from mercury in the treatment of acute disease ; and that, without any of the injurious consequences that so frequently ensue from the exhibition of the last-named agent. Persons of anæmic or of scrofulous habit are liable to serious injury from the use of mercury, whether given in large doses, during a few days, or in alterative doses during weeks or months. It is quite otherwise in respect to the acids, the most marked and lasting improvement of the general health being the ordinary result of their exhibition.

The rule, says Dr. Bence Jones, is, sulphuric acid to astringe, hydrochloric acid to promote digestion, nitric acid to promote secretion.

The good effects of nitric and muriatic acids in the treatment of some kinds of stomach disorder, are stated by Dr. Budd to have " been fully established by Dr. Prout."

" Prout found them of especial efficacy in the gastric disorder that occurs in what is termed the oxalic diathesis, and that is marked chiefly by distressing flatulence and palpitation, or irregular action of the heart, occurring some time after meals, and by the presence of oxalate of lime in the urine.

The mineral acids are often useful to persons in whom digestion is habitually slow and feeble, from a scanty secretion of gastric juice, and who have a sense of weight or oppression at the stomach after meals.

They are often useful also, as Pemberton showed, in the indigestion, attended with excessive formation of lactic acid, that occurs in weak and nervous persons, and when the stomach has been for some time disordered and weakened by a source of irritation elsewhere."

Dr. Prout is then quoted on the proper regulation and use of the mineral acids. " In cases of oxalic diathesis, where the patient lives at a distance in the country, I commonly recommend the use of the muriatic acid, or nitro-muriatic acid, as the case may be, to be persisted in, till the lithate of ammonia, or the lithic acid, begins to appear in the urine, or for *a month ;* and by adopting such a course of acids three or four times in the year, and by a carefully regulated diet, I have seen the diathesis gradually subdued, and at length removed altogether." This authority adds that the best time for exhibiting the acids is half an hour or so before meals.

CASE I.—Major ——, aged forty-two, originally of powerful constitution, has served twenty-five years in India, and has never till now been absent from duty. He has been a keen sportsman, and been therefore much exposed to direct solar influence, independently of the exposures incident to active service. His habits of life have been "free," but with the exception of one severe attack of jungle (remittent) fever, followed by a protracted ague, in the early period of his service, his health has been generally good. Three years ago, while serving in a low malarious district, he became severely dyspeptic, falling off rapidly in appetite and in condition. He became pale and sallow, suffering great distress from oppressive distension after meals. At length he became so enfeebled that he was ordered home.

There is now much debility, emaciation, and mental depression, the general appearance indicating premature old age. The complexion is of a lemon yellow ; the integument is dry, loose, and inelastic, as if wanting in vitality, and feels like chamois leather : the abdomen is flattened ; the state of the general habit is anæmic ; the appetite is very defective, the dyspeptic symptoms, accompanied by excessive acidity, having greatly increased during the cold of the last ten days. There is cough, with a sense of dull pain and weight in the head. He suffers from what he terms "a dry state of the bowels," the excretions being pale, sometimes white, and always scanty. The tongue is foul, with bitter taste in the mouth. The urine is now pale and abundant, but it is sometimes high-coloured and surcharged. There is no organic disease discoverable; the pulse is feeble and slow.

He was ordered to take a pill every night, composed of watery extract of aloes, with a grain each of the sulphates of quinine and iron. The gentle action of the bowels being thus obtained, he took, during nearly two months, the fluid extract of taraxacum, with bicarbonate of soda, using a light but nutritious diet, and taking exercise on horseback daily. The warm bath, at 96°, was used twice a week, at the bed-side and just before retiring to rest, while active friction with the Indian hair-glove* was applied to the surface of the body, great care being observed at the same time to avoid exposure to the cold and damp of our winter and spring seasons. All these directions were rigorously attended to by the patient, but the progress towards recovery was slow. On the return of warmer weather, however, in April, the digestive power improved, along with the secretions, the complexion having assumed more of the European hue. The weight of the body, though much under the average of health, was gradually augmenting, while the power of increasing his exercises, with the enjoyment in them, steadily returned. Mild chalybeates were now ordered, and these, along with an improved diet and increased exercise, brought a more rapid increase of health. The hepatic and digestive functions acquired tone perceptibly under this course of treatment, and in the month of August Major —— went to the moors. In October he returned to London, on his way to travel on the continent, and if his weight was still some pounds under his Indian standard of health, he nevertheless admitted that he was more muscular and energetic than when he last enjoyed tiger-hunting.

Remarks.—In this case, as in many others of the like nature, the anæmic condition was the pervading injury, and the liver partook largely of it; indeed, I believe that the proper pathology of torpor of the liver, in the instance of tropical invalids in general, and where actual disease is not present, may more justly be expressed by anæmia of the organ than any other phrase; and the term becomes important if, as I conceive, it represents a true condition. Certain it is, that in the case of Major ——, the most

---

* This glove, made from goat-hair cloth (very superior to the common horse-hair glove, which frets the skin severely), is manufactured by Mr. Savory, of New Bond-street, at my suggestion, after the pattern of those in universal and immemorial use in Hindustan, the country of all others where the purification of the skin is most and best attended to.

marked and decided improvement took place under the appropriate operation of chalybeates, and so I continually find it to be in such cases.

The benefits derivable from the persistent use of the natural saline and chalybeate waters can only be referred to their joint operation, as alteratives and diluents, in exciting the action of the depurative functions while they improve the quality of the blood by the iron contained in them. There can be no doubt, also, that the important accessories of the warmer season of the year—pure air, regulated diet, exercise, and mental relaxation, tend materially to promote the remedial actions of all the mineral waters so much resorted to of late years.

CASE II.—Captain ——, of a delicate and dyspeptic habit, has served twenty-one years in India. During his service, he had two attacks of remittent fever, for which he was moderately bled, generally and locally, and used calomel and purgatives. His recovery from the first was slow, and on the last occasion his debility was so great, that he was ordered to the Cape of Good Hope for change of air. He returned to his duty, after an absence of eighteen months, in his ordinary state of health, and continued so during three years, when the bowels became irregular, with alternate states of constipation and diarrhœa. From this time his health sank, and, notwithstanding a voyage to Prince of Wales' Island, and a short residence in the mountain ranges, dyspeptic symptoms and diarrhœa increased upon him, so that at length he was ordered to Europe, and arrived in England in the month of August. Captain —— visited me in the end of October, having since his arrival been under alterative mercurial treatment, which has induced a painful and irritable recurrence of diarrhœa. He is pale and exsanguine, his general appearance giving the impression of very defective nutrition. The muscular system is flattened, relaxed, and extremely enfeebled, the integument being harsh and cold to the touch. The abdomen is tumid, but there is no enlargement of either liver or spleen. The pulse is frequent (eighty-six) and feeble. He complains of severe headache, loss of appetite, and of want of power to digest other than farinaceous food, on which he has principally subsisted on the voyage home round the Cape of Good Hope. The diarrhœa had ceased by the time of his arrival in England, but his dyspeptic symptoms had increased, accompanied by excessive flatulence, short dry cough, and swelling of the feet and ankles. The excretions from the bowels are pultaceous, clay-coloured, and sometimes chalky, the urine being clear and scanty. The mental despondency is most distressing. Ordered to take, three times a day, a mixture composed of the fluid of taraxacum, with dilute nitric and hydrochloric acid, with aromatics. It became necessary, on three occasions, to add tincture of opium to this preparation, the bowels being still irritable. A warm bath at night twice a week, with frictions to the surface night and morning, were ordered, and gentle horse-exercise was used on fair days, while a moderate allowance of animal food and stale bread composed his dinner. In little more than a month under this treatment, the discharges from the bowels became so consistent as to amount to constipation, when a pill, containing a small quantity of aloes, with the sulphates of iron and quinine, was taken every night. Captain —— then proceeded to the country, whence he wrote me, in January, that his digestive power and the alvine secretions had much improved. He was now directed to use a weak solution of quinine and sulphate of iron, with dilute sulphuric acid, while the diet and exercise were increased.

During the spring and summer months, pure chalybeates, gradually increased in quantity, were exhibited, and by the middle of autumn he was so much improved in health and strength as to proceed on his travels. It required three years' residence in England to restore this officer to health, when he returned to India full of high hope and expectation; and after four years he writes me that his health continues excellent.

Remarks.—Looking to the previous fevers, and the diarrhœa that followed them, and also to the existing febrile condition (which latter state I considered as referable to intestinal irritation) I directed the use of the nitro-muriatic acid treatment, as being febrifuge, emulgent, tonic, and refrigerant. In such cases it also proves, along with the taraxacum, an excellent preparative for more active tonics. Captain ——'s condition appeared at first to promise an unfavourable result.

Torpor of the liver, like congestion of that organ, is frequently associated with very severe cerebral disturbance. Of this fact the two following cases will afford illustrations :—

CASE III.—Lieut.-Col. —— served twenty-eight years in India, and has been throughout of careful and regular habits. In 1831 he came to England at my recommendation, suffering dangerously from remittent fever, and consequent enlargement of the liver. He remained two years at home, and regained health despite an attack of bronchitis. Colonel —— returned a second time to England, on sick leave, in 1849. The official statement of his case, from the surgeon of his regiment, sets forth that, for some years after his first sick furlough to Europe, "he had enjoyed good health," but that latterly he became "subject to frequent attacks of pain in the head, the slightest irregularity in diet producing it." On the 6th of January, 1849, the weather being cold, and his corps encamped before Moultan, Colonel —— became jaundiced, his urine being of a blood-red appearance, and the head heavy and oppressed. While under the influence of active purgative treatment he was, on the 8th of January, seized with a fit. "He suddenly fell back in his chair in a state of insensibility," and was found by his surgeon lying on the floor of his tent, "his face tinged of a leaden hue, pupils dilated, breathing oppressed and laboured, skin cold and clammy, and his pulse slow and full. He was immediately bled in the right arm, but the blood not flowing very freely the vein of the other arm was opened, and a large quantity of blood was abstracted, when his pulse became small, soft, and more frequent. During the bleeding he had two very severe attacks of convulsive movements of the right side, with throbbings of the right corner of the mouth and winking of the eye of that side, the pupils becoming very much contracted. These convulsive fits lasted three minutes."

For three hours he remained insensible, after which, sinapisms, fomentations, large doses of calomel, followed by purgatives, were used, and he recovered. Though but forty-seven years of age he now appeared (September, 1849) prematurely old, and much emaciated. Hepatic torpor, and torpor of all the functions of the body, accompanied by severe headaches, were now the symptoms complained of. He was completely anæmic, and no wonder, for the blood-letting he declared to have been enormous. In the first winter and spring seasons after his arrival at home he suffered severely after meals from sleepiness, uneasiness, and occasional pain in the head, accompanied by sense of weight and oppression of the epigastric region, and fits of coughing. These symptoms after four or five hours disappeared; but it was long before he regained proper digestive power, healthy secretions, or muscular condition, sufficient to enable him to take exercise without fatigue.

Remarks.—This officer was seen by many physicians in various quarters, and various remedies were prescribed. I directed the use of the mineral acids, chalybeates, and latterly of the cod-liver oil. All three were followed by some improvement; but two years and a half of furlough proved insufficient to restore the vigour of the digestive functions, and he returned to India in a condition which did not promise that he could render effective service.

CASE IV.—Major ——, ætatis fifty, served thirty years in India, and had enjoyed an average degree of good health until within the last six or seven years, when, according to the statement of his surgeon, he suffered, "at periods varying from a week to a month, from severe headaches of a most intense character. The affection commences primarily with a weight and heaviness in the head, which gradually increasing, ceases not until it assumes a degree almost insupportable. During the attack, and until the operation of medicine, he is incapable of moving, and often of lying down, the only relief experienced being in the sitting posture. From the previous history, present state, and observing the action of medicine on the case, I came to the conclusion that the disordered functions of the brain are entirely caused by torpidity of the liver, and derangement of the digestive organs generally, the retention, in fact, of some of the component parts of the secretion of bile, which are not eliminated from the blood under deficient action of the hepatic apparatus.

"In the intervals between the attacks, irregularity of the bowels and extreme torpidity of the liver have always been present, evinced by great dryness of the skin, sallow countenance with loaded conjunctivæ, occasional pains in the right shoulder, and heaviness in the hepatic region, &c.

"The disposition to torpor, and consequent disturbance in the sensorium, has always been here increased, and brought on, by the slightest change in the seasons or weather, by change of habits from cantonments to camp, and *vice versâ*, while the slightest irregularity of diet, or even a change of the dinner-hour, has always produced its punishment."

Such is the statement of the able surgeon of Major ——'s corps. "The treatment," he says, "was in the first instance, and between the attacks, to restore due actions of the hepatic system, by mercurial alteratives and purgatives, particular attention being paid to the habits and mode of living; but the treatment during the attack has never been altered. On the warning of his headache approaching, pills, containing a large dose of calomel and colocynth, were immediately taken, followed, some hours after, by an aperient draught of salts and senna, and after copious dark evacuations the headache has generally subsided, leaving him, however, pallid and depressed in spirits for some days. The action of mercurial purgatives in this case was remarkable; the earlier their operation on the biliary system was effected, the less severe the attack; and if by any delay the medicine was not directly taken, the more severe the affection." Seeing that length of residence in India produced "increased severity and frequency" in the disease, and that a return to Europe was deemed "the only means now in his power for the due restoration of the hepatic function," Major —— obtained sick leave, and arrived in England in the spring season.

Remarks.—Major —— came under my observation only at intervals. He visited Brighton, Bath, Cheltenham, and other places, and sought various opinions. For the first year he continued exactly as described in India, headache attacking him on an average once a month. The fluid extract of taraxacum with alkalies appeared to me to be of much service to him, and had he persevered in their use, his recovery, I think, would have been more rapid and progressive.

In the treatment of all the disorders and diseases affecting persons who have resided in hot climates, I endeavour to impress on the patient the vast importance of attention to the habits of life—to the diet, to the clothing, especially in the winter and spring seasons, to exercise in a pure air, to the functions of the skin, &c.;

and that without such care no medical treatment whatever can avail them ; in short, that all those means which are preventive of disease are also curative.

Dr. Budd, in his admirable treatise on Diseases of the Liver, speaking of the injurious effects of indulgence at table, and of the neglect of exercise, especially in persons of middle age, in whom respiration has therefore become less active, says :—

" We may often see inverse evidence of those relations in the effect of pure air and active exercise in relieving various disorders that result from repletion and from the retention of principles which, if burnt out in respiration, should pass off by the liver as bile. Every sportsman must have remarked the effect of a single day's hunting in clearing the complexion. It has no doubt much the same effect on the liver as on the skin."

If the truth and force of these important observations were more generally appreciated in practice, we should have fewer hepatic disorders, and fewer still of those hepatic diseases, which, taken together, render the days of many amongst us presently as miserable as they are sure ultimately to shorten them. Exercise in the open air must also prove powerfully beneficial in another manner —viz., by accelerating the actions of respiration, it thus increases the power of the circulation, and thereby promotes a more active return of blood from the liver, spleen, and other important organs, so often engorged and oppressed in the instances of invalids from hot climates.

"Exercise on horseback," says Dr. Billing, "has innumerable advantages over every other kind, as it gives motion to the viscera without fatiguing the limbs ; very little motion is given to the viscera in walking or in carriages."

If it be true that "the portal circulation is carried on in a great measure by the pressure of the abdominal muscles," how great must be the benefits resulting from well-regulated exercises in the open air in such cases. The quantity of carbonic acid exhaled from the lungs is proved to be greatly increased under active exercise, and thus we possess another channel of powerful depuration, the active promotion of which should never be neglected. The same result under exercise is found by Lehmann in the depuration by the kidneys ; for, while the proportion of uric acid to urea in a state of rest was 1 to 38, after active exercise it fell to 1 in 77. The truth is that the amount of good that may be effected, in the way of prevention and cure of disease, by pure air and water, proper diet and active exercise, is a matter which up to this day has not received all the attention that is due to it.

In no class of disease is the most rigid adherence to strict rule of diet more necessary than in such as affect the function and structure of the liver ; and this truth should be strenuously impressed on the attention of the returned Indian : he should be made to understand that no cure can be effected without it.

Dr. Budd observes justly, with respect to increasing the activity and effect of the respiratory process, that in the vast power we have in modifying them by regulations having reference to the great conditions of air, exercise, temperature, and food, we have means much more effectual than any other of dealing with biliary disorders.

Patients, in their ignorance of their present condition, and referring only to our heroic measures of cure, under directly opposite circumstances, in India, will sometimes look anxiously to "active treatment," and to speedy and substantive results. They must be made to understand that there are many morbid conditions for which we cannot pretend to find any *direct* and *immediate* remedies; and that even in withdrawing things that tend to injury, or to retard the curative operations of nature, the physician does much;—much more than can be hoped for by random attempts at rapid or "decided" measures of cure, by powerful medicinal agents applied to an exhausted constitution. They must, in short, be induced to look hopefully to the future, and to judge of the power and value of their medical management by the result—by the gradual restoration of health. It is seldom, indeed, that we shall find reasoning such as this disregarded.

CHRONIC ENLARGEMENT OF THE LIVER.

NEXT to the liability to periodical fever and bowel complaints, such as dysentery and diarrhœa, engendered by residence in malarious countries, stands the liability to disorder and disease of the liver, engendered by antecedent circumstances of climate and of habit of life. It is well known to such as are acquainted with the health history of the British army, that the soldiers employed on the expedition to Walcheren never afterwards proved serviceable in the Spanish campaigns, or when sent to the intertropical colonies.

The least exposure to malaria, to cold and damp, night duties, a shower of rain, or wet feet, was sure to induce fever of an intermittent character. The same latency of disposition, and subsequent liability to fever on the application of slight causes, has at all times been remarked, in the East Indies, in Europeans who have once been affected with remittent (jungle) fever.

The chronic enlargement of the liver will generally be found in persons who have suffered from previous acute inflammation, or from repeated congestions of that organ, from fevers, both remittent and intermittent, and from dysentery and diarrhœa. This form of hepatic disease is often associated also with dysentery, acute and chronic, and with diarrhœa; so that, in fact, it may be said to precede, to accompany, and to follow those bowel diseases.

3 c

In the East Indies we find that acute hepatic disease stands in the hospital returns as third in order of frequency, fevers and dysenteries being in the first and second relations.   But though this order will be found generally correct, it must be remembered .in addition that, in the course of fevers, dysenteries, and diarrhœas, hepatic diseases are very apt to arise, and to follow upon them, so as, in fact, to render the total amount of cases of hepatic disease which occur in the East very great in the aggregate—far greater than can be exhibited in any hospital returns.*   Out of an aggregate European force of 25,431 men of Her Majesty army, serving during ten, eight, and ten years respectively, between 1823 and 1826, at the stations of Calcutta, Chinsurah, and Berhampore, all in Bengal Proper, there occurred, according to Sir A. Tulloch, 1354 cases of original and uncomplicated hepatitis ; but if we could to this enumeration add the amount of consecutive hepatic disease, the grand total would be very great.   Whether the returns made from the Madras Presidency be more accurate than those of Bengal, I know not ; but we find that out of an aggregate British force of 82,342 men, serving in the former Presidency, from 1842 to 1848, there occurred 5911 cases of liver diseases.   " In India," says Sir James M'Grigor, "the liver seems to be the seat of disease, in nearly the same proportion that the lungs are in England."

I have, on the other hand, treated numerous cases of hepatic enlargement at home, in persons who had never suffered from any tropical disease, nor yet from any functional disorder, or from structural disease of the organ in question, so far as could be ascertained, but who had nevertheless been exposed in India to the general influences explained in the opening chapter of this part.

The history of these latter instances is very generally as follows : —The patient has been enfeebled by many years of residence in hot climates : he comes to England in an impaired state of general health, with torpor of the liver : he is exposed to cold; and along with this, perhaps, are associated excesses in food and drink. Passive congestion results from all these influences ; and years may intervene before alteration of structure, with enlargement of the liver, calls for the notice of the patient or his friends ; and then too frequently the organ will be found on percussion to be enlarged in all directions—upwards yielding a dull sound far above the sixth rib, extending sometimes so high as the nipple ; and downwards far below the ribs, extending sometimes even below the umbilicus.

---

* Fever is a most efficient cause, especially when treated on the exclusive tonic plan ; and the result is sometimes many years in being manifested. I have at this moment, September, 1861, under my care, a gentleman who was treated in Persia during convalescence from a remittent by port wine, and during the fever by quinine alone.   This occurred in 1835 ; and now he has an enormous enlargement of the liver with induration, which he regards as having crept on him during several years past.

Where, as in the disease before us, actual enlargement is so easily recognisable by the senses, it seems hardly necessary here to dwell on a minute detail of the symptoms, especially as most of them are common to the disease under consideration, and to the hepatic affections noticed in the two last sections. But I would mention that an excited or a disturbed state of the heart's action is frequently present, as a complication, in the chronic enlargement of the liver, and albumen is likewise occasionally discoverable in the urine; but, according to my experience, these derangements disappear on the removal of the hepatic disease; thus showing that the functions of the heart and kidneys are but temporarily disturbed in these cases.

In chronic enlargement, with induration of the liver, the heart becomes excited, apparently through the constant exertion of its muscular textures in propelling the blood through an indurated mass so near to the heart, and of so large a size as the liver. This state of the heart's action, unless relieved by the removal of its cause, terminates in disease of the cardiac structure. In such cases there will likewise be found a hurried and imperfect respiration; and it will necessarily follow, from all these impediments to the operation of the vital functions, that dropsies shall often ensue.

The influence of antecedent climatic circumstances of preceding seasons, prolonged into succeeding seasons, and even into years, is pointedly commented on by Hippocrates, as influencing morbid manifestations. It is a sort of latent disposition, created by a cause which has operated in previous force or by previous duration. "At the same time," says M. Boudin, "that a certain time intervenes between the introduction into the system of the morbid cause and its manifestation in the form of disease, it happens, also, that certain diseases are developed far from the places where they were contracted, and long after the action of the causes which gave them birth." Applying these doctrines to facts, this eminent military surgeon instances regiments which have passed into Africa, carrying along with them for a certain time, varying in duration, a disposition to be afflicted by the fevers and intestinal diseases that had prevailed amongst them in France; and, conversely, of other corps returned from Africa, and which exhibited, for a longer or shorter period, according to length of residence or to circumstances of exposure during active service, the fevers and fluxes of hot and malarious regions, thus preserving for a time, in both cases, the dominant medical constitution of the previous seasons, and of the countries from which they had taken their departure. The utility of such diagnostic considerations must be evident; for, in a practical point of view, "it is of the highest importance," he observes, "never to lose sight of the pathology proper to the localities to which masses of men have been previously habituated, and to observe, in relation to places, the celebrated precept of Celsus in relation to time, 'Neque solum interest quales dies sint, sed etiam quales præcesserint.' "*

All our experiences derived from the intertropical possessions of the British empire go to confirm the doctrines and facts here referred to ; and to no diseases do they apply with more justice than to those of the liver.

The actions of the nitro-muriatic acid, the manner of preparing and using the bath, &c., have already been detailed. The late Dr. Helenus Scott, of the Bombay army, was the first to use this remedy in its most powerful form of bath, in chronic diseases of the liver. He says that, in a constitution broken down by disease, by the use of powerful remedies, such as mercury, or by the long-continued action of the poison of syphilis, the acid treatment was quite as beneficial in this climate as in that of India. " I know of no other means that are capable of producing effects at once so salutary and so considerable, so free from injury, with so little inconvenience or disturbance. . . . As with mercury, the system should be charged with it for a longer or shorter time, according to circumstances. In short, and as a general rule, I have found the acid bath advantageous and salutary in all cases where mercury is useful, and with the additional advantage that the acid treatment is attended by neither injury nor disadvantage." Dr. Scott adds : " *By the harmless remedies that I now recommend much good may be done in some diseases that are acknowledged to be beyond the ordinary means of relief;*" and my personal experience in India and in England amply confirms this able and excellent officer's declaration. " Even in irremediable cases of chronic enlargement of the liver," says Dr. Christison, " it proves useful in cleaning the tongue, improving the appetite, abating thirst, and sometimes in retarding the progress of disease." For the dispersion of the products of inflammatory effusion into the viscera, in anæmic subjects, the use of the nitro-muriatic acid, whether internally or externally exhibited, proves of excellent effect ; and its resolvent power is accelerated and increased by alternating its use with the renal depurants. The external application of the acids in the form of bath is, I repeat, by far the most effective mode of using this very valuable remedy.†

The disuse of this powerful means must be mainly ascribed to the imperfect, brief, and desultory manner in which it has generally been used, whether internally or externally prescribed. It is only by those who have attentively observed the effects of this remedy, whether exhibited internally or externally, during months together in many cases, that its powerful influences in bringing

---

* " Œuvres complètes d'Hippocrate," par E. Littré.

† Dr. Jephson, of Leamington, has stated to me that, in diseases of the mesentery, and of swellings of the cervical glands also, he has found the swathing the abdomen and the neck with muslin soaked in the warm solution of the acids, as used by me for the bath, of surprising efficacy, covering the wetted muslin with gutta-percha cloth.

about the removal of chronic disease, and in maturing convalescence, can be justly appreciated. Certainly, had mercury been used in the desultory and irregular manner spoken of, in the treatment of acute and chronic disease, without regard to rational persistence or to curative effect, it never could have attained to any repute in the practice of medicine. The nitro-muriatic acid, like mercury, when used internally, is apt, after a time, to irritate the mucous surfaces ; but, like mercury again, when exhibited through the channel of the skin, it generally agrees thoroughly and acts beneficially on all the secreting organs; irritation of the gums and the mucous membranes occurring only after a protracted use of the acid bath, and often not at all.

Three remarkable cases have recently come to my notice in which patients, after using the baths for months, abandoned it in despair ; but in each case, some weeks after discontinuance of the remedy, the biliary secretion was restored and the hepatic enlargement disappeared—health being in each instance completely restored.

N.B.—Should the bowels not act with sufficient freedom of themselves, or should the bath not excite them to sufficient action, I am in the habit of ordering a mild aperient draught of Epsom salts in some bitter infusion every other morning, so long as the use of the bath may be in progress.

Case I. ——, Esq., had served thirty-eight years in India, and there enjoyed excellent health, terminating his official career as member of one of the medical boards. His constitution had been robust ; but he was now seventy years of age. He had never suffered from fever, dysentery, or hepatitis, though his habits had always been those of one who is said to " live well." He had retired from the service, and resided in England twelve years, and until eight months previously to his consulting me his health had continued good. At the time now stated he began to fall off in condition, was observed to look sallow, and complained of dyspeptic ailments with fulness in the epigastrium ; but there was no pain. Latterly tumidness of the whole abdomen attracted his notice, and that of his family. I found the liver enormously enlarged, and extending down to the umbilicus, accompanied by considerable serous effusion into the abdominal cavity, and by œdema of the lower extremities. The bowels were constipated, the excretions being clay-coloured, the urine turbid and scanty. There was no disturbance of the heart's action.

In consultation with Dr. Chambers it was determined to use the nitro-muriatic acid bath by sponging the limbs and abdomen, using a mild aperient draught every second morning. The sponging was done by the patient's wife and her female attendant; but after ten days they were obliged to desist, both of them being seized with bilious diarrhœa. The person next employed in sponging used gloves of oiled cloth, and the remedy was continued for more than three months, with a powerful effect on the secretions of the liver, bowels, and kidneys. The liver was now not to be felt under the margin of the ribs, and the patient rapidly acquired appetite, condition, and strength. Mr. —— now proceeded to his country residence, returning to London for the winter season, and enjoying excellent health, which he retained for upwards of two years. At the expiration of this time he complained of nausea after meals, accompanied by great languor and distress at the stomach. Vomitings after meals soon succeeded, the matters rejected being latterly of a dark coffee colour, and he died greatly emaciated, three months from the accession of his latter illness, in his seventy-third year.

The contents of the abdomen were examined by Mr. Pollock, of St. George's Hospital, thirty hours after death. He describes the liver as "quite healthy in structure and appearance; rather smaller than natural; the diminution of size appeared as if occasioned by the viscus being less congested than is generally the case. The cells of the liver, when examined under a high power, were found to be very distinct and almost empty—much more so than is generally seen. The gall-bladder was filled with small pieces of black matter, which crumbled easily under the pressure of the finger, and were found to be composed of pure bile."

The stomach was quite healthy, but "distended with fluid of a dark blackish colour. An ulcer, about the size of a shilling, was found in the duodenum where it lies in contact with the head of the pancreas, its edges much thickened and elevated. Spleen healthy."

Remarks.—This case shows how, after the lapse of many years of residence in a temperate climate, disease will arise in the liver, and that in persons who have never suffered in hot climates either from functional or structural affections of that organ. It was long before the latent disposition was here roused into actual disease; but more generally it happens otherwise, and within a few years—sometimes within a few months from arrival in England. In respect of the treatment, we perceive, first, the power of the nitro-muriatic acid on those whose hands merely were, while in a state of good health, wetted by it; and secondly, its power to remove an enormous enlargement of the liver, and the consequent dropsy, in the instance even of an aged person. His general health remained excellent during two years and upwards from this point of time; and but for the ulcer in the duodenum, his life might have been extended for a term of years.

CASE II. ——, Esq., aged thirty-eight, originally of a robust habit, had resided nineteen years in India, and chiefly in the upper and healthier parts of the Bengal Presidency. He had not suffered from tropical disease up to the time referred to in his statement. "I was first taken ill in the hot weather of 1840, with indigestion, nervousness, and very slight fever, and was sent to the Himalayan mountains. I returned in November, well. In the hot weather of the following year I was again seized, and again returned to the Himalaya. I remained over the winter in the hills, and also in the summer of 1842, in tolerable health. Towards the close of it, however, I suffered very much from indigestion and nervousness, stoppage of the pulse, out of spirits, no appetite, cross and unhappy with myself and everybody else. On coming down the country in November, 1842, I was ordered home. Up to this time I had taken very little medicine—merely small doses of opening stuff occasionally. Now my legs began to swell, my breathing to be difficult, and I got alarmed. In coming down the Ganges I had but little advice. A medical man I saw at —— said there was not much the matter with me, and I wanted a change to sea. On reaching Calcutta, Mr. Nicolson said my liver was much enlarged. I was now almost unable to leave my room—almost my bed. Mr. Nicolson gave me, I believe, calomel and opening medicines, and something to operate upon my kidneys. I did not get worse in Calcutta, and was put on board ship. Here I took lots of calomel three times a day, and digitalis. On reaching the Cape of Good Hope I was much better, and a month afterwards very much improved indeed ; in fact, I considered myself well. On board ship, Dr. —— latterly gave me some sort of acid to rub into my side, but he had not much in store, and I used it sparingly. On reaching England I consulted ——, who attended me for three months, and during that time I grew as bad, or worse than I had been on leaving Calcutta. I had calomel and digitalis. After that I was treated by Mr. J. R. Martin with acid baths, and occasional medicine at night, and in three months grew very much better, with the constant use of the bath night and morning, and in about six months became a sound man, I hope. My internal organization has worked soundly for about two years, and I embark to-morrow, July 30th, 1846, again for India, without apprehension of a return of my disease. I think I took eight hundred grains of calomel between November, 1842, and August, 1843 !"

At the time here last referred to, this gentleman's condition was most unpromising. The abdomen was full of serum, and there were signs of commencing effusion into the cavities of the pleura and pericardium, the heart being slightly enlarged. The liver was of enormous size, and anasarca had extended to the face and eyelids.

It was under these circumstances that the nitro-muriatic acid bath was commenced, using daily various diuretics, and a draught composed of compound powder of jalap in aromatic water, every other morning.

The result of this plan of treatment is stated above by the patient.

He landed in Calcutta in November, 1846, as he wrote to me,

"in excellent health." During the voyage by the Cape of Good Hope from England, he added, that he had been "remarkably well, and never troubled the doctor or his chest."

Unhappily, Mr. —— remained for months in Lower Bengal, where he was seized with remittent fever. The result was ruinous to his general health. The abdominal functions became torpid and depraved; the heart became perceptibly enlarged, with a return of dropsy of the abdominal cavity, and general anasarca. He died in August, 1847—nine months from the date of his return to Bengal.

On examination after death, the heart was found by Dr ——, of Calcutta, to be enlarged, but all the valvular structures were sound. The abdomen "contained an enormous quantity of fluid." The liver was "small, hard, tuberculated; studded in its whole surface with white cartilaginous deposits of very old formation, giving it quite a rough granular feel; adherent for about a hand's breath to the diaphragm by a horny cicatrix, as if from an old abscess. The spleen small, hard, and heavy; its outer coat of a dirty white colour, and a cartilaginous appearance, tough and hard, like the sole of a shoe; the inner structure fleshy and firm, hepatized, and almost black. Kidneys of a natural appearance in every respect, except a few small granulations in the pelvis of one; not larger than pin-heads, of a soft cheesy character."

Remarks.—The interest attaching to this case is great on various points—especially as showing how insidiously the most dangerous hepatic diseases may arise, when they assume the passive form; but I must here confine my observations to the results of treatment. Mercury during the homeward voyage, and during the first three months' residence in England had its full trial—in the first instance, with some temporary benefit, but in the second with none.

With a view to obtain a rapid and powerful effect, I desired that the nitro-muriatic acid bath should be used by immersion; but the patient was too feeble to bear the exertion, faintness being produced by any sudden effort or change of posture. The more tedious course of sponging was therefore used. In about five weeks darting pains were experienced in the region of the liver; and this result of the bath I have always viewed as a favourable indication; for here, as in other cases, the pains were coincident with increase and activity of the hepatic function, as evidenced by a great discharge of vitiated bile. From this extreme state of disease and of depression he gradually and steadily regained health, and for two years he remained stout, ruddy-faced, and capable of using active exercise. Had this estimable officer escaped fever, he might have completed the object of his desire—three years of additional service—with safety to his health.

In both the cases now related atrophy of the liver had succeeded to previous enlargement, and several instances of cirrhosis from this cause have come under my observation. Such, indeed, we may infer to be a necessary consequence of inflammatory and congcstive states of long standing,—the matters effused, according to Dr. C. J. B. Williams, swelling some parts, compressing others of the textures, and by preventing a due supply of blood, and by interfering with the nutrition and other functions, causing a subsequent atrophy. Contraction and condensation of the natural textures are the necessary consequences, "whilst the new deposit itself forms a granular or nodulated texture, of low vitality. . . . . This is the chief mode in which contractile diseases of the liver and kidneys gradually infringe on the circulation and secretion of these organs, and thus may eventually prove fatal."

Professor Bennett states, that this morbid change in the liver consists of hypertrophy of the fibrous element between the lobules of the organ, and its subsequent contraction, whereby its volume is diminished, and the secreting cells compressed and atrophied. As a further result, the large venous trunks are also compressed, and their commencing ramifications so congested that effusion into, or dropsy of the peritonæal cavity is induced.

Dr. Handfield Jones, on the other hand, regards the thickening and condensation of the fibrous tissue of the liver, not so much the effect of inflammatory action, as of a low degenerative process. He states that there are two forms of cirrhosis ; " the one depending on thickening of the Glissonian capsule, and the other, in which the capsules themselves are involved in fibroid degeneration, the abolition of tissue, and of function being much more complete in the latter !"

More than sixty years ago, Dr. Dick, an intelligent physician of Calcutta, noted that, " In chronic cases, where there is no fever, but only an obtuse pain in the side and shoulder, with a fulness in the side and about the pit of the stomach, keeping up a constant uneasiness, mercury seems to me to have but little good effect. When used freely it removes the symptoms for the time, but they generally return as soon as the mercury is left off." Dr. Dick states, also, that "such liver attacks very often succeeded long courses of mercury." Mercury, in the case here last related, as in other similar cases, did no good, but, on the contrary, much harm, though tried in various ways, and for longer and shorter continuance.

Dr. Girdlestone made the same observation in Madras in 1781-83. He ascribes hepatic disease to the abuse of calomel, even when used " as a prophylactic," but not so in any degree to mercurial frictions, which, however long-continued, did not, he thought, produce such results. He also declares that " after the hepatitis is removed, the constant but cautious use of acids, in hot climates, proves the best means of preventing a relapse."

Dr. —— had never been in a hot climate, and he stated that his case had originally been one of syphilitic ulceration, treated without mercury. Secondary and tertiary forms of syphilis followed, and for these three protracted courses of mercury were

had recourse to, with no benefit.   When I saw him his constitution
was entirely destroyed, and his liver was of enormous size, having
become so after the last mercurial course.

Enlargement of the liver was a very frequent occurrence in the
Lock hospitals of old, in which mercury was used to a very destructive effect.

Cases of hepatic torpor and subsequent enlargement of the organ,
from the abuse of mercury, have so often come under my observation in this country, far exceeding in obstinacy and suffering,
mental and bodily, anything which I have ever witnessed in tropical
invalids, that I think it proper to allude to two of them.   Both
were women of rank, who had never been out of England : the first,
married and a mother, used calomel once, and often twice a week
for five-and-twenty years ; and the other, unmarried, had done the
same for fifteen years.   Headaches of indescribable severity, which
overwhelmed the mental and bodily functions for a time, were in
each case of frequent recurrence ; and fully conscious of the results,
five grains of calomel were yet had recourse to, again and again,
as the only means of relief—thus dramming the liver into excitement, only to become more and more torpid thereafter.   Torture
from the use of animal food, or of any kind of food in the required
quantity, chronic ptyalism, with distressing irritability of the
entire mucous surface, and loss of all the teeth, were amongst the
least of the sufferings entailed by this terrible course.   In truth, it
is hard to say which suffered most—the mind or the body; the
lives of both persons being nothing but a hopeless misery.

For the following interesting case I am indebted to Mr. Pollock,
of St. George's Hospital :—

"27, Grosvenor-street, January 5, 1850.

CASE III.—" I send you the particulars of the case I mentioned
to you of scrofulous disease of the hip-joint and enlarged liver, the
recovery from which I attribute solely to the use of the nitro-
muriatic-acid bath, used as recommended by yourself.

" In July, 1848, I was requested to see a boy (Walter M——),
fifteen years of age, with extensive scrofulous disease of the hip.
The region of the joint was externally marked by numerous deep
cicatrices, and several sinuses still discharged their pus from the
interior.   The thigh was contracted on the body, and the pelvis
much distorted.   His aspect was very unhealthy; countenance
delicately pallid.   It was impossible to ascertain the exact condition of the joint, or position of the head of the femur, from the
consolidation of the surrounding soft parts, and also from the
suffering any movement of the parts produced in the child, but
there was no doubt that considerable mischief had occurred in the
joint, and had been going on for some time.

" The abdomen was also found to be very large ; there was a
small quantity of fluid in the cavity of the peritonæum, but the

enlargement was chiefly dependent on the great size of the liver, which was very prominent, reached down below the crest of the ileum, and filled up the greater part of the abdomen. He was unable to sit up, and moved with difficulty.   Pulse weak and quick ; appetite good ; tongue clean ; but every structure marked his *ex-sanguine* condition.

"When six years of age, and nine years before I was consulted, he had a fall downstairs. Some months subsequently, his parents observed him walking lame, and, as they describe it, 'he was attended by a doctor for the disease of the hip.' He became worse by degrees, and for the symptoms referred to the hip ; he had an issue made in the back part of the thigh, which was kept open for some eighteen months. He appeared to improve under the treatment, but soon after an abscess formed in the side of the thigh, which was opened, allowing the escape of much pus. From this time until I saw him many abscesses opened and healed, but a constant discharge continued from the hip, and occasionally pieces of carious bone came through the openings. Within twelve months of my seeing him his parents observed the increased size of the abdomen. About a week after I saw him, he commenced using the nitro-muriatic-acid foot-bath, and sponging the body with the nitro-muriatic acid, as recommended by you. *In the first week* of its application, the size of the abdomen, by measure, *diminished one inch and a half*, and during the four subsequent weeks, *one inch every week*. After this the parents ceased to keep the measure accurately ; but during the whole of the time, from the commencement of the use of the bath, he rapidly improved in every respect ; he gained strength, and health, and colour, and all the sinuses healed up rapidly ; and he was shortly afterwards able to move about upon crutches. I saw him again in April, 1849, so much improved that I did not know him again. Every sinus was closed round the joint, and quite sound ; he could place his foot to the ground, and even bear some weight upon it. He had gained flesh, and could walk about with the help of one crutch only, and wished much to have a high-heeled shoe, which, however, I recommend not to be tried too soon. The liver could not be detected larger than natural. The bath was used for some three or four months, being omitted for the interval of a week or a fortnight occasionally ; and in the interval he took internally small doses of the nitro-muriatic acid. The entire treatment consisted in this ; and to the use of the bath I cannot but attribute the favourable result of the case.

"I enclose you a letter from the parents, of which you can make any use you may think proper.

(Signed)   " GEORGE D. POLLOCK.

"To J. R. Martin, Esq."

Case IV.—Mr. ——, a surgeon of eminence, states that, when fourteen years of age, he had an attack of jaundice. In January, 1840, " after being much worried and fatigued," he had a severe bilious attack, with incessant vomiting of bile, followed by jaundice. During a month, his health was not " improved by any sort of treatment;" but on his " mind being powerfully acted on by agreeable intelligence, and stimulated by hope, the jaundice, from that day, began to give way, and in a week it disappeared."

With exception of occasional bilious attacks, one of which was caused by anxiety, he enjoyed good health from this time till March, 1849, when he was " worried about professional matters, and underwent great fatigue."

On the 29th of April of this year he was seized with rigors, and sense of cold in the back, headache, and tenderness of the eyes, followed by much fever ; and while still suffering from anxiety and depression of mind, he had profuse and offensive perspirations. From this time till the 18th of October, 1849, when I first saw the patient, the "wave chills," as he calls them, increased, followed by fever, pain of the right hypochondrium and epigastrium. The bowels were constipated, the excretions depraved. For this he took purgatives, and large doses of quinine, which removed the rigors; but fever, followed by profuse and offensive night-sweats, harassed him. The abdomen had for some time been much enlarged, and " a hard, ill-defined swelling at the epigastrium" was perceived by his friends (16th of September). By this time, great emaciation had taken place; the pulse ranged from 84 to 90 ; the complexion was "of a dusky yellowish white; the lips were pale and dusky; the tongue covered with white pasty fur; urine, like porter dregs." There were lancinating pains of the abdomen, but especially of the epigastric region. "The countenance had assumed a drawn, haggard look, the *scaffolding* of his face standing out in bold relief." Quinine had been largely used, and when "congestion of the left lobe of the liver" became apparent, "and that the rigors *might* indicate suppuration," the nitro-muriatic acid with taraxacum was exhibited, and he took blue pill, with henbane, every other night. Two leeches were applied to the epigastric region, "and the swelling was painted over with tincture of iodine ;" but this last produced increase of "febrile excitement ; the pulse, which was never under 85, frequently rose to 100." Mr. —— had, since his first illness, sought relief in change of air at Brighton, Ramsgate, Derbyshire, and Berkshire, but, after the last trip, he " decidedly retrograded." The liver was now ascertained by two eminent surgeons, friends of the patient, to be greatly increased in volume, extending plainly downwards and forwards for many inches ; and there was a hard tumour in the left hypochondrium; fever and emaciation, with great mental depression, having acquired a distressing height.

I saw the patient on the 18th of October, 1849, and on careful examination I perceived the tumour in the left hypochondrium to arise from enlargement and induration of the spleen. By pressing the fingers in a vertical direction they fell into a sulcus, marking a separation between the two masses, that of the liver and the spleen. Both organs occupied two-thirds of the abdominal cavity, and the hand could be made to slip off their margins as from the rounded-off corner of a table; the spleen was more painful on pressure than the liver.

Mr. —— was recommended to use the nitro-muriatic-acid bath, by immersion of the whole body, night and morning, for fifteen minutes. This course was commenced on the 23rd of October, and on the 27th a very copious discharge took place from the bowels. " On the 29th, the effect of the baths was made manifest by a smart diarrhœa, the bowels being acted on seven times in twelve hours. On the 30th, the bowels were acted on four times before 10 A.M." The effect being thus powerful, and Mr. —— having duties to perform, the use of the bath was omitted till November 3, when it was resumed once only in the twenty-four hours, in the morning. A draught containing forty grains of compound powder of jalap was the only medicine exhibited internally, and that but on the first day of using the bath. On the 12th of November, when suffering from inflamed hæmorrhoids, he took a drachm of confection of senna, and by 10 A.M. of the following morning he passed six copious motions of vitiated bile, "like molten lead." On the 17th of November, I made a careful examination of Mr. ——'s abdomen, and found the liver and spleen softened and flattened, but still nearly of the same extent as before. The tumour of the abdomen had much subsided; the complexion had improved ; the urine had become less turbid ; and the frequency of the pulse was reduced. The circumference of the body had undergone " a diminution of four and a half inches in less than a month, and this in spite of a considerable increase of fat, for his ribs were now decently covered, and his arm measured an inch more in circumference. The excretions were now nearly natural, with exception of an abundant deposit of lithates in the urine, which was passed in very large quantities. The sleep was good, and the appetite excellent."

Dec. 4th.—Had slight bilious diarrhœa. The spleen scarcely perceptible, and the liver greatly diminished.

Dec. 7th.—Took a seidlitz powder, which was followed by "a copious discharge of pure, honest, laudable bile."

Dec. 28th.—" During the last few days I have felt some irritability and depression of spirits; my gums are red and turgid, and bleed on the least suction. Mr. Martin made a careful examination, and finding that the spleen is no longer perceptible, and that the liver has also recovered its natural size, and being of opinion that malaise, and the condition of the gums, indicated that the system was fully under the influence of the nitro-muriatic acid, permitted me to leave off bathing, which has been steadily pursued day after day, with one or two exceptions only, since the 23rd October.

" January 5th, 1850.—I now feel in every respect in excellent health; stronger in body and more cheerful than I have been for many months; I may almost say for twelve months. I have gained considerably in bulk; the functions of the alimentary canal are healthily performed; the pulse is firm and natural; the skin soft and healthy; the muscles firm; and I am equal to a great amount of exertion.

" I cannot conclude without expressing my conviction that, under Providence, I owe my life to the treatment directed by Mr. Martin. On reviewing my case, it will be seen that there was a steady progress from bad to worse. There were amendments from time to time, but each amendment was succeeded by symptoms more severe and more intractable than had before appeared. It will be further seen that the ordinary treatment, under the direction of most able physicians (whose friendly attention I can never forget), although producing temporary lull, quite failed in removing the cause of the mischief. The state of debility to which I was reduced by the fearful night-sweats forbade depletion. The enlarged and tumid spleen put mercury out of the question. Quinine had been tried most fully, and had disappointed us. The mineral acid and taraxacum, though affording some relief at first, soon ceased to produce a beneficial effect, and iodine absolutely disagreed. Thus the line of treatment still open was so circumscribed that the most skilful physician to whom the endermic use of the nitro-muriatic acid was not familiar might well be embarrassed; and the patient, keenly alive to his condition, might well regard the prospect before him with dismay. Happily for me the one remedy appropriate was employed, and by the blessing of God I have been restored to health in the brief period of two months."

One of the medical friends, already mentioned, who saw Mr. —— just before my return to town in October, writes as follows:—

" The countenance was anxious; he had emaciated a good deal of late, and his appearance was that of a man *seriously* ill. The tongue was red at the edges, and covered with a white thick fur, and but slightly moist. Pulse quick; no appetite, and much languor. He complained chiefly of pain in the region of the liver, but pain also was referred to the epigastrium and left hypochondrium. On examination, the abdomen appeared very full; considerable enlargement of the liver was felt, not extending downwards to the pelvis, but pressing forwards as if it was greatly and generally enlarged from congestion. The enlargement extended so much to the left side, that I imagined the left lobe was occupying a large space in the left hypochondrium. This was, however, what you considered to be the spleen considerably enlarged.

" The pain over all this enlarged mass was so great, and so little able to submit to pressure, that I was almost afraid, that if abscess had not already commenced, there was sufficient reason to anticipate such might very probably be the result. I was especially more fearful of this, as Mr. —— had suffered from recent rigors.

"The case was of so anxious a nature that I asked Mr. —— to see him with me till you returned. We agreed to give him small doses of blue pill daily, and attend to the bowels with gentle aperients ; on your return to town a few days after, you took charge of the case. When I recollect what was his condition when he first came to me, and the rapid improvement that took place under the use of the nitro-muriatic-acid bath, under your advice, and from what I have seen of the efficacy of the bath in some other instances, I cannot but consider the use of it as one of the most important modes of treatment in a vast number of cases both medical and surgical."

This gentleman's case had some points of great interest in it. The rigors in his, as in Major ——'s case (page 729), were arrested by the quinine ; but the fever only assumed a more continued form, with increased tumidness and tenderness of the abdomen generally, and of the liver in particular. More than seventy years ago it was observed by the medical officers in India, and by Curtis amongst others, that the Peruvian bark changed the fevers symptomatic of jaundice, and other affections of the liver, "into a continued fever."

Mr. —— also used the acid bath under grave disadvantages. He commenced this course of treatment in the end of October, and continued it through winter cold of the two following months ; and with all this he was in continual and active professional exercise, exposed to weather and other injurious influences ; yet, despite such serious disadvantages, the result was complete in curative effect ; and he is now, October, 1861, in perfect health.

Case V.—Through the kindness of the late Mr. Dalrymple, the following case has been brought to my recollection :—

"I have great pleasure in giving you an account of the case of hepatic disease about which I consulted you some few years ago ; although the relation wants the precision of accurate notes taken at the time.

"Captain W——, then about thirty-six years of age, had already made several voyages to India and China, and had usually enjoyed excellent health. He was a well-built, muscular man, exceedingly temperate, and of very active, energetic habits. During his last voyage to the East, he had suffered from bilious fever and dysentery, which had been checked, though not cured, by some American physician whom he consulted in his voyage back round Cape Horn, in the Brazils.

"On his arrival in London I was called to see him, and I found him greatly emaciated in his limbs, but protuberant in the abdomen. His complexion was that of a pale lemon, no red blood even in his lips. His bowels were obstinately costive; the evacuations clay-coloured, without a trace of bile. He suffered grievous pain all over the upper part of the abdomen; his strength was gone; and his spirits, in spite of his natural firmness and energy, depressed to the last degree.

" On examination of his abdomen, I found the hypochondria expanded, the epigastric region bulging, the liver extending upwards, as determined by percussion, and invading the right thoracic space. The pain produced by even moderate pressure over the hepatic region was exquisite. Under these circumstances, I believed he had acute inflammation of the liver, and that mercury energetically given was indispensable to his recovery. It was fortunate, however, for my patient, that I determined to fortify myself by the advice of another, and before beginning the treatment I asked the opinion of the late Dr. James Johnson. On his first examination of the patient's abdomen, and from observing pressure and percussion produced pain amounting to agony, he told me he feared that abscess of the liver had already formed; but he declined to prescribe, and advised us to consult you, giving me an introduction to yourself for that purpose.

" After you had heard our history, and had made a careful examination, you gave as your opinion that the case was one of active congestion of the liver; that no suppuration had probably taken place, though disorganization was threatened, unless means could be found to emulge this great viscus. Mercury you denounced, saying you believed it would produce the very consequences we were anxious to avert. Captain W—— was advised to use the nitro-muriatic acid sponging-bath twice a day; and I well remember the only medicine he was directed to take was some simple aloetic aperient, to maintain a free state of the bowels. The recital of the rest of the case need require but few words. No other means were used from first to last, but the bath was most honestly persevered in, and a few short weeks sufficed to render the stools again bilious. The pale yellow gave place to a more healthy colour in the cheeks, as the food once more became assimilated, and red blood again elaborated. In less than three weeks all pain had vanished, even on firm pressure. His appetite increased ; his spirits became elastic; his limbs were evidently more muscular, and a remarkable diminution in the size and prominence of the upper part of the abdomen took place. In six weeks he was well, and required only that additional vigour that change of air gives to the convalescent.

" Since the period I have referred to, Captain W—— made two voyages to China and returned in perfect health. He has been for the last three years, and is now, in China, and I heard of him only a few days back, from Hong-Kong, stating that he has been uniformly well during this his last residence in these climates.

" In this history I have not dwelt upon any but the more promi. nent symptoms, nor have I thought it necessary to state the day-by-day progress.   The case is mainly valuable as showing the exact adaptation of the treatment to the exigencies of the case; for like as a ship once within the influence of the trades has no need to trim her sails for weeks perhaps together, so, here, no alteration of treatment was required from the time Captain W—— set out upon his voyage of recovery until he arrived at the haven of health.

(Signed)   " J. DALRYMPLE.

"60, Grosvenor-street, Jan. 22, 1850."

CASE VI.—For the following interesting case I am indebted to Dr. Donald Dalrymple, of Norwich :—

"The Rev. T. C——, aged fifty, the subject of this case, is a tall, bony man, nearly six feet high.   His father is alive, and very vigorous, at an advanced age; his mother suffered from, and died of gall-stones.   He has lost some of his family from phthisis. He was very active in his habits, a teetotaller by habit and convietion, and in addition to his clerical duties, earnestly and energetically performed, kept a school, and has been unremittingly overworked.   As a youth, while at college and since, he was subject to bilious headaches, and about five years ago, having previously suffered from indigestion (so-called), had a regular fit of gall-stones. These attacks recurred at longer or shorter intervals, with greater or less intensity and frequency, but always yielded to calomel and opium, warm baths, &c.; yet, though during the attack there was a total suppression of bile, no biliary calculus was detected, though very accurate search was made, and nothing more than a dark *débris* could be found in the stools.   On the 19th of March, 1849, he was seized with one of his usual attacks; the pain, sickness, &c., yielded, as before, to the ordinary remedies, but he quickly became jaundiced, attended with fever, high pulse, and great prostration.   He was put on a course of calomel, with mercurial liniment rubbed in over the liver, and this was persisted in till the 7th of April, when bile re-appeared in the stools, and his jaundice lessened.

For a week he improved, but on the 16th all his symptoms returned, beginning as before; from this time his condition was as follows : he was universally jaundiced; skin a yellow brown; nails and conjunctivæ orange; urine, deep mahogany colour; pulse 130 ; tongue dry and cracked; respiration rapid, abdomen distended, but not painful, even on deep pressure; brain confused, occasionally delirious; great emaciation, and he presented the appearance of a man poisoned with bile.

3 D

On the 30th of April I wrote to Mr. Martin, who, taking a very unfavourable view of the case, advised the use of croton-oil purgatives, to emulge the bile-ducts; this advice was, at a consultation held with Dr. Hull, Mr. Cope, my brother, and myself, rejected, on the ground that the patient was not strong enough to bear it. Medicines were confined to obtaining an evacuation daily, which was *perfectly white;* and he was freely supplied with stimulants, and the most nutritious food, in spite of which he got worse, till the 20th of May, when he appeared to be sinking. From this period, when all prospect of recovery seemed lost, he gradually improved, and it is needless to occupy time and space in describing it; but in one, and the most essential point, no alteration took place—no bile appeared in his stools, they were as white as ever. About this time he began to cough, and, knowing his family tendencies, I became very uneasy about this new symptom.

On June 3rd, Dr. C. J. B. Williams, being in Norwich to see a patient of ours, he kindly visited this case, and, though unable to detect the existence of pulmonary disease, entertained serious fears that, in a system so shattered, such might be developed, and that possibly there existed tuberculous disease of the liver; at that time the right thoracic cavity was encroached upon by the liver very much, and the air with some difficulty permeated the inferior lobe. The doctor's suggestion was the use of cod-liver oil, a sustaining but non-stimulant diet, and occasional aperients, but no mercurials. The same gradual improvement took place as had been witnessed before, till the 20th of June, when all his worst symptoms returned, and on the 25th of June he was nearly, if not quite, as bad as ever.

Our patient ran through, as nearly as possible, the same course, and again, without any obvious reason, rallied and continued to improve. His pulse, which never had been under 110, and commonly 115, fell to 105 or 100; his tongue cleaned, his strength returned to a certain degree, and he regained his appetite. He continued to improve till he was able to ride in a pony-chaise, but yet no signs of bile appeared in his stools, which were either of a white chalk or a dull putty colour. On or about the 15th of August he was well enough to go to London, to consult Mr. Martin, and at the time he went this was his condition: He was greatly emaciated, weighing scarcely nine stone (fourteen pounds to the stone); his skin was of a dusky, tawny hue; his pulse from 100 to 106 in the minute; his tongue white, pasty, and fissured; his abdomen, between the umbilicus and ensiform cartilage, distended and drum-like, only slightly tender, however (nor, indeed, throughout was there much tenderness on pressure), below the umbilicus, and the abdomen was hardly more prominent than natural; the feeling conveyed to the touch was that of a bladder distended to the verge of bursting.

Mr. Martin ordered him to begin the nitro-muriatic acid bath daily, and to procure, by means of the croton oil, one or two daily evacuations, which system he commenced about the 20th of August, and in addition he kept on the use of the cod-liver oil. From this time, for six weeks, he continued steadily to improve, his skin became brighter, bile gradually appeared in his stools, first scantily, latterly more abundantly; his pulse fell to 95, and then to 90 ; his cough abated, his feet, which I had forgot to mention as swollen, became less so, and, above all, he made fifteen pounds of flesh in seven weeks. At this time, still continuing his treatment, he received, as the reward of his long and zealous Christian labours in the ministry, a living from the Crown, which raised him from the difficulties which had terribly weighed upon him, to a state of humble though comparative competence.

This good fortune had an evident and considerable influence upon him, and he continued to improve in all points, and was able to superintend in great measure the removal of his family and household to his new abode, in October; since when I have not seen him.

In conclusion I would add, that during the course of this long and interesting case, no remedy or plan of treatment that could be devised was left untried, though it would be impossible, in the limits of a case, to detail it at length."

The patient reports, on the 30th of Jan., 1850, that his eyes and skin are clear of all yellow tinge, and that his urine is of a healthy appearance, the intestinal secretions having the same character. "The abdominal enlargement, as far as visible to the eye, is quite gone."

" I attribute the improvement in our patient's health," says Mr. Dalrymple, "to the action of the acid bath, and to the emulgent effect of the croton oil."

Mr. C——, on my recommendation, used the bath again during part of June and July, and he now writes :—" I feel as if I never was in better bodily health," while the weight of the body has increased from nine stone four pounds to about twelve stone.

This gentleman is now reported to be " stout and well."

CASE VII.—April 6th, 1853.—I was requested by Mr. Fergusson, of King's College Hospital, to visit Colonel ——, of the Indian army, an officer of about sixty-five years of age, having gone to India in 1805. During his course of service, which exceeded thirty-five years of actual residence in India, he had been a keen sportsman, and had consequently been continually exposed to direct solar influence, while his habits were what is called free. He had had three severe attacks of remittent jungle fever, which were followed by often-repeated attacks of intermittent fever. He also suffered from severe rheumatism, for the cure of which he came to England in 1812, returning to his duty in good health, after fourteen months' residence at home. By constitution he was gouty, his mother having died of that disease.   He came home again on sick leave in 1842, suffering from emaciation and debility, and returned to his duty in India in November, 1846.

While at his Presidency he was nearly destroyed by a large quantity of arsenic, administered by one of his servants, with a view to murder and robbery.   From this poisoning he recovered rapidly, and returned to England finally, in March, 1847.   From this time he describes his health as always indifferent ; but it has been more especially so during the last three years.   In India, from 1835, he had occasional slight attacks of gout, but in England they have become more severe and more frequent of occurrence, especially since exposure to wet and cold, while shooting in the Highlands of Scotland two years ago.

In January, 1853, Colonel —— became seriously indisposed, and confined altogether to his house.   His skin became of a lemon yellow, hard and dry to the touch.   The pulse became rapid, and he had no natural sleep ; the appetite failed, accompanied by a most violent "burning pain" in the epigastric region, increased, even on swallowing the most bland food, as milk, sago, or arrow-root.   The urine was scanty and blood-red, the alvine excretion being clay-coloured.   He had greatly emaciated since January. The liver was, on April 6th, found greatly enlarged, extending down to near the umbilicus, hard, and very painful on pressure, . especially in the epigastric region ;—pulse one hundred ; tongue much coated.   Ordered, in consultation with Mr. Fergusson, the nitro-muriatic acid bath for the whole body, to be used night and morning, followed every other morning by a mild aperient draught. To secure sleep, a mild anodyne of solution of morphia was used every night, while the dilute nitro-muriatic acid was exhibited internally three times a day in bitter infusion.   By this means the fever, pain, and restlessness were in some degree relieved ; but on the fifth day the treatment was discontinued, owing to a violent gouty inflammation in the knee-joint : on April 25th the bath was resumed, and about May 12th its action on the liver and bowels became perceptible in two or three large bilious motions from the bowels in twenty-four hours, and in a copious excretion of straw-coloured urine.   By this time, also, the pulse had become natural, the tongue clean, the skin perspirable and free from jaundice ; and food of every kind was borne, not only without pain, but it was taken with appetite.   The anodyne and aperient draughts were now discontinued, as were the internal doses of dilute acid, and the bath was used only once in the twenty-four hours—viz., at bed-time.   The fever had now been subdued, and there was but slight uneasiness in the hepatic region on pressure, none in the epigastrium.   After a few more days the flow of green and yellow bile became more copious, the number of motions averaging from five to six in the twenty-four hours, accompanied by slight malaise, with redness and tenderness of the gums and tongue, so that on May 23rd all treatment was discontinued. By this date, Colonel —— had used thirty-seven baths.

May 26th.—Owing to the frequent passage of acrid green bile he felt griped and uneasy, and had but little inclination for food. Ordered—bicarbonate of soda in bitter infusion, and a magnesian aperient in the morning.

28th.—Draught acted twice, and he now feels much better, appetite returning; has improved in condition.

June 6th.—Has continued improving in all ways until to-day, when, owing to overloading of the stomach, he was seized with epigastric pains of a severe character : the bowels have continued open twice or thrice a day, without medicine, the discharges containing a greenish-yellow bile ; urine high coloured, tongue furred. Ordered a repetition of the bath every night, and a magnesian draught in the morning.

June 7th.—Two dark green motions followed by much relief from pain. Urine examined carefully, and found nothing unnatural.

June 8th.—Much better. Had three dark green motions, followed by much relief from pain. Urine abundant and straw-coloured. To continue the bath at bedtime only.

Towards the end of June, Colonel —— had so far recovered in condition and strength as to take regular and daily active exercise, and he then went into the country. I saw no more of him till the 10th September. He stated that for some three weeks previously, the epigastric pain had returned, with frequent vomiting, and some tendency to diarrhœa. All food, even the most bland, caused excessive pain. He had again fallen off in condition; the pulse was frequent, and the countenance had become extremely pallid.

Sept. 12th.—Visited Colonel —— in company with Mr. Pollock. The patient was now much exhausted from constant vomiting and pain, the matter vomited being streaked with blood, as were the contents of the bowels. Having left London at this time, I saw no more of the patient, who died on the 11th October, 1853.

For the following report of the *post-mortem* examination by Dr. Quain, I am indebted to Mr. Fergusson :—

"*Stomach.*—There was no disease of this organ, save some thickening of the coats over the pylorus. The mucous membrane was everywhere sound.

"*Liver.*—The whole of this organ was throughout paler than natural—the tissue was tolerably firm—towards the anterior margin there was some contraction, rounding and puckering, giving it to a limited extent, the appearance of cirrhosis.

"*Spleen.*—This organ was small, firm, and traversed by an unusual number of fibres, or trabeculæ.

"*Kidneys.*—These organs appeared healthy.

"*The small intestines* were healthy.

"*Large Intestine.*—This bowel appeared elongated—much convoluted—distended at some points, contracted at others. On laying the bowel open, it was found filled with a chocolate-coloured viscid substance, about the consistence of treacle. This substance was bounded above by the ileo-cæcal valve, and occupied the bowel to the anus. On washing the surface of the intestine, the mucous membrane was seen to be of a deep chocolate colour—the follicular structure of the cæcum was particularly well marked—the membrane in some parts was extremely thin, in others presenting marked vascularity. There were seen also the perfect cicatrices of some old ulcers."

Remarks.—The subject of this very interesting record would seem to have died, after all, from the depressing influences of irritation, pain, and vomiting, on a worn-out, gouty, and anæmic constitution. Separated from the general ill habit, there was no structural disease to cause death—or indeed, under more favourable circumstances, to preclude the recovery of health. The restored health of the liver, under the use of the acid bath, is here again remarkable, as occurring after great previous enlargement with induration. The appearance of cirrhosis, in cases where the liver had previously been much enlarged, has already been commented on, and at page 761, it is stated on the authority of Professor Bennett, that hypertrophy of the fibrous element exists between the lobules of the organ, and its subsequent contraction, whereby its volume is diminished and the secreting cells compressed and atrophied, necessarily results.

The perfect cicatrices of some old ulcers, too, exhibited the reparative power of nature in tropical dysentery, in which disease extensive portions of the large intestines are known to be abraded and ulcerated.

The disappearance of gout, and of epigastric pain, under the influence of the acid bath, is another feature in this case worthy of notice.

The following case is presented in conclusion :—

MEMORANDUM ON THE HEALTH OF MR. DE C——L.

"The patient came under my observation during the voyage from Calcutta to England, on board the ship *Hotspur;* his aspect was anæmic to the greatest extent, besides being jaundiced. I learned from him that for the latter disease he had undergone most active treatment in the shape of purgatives, mercurials, nitro-muriatic acid baths, taraxacum, &c. &c. ; that he had lost four stone in weight. Examination of the abdomen gave me clear indication of induration and great enlargement of the liver, the organ extending below the ribs very considerably. The tongue was flabby, gums scorbutic, bowels uncertain in their action, the colour of the evacuations light, the urine deeply tinged with bile.

(Signed) " H. D——N, M.D.

"British Channel, April 13, 1855."

Eugène de C——l, ætatis 40, resided all his life in India, in Bengal Proper, and chiefly in the district of Moorshedabad. The following is his own account of his case :—

" I enjoyed tolerable health until March, 1854, when I became suddenly jaundiced, a state of health which had been preceded during two years by occasional spasms in the pit of the stomach. In October, 1854, I came down to Calcutta for medical advice, when a great enlargement of the liver was discovered, the jaundice having by this time become intense, the spasms recurring monthly, and the complexion being a deep green and yellow. Treatment having failed of doing me good, I embarked, by the advice of my medical attendant, for England in January, 1855. During the voyage round the Cape I had partly the assistance of the surgeon of the vessel, but without any avail; and in April of the same year I arrived in England, and on the 26th of that month consulted Mr. J. R. Martin, of Grosvenor-street, and formerly of Calcutta. At this time I was emaciated and enfeebled to the last degree; my stomach was large and tumid; my urine was like porter, thick and dark, and the motions from my bowels were white. I was instantly put under a course of acid baths, which I continued without intermission for four months. I am now in a state of feeling of comfort and health, such as I have not experienced for a couple of years; I eat with an appetite and sleep well; my complexion is very clear, and the urine apparently healthy looking. The liver, my medical adviser in the country says, is not now to be felt, and my strength is rapidly returning, so much so that I can walk six and seven miles with ease. Formerly, my friends and medical attendant, who had not seen me for some years, did not recognise me, so emaciated and altered had I become in every way; my sister, whom I had not met for eight months, received me as a stranger; and even my wife declared she would have passed me in the street without recognition. When I first put myself into Mr. Martin's hands, which was at the end of April last, as above stated, I weighed only nine stone (my original weight in health having been thirteen stone ten pounds), and in August last, when I again weighed myself, I weighed ten stone. I now weigh about eleven stone, November 15th, 1855."

This gentleman, writing from Mirzapore, June 17th, 1858, says :—" I am now feeling better, and am in better actual health than I have enjoyed at any time during the last twelve years; and I both eat and drink things which formerly I could not touch without suffering."

CONCLUSION.

It will be seen that in the management of convalescence from acute diseases, and for the treatment of those of a chronic kind, I have seldom had recourse to mercury as a therapeutic agent; believing that the powerful actions of this mineral are most appropriately applied to acute and dangerous maladies. To use mercurials perseveringly for disorders of the health, or for the cure of chronic affections, is to confound that which is appropriate to acute, with what is applicable to protracted forms of organic lesion. In this our climate a sparing application of the means in question, for a short time, may be justly made where congestion threatens greatly to disturb the function, or to affect the structure of the liver; but I know nothing so greatly to be reprehended as the indiscriminate or inconsiderate use of so powerful a class of remedies.

In India, whether we have to treat an European suffering from remittent fever, dysentery, hepatitis, or cholera, the symptoms and progress of disease are so acutely violent as to leave but a very few days between recovery and death: the means of cure, therefore, to be effective must be energetic, that is, if we would save life, and prevent the occurrence of dangerous organic diseases. In fever, dysentery, and hepatitis, the patient, as a first measure, is bled to an extent proportioned to the severity of the disease, reference being had to age, constitution, habits of life, and length of residence in India; and blood-letting is repeated, generally or locally, or in both forms, until a sufficient abatement is obtained in the force and frequency of the actions of the heart and arteries. The disease still proceeding with dangerous force and rapidity, we have next to employ calomel in aid of blood-letting, followed by purgatives, sudorifics, and diuretics, so as to excite all the depurative functions, and thus bring about a solution of acute and dangerous disease. These means we gradually abate as symptoms yield, and generally no injury is done to the patient's constitution, couvalescence being rapid; but they are heroic remedies nevertheless, which demand much knowledge, discernment, and experience, for their just scientific application, and even for their withdrawal. In the present state of our knowledge we possess no other means of cure than those here briefly described, aided by antiperiodics and tonics.

Under the sanction of the Royal Medical and Chirurgical Society of London, in its thirty-eighth volume, Dr. Garrod, in contrasting the actions of alkalies and mercurials in the treatment of acute rheumatism, expresses his belief that mercurials " have more power in causing absorption of recently deposited lymph, than alkalies or any other known remedies. This point he has recently had opportunities of testing in cases of pleuritis, in which it appeared that the alkaline treatment by the bicarbonate of potash possessed great influence in preventing deposition, but that when the lymph was already deposited, its value in causing its absorption was far inferior to that of mercurials; he believes that the same holds good in peri- and endocarditis of a rheumatic character."

I believe this statement to be essentially true; and I quote it here as being altogether confirmatory of what is set forth in page 480 of the present work. The day may come when we shall be enabled effectually to cure acute tropical and other diseases, without the assistance of mercury; but it has not as yet arrived. In the meantime, and in the absence of a better knowledge, what we should try to obviate is—not the use of mercury, but its abuse. "But the more explicit knowledge we possess," says Sir H. Holland, "of the effects of calomel, and its undoubted efficacy, for all the most important purposes in practice, must ever sustain its repute, whatever equivalents may hereafter be acquired for the results we now obtain through its agency."

Of the sufferers who have passed through the storms of tropical disease described in this work, it will be seen that many recover immediately on the spot, a certain proportion sinks, while others come to their native country for the restoration and confirmation of health. In the cases of these last, it is evident that a careful consideration of all their antecedent circumstances is absolutely necessary to their just management, and that we must understand the nature of their acute diseases in India, and their treatment there, to appreciate aright their chronic ailments on their return to Europe. Such a review will, I think, generally satisfy the medical observer at home, that with mercury in any form his emaciated, relaxed, enfeebled, and generally anæmic tropical patient need now have but little to do.

I have seen more mercury administered in this country in chronic diseases, or for what may be termed the disorders of health in adults, and more "gray powder" given persistently to children, sometimes by female relatives, governesses, and even by nurses, than is ever seen in India under acute diseases treated by medical officers; and in many instances the results have been more lasting and lamentable than anything I witnessed in the East. It ought to be made a rule in families that no preparation of mercury should be used excepting under competent and careful medical advice; and I feel assured that the carrying out so salutary a domestic reform would confer a greater benefit, on young women especially, than all those lighter accomplishments with the acquisition of which their earlier years are teased.

These circumstances I think it right to mention; and certainly I do so in no arrogant controversial spirit, nor with a view to finding fault.

Angry criticisms and unseemly wranglings on the subject of the efficacy, or otherwise, of certain remedies, and on the merits of certain kinds of practices, I have ever seen to be prejudicial at once to the character of the profession of medicine and to individual credit and reputation for usefulness.

If we cannot carry our point by justice, truth, and reason, we must wait till they come to our aid, as eventually they are sure to do. Cabanis said, more than half a century ago:—" Let us unite our efforts, and endeavour to introduce into the study and practice of our art that superior reason and philosophy without which, so far is it from affording useful aid, that it becomes a real public scourge."

THE END.

OPINIONS OF THE PRESS.

"WE can safely and heartily recommend this work as containing a mass of information of the most valuable kind, and relieving a want which no one, probably, now living, except Mr. Martin, could so adequately and efficiently supply."—*Medical Times and Gazette.*

"It is gratifying to find a man who, after passing a life of active practice in the East, sits down, in the midst of laborious professional occupations here, to give to the profession the results of his extended observation. We feel sure nothing we can say adds value to this work; nothing we can say will render it too highly appreciated."—*Association Medical Journal.*

"Mr. Martin's volume is a most valuable contribution to medical science. To the young practitioner about to depart to the tropics, and to those already settled in hot countries, this work must prove invaluable. To the sanitarian it offers a mine of knowledge and experience. It must prove of very great service indeed to medical practitioners in this country, who have to treat those who have resided in India, or in any other of our tropical colonies." . . . . "The testimony of such a man as Dr. Borland furnishes the best evidence of the value of Mr. Martin's services to the science of the prevention and cure of disease within the tropics—services, the highest praise of which is to say that they were equal to the long and ample opportunities which Mr. Martin enjoyed."—*Lancet.*

"We take leave of this book, congratulating Mr. Martin as the author, and Mr. Churchill as the publisher of a work, for which we can most certainly prognosticate a large and continuous sale. We have no hesitation in regarding it as the standard work upon the many important subjects of which it treats."—*Dublin Quarterly Journal.*

"Mr. Martin's observations throughout are so true, so clear, and so correct, that it is difficult to select any one passage in particular for consideration. The whole chapter bearing on this head" (the preservation of the soldier's health by proper selection of localities) "should be printed at the public expense, and distributed on the benches of the House of Commons.

"We quit Mr. Martin's book with these words—viz., that its circulation cannot be too general, since it is the result of an experience that few have ever similarly enjoyed, and none turned to equal account."—*Dublin Medical Press.*

OPINIONS OF THE PRESS.

"It is not necessary for us to say anything to secure a favourable notice of a work which has become so established a text-book upon the subject of which it treats—a work which is read by every one, both at home and abroad, who is wishful to gain a thorough knowledge of the science of medicine; for every one who has read the old will assuredly make a point of seeing for himself wherein the new edition differs from it. For our own part, we have read the work with much additional pleasure and profit."—*The Half-Yearly Abstract of the Medical Sciences.* By Drs. RANKING and RADCLIFFE.

The reviewer, after stating that Mr. Martin's work is based on a sound physiology, and that he observes extreme care to adapt his remedies to the nature and stage of the diseases which he describes, adds that he impresses the importance and points out the means of preventing disease.

"We are obliged to close our task, feeling that we have been unable to do Mr. Martin full justice in our remarks upon his valuable contribution to medical literature. Our object has been more to present the results of the author's observations and experience than to criticise his views; more to cull what he has learned during a life spent among a certain class of diseases, than to compare his doctrines with those of other authors who have written upon the same subjects. If, in accomplishing this task, we have imparted a tithe of the information and pleasure we have derived from perusing the volume, we shall be satisfied. It is a work which cannot fail deeply to interest every scientific physician, while it will prove a most valuable addition to the library of the army and navy surgeon."—*North American Medico-Chirurgical Review* for July, 1857.

"The work of Mr. Martin, being a summary of all that has been written in England on the subject, gives for the solution of scientific and practical questions a considerable addition of very elaborate matter; and the reader will always consult them with advantage on the questions referred to. The author exhibits thoughtful and profound knowledge of facts, a sound judgment, and a desire to be useful."—*Gazette Medicale de Paris.*

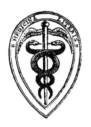

London, New Burlington Street,
October, 1873

SELECTION

FROM

MESSRS J. & A. CHURCHILL'S

𝕲eneral 𝕮atalogue

COMPRISING

ALL RECENT WORKS PUBLISHED BY THEM

ON THE

ART AND SCIENCE

OF

MEDICINE

INDEX

THE PRACTICE OF SURGERY:

A Manual by THOMAS BRYANT, F.R.C.S., Surgeon to Guy's Hospital.
Crown 8vo, with 507 Engravings on wood, 21s. [1872]

DIAGRAMS OF THE NERVES OF THE HUMAN BODY,

Exhibiting their Origin, Divisions, and Connexions, with their Distribution, by WILLIAM HENRY FLOWER, F.R.S., Conservator of the Museum of the Royal College of Surgeons. Second Edition, roy. 4to, 12s. [1872]

OUTLINES OF SURGERY

and Surgical Pathology, including the Diagnosis and Treatment of Obscure and Urgent Cases, and the Surgical Anatomy of some Important Structures and Regions, by F. LE GROS CLARK, F.R.S., Consulting Surgeon to St. Thomas's Hospital. Second Edition, Revised and Expanded by the Author, assisted by W. W. WAGSTAFFE, F.R.C.S., Assistant-Surgeon to, and Joint-Lecturer on Anatomy at, St. Thomas's Hospital. 8vo, 10s. 6d. [1872]

DISEASES OF THE OVARIES;

their Diagnosis and Treatment. By T. SPENCER WELLS, F.R.C.S., Surgeon to the Queen's Household and to the Samaritan Hospital. 8vo, with about 150 Engravings, 21s. [1872]

THE INFLUENCE OF THE MIND UPON THE BODY

in Health and Disease (Illustrations of), designed to elucidate the Action of the Imagination, by DANIEL HACK TUKE, M.D., M.R.C.P. 8vo, 14s. [1872]

FISTULA, HÆMORRHOIDS, PAINFUL ULCER,

Stricture, Prolapsus, and other Diseases of the Rectum: their Diagnosis and Treatment. By WM. ALLINGHAM, F.R.C.S., Surgeon to St. Mark's Hospital for Fistula, &c., late Surgeon to the Great Northern Hospital. Second Edition, enlarged, 8vo, 7s. [1872]

SYMPATHETIC SYSTEM OF NERVES

as a Physiological basis for a rational System of Therapeutics (On the Functions of the), by EDWARD MERYON, M.D., F.R.C.P. 8vo, 3s. 6d. [1872]

THE GRAFT THEORY OF DISEASE,

being an Application of Mr. DARWIN's Hypothesis of Pangenesis to the Explanation of the Phenomena of the Zymotic Diseases by JAMES ROSS, M.D., Waterfoot, near Manchester. 8vo, 10s. [1872]

FUNCTIONAL DISEASES

of the Renal, Urinary, and Reproductive Organs (On the), by D. CAMPBELL BLACK, M.D., L.R.C.S. Edin., Member of the General Council of the University of Glasgow. 8vo, 10s. 6d. [1872]

A MANUAL FOR HOSPITAL NURSES

and others engaged in Attending on the Sick by EDWARD J. DOMVILLE, L.R.C.P., M.R.C.S. Crown 8vo, 2s. 6d. [1872]

CANCER:

its varieties, their Histology and Diagnosis. By HENRY ARNOTT, F.R.C.S., Assistant-Surgeon to, and Lecturer on Pathology at, St. Thomas's Hospital. 8vo, with 5 Lithographic Plates and 22 Wood Engravings, 5s. 6d. [1872]

ON DISEASES OF THE LIVER:

Lettsomian Lectures for 1872 by S. O. HABERSHON, M.D., F.R.C.P., Physician to Guy's Hospital. Post 8vo, 3s. 6d. [1872]

ON SOME AFFECTIONS OF THE LIVER

and Intestinal Canal; with Remarks on Ague and its Sequelæ, Scurvy, Purpura, &c., by STEPHEN H. WARD, M.D. Lond., F.R.C.P., Physician to the Seamen's Hospital, Greenwich. 8vo, 7s. [1872]

ON CEREBRIA

and other Diseases of the Brain by CHARLES ELAM, M.D., F.R.C.P., Assistant-Physician to the National Hospital for Paralysis and Epilepsy. 8vo, 6s. [1872]

HANDBOOK OF LAW AND LUNACY;

or, the Medical Practitioner's Complete Guide in all Matters relating to Lunacy Practice, by J. T. SABBEN, M.D., and J. H. BALFOUR BROWNE. 8vo, 5s. [1872]

FOURTEEN COLOURED PHOTOGRAPHS OF LEPROSY

as met with in the Straits Settlements, with Explanatory Notes by
A. F. ANDERSON, M.D., Acting Colonial Surgeon, Singapore. 4to,
£1 11s. 6d. [1872]

LECTURES ON WINTER COUGH

(Catarrh, Bronchitis, Emphysema, Asthma) by HORACE DOBELL,
M.D., Senior Physician to the Royal Hospital for Diseases
of the Chest. Second Edition, with Coloured Plates, 8vo,
8s. 6d. [1872]

BY THE SAME AUTHOR,

TRUE FIRST STAGE OF CONSUMPTION

(Lectures on the). Crown 8vo, 3s. 6d. [1867]

A HANDBOOK OF UTERINE THERAPEUTICS

and of Diseases of Women by E. J. TILT, M.D., M.R.C.P. Third
Edition, post 8vo, 10s. [1868]

BY THE SAME AUTHOR,

THE CHANGE OF LIFE

in Health and Disease : a Practical Treatise on the Nervous and
other Affections incidental to Women at the Decline of Life. Third
Edition, 8vo, 10s. 6d. [1870]

THE ORIGIN OF CANCER

considered with Reference to the Treatment of the Disease by
CAMPBELL DE MORGAN, F.R.S., F.R.C.S., Surgeon to the Middlesex
Hospital. Crown 8vo, 3s. 6d. [1872]

THE ANATOMICAL REMEMBRANCER;

or, Complete Pocket Anatomist. Seventh Edition, carefully Revised, 32mo, 3s. 6d. [1872]

ZYMOTIC DISEASES:

their Correlation and Causation. By A. WOLFF, F.R.C.S. Post
8vo, 5s. [1872]

THE URINE AND ITS DERANGEMENTS

(Lectures on), with the Application of Physiological Chemistry to the Diagnosis and Treatment of Constitutional as well as Local Diseases by GEORGE HARLEY, M.D., F.R.S., F.R.C.P., formerly Professor in University College. Post 8vo, 9s. [1872]

ADVICE TO A MOTHER

on the Management of her Children, by PYE H. CHAVASSE, F.R.C.S. Eleventh Edition, fcap 8vo, 2s. 6d. [1872]

BY THE SAME AUTHOR,

COUNSEL TO A MOTHER:

being a Continuation and the Completion of 'Advice to a Mother.' Second Edition, fcap 8vo, 2s. 6d. [1872]

ALSO,

ADVICE TO A WIFE

on the Management of her own Health. With an Introductory Chapter, especially addressed to a Young Wife. Tenth Edition, fcap 8vo, 2s. 6d. [1873]

ALSO,

MENTAL CULTURE AND TRAINING OF A CHILD

(Aphorisms on the), and on various other Subjects relating to Health and Happiness. Fcap. 8vo, 2s. 6d. [1872]

WORMS:

a Series of Lectures delivered at the Middlesex Hospital on Practical Helminthology by T. SPENCER COBBOLD, M.D., F.R.S. Post 8vo, 5s. [1872]

CANCEROUS AND OTHER INTRA-THORACIC

Growths, their Natural History and Diagnosis. By J. RISDON BENNETT, M.D., F.R.C.P., Member of the General Medical Council. Post 8vo, with Plates, 8s. [1872]

FRACTURES OF THE LIMBS

(On the Treatment of) by J. SAMPSON GAMGEE, Surgeon to the Queen's Hospital, Birmingham. 8vo, with Plates, 10s. 6d. [1871]

WINTER AND SPRING

on the Shores of the Mediterranean; or, the Riviera, Mentone, Italy, Corsica, Sicily, Algeria, Spain, and Biarritz, as Winter Climates. By HENRY BENNET, M.D. Fourth Edition, post 8vo, with numerous Plates, Maps, and Wood Engravings, 12s. [1869]

BY THE SAME AUTHOR,

TREATMENT OF PULMONARY CONSUMPTION

(On the) by Hygiene, Climate, and Medicine. Second Edition, enlarged, 8vo, 5s. [1871]

CLINICAL USES OF ELECTRICITY

(Lectures on the) delivered at University College Hospital by J. RUSSELL REYNOLDS, M.D. Lond., F.R.C.P., F.R.S., Professor of Medicine in University College. Second Edition, post 8vo, 3s. 6d. [1873]

THE SCIENCE AND PRACTICE OF SURGERY:

a complete System and Textbook by F. J. GANT, F.R.C.S., Surgeon to the Royal Free Hospital. 8vo, with 470 Engravings, £1 4s. [1871]

BY THE SAME AUTHOR,

THE IRRITABLE BLADDER:

its Causes and Treatment. Third Edition, crown 8vo, with Engravings, 6s. [1872]

THE LAWS AFFECTING MEDICAL MEN

(A Manual of) by ROBERT G. GLENN, LL.B., Barrister-at-Law; with a Chapter on Medical Etiquette by Dr. A. CARPENTER. 8vo, 14s. [1871]

THE MEDICAL JURISPRUDENCE OF INSANITY.

By J. H. BALFOUR BROWNE, Barrister-at-Law. 8vo, 10s. 6d. [1871]

OBSTETRIC APHORISMS

for the Use of Students commencing Midwifery Practice by J. G. SWAYNE, M.D., Physician-Accoucheur to the Bristol General Hospital. Fifth Edition, fcap 8vo, with Engravings on Wood, 3s. 6d. [1871]

GROWTHS IN THE LARYNX,

with Reports and an Analysis of 100 consecutive Cases treated since the Invention of the Laryngoscope by MORELL MACKENZIE, M.D. Lond., M.R.C.P., Physician to the Hospital for Diseases of the Throat. 8vo, with Coloured Plates, 12s. 6d. [1871]

BY THE SAME AUTHOR,

HOARSENESS, LOSS OF VOICE,

and Stridulous Breathing in relation to Nervo-Muscular Affections of the Larynx. Second Edition, 8vo, fully Illustrated, 3s. 6d. [1868] .

ALSO

THROAT HOSPITAL PHARMACOPŒIA,

containing upwards of 150 Formulæ. Second Edition, fcap 8vo, 2s. 6d. [1873

A MANUAL OF PRACTICAL THERAPEUTICS

by E. J. WARING, M.D., F.R.C.P. Lond. Third Edition, fcap 8vo, 12s. 6d. [1871]

DISCOURSES ON PRACTICAL PHYSIC

by B. W. RICHARDSON, M.D., F.R.C.P., F.R.S. 8vo, 5s. [1871]

THE SURGERY OF THE RECTUM:

Lettsomian Lectures by HENRY SMITH, F.R.C.S., Surgeon to King's College Hospital. Third Edition, fcap 8vo, 3s. 6d. [1871]

HANDBOOK OF DENTAL ANATOMY

and Surgery for the Use of Students and Practitioners by JOHN SMITH, M.D., F.R.S. Edin., Surgeon-Dentist to the Queen in Scotland. Second Edition, fcap 8vo, 4s. 6d. [1871]

ORGANIC STRICTURE OF THE URETHRA

(An Analysis of 140 Cases of), by JOHN D. HILL, F.R.C.S., Surgeon to the Royal Free Hospital. 8vo, 3s. [1871]

§

THE REPRODUCTIVE ORGANS

in Childhood, Youth, Adult Age, and Advanced Life (The Functions and Disorders of), considered in their Physiological, Social, and Moral Relations, by WILLIAM ACTON, M.R.C.S. Fifth Edition, 8vo, 12s. [1871]

BY THE SAME AUTHOR,

PROSTITUTION:

Considered in its Moral, Social, and Sanitary Aspects. Second Edition, enlarged, 8vo, 12s. [1869]

NOTES AND RECOLLECTIONS

of an Ambulance Surgeon, being an Account of Work done under the Red Cross during the Campaign of 1870, by WILLIAM MacCORMAC, F.R.C.S., M.R.I.A., Surgeon to St. Thomas's Hospital. 8vo, with 8 Plates, 7s. 6d. [1871]

A TREATISE ON GOUT, RHEUMATISM

and the Allied Affections by P. HOOD, M.D. Crown 8vo, 10s. 6d. [1871]

LECTURES ON OBSTETRIC OPERATIONS,

including the Treatment of Hæmorrhage, and forming a Guide to the Management of Difficult Labour, by ROBERT BARNES, M.D., F.R.C.P., Obstetric Physician to, and Lecturer on Midwifery at, St. Thomas's Hospital. Second Edition, 8vo, with 113 Engravings, 15s. [1871]

PRACTICAL MIDWIFERY AND OBSTETRICS,

including Anæsthetics. By JOHN TANNER, M.D., M.R.C.P. Edin. Fcap 8vo, with numerous Engravings, 6s. 6d. [1871]

A TRANSLATION OF DR. DILLNBERGER'S

Handy-Book of the Treatment of Women's and Children's Diseases according to the Vienna Medical School, with Prescriptions, by PATRICK NICOL, M.B. Fcap 8vo, 5s. [1871]

OPERATIVE SURGERY
by C. F. MAUNDER, F.R.C.S., Surgeon to the London Hospital, formerly Demonstrator of Anatomy at Guy's Hospital. Second Edition, post 8vo, with 164 Wood Engravings, 6s.   [1872]

ON DEFORMITIES OF THE HUMAN BODY:
a System of Orthopædic Surgery, by BERNARD E. BRODHURST, F.R.C.S., Orthopædic Surgeon to St. George's Hospital. 8vo, with Engravings, 10s. 6d.   [1871]

A COMPENDIUM OF DOMESTIC MEDICINE
and Companion to the Medicine Chest; intended as a Source of Easy Reference for Clergymen, and for Families residing at a Distance from Professional Assistance by JOHN SAVORY, M.S.A. Eighth Edition, 12mo, 5s.   [1871]

SYPHILITIC DISEASES
(The Modern Treatment of), both Primary and Secondary; comprising the Treatment of Constitutional and Confirmed Syphilis, by a safe and successful Method, by LANGSTON PARKER, F.R.C.S. Fifth Edition, 8vo, 10s. 6d.   [1871]

METHOD AND MEDICINE:
an Essay on the Past, Present, and Future of Medicine by BALTHAZAR W. FOSTER, M.D., Professor of Physic in Queen's College, Birmingham. 8vo, 2s. 6d.   [1870]

THE TREATMENT OF SURGICAL INFLAMMATIONS
by a New Method, which greatly shortens their Duration, by FURNEAUX JORDAN, F.R.C.S., Professor of Surgery in Queen's College, Birmingham. 8vo, with Plates, 7s. 6d.   [1870]

ATLAS OF OPHTHALMOSCOPY:
representing the Normal and Pathological Conditions of the Fundus Oculi as seen with the Ophthalmoscope: composed of 12 Chromolithographic Plates (containing 59 Figures), accompanied by an Explanatory Text by R. LIEBREICH, Ophthalmic Surgeon to St. Thomas's Hospital. Translated into English by H. ROSBOROUGH SWANZY, M.B. Dub. Second Edition, Enlarged and Revised, 4to, £1 10s.   [1870]

THE PRINCIPLES AND PRACTICE OF SURGERY

by WILLIAM PIRRIE, F.R.S.E., Professor of Surgery in the University of Aberdeen.   Third Edition, 8vo, with 490 Engravings, 28s.   [1873]

A SYSTEM OF PRACTICAL SURGERY

by Sir WILLIAM FERGUSSON, Bart., F.R.C.S., F.R.S., Serjeant-Surgeon to the Queen.   Fifth Edition, 8vo, with 463 Illustrations on Wood, 21s.   [1870]

OPERATIVE SURGERY OF THE FOOT AND ANKLE

(The) by HENRY HANCOCK, President of the Royal College of Surgeons of England.   8vo, 15s.   [1873]

ON DISEASES OF THE SKIN:

a System of Cutaneous Medicine by ERASMUS WILSON, F.R.C.S., F.R.S.   Sixth Edition, 8vo, 18s, with Coloured Plates, 36s.

BY THE SAME AUTHOR,

THE ANATOMIST'S VADE-MECUM:

a System of Human Anatomy.   Ninth Edition, by Dr. G. BUCHANAN, Professor of Anatomy in Anderson's University, Glasgow.   Crown, 8vo, with 371 Engravings on Wood, 14s.   [1873]

ALSO,

LECTURES ON EKZEMA

and Ekzematous Affections; with an Introduction on the General Pathology of the Skin, and an Appendix of Essays and Cases.   8vo, 10s. 6d.   [1870]

ALSO,

LECTURES ON DERMATOLOGY

delivered at the Royal College of Surgeons, 1870, 6s.; 1871-3, 10s. 6d.

CLINICAL AND PATHOLOGICAL OBSERVATIONS

in India by J. FAYRER, C.S.I., M.D., F.R.S.E., Fellow of the Royal College of Physicians of London, Honorary Physician to the Queen.   8vo, with Engravings on Wood, 20s.   [1873]

A TREATISE ON RHEUMATIC GOUT,

or Chronic Rheumatic Arthritis ? all the Joints, by ROBERT ADAMS, M.D., M.R.I.A., Surgeon . H.M. the Queen in Ireland, Regius Professor of Surgery in the University of Dublin. Second Edition, 8vo, with Atlas of Plates, 21s. [1872]

THE SURGERY, SURGICAL PATHOLOGY,

and Surgical Anatomy of the Female Pelvic Organs, in a Series of Coloured Plates taken from Nature: with Commentaries, Notes, and Cases by HENRY SAVAGE, M.D. Lond., F.R.C.S., Consulting Physician to the Samaritan Free Hospital. Second Edition, greatly Enlarged, 4to, £1 11s. 6d. [1870]

ON HERNIAL AND OTHER TUMOURS

of the Groin and its Neighbourhood with some Practical Remarks on the Radical Cure of Ruptures by C. HOLTHOUSE, F.R.C.S., Surgeon to the Westminster Hospital. 8vo, 6s. 6d. [1870]

PRACTICAL PATHOLOGY:

third Edition, in 2 Vols., containing Lectures on Suppurative Fever, Diseases of the Veins, Hæmorrhoidal Tumours, Diseases of the Rectum, Syphilis, Gonorrhœal Ophthalmia, &c., by HENRY LEE, F.R.C.S., Surgeon to St. George's Hospital. 8vo, 10s. each vol. [1870]

RENAL DISEASES;

a Clinical Guide to their Diagnosis and Treatment by W. R. BASHAM, M.D., F.R.C.P., Senior Physician to the Westminster Hospital. Post 8vo, 7s. [1870]

ALSO,

THE DIAGNOSIS OF DISEASES OF THE KIDNEYS

(Aids to). 8vo, with 10 Plates, 5s. [1872]

ON DISEASES AND INJURIES OF THE EAR

by W. B. DALBY, F.R.C.S., M.B., Aural Surgeon and Lecturer on Aural Surgery at St. George's Hospital. Crown 8vo, with 21 Engravings, 6s. 6d. [1873]

ON THE PRESENT STATE OF THERAPEUTICS;

with some Suggestions for placing it on a more scientific basis by
JAMES ROGERS, M.D.   8vo, 6s. 6d.   [1870]

STUDIES ON FUNCTIONAL NERVOUS DISORDERS

by C. HANDFIELD JONES, M.B., F.R.C.P., F.R.S., Physician to St.
Mary's Hospital.   Second Edition, much enlarged, 8vo, 18s.   [1870]

PRINCIPLES OF SURGICAL DIAGNOSIS

(Lectures on the) especially in Relation to Shock and Visceral
Lesions, delivered at the Royal College of Surgeons by F. LE GROS
CLARK, F.R.C.S., Senior Surgeon to, and Lecturer on Surgery at,
St. Thomas's Hospital.   8vo, 10s. 6d.   [1870]

IMPERFECT DIGESTION:

its Causes and Treatment.   By ARTHUR LEARED, M.D., F.R.C.P.,
Senior Physician to the Great Northern Hospital.   Fifth Edition,
fcap 8vo, 4s. 6d.   [1870]

STRICTURE OF THE URETHRA

and Urinary Fistulæ; their Pathology and Treatment: Jacksonian
Prize Essay by Sir HENRY THOMPSON, F.R.C.S., Surgeon-Extra-
ordinary to the King of the Belgians.   Third Edition, 8vo, with
Plates, 10s.   [1869]

BY THE SAME AUTHOR,

PRACTICAL LITHOTOMY AND LITHOTRITY;

or, An Inquiry into the best Modes of removing Stone from the
Bladder.   Second Edition, 8vo, with numerous Engravings, 10s.   [1871]

ALSO,

DISEASES OF THE URINARY ORGANS.

(Clinical Lectures on).   Third Edition, crown 8vo, with Engravings, 6s.   [1872]

THE DISEASES OF THE PROSTATE:

their Pathology and Treatment.   Fourth Edition, 8vo, with numerous Plates, 10s.

MENTAL DISEASES

(The Pathology and Therapeutics of). By J. L. C. Schroeder Van
der Kolk. Translated by Mr. Rudall, F.R.C.S. 8vo, 7s. 6d. [1869]

THE CLIMATE AND RESOURCES OF MADEIRA,

as regarding chiefly the Necessities of Consumption and the Welfare
of Invalids. By Michael C. Grabham, M.D., M.R.C.P. Crown
8vo, with Map and Engravings, 5s. [1869]

A MANUAL OF THE DISEASES OF THE EYE

by C. Macnamara, Surgeon to the Calcutta Ophthalmic Hospital.
Second Edition, fcap 8vo, with Coloured Plates, 12s. 6d. [1872]

CLUBFOOT:

its Causes, Pathology, and Treatment; being the Jacksonian Prize
Essay by Wm. Adams, F.R.C.S., Surgeon to the Great Northern
Hospital. Second Edition, 8vo, with 106 Wood Engravings and
6 Lithographic Plates, 15s. [1873]

PHTHISIS AND THE STETHOSCOPE;

or, the Physical Signs of Consumption. By R. P. Cotton, M.D.,
F.R.C.P., Senior Physician to the Hospital for Consumption,
Brompton. Fourth Edition, fcap 8vo, 3s. 6d. [1869]

PRACTICAL ANATOMY:

a Manual of Dissections by Christopher Heath, F.R.C.S., Surgeon
to University College Hospital. Second Edition, fcap 8vo, with
226 Engravings, 12s. 6d. [1869]

BY THE SAME AUTHOR,

MINOR SURGERY AND BANDAGING

(A Manual of) for the Use of House-Surgeons, Dressers, and Junior
Practitioners. Fourth Edition, fcap 8vo, with 74 Engravings, 5s. 6d.
[1870]

ALSO,

INJURIES AND DISEASES OF THE JAWS:

Jacksonian Prize Essay. Second Edition, 8vo, with 164 Engravings, 12s. [1872

ON MEGRIM, SICK-HEADACHE,

and some Allied Disorders: a Contribution to the Pathology of
Nerve-Storms by EDWARD LIVEING, M.D. Cantab., Hon. Fellow of
King's College, London.　8vo, with Coloured Plate, 15s.　　[1873]

HUMAN OSTEOLOGY:

with Plates, showing the Attachments of the Muscles.　By LUTHER
HOLDEN, F.R.C.S., Surgeon to St. Bartholomew's Hospital.　Fourth
Edition, 8vo, 16s.　　[1869]

BY THE SAME AUTHOR,

THE DISSECTION OF THE HUMAN BODY

(A Manual of).　Third Edition, 8vo, with Engravings on Wood,
16s.　　[1868]

MANUAL OF THE DISEASES OF CHILDREN

(A Practical), with a Formulary, by EDWARD ELLIS, M.D., Physician
to the Victoria Hospital for Children.　Second Edition, crown 8vo,
7s.　　[1873]

INJURIES AND DISEASES OF THE KNEE-JOINT

and their Treatment by Amputation and Excision Contrasted:
Jacksonian Prize Essay by W. P. SWAIN, F.R.C.S., Surgeon to the
Royal Albert Hospital, Devonport.　8vo, with 36 Engravings, 9s.

[1869]

A TREATISE ON SYPHILIS

by WALTER J. COULSON, F.R.C.S., Surgeon to the Lock Hospital.
8vo, 10s.　　[1869]

BY THE SAME AUTHOR,

STONE IN THE BLADDER:

Its Prevention, Early Symptoms, and Treatment by Lithotrity.
8vo, 6s.　　[1868]

PRINCIPLES OF HUMAN PHYSIOLOGY.

By W. B. CARPENTER, M.D., F.R.S.　Seventh Edition by Mr.
HENRY POWER, 8vo, with nearly 300 Illustrations on Steel and
Wood, 28s.　　[1869]

A MANUAL OF PRACTICAL HYGIENE
by E. A. PARKES, M.D., F.R.C.P., F.R.S., Professor of Hygiene in the Army Medical School. Fourth Edition, 8vo, with Plates and Woodcuts, 16s. [1873]

ON KIDNEY DISEASES, URINARY DEPOSITS
and Calculous Disorders by LIONEL S. BEALE, M.B., F.R.S., F.R.C.P., Physician to King's College Hospital. Third Edition, much Enlarged, 8vo, with 70 Plates, 25s. [1868]

BY THE SAME AUTHOR,

DISEASE GERMS;
and on the Treatment of the Feverish State. Second Edition, crown 8vo, with 28 Plates, 12s. 6d. [1872]

PHYSIOLOGICAL LABORATORY
(Handbook for the). By E. KLEIN, M.D., formerly Privat-Docent in Histology in the University of Vienna, Assistant Professor in the Pathological Laboratory of the Brown Institution, London; J. BURDON-SANDERSON, M.D., F.R.S., Professor of Practical Physiology in University College, London; MICHAEL FOSTER, M.D., F.R.S., Fellow of, and Prælector of Physiology in, Trinity College, Cambridge; and T. LAUDER BRUNTON, M.D., D.Sc., Lecturer on Materia Medica in the Medical College of Bartholomew's Hospital; edited by J. BURDON-SANDERSON. 8vo, with 123 Plates, 24s. [1873].

THE SURGEON'S VADE-MECUM
by ROBERT DRUITT. Tenth Edition, fcap 8vo, with numerous Engravings on Wood, 12s. 6d. [1870]

HOOPER'S PHYSICIAN'S VADE-MECUM
or, Manual of the Principles and Practice of Physic, Ninth Edition by W. A. GUY, M.B., F.R.S., and JOHN HARLEY, M.D., F.R.C.P. Fcap 8vo, with Engravings. 12s. 6d. [1874]

THE APPLICATIONS OF CHEMISTRY
and Mechanics to Pathology and Therapeutics (Lectures on some of) by H. BENCE JONES, M.D., F.R.C.P., D.C.L., F.R.S. 8vo, 12s. [1867]

MEDICAL ANATOMY.

By FRANCIS SIBSON, M.D., F.R.C.P., F.R.S., Consulting Physician to St. Mary's Hospital. Imp. folio, with 21 coloured Plates, cloth, £2 2s.; half-morocco, £2 10s.   [Completed in 1869]

LECTURES ON MADNESS

in its Medical, Legal, and Social Aspects by EDGAR SHEPPARD, M.D., M.R.C.P., Professor of Psychological Medicine in King's College; one of the Medical Superintendents of the Colney Hatch Lunatic Asylum. 8vo, 6s. 6d.   [1873]

TEMPERATURE OBSERVATIONS

containing (1) Temperature Variations in the Diseases of Children, (2) Puerperal Temperatures, (3) Infantile Temperatures in Health and Disease, by WM. SQUIRE, M.R.C.P. Lond. 8vo, 5s.   [1871]

A DICTIONARY OF MATERIA MEDICA

and Therapeutics by ADOLPHE WAHLTUCH, M.D. 8vo, 15s.   [1868

DIABETES:

Researches on its Nature and Treatment by F. W. PAVY, M.D., F.R.S., F.R.C.P., Physician to Guy's Hospital. Second Edition, 8vo, with Engravings, 10s.   [1868]

BY THE SAME AUTHOR,

DIGESTION:

its Disorders and their Treatment. Second Edition, 8vo, 8s. 6d.
                                                           [1869]

A MEDICAL VOCABULARY;

or, an Explanation of all Names, Synonymes, Terms, and Phrases used in Medicine and the relative branches of Medical Science by R. G. MAYNE, M.D., LL.D. Third Edition, fcap 8vo, 8s. 6d.
                                                           [1868]

IRRITATIVE DYSPEPSIA

and its Important Connection with Irritative Congestion of the Windpipe and with the Origin and Progress of Consumption. By C. B. GARRETT, M.D. Crown 8vo, 2s. 6d.   [1868]

MEDICAL JURISPRUDENCE

(The Principles and Practice of) by ALFRED S. TAYLOR, M.D., F.R.C.P., F.R.S. Second Edition, 2 vols., 8vo, with 189 Wood Engravings, £1 11s. 6d.   [1873]

SCHROEDER'S MANUAL OF MIDWIFERY,

including the Pathology of Pregnancy and the Puerperal State. Translated by CHARLES H. CARTER, B.A., M.D. 8vo, with Engravings, 12s. 6d.   [1873]

THE PARASITIC AFFECTIONS OF THE SKIN.

By McCALL ANDERSON, M.D., F.F.P.S., Professor of the Practice of Medicine in Anderson's University, Glasgow. Second Edition, 8vo, with Engravings, 7s. 6d.   [1868]

STRICTURE OF THE URETHRA

(On the Immediate Treatment of) by BARNARD HOLT, F.R.C.S., Consulting Surgeon to the Westminster Hospital. Third Edition, 8vo, 6s.   [1868]

OXYGEN:

its Action, Use, and Value in the Treatment of various Diseases otherwise Incurable or very Intractable. By S. B. BIRCH, M.D., M.R.C.P. Second Edition, post 8vo, 3s. 6d.   [1868]

BY THE SAME AUTHOR,

CONSTIPATED BOWELS:

the Various Causes and the Different Means of Cure. Third Edition, post 8vo, 3s. 6d.   [1868]

OBSCURE DISEASES OF THE BRAIN AND MIND.

By FORBES WINSLOW, M.D., D.C.L. Oxon. Fourth Edition, post 8vo, 10s. 6d.   [1868]

ULCERS AND CUTANEOUS DISEASES

(A Manual of the Pathology and Treatment of) of the Lower Limbs by J. K. SPENDER, M.D. Lond. 8vo, 4s.   [1868]

A COMPENDIUM OF PRACTICAL MEDICINE
and Morbid Anatomy by WILLIAM DALE, M.D. LOND.   12mo,
with Plates, 7s.   [1868]

GERMINAL MATTER AND THE CONTACT THEORY:
an Essay on the Morbid Poisons by JAMES MORRIS, M.D. Lond.
Second Edition, crown 8vo, 4s. 6d.   [1867]

BY THE SAME AUTHOR,

IRRITABILITY:
Popular and Practical Sketches of Common Morbid States and
Conditions bordering on Disease; with Hints for Management,
Alleviation, and Cure.   Crown 8vo, 4s. 6d.   [1868]

A MANUAL OF MATERIA MEDICA
by J. F. ROYLE, M.D., F.R.S., and F. W. HEADLAND, M.D., F.R.C.P.
Fifth Edition, fcap 8vo, with numerous Engravings on Wood,
12s. 6d.   [1868]

DISEASES OF THE CHEST:
Contributions to their Clinical History, Pathology and Treatment
by A. T. H. WATERS, M.D., F.R.C.P., Physician to the Liverpool
Royal Infirmary.   8vo, with Plates, 12s. 6d.   [1868]

NEURALGIA AND KINDRED DISEASES
of the Nervous System : their Nature, Causes, and Treatment, with
a series of Cases, by JOHN CHAPMAN, M.D., M.R.C.P., Assistant-
Physician to the Metropolitan Free Hospital.   8vo, 14s.   [1873]

THE STOMACH AND DUODENUM
(The Morbid States of) and their Relations to the Diseases of oth
Organs.   By SAMUEL FENWICK, M.D., F.R.C.P., Assistant-Physi-
cian to the London Hospital.   8vo, with 10 Plates, 12s.   [1868]

BY THE SAME AUTHOR,

THE STUDENT'S GUIDE TO MEDICAL DIAGNOSIS.
Third Edition, fcap 8vo, with 87 Engravings, 6s. 6d.   [1873]

REVIEW OF THE HISTORY OF MEDICINE

among Asiatic Nations by T. A. WISE, M.D., F.R.C.P. Edin. Two
Vols., 8vo, 16s.   [1868]

DISEASES OF THE EYE

(Illustrations of some of the Principal), with an Account of their
Symptoms, Pathology, and Treatment, by HENRY POWER, F.R.C.S.,
M.B. Lond., Ophthalmic Surgeon to St. Bartholomew's Hospital.
8vo, with twelve Coloured Plates, 20s.   [1867]

HANDBOOK OF MEDICAL ELECTRICITY

by HERBERT TIBBITS, M.D., L.R.C.P.L., Medical Superintendent
of the National Hospital for the Paralysed and Epileptic. 8vo,
with 64 Wood Engravings, 6s.   [1873]

OBSTETRIC MEDICINE AND SURGERY

(The Principles and Practice of). By F. H. RAMSBOTHAM, M.D.,
F.R.C.P.. Fifth Edition, 8vo, with One Hundred and Twenty
Plates on Steel and Wood, 22s.   [1867]

DISEASES OF THE EYE

(A Treatise on the) by J. SOELBERG WELLS, F.R.C.S., Ophthalmic
Surgeon to King's College Hospital and Surgeon to the Royal
London Ophthalmic Hospital. Third Edition, 8vo, with Coloured
Plates and Wood Engravings, 25s.   [1873]

THE INDIGESTIONS

or Diseases of the Digestive Organs Functionally Treated, by T. K.
CHAMBERS, M.D., F.R.C.P., Lecturer on Medicine at St. Mary's
Hospital. Second Edition, 8vo, 10s. 6d.   [1867]

THE LUNGS AND AIR PASSAGES

(On Diseases of) by W. H. FULLER, M.D., F.R.C.P., Senior
Physician to St. George's Hospital. Second Edition, 8vo, 12s. 6d.
                                                                   [1867]

THE MEDICAL REMEMBRANCER;

or, Book of Emergencies. Fifth Edition by JONATHAN HUTCHINSON,
F.R.C.S., Senior Surgeon to the London Hospital. 32mo, 2s. 6d.
                                                                   [1867]

ESSAYS ON THE DISEASES OF CHILDREN

by WILLIAM HENRY DAY, M.D., Physician to the Samaritan Hospital for Diseases of Women and Children. Fcap. 8vo, 5s.   [1873]

A HANDBOOK OF HYGIENE

for the Use of Sanitary Authorities and Health Officers by GEORGE WILSON, M.D. Edin., Medical Officer of Health for the Warwick Union of Sanitary Authorities. Second Edition, crown 8vo, with Engravings, 8s. 6d.   [1873]

ON THE ACTION OF MEDICINES

in the System by F. W. HEADLAND, M.D., F.R.C.P., Professor of Medicine in Charing Cross Medical College. Fourth Edition, 8vo, 14s.   [1866]

A MANUAL OF MEDICAL DIAGNOSIS

by A. W. BARCLAY, M.D., F.R.C.P., Physician to, and Lecturer on Medicine at, St. George's Hospital. Third Edition, fcap. 8vo, 10s. 6d.   [1870]

EPIDEMIOLOGY;

or, the Remote Cause of Epidemic Disease in the Animal and in the Vegetable Creation, by JOHN PARKIN, M.D., F.R.C.S. Part I, 8vo, 5s.   [1873]

THE ACTION AND SOUNDS OF THE HEART

(Researches on). By GEORGE PATON, M.D., author of numerous papers published in the British and American Medical Journals. 8vo, 3s. 6d.   [1873]

MICROSCOPIC STRUCTURE OF URINARY CALCULI

(On the) by H. V. CARTER, M.D., Surgeon-Major, H.M.'s Bombay Army. 8vo, with Four Plates, 5s.   [1873]

HANDBOOK FOR NURSES FOR THE SICK

by Miss VEITCH. Crown 8vo, 2s. 6d.   [1870]

ON THE WASTING DISEASES OF CHILDREN

by EUSTACE SMITH, M.D. Lond., Physician to the King of the Belgians, Physician to the East London Hospital for Children. Second Edition, post 8vo, 7s. 6d.   [1870]

A SYSTEM OF DENTAL SURGERY

by JOHN TOMES, F.R.S., and CHARLES S. TOMES, M.A., Lecturer on Dental Anatomy and Physiology, and Assistant Dental Surgeon to the Dental Hospital of London. Second Edition, fcap. 8vo, with 268 Engravings, 14s.   [1873]

A MANUAL OF DENTAL MECHANICS,

with an Account of the Materials and Appliances used in Mechanical Dentistry, by OAKLEY COLES, L.D.S.R.C.S., Surgeon-Dentist to the Hospital for Diseases of the Throat. Crown 8vo, with 140 Wood Engravings, 7s. 6d.   [1873]

NOTES ON ASTHMA;

its Forms and Treatment, by JOHN C. THOROWGOOD, M.D. Lond., Physician to the Hospital for Diseases of the Chest, Victoria Park. Second Edition, Revised and Enlarged, crown 8vo, 4s. 6d.   [1873]

ENGLISH MIDWIVES:

Their History and Prospects, by J. H. AVELING, M.D., Physician to the Chelsea Hospital for Women, Examiner of Midwives for the Obstetrical Society of London. Crown 8vo, 5s.   [1872]

A TOXICOLOGICAL CHART,

Exhibiting at one View the Symptoms, Treatment, and mode of Detecting the various Poisons—Mineral, Vegetable, and Animal : with Concise Directions for the Treatment of Suspended Animation, by WILLIAM STOWE, M.R.C.S.E. Thirteenth Edition, 2s.; on roller, 5s.   [1872]

DICTIONARY OF PRACTICAL SURGERY

and Encyclopædia of Surgical Science, by SAMUEL COOPER. New Edition, brought down to the present Time by SAMUEL A. LANE, Consulting Surgeon to St. Mary's and to the Lock Hospitals; assisted by various Eminent Surgeons. 2 vols. 8vo, 50s.   [1861 and 1872]

The following Catalogues issued by Messrs Churchill will be forwarded post free on application:

1. *Messrs Churchill's General List of* 400 *works on Medicine, Surgery, Midwifery, Materia Medica, Hygiene, Anatomy, Physiology, Chemistry, &c., &c.*

2. *Selection from Messrs Churchill's General List, comprising all recent Works published by them on the Art and Science of Medicine.*

3. *A descriptive List of Messrs Churchill's Works on Chemistry, Pharmacy, Botany, Photography, and other branches of Science.*

4. *Messrs Churchill's Red-Letter List, giving the Titles of forthcoming New Works and New Editions.*

[Published every October.]

5. *The Medical Intelligencer, an Annual List of New Works and New Editions published by Messrs J. & A. Churchill, together with Particulars of the Periodicals issued from their House.*

[Sent in January of each year to every Medical Practitioner in the United Kingdom whose name and address can be ascertained. A large number are also sent to the United States of America, Continental Europe, India, and the Colonies.]

Messrs CHURCHILL have concluded a special arrangement with Messrs LINDSAY & BLAKISTON, of Philadelphia, in accordance with which that Firm will act as their Agents for the United States of America, either keeping in Stock most of Messrs Churchill's Books, or reprinting them on Terms advantageous to Authors. Many of the Works in this Catalogue may therefore be easily obtained in America.

PRINTED BY J. E. ADLARD, BARTHOLOMEW CLOSE.